Seminars in General Adult Psychiatry

Edited by
George Stein & Greg Wilkinson

with the assistance of
Rosalind Ramsay

Volume 2

GASKELL

British Library Cataloguing-in-Publication Data
A catalogue record for this book is available from the British Library.
ISBN 0 902241 91 5 (Boxed set of 2 volumes)
ISBN 1 901242 12 9 (Vol. 2)

Distributed in North America
by American Psychiatric Press, Inc.
ISBN 0 88048 577 9

Gaskell is an imprint of the Royal College of Psychiatrists,
17 Belgrave Square, London SW1X 8PG
The Royal College of Psychiatrists is a registered charity, number 228636

The views presented in this book do not necessarily reflect those of the
Royal College of Psychiatrists, and the publishers are not responsible for
any error of omission or fact. College Seminars are produced by the
Publications Department of the College; they should in no way be
construed as providing a syllabus or other material for any College
examination.

Printed by Bell & Bain Ltd., Thornliebank, Glasgow

Contents

Contributors

Dr Morris Bernadt, Department of Psychological Medicine, Kings College Hospital, Denmark Hill, London SE5 9RS

Dr Jonathan Bird, Burden Neurological Hospital, Stoke Lane, Stapleton, Bristol, Avon BS16

Sharon Borrows, Sleep Centre, Papworth Hospital, Papworth Everard, Cambridge CB3 8RE

Dr Tom Brown, St John's Hospital at Howden, Howden Road West, Livingston, West Lothian EH54 6PP

Professor Patricia Casey, Department of Psychiatry, Mater Hospital, 62–63 Eccles Street, Dublin 7, Republic of Ireland

Dr John Cookson, The Royal London Hospital, 2A Bow Road, London E3 4LL

Dr Lynne M. Drummond, Department of Psychiatry, St George's Hospital Medical School, Cranmer Terrace, Tooting, London SW17 0RE

Dr Tom Fahy, The Maudsley Hospital, Denmark Hill, London SE5 8AZ

Professor Nicol Ferrier, Department of Psychiatry, School of Neurosciences, The Royal Victoria Infirmary, Queen Victoria Road, Newcastle upon Tyne, Tyne and Wear NE1 3LP

Dr Alistair G. Hay, Craig Dunain Hospital, Inverness IV3 6JU

Dr Frank Holloway, Maudsley Hospital, Denmark Hill, London SE5 8AZ

Dr Roger Howells, Maudsley Hospital, Denmark Hill, London SE5 8AZ

Dr Robin Jacobson, Department of Psychiatry, Jenner Wing, St George's Hospital Medical School, London SW17 0RE

Dr Michael Kopelman, Academic Unit of Psychiatry, United Medical and Dental Schools, St Thomas's Hospital, Lambeth Palace Road, London SE1 7EH

Dr Alan Lee, Department of Psychiatry, University Hospital, Queen's Medical Centre, Nottingham NG7 2UH

Dr Peter F. Liddle, Department of Psychiatry, University of British Colombia, 2255 Westbrook Mall, Vancouver, British Colombia V6T 2A1, Canada

Professor Clive Mellor, PO Box 399, Chilliwack, British Colombia V2P 6J7, Canada

Professor Harold Merskey, London Psychiatric Hospital, 850 Highbury Avenue, PO Box 2532, London, Ontario N6A 4H1, Canada

Dr Stirling Moorey, Hackney Hospital, Homerton High Street, London E9 6BE

Professor Gethin Morgan, Department of Mental Health, University of Bristol, 41 St Michael's Hill, Bristol, Avon BS2 8DZ

Dr John Owen, Cossham Hospital, Lodge Hill, Kingswood, Bristol, Avon BS15 1LF

Dr David Cunningham Owens, Royal Edinburgh Hospital, Kennedy Tower, Morningside Park, Edingurgh, Lothian EH10 5HF

Dr Jeremy Pfeffer, Department of Psychiatry, London Hospital, Whitechapel, London E1 1BB

Dr Rosalind Ramsay, St Thomas's Hospital, Lambeth Palace Road, London SE1 7EH

Dr Mary Robertson, Academic Department of Psychiatry, Wolfson Building, The Middlesex Hospital, London W1N 8AA

Professor Jan Scott, Department of Psychiatry, School of Neurosciences, The Royal Victoria Infirmary, Queen Victoria Road, Newcastle upon Tyne, Tyne and Wear NE1 3LP

Dr Philip Sedgwick, St George's Hospital Medical School, Cranmer Terrace, London SW17 0RE

Dr George Stein, Kings College Hospital, Farnborough Hospital, Farnborough Common, Orpington, Kent BR6 8ND

Dr Richard Stern, Springfield Hospital, 61 Glenburnie Road, London SW17 7DJ

Professor Michael Stone, Suite 114, 225 Central Park West, New York City, NY 10024, USA

Dr George Szmukler, The Maudsley Hospital, Denmark Hill, London SE5 8AZ

Dr Mark Tattersall, Huntercombe Manor Hospital, Huntercombe Lane South, Taplow, Berkshire SL6 0PQ

Dr Janet Treasure, Institute of Psychiatry, Denmark Hill, London SE5 8AF

Dr Christopher Vassilas, Department of Old Age Psychiatry, Wedgwood Unit, West Suffolk Hospital, Bury St Edmunds, Suffolk IP33 2QZ

Professor Greg Wilkinson, Academic Department of Psychiatry, Royal Liverpool University Hospital, Liverpool L69 3BX

Dr Peter Woodruff, Institute of Psychiatry, De Crespigny Park, London SE5 8AF

Foreword

Series Editors

The publication of *College Seminars*, a series of textbooks covering the breadth of psychiatry, is very much in line with the Royal College of Psychiatrists' established role in education and in setting professional standards.

College Seminars are intended to help junior doctors during their training years. We hope that trainees will find these books useful, on the ward as well as in preparation for the MRCPsych examination. Separate volumes will cover clinical psychiatry, each of its subspecialities, and also the relevant non-clinical academic disciplines of psychology and sociology.

College Seminars will make a contribution to the continuing professional development of established clinicians.

Psychiatry is concerned primarily with people, and to a lesser extent with disease processes and pathology. The core of the subject is rich in ideas and schools of thought, and no single approach or solution can embrace the variety of problems a psychiatrist meets. For this reason, we have endeavoured to adopt an eclectic approach to practical management throughout the series.

The College can draw on the collective wisdom of many individuals in clinical and academic psychiatry. More than a hundred people have contributed to this series; this reflects how diverse and complex psychiatry has become.

Frequent new editions of books appearing in the series are envisaged, which should allow *College Seminars* to be responsive to readers' suggestions and needs.

Hugh Freeman
Ian Pullen
George Stein
Greg Wilkinson

Preface

Psychiatry, according to Johann Christian Reil (1759–1813) the German anatomist who first coined the term, consists of the meeting of two minds, the mind of the patient with the mind of the doctor. As patients tell their story, it is the task of the doctor to recognise the tale, and to do so with some compassion. Pattern recognition lies at the heart of the diagnostic process; common trends in the rich tapestry of the patient's experiences are summarised in the many clinical syndromes and disorders of psychiatry. This book, intended for doctors in training beginning their career in psychiatry, places its greatest emphasis on detailed descriptions of the common psychiatric disorders. We hope such a clinical descriptive approach will help the doctor recognise patterns and so make a sound psychiatric diagnosis. Our intention is that this book will serve as a useful basis for trainees preparing for their Membership examinations, but in addition it should engage those who have passed that hurdle.

Diagnostic acumen separated from therapeutic skill is of little use to patients or their families. When Reil first introduced the word psychiatry, he meant it in a therapeutic sense, in that the psyche of the doctor would act as a healing agent on the mind of the patient. While the initial meetings between doctor and patient usually have a diagnostic purpose, later contacts involve treatment. Throughout the book we have tried to provide guidelines on the management of common disorders. Our approach to treatment has been eclectic, but at the same time we have tried to describe each of the many treatments now available in some depth. The more specialised psychotherapies, once shrouded in a mystique requiring years of specialised training, are now gradually being replaced by briefer, less intensive treatment more readily grasped by trainees. We have described these newer treatments in some detail (for example, with behaviour therapy for the treatment of phobias, or cognitive therapy for depression). Physical treatments are accorded equal weight and separate chapters describe the physical treatments of both depression and schizophrenia.

Our hopes for better understanding and new treatments lie in scientific research. Sometimes, the scientific advances of the previous decades have been spectacular, such as the introduction of new drugs to treat depression or schizophrenia; in other cases developments have been less dramatic but as important, such as the gradual realisation that much of the depression found in the community is socially determined. At one time, a medical advance was deemed to have occurred if a charismatic professor at an ancient university announced a new classification; if another professor, perhaps from a different school of psychiatry, disagreed, it was hailed as a medical controversy. Today, this is no longer possible and rigorous scientific evidence is required before any new information can be incorporated into the fabric of existing knowledge. This applies to both the biological and psychosocial dimensions of the spectrum of knowledge.

We have tried to balance the essential clinical descriptive information and its supporting scientific evidence, with some of the more interesting but still speculative recent findings, hopefully without overwhelming the reader with too many studies. In this lies a dilemma, because the needs of the beginner and those with experience can be at variance. The novice must assimilate the body of existing knowledge while the established clinician is more interested in the advancing front of knowledge, even if many of the new findings eventually prove ephemeral.

Our guiding principle in editing the book has been to remain close to clinical issues and to answer the two questions "What disorder is it?" and "How can we help?" The third and often the most tantalising question "Why is it" remains unanswered, at least for most conditions, and so we have tended to focus less on aetiological considerations.

An era is now passing when doctors bear sole responsibility for the treatment of patients under their care. Modern psychiatric treatment is a team effort and this change is to be welcomed, not least because it helps to ease the burden on the doctor. Medical authority no longer rests on a position in the hierarchy, but rather on greater knowledge and wider clinical experience. Increasingly patients, relatives, carers, managers and other members of the psychiatric team question the doctor's decisions and treatment, and as a consequence of these wider changes this book is rooted in an evidence base and comprehensively and extensively referenced.

The *College Seminars* series has separate volumes for each of the sub-specialities of psychiatry, and this structure has given the editors and contributors considerable freedom, permitting us to concentrate solely on general psychiatry. General psychiatry is now too vast a subject for a single person to be an expert in all its aspects and this inevitably means a comprehensive text must be multi-authored. We believe that many of the chapters are works of great scholarship by leading experts in their fields, and their length and detail bear witness to long hours of toil. For this the editors express their deepest gratitude. In other chapters the clinical acumen, diagnostic nuances and imaginative therapeutic strategies have an immediacy which brings the whole book to life, while offering the clinician new ways to help patients and their families. We hope our readers will derive both pleasure and wisdom from this book.

We would like to thank the American Psychiatric Association and the World Health Organization for permission to publish tables from DSM–IV and ICD–10. The editors are particularly grateful for the assistance of Dr Rosalind Ramsay throughout the preparation of this book, first for keeping the editors in touch with the needs of the readership, and second for critically scrutinising the text. Much of this book was edited in the library of the Maudsley Hospital, which houses a unique collection of psychiatric journals and books; we would like to thank the librarian, Mr Martin Guha, and his staff for their unfailing support. Numerous junior doctors from Farnborough Hospital, the London Hospital and the University of Liverpool have read earlier drafts of the chapters in this book and their comments have helped us greatly to sharpen the focus of the text. Special thanks are due to Penny Nicholson at Farnborough Hospital who typed and re-typed many of the manuscripts as well as coordinating the whole project, ably assisted in this task by Christine Scotcher. The technical and publishing expertise of Lesley Bennun, Dinah Alam and Andrew Morris at the College is also acknowledged with much gratitude.

George Stein
Greg Wilkinson

18 Personality disorders

Patricia Casey

Concept of personality disorders • *A critique of the concept* •
Epidemiology • *Aetiology* • *Categories of personality disorder* •
Miscellaneous disorders • *Comorbidity in the personality disorders* •
Assessment • *Impulse and habit disorders*

The history of the personality disorders is among the lengthiest in psychiatry, going back to Hippocrates. It is a tale of ever-changing approaches to classifying and redefining the same morbid group of people, combined with recurrent speculations on the nature of the human character, and, until recently, very little in the way of scientific enquiry.

The scheme of Hippocrates for describing personality disorders held sway for more than two millennia. He believed that all diseases stemmed from an excess or imbalance of the four humours: yellow bile from the liver which corresponded to the choleric humours; black bile from the spleen, secreted under the influence of the planet Saturn, corresponding with the melancholic; blood corresponding with the sanguine; and phlegm with the phlegmatic. According to the Greek philosopher Empedocles, the humours themselves were the embodiments of the four basic elements of the universe: earth, water, fire and air. Theophrastus, a pupil of Hippocrates, went on to describe systematically some 30 or more different personality types, some of which show a resemblance to those outlined in modern schemes. Many centuries later Galen modified this scheme and associated the choleric temperament with irascibility; the melancholic with sadness; the sanguine with a tendency towards optimism; and the phlegmatic with a tendency to apathy. The modern use of these words (e.g. sanguine meaning good-humoured and melancholic meaning pessimistic) are relics of this ancient formulation.

The idea that differences in the composition of body fluids were the cause of variations in human character later gave way to the notion that the shape of the brain and body were responsible. In the late 18th century, Franz Joseph Gall developed the science of phrenology. He started to map in detail the shapes of people's skulls and tried to link them with the shape of the brain, and hence the person's character. He argued that, in the same way that a large biceps predicts strength, a person with a large cranial protuberance would have some correspondingly well-developed psychological characteristic. Although we know very much more today about neuroanatomy, phrenology represents an early scientific attempt to link the size and shape of the brain to mental disorder, and so perhaps was a forerunner of modern brain-scanning studies.

Kretschmer (1922) provided excellent descriptions of personality *types*, but his aetiological classification was based on physique. Stocky individuals were described as pyknic, and were prone to manic–depression, while thin asthenic individuals were more liable to schizophrenia. His American disciple, Sheldon (1940), tried to correlate three bodily types with different temperaments. Endomorphy (predominance of body roundness and softness) was associated with a viscerotonic temperament, with gregariousness, the love of comfort, relaxation, and avoidance of pain. Mesomorphy (muscular and connective tissue dominance) was associated with a somatotonic temperament, with assertive, physical, energetic individuals who were indifferent to pain and were callous. The third group had ectomorphy (linearity and fragility of structure) and were cerebrotonic, with a tendency to restraint, introversion, social awkwardness and a desire for solitude. Needless to say, this scheme has few adherents today.

Personality, character, temperament and traits

The origins of the word 'personality' came from the amphitheatres of ancient Greece and Rome. *Persona* is the Latin word for mask. The Romans took the word from the Greek theatre where the actors wore masks and held a megaphone at the mouth opening, through (*per*) which the sound (*sona*) was magnified. *Personality* therefore represented an amplification of the voice and individual features that the actor was trying to portray (Stone, 1993). The word 'character' is derived from the Greek word *charasso*, which means to dig in or engrave, and refers to those characteristics which have been acquired earlier in life or during childhood. A rather more narrow definition of character with social and moral connotations describes how closely a person endorses the values of his or her society (as in a good or bad character).

More innate or constitutional aspects of behaviour are sometimes referred to as the person's 'temperament' (Latin *temperare* = mixture, due measure; *mens* = mind). The term is more often used in child psychiatry to describe the manner in which a child behaves rather than the specific behaviours themselves.

The term 'trait' also describes the manner of behaviour but is applied in adult psychiatry to describe more specific features of the personality, and the modern concept of personality disorder is firmly rooted in trait psychology. An early example of trait-based typology was given by the French psychologist Ribot (1890). He formulated the different character types by varying the intensity of two primary traits, sensitivity and activity. He described humble characters who had excess sensitivity but limited energy, and emotional types who had excessive sensitivity and high degrees of energy. The best known of these 'trait' approaches is that of Jung (1921), who described introversion and extroversion, traits which were later extensively studied by Eysenck. He described three separate trait dimensions;

extroversion–introversion, neuroticism–stability and psychoticism–stability. This formulation has generated a huge amount of research in psychology, but has had a rather lesser impact in the clinical world. Other trait formulations are reviewed by Millon (1981).

Psychiatrists such as Kraepelin were more interested in exploring the causes of the functional psychoses. In an attempt to trace their origins he described cyclothymia which he believed predisposed to manic–depression; and the autistic temperament which might predispose to schizophrenia. Kraepelin (1913) also distinguished "psychopathic inferiority" from other psychiatric disorders, and provided clinical descriptions of the personality disorders, including individuals who were shiftless, liars, swindlers and trouble-makers.

The modern era begins with Schneider who published *Psychopathic Personalities for Modern Classificatory Schemes* in 1923, which was translated into English in 1950. He stressed that a personality disorder must always be judged by its effects on others, whether they were friends, relations, colleagues, or society as a whole. His types included the hyperthymic, depressive, explosive, insecure, insensitive, anankastic, fanatic, attention-seeking, labile, and affectionless. With some modification, most of these types have appeared in all the various DSM and ICD schemes, and also form the basis for the current DSM–IV (American Psychiatric Association, 1994) and ICD–10 (World Health Organization, 1992).

Psychoanalytical contributions

The analytical contribution has also been important, particularly in the US, and this is reflected in DSM–IV. The early analysts, such as Freud and especially Abraham (1925), linked the different character types to the oral, anal and phallic phases of development. The oral phase was divided into two. The first was an oral sucking phase in which all food is accepted indiscriminately. Excessive indulgence during this phase was said to result in an oral dependent type: excessively dependent, gullible or "able to swallow anything". Later there is an oral biting phase when food is sometimes aggressively chewed or rejected and then spat out. Frustration at this phase may lead to oral sadistic character formation, a pattern of pessimistic distrust, sarcasm, and a tendency to be cantankerous. The anal phase was concerned with the acquisition of sphincter control, and frustration during this phase was thought to lead to later difficulties in areas of control and authority as well as obsessional features, or the anankastic personality.

Difficulties during the phallic phase were thought to result in sexual impulses being excessively self-orientated, rather than directed towards others of the opposite sex. Such self-love would result in phallic narcissistic character formation, and traits of being vain, brash or arrogant. Hysterical and masochistic types may also fail to mature appropriately through the genital phase of development. Alexander (1930) believed that abnormal personalities were often the sufferers of neuroses and advanced the concept of the neurotic character, which has been echoed more recently in the "general neurotic syndrome" of Tyrer (1989).

Reich (1933) believed that the neurotic solution to psychosexual conflict for those with character disorders was achieved through a pervasive restructuring of the individual's defensive style. This ultimately crystallised into a very rigid structure, the "character armour", which like the armour of a soldier was difficult to dent or bend and protected the individual from threats arising from both the external and internal world. More recently, Vaillant (1977) suggested that identification of the defence mechanism used by a patient might form a basis for the classification of abnormal personality. Millon (1981) argued that the personality served as a host mechanism, comparable to the immune system, offering protection against the many psychological and interpersonal stresses of living, and in this way acted as a barrier to prevent symptom formation and breakdown. In common parlance the terms 'thin-skinned' and 'thick-skinned' neatly describe this aspect; that is, a person's sensitivity to external stress. Stone (1993) has also emphasised the role of the *facade*, a false self outside the true personality that enhances survival in a potentially hostile world, and includes the ability to say nothing or to smile in the presence of adversity or humiliation, to be tactful, and so forth. There is a danger, however, for a few individuals who suppress their emotions and personality so greatly that the facade assumes the role of the true personality, and the mask becomes the face.

The notion that a subject's defence mechanism may be of diagnostic importance is more widely accepted in the US than elsewhere. A new scale and possibly a new axis, the "Defense functioning scale", is described in DSM–IV, where the individual's defence mechanisms and coping styles are recorded. Because this scale appears in a section entitled "Proposed axes for further study", its use at present is regarded as experimental.

Other analysts have emphasised "ego psychology", the notion that the unconscious and the id are rather less important than the patient's ego and the experience of reality. Sullivan (1947) emphasised the role of anxiety and the need for security as well as the style of interpersonal relationships. Character types were described almost exclusively in terms of their relationships with others; for example, "ambition-ridden" personalities were noted for their exploitiveness, competitiveness and unscrupulous manipulations. Adler (1964) emphasised *over-compensation*, an inborn tendency to counteract deficiencies and inadequacies through reparative striving. Undoing this over-compensation plays a key role in therapy. In Horney's (1945) typology there were those who "move towards people" in their relationships and who were compliant and self-effacing, with their self-esteem being determined by others (dependent types). Those who "moved against others" in relationships were aggressive, saw life as a struggle, sought power and exploited others (sociopathic types). A third group who "moved away" from other people became detached and so avoided relationships, leading to restricted lives (avoidant and schizoid types).

More recently, Kernberg (1967) broke away from the former rigid adherence to the psychosexual developmental model, and suggested a different structural model based on the level of functioning. At the lowest and most primitive level were the antisocial characters who have little or no concept of the existence or needs of other people. At an intermediate level were those who function at an infantile level, mainly borderline and narcissistic types. At a higher level were hysterical, obsessive–compulsive and depressive types who were able to relate to others, although not quite at the mature level.

Concept of personality disorders

The topic of personality disorders does not lend itself easily to the medical model. Everyone has a personality, and defining precisely where, in the continuum, normal personality changes into a personality problem, and the latter becomes sufficiently severe to be a clinical personality disorder, is necessarily arbitrary. The dividing line is usually taken as when the personality disturbance results in impaired relationships and reduced social or occupational functioning. Schneider (1923) defined personality as the stable composite of feelings, values, tendencies and volitions. He excluded cognitive functions. Abnormal personality was defined simply as a state of divergence from the mean. Clinically abnormal personalities (Schneider used the term "psychopathic") were only one subclass of all the abnormal personalities, and were designated as those "who suffer, or make society suffer on account of their abnormality".

The modern concept of personality disorder derives from trait psychology. According to DSM–IV, personality traits are enduring patterns of perceiving, relating and thinking about the environment and oneself, and are exhibited in a wide range of important social and personal contexts. They describe the 'how' that underlies the behaviour pattern, but not specific behaviours themselves. Maladaptive traits are designated as abnormal and these are combined to form a limited number of categories of personality disorder; there are 11 categories in the ICD–10 and DSM–IV schemes. Such a limited number of categories fails to do justice to the rich tapestry of morbid human personality, but probably provides the best available scheme in the light of present knowledge.

Personality tends to be stable over time, although the psychologist, William James (1890), may have overstated the case when he said "by age 30 . . . our characters are as set in concrete". Disorders of personality are usually recognisable in adolescence or early adult life, and persist until middle age, when they seem to wane or at least become less obvious. Defining exactly what constitutes a personality disorder is an almost impossible task, but ICD–10 provides a lucid statement encompassing most of the main features:

> These types of condition comprise of deeply ingrained and enduring behaviour patterns manifesting themselves as inflexible responses to a broad range of personal and social situations. They represent either extreme or significant deviations from the way the average individual in a given culture perceives, thinks, feels and particularly relates to others. Such behaviour patterns tend to be stable and become multiple domains of behaviour and social functioning. They are frequently, but not always, associated with various degrees of subjective distress and problems in social functioning and performance. (World Health Organization, 1992)

Differences between ICD–10 and DSM–IV

Although both schemes now share a considerable area of agreement, there are a number of differences between the two systems of classification. For diagnostic assessment, DSM–IV tends to favour the clinician's interview with the patient, while ICD–10 emphasises the role of informants, but data from informants may also be used in making a DSM–IV diagnosis.

A second difference lies in the type and number of categories included in each classification, as shown in Table 18.1. DSM–IV also describes criteria for narcissistic personality disorder, which is not represented in ICD–10. This reflects the ongoing influence of the psychodynamic schools in the US compared with Europe where their influence has been rather more limited. Due to its close genetic connection with schizophrenia, schizotypal disorder is classified with schizophrenic disorders in ICD–10, but it remains within the personality disorder section in DSM–IV. Both schemes have removed cyclothymic personality from the personality disorders section and included it with the affective disorders. Borderline personality disorder, which has an extensive section in DSM–IV, was not included in ICD–9, but ICD–10 incorporates it as a subtype of the emotionally unstable personality.

DSM–IV groups the personality disorders into three groups. The first cluster, known as cluster A, or the eccentric disorders, includes paranoid, schizoid and schizotypal disorder. Cluster B, the dramatic group, includes antisocial, borderline, histrionic and narcissistic personality disorders. The third group, cluster C or the fearful group, includes avoidant, dependent, obsessive–compulsive, and passive aggressive personality disorders.

A final difference is the way in which the two schemes meet the problem of patients who cannot be easily placed into the existing categories. Some patients meet the criteria for several categories of personality disorder, and in these cases DSM–IV directs the clinician to record all the possible diagnoses (e.g. if borderline and schizotypal criteria are both met, then both conditions should be diagnosed), while ICD–10 has a category called "mixed personality disorder". DSM–IV also has a category "personality

Table 18.1 DSM–IV and ICD–10 personality disorders

	DSM–IV	ICD–10	Main features
Cluster A	Paranoid	Paranoid	Suspicious, feelings of perception, sensitivity
	Schizoid	Schizoid	Cold, detached, isolated
	Schizotypal	–[1]	Isolated, eccentric ideas
Cluster B	Antisocial	Dissocial	Behaviour disorder, callous, antisocial acts
	–	Emotionally unstable	Instability of mood, behaviour, relationships
	–	a. impulsive[3]	
	Borderline	b. borderline	
	Histrionic	Histrionic	Shallow, dramatic, egocentric
	Narcissistic	–[2]	Self-centred, grandiosity, entitlement
Cluster C	Avoidant	Anxious	Hypersensitive, timid, self-conscious
	Dependent	Dependent	Submissive, helplessness
	Obsessive–compulsive	Anankastic	Doubt, caution, obsessional
Additional categories	Personality disorder not otherwise specified	Mixed and other personality disorders	No predominant pattern of any of the above, but still impaired

1. Schizotypal disorder is classified in the section on schizophrenia.
2. Narcissistic personality disorder is not included in ICD–10.
3. Impulsive personality disorder is in ICD–10 but not DSM–IV, which instead includes intermittent explosive disorder as one of the habit disorders.

disorder not otherwise specified" which includes subjects who are socially impaired with relationship difficulties, yet fail to meet the diagnostic criteria of any one subtype. This category is also used to include other subtypes such as impulsive or immature types. Finally, ICD–10 includes a category of "troublesome personality changes" in which the personality changes are regarded as being secondary to coexisting affective or anxiety disorder.

A critique of the concept

Many criticisms have been levelled at the concept of personality disorder from sources as varied as philosophy and psychology, but mainly from within psychiatry itself. Blackburn (1988) pointed out how ICD–9 and ICD–10 almost reify the concept of normal personality on which the whole edifice of personality disorder is built. However, social psychologists are increasingly abandoning this concept of a normal and fixed personality, giving evidence that people do not behave similarly in particular situations (Mischel, 1968). Until recently the definitions of the various personality disorders and their subtypes were little more than literary descriptions by eminent psychiatrists, without evidence for acceptable degrees of either validity or reliability. Reliability is poorest for the trait-based definitions because traits are difficult to rate. For example, Thompson & Goldberg (1987) found that core traits of histrionic personality disorder (seductiveness, being dramatic, and labile) had very poor interrater reliability. Reliability may be better for definitions which incorporate specific symptoms or behaviours among their criteria. Thus, the DSM–IV categories of borderline and antisocial personality disorders have acceptable levels of interrater reliability because their definitions include certain observable behavioural items. None of the other DSM–IV subtypes have been studied sufficiently or shown to have acceptable levels of reliability. It is commonly assumed that reliability also signifies validity, but for the personality disorders there is no proof that the current definitions provide a valid description of those abnormal types met in clinical practice.

The construct of the present definitions of personality disorders has also been criticised on logical grounds (Blackburn, 1988). Traits describe inferred tendencies, the "manner" or the "how" of behaviour, and they fall into a different logical class to occurrences and behaviours. Blackburn pointed out that the DSM–III (American Psychiatric Association, 1980) definition of antisocial personality disorder (ASPD) almost wholly comprised a catalogue of the patient's crimes rather than a description of a type of personality. The more recent DSM–IV definition is more trait-orientated. The DSM–III definition of borderline personality disorder was even more inconsistent, comprising an unholy alliance of some traits (such as impulsiveness), some mental symptoms (such as lability of mood, anxiety and irritability), a few specific behaviours such as self-mutilation, as well as certain psychodynamic concepts (such as identity disturbance, over-idealisation and devaluation). It is not surprising that European psychiatrists have failed to warm to the concept, even though it remains popular in the US where the analytical influence remains strong.

Trait psychologists have also criticised the categorical approach and favour a dimensional one because this is less arbitrary, and therefore there is less loss of information. Eysenck is perhaps the best-known exponent of this approach and he described three dimensions (extroversion, neuroticism and psychoticism) which he derived from Jung. The status of the patient can be plotted graphically in each of these dimensions. The Minnesota Multiphasic Personality Inventory (MMPI) also uses a dimensional approach. Unfortunately, dimensions are of little value in the clinical situation where decisions need to be made quickly, and communicated to other clinicians or the court. A dimensional approach may have more accuracy, but deciding the cut-off between the normal and the pathological may not be possible.

A further criticism of current categories is that there are many hundreds of different traits and probably an enormous variety of abnormal personalities, which the present limited number of categories could not possibly describe adequately. The present definitions may be too restrictive and share too many common items, with resultant overlap. Studies have shown that many individuals are often comorbid for two or three different personality disorders and up to a third of patients cannot be diagnosed at all. This makes subtyping an almost meaningless exercise. The majority of clinicians content themselves with a diagnosis of personality disorder and make no attempt at subtyping unless the picture is easily recognised as one of the classical subtypes. Rutter (1987) went so far as to suggest that even though the concept of personality disorder should be retained, all the individual categories, with the exception of antisocial personality disorder, should be jettisoned.

Are personality disorders illnesses or not?

Disorders which are almost impossible to define, may have no actual symptoms, are of unknown cause, and also lack any specific treatment, barely fit into the medical concept of disease. However, they are serious conditions that can cause a considerable amount of damage, and are associated with an elevated mortality and morbidity. Doctors who continue to diagnose and treat personality disorders implicitly accept the notion of illness and are positing themselves as arbiters of social behaviour. On the other hand, a complete negation of the illness concept may not be helpful either. It may result in legal conundrums such as the "irresistible impulse" which has been used to explain the behaviour of some violent psychopathic individuals in forensic settings. Lewis & Appleby (1988) pointed to the more serious hazard of separating the personality disorders from the mental illnesses, in that it results in therapeutic neglect of those assigned a diagnosis of personality disorder, and they suggested the term should be abandoned. As Gunn (1988) pointed out, being "ill" entitles a patient to certain types of medical care, hospitalisation and degrees of tolerance not normally accorded to other people. On the other hand, not being ill means "being well", implying responsibility for one's actions, and if these are behaviourally disordered it is tantamount to being "bad". This leads to rejection by health services, withdrawal of patient privileges, and a lack of mitigation in legal circumstances.

Another concern within the profession is that whatever term is used eventually becomes a term of opprobium (Chodoff & Lyons, 1958). An early example of this is given by Kretschmer (1922) who felt at the time that the term 'hysterical' had acquired bad moral connotations, and so proposed the new and, at least initially, neutral term 'attention-seeking' to describe such individuals, but this term also rapidly fell into disrepute. The diagnosis is also often applied to patients on inadequate grounds. For example, Thompson & Goldberg (1987) found that over half of those diagnosed as having hysterical personality disorder had none of the DSM–III diagnostic features of histrionic personality disorders. Instead, the label was used to describe a group of difficult, hostile and manipulative individuals, with the presumed purpose of ejecting them from hospital. It is curious that most of the criticisms in relation to the definition of personality disorders have focused on borderline, antisocial and histrionic types – those in the dramatic cluster where disorders of behaviour are prominent features – while the definitions of personality disorders within the anxious and eccentric clusters have been generally accepted with little debate.

Epidemiology

Early studies

The early studies which used community samples had serious flaws in the methodology. The classification of personality disorder was vague, the disorder was generally equated with psychopathy, and non-clinicians were used to make the psychiatric assessments with the possibility of misdiagnoses and over-reporting. One of the earliest community studies of psychiatric illness conducted by a psychiatrist was in 1956 when Essen-Moller personally interviewed 2550 people in the community using predetermined clinical criteria to investigate the prevalence of psychiatric disorder. This study was a landmark as it was one of the first to incorporate both axis I and axis II diagnoses. Essen-Moller (1956) found that 29% of men and 19% of women had a definite or probable personality disorder, a further 13% and 38% respectively had asthenic (dependent) personalities, while 14% and 2% had "asociality". In the well-known Midtown Manhattan study, Srole *et al* (1962) found that 10% had a personality disorder. Leighton *et al* (1963) in Canada showed that 11% of men and 5% of women had sociopathy, and 7% and 6% respectively had other types of personality disorder. Self-report questionnaires usually give much higher rates of personality disorder than interview methods. Reich *et al* (1989) measured personality disorder using a self-administered questionnaire and found that 28.9% of a randomly selected community sample and 20% of a 'normal' volunteer group met the criteria for any category of personality disorder.

Before the publication of the Feighner criteria (Feighner *et al*, 1972), there were few reliable definitions even for the major mental disorders, let alone the rather more vague conditions like the personality disorders. Because severe personality disorders are usually ego-syntonic, self-report may be unreliable, and so interviews with informants (usually relatives) may give a more accurate picture. Case registers tend only to record axis I diagnoses, and are therefore less useful for studying axis II disorders. An epidemiological study of personality disorder should therefore use a structured interview, obtain data from informants, and the diagnosis should be based on one of the currently accepted definitions, preferably from DSM–IV or ICD–10.

The application of modern diagnostic criteria to the study of personality disorder started with Weissman *et al* (1978) who applied the Research Diagnostic Criteria (RDC; Spitzer *et al*, 1978) and demonstrated that 4.5% had depressive personality disorder, but less than 1% met criteria for cyclothymic or antisocial personality disorder. Casey & Tyrer (1986), using the Personality Assessment Schedule (PAS), found that 13% of subjects drawn from a GP's list had a personality disorder. Explosive and anankastic types were most common, with the explosive type being more common in men, and the asthenic (dependent) type in women. Maeir (1992) applied DSM–III–R (World Health Organization, 1987) criteria to a German community sample and found a prevalence of personality disorder of 10.3%. There is a trend for individuals with personality disorders to congregate in inner cities, particularly in disintegrated areas (Leighton *et al*, 1963), and this probably explains the urban/rural differences. The natural history of most personality disorders, particularly the flamboyant types, is to attenuate with advancing years. The excess of those who are under 45 has been replicated in many studies (Spitzer *et al*, 1979; Myers *et al*, 1984).

Special populations

Parasuicide population

The parasuicide population has a high rate of personality disorder. Investigations using clinical criteria have found a range of figures: 15.4% for men and women combined (Hanson & Wang, 1984); 42% for men and 22% for women (Morgan *et al*, 1975); 52% for men and 44% for women (Ovenstone, 1973). Using the Present State Examination, Urwin & Gibbons (1979) found that 26% of men and 16% of women had a personality disorder. Using the PAS, Casey (1989) found that 75–83% of men and 54–64% of women had a personality disorder, mainly of the explosive type. Applying the DSM–III–R scheme, Ennis *et al* (1989) showed that 56% had a diagnosis of personality disorder, mainly of the borderline or antisocial type.

General practice populations

Kessel (1960) and Shepherd *et al* (1966) found that 5% of primary care attenders were assessed by their general practitioners (GPs) as having abnormal personalities. According to Casey *et al* (1984), of those identified by their GP as having "conspicuous morbidity", the GP diagnosed 8.9% as having a personality disorder, while 6.4% were given this diagnosis by the research psychiatrist. When personality was assessed independently of mental state diagnosis using the PAS, 33.9% had an axis II diagnosis, of which the explosive type was the most common. A much lower figure of 3.3% was given by Dilling & Weyerer (1989), using rather stricter criteria.

Psychiatric out-patients

High rates of personality disorder occur among psychiatric out-patients. Alnaes & Torgersen (1988) applied the Structured Interview for DSM–III Personality Disorders (SIDP) (see below) to assess personality in consecutive out-patient attenders, showing that 81% met DSM–III criteria for personality disorder, and over half met criteria for more than one category. For new out-patients in the US, Jackson *et al* (1991) gave a figure of 67% and Kass *et al* (1985) of 51%, with borderline type being the most frequent. Tyrer *et al* (1983), using the PAS and applying ICD–9/10 criteria, found that 39% of non-psychotic out-patients had a personality disorder.

Psychiatric in-patients

Over ten years ago 7.6% of all admissions to psychiatric hospitals in England and Wales had a primary diagnosis of personality disorder (Department of Health and Social Security, 1985). The publication of multi-axial diagnostic schemes such as DSM–III, which have easily understood and explicit definitions, led to a substantial increase in the frequency with which the diagnosis of personality disorder was made among in-patients. Loranger (1990) compared the last five years of the DSM–II era (1975–1980) with the first five years of the DSM–III era (1980–1985) and showed that the rate of personality disorder diagnoses rose from 19% to 49%, with no change in admission policy for the unit studied. The most common categories were the borderline and "mixed group", as shown in Table 18.2. Pfohl (1986) also found that 51% of non-psychotic in-patients met the SIDP criteria for personality disorder, with the borderline and histrionic types being most frequent. Among unipolar depressed in-patients, Baxter *et al* (1984) found that 50% had borderline personality disorders.

Eating disorders

An association between personality disorders, particularly borderline personality disorder (BPD), and eating disorders is well-established, but published figures vary widely; the literature is reviewed by Skodol *et al* (1993). Rates are higher for eating disorder subjects who are in-patients (93% comorbid for any personality disorder; 55% combined with BPD)

(Piran *et al*, 1988) than for out-patients (27% comorbid for personality disorders, 9% BPD) (Herzog *et al*, 1992). Bulimia is more often associated with cluster B, the dramatic personality disorders, especially BPD, but it should be noted that the symptom of binge eating is one of the diagnostic criteria of BPD. In particular, the bulimic subtype of anorexia nervosa is particularly associated with high rates of BPD (55%), as compared with only 7% for the pure restricting subtype of anorexia, which tends to be more associated with avoidant personality disorder. A history of sexual abuse in childhood may be common to both the personality disorder and the eating disorder, but Waller (1993) concluded that the relationship was relatively non-specific and only present among BPD subjects with both anorexia nervosa and bulimia. Whatever the aetiological significance of the association, patients with combined disorders seem to have a more chronic course and are more difficult to treat. The topic is also discussed on page 864.

Prison populations

Studies in prison settings have shown a high prevalence of antisocial personality disorder (39–76%) (Hare, 1983; Bland *et al*, 1990; Cote & Hodgins, 1990). The variation may be due to differences in the concentration of hardened career criminals in the various prisons. Among prisoners with recurrent and serious disciplinary problems, 86% had antisocial personality disorder, the remainder being psychotic. Patients who are legally detained

Table 18.2 Frequency of different DSM–III personality disorders in psychiatric in-patients (*n* = 2916)

Personality disorder type	%
Paranoid	2.4
Schizoid	3.3
Schizotypal	4.1
Compulsive	2.9
Histrionic	2.3
Dependent	9.1
Antisocial	4.6
Narcissistic	5.9
Avoidant	2.4
Borderline	26.7
Passive aggressive	3.5
Atypical/mixed/other	32.6

After Loranger (1990). 10 914 admissions were screened, and 2916 fulfilled criteria for personality disorder. Note the residual category of atypical/mixed/other accounts for more cases than any specific type.

on the grounds of psychopathic behaviour comprise 0.24% of the general psychiatric hospital population, but as many as 25% of the population of the special hospitals (Coid, 1993).

Aetiology

The personality disorders are conditions of unknown aetiology. In the absence of much reliable information, the nature–nurture dichotomy has attracted considerable speculation, but it is likely that both make an important contribution. A hereditary contribution for some types of adult personality disorder has been established, and there are links with certain childhood psychiatric disorders. Clearest evidence for a hereditary contribution has been found for antisocial and schizotypal personality disorders, and to a lesser extent for obsessional and borderline types. Milder types of personality disorder that only occasionally reach clinical attention have not been studied to the same extent. Personality disorders are composites of several traits, and it is likely that these represent the inherited element rather than the clinical personality disorders themselves. Studies based on the MMPI show that social introversion, depression, psychopathic deviance and some schizophrenia-like traits in particular may be heritable, but there is little evidence for other traits (McGuffin & Gottesman, 1984). Twin studies based on the Eysenck Personality Inventory suggest that hereditability accounts for 35–50% of the variance for the traits of neuroticism and extroversion, and there is also evidence that obsessional traits may be partially genetic in origin (Clifford *et al*, 1984). The neural substrate for abnormal traits is not known, but Eysenck (1979) has suggested that differences in extroversion and neuroticism may be explained by variations in the level of arousal of the limbic system and the ascending reticular formation.

A biological basis to the personality disorders has been suggested for centuries, most notably in the humoural theory of Hippocrates which was quintessentially biological. A more modern expression of this idea occurs in neurochemistry, with the humours of today being the neurotransmitters such as serotonin, but whether these are more relevant to the human character than the yellow bile or phlegm of Hippocrates remains to be seen. Cloninger (1987) has speculatively suggested that novelty-seeking is linked to dopamine, harm-avoidance to serotonin, and reward-dependence to noradrenaline. There is also the repeated suggestion in the literature going back to Kraepelin that some personality disorders, such as the schizoid and schizotypal, might be related to schizophrenia, while others, such as the borderline, depressive and cyclothymic, are related to affective disorder, and that similar biochemical mechanisms are responsible for both the functional psychoses and their corresponding personality disorders.

Learning theory has been used to explain the development of both normal and abnormal personality. It is hypothesised that faulty learning exaggerates genetically predetermined traits, which results in clinical disturbances of the personality. A child with an extrovert temperament reared in a violent household may later develop violent tendencies, but a shy child in similar circumstances would not do so (Farrington *et al*, 1990). Psychoanalysts, such as Bowlby (1977), have focused on early attachments to the mother. Rejection by the parents and violence or abuse in the formative years may all lead to later personality difficulties. Coercive patterns of child-rearing are thought to be particularly harmful as they evoke counter-aggression in the child, so that a mutually coercive pattern is set up. By contrast, over-protective parenting may lead to later dependent patterns. In this respect, the so-called difficult child syndrome may contribute later to adult maladjustment. This comprises irregularity of biological functions, withdrawal from novel stimuli, poor adaptability, intense responses and negative mood (Thomas & Chess, 1982). Another long-lasting constitutional trait is shyness, which is probably linked to avoidant personality disorder both in childhood and in adult life.

It would be an over-exaggeration to suggest there was a close one-to-one link with childhood temperamental difficulties and adult personality disorder; most children with difficulties of temperament will develop normally and do not suffer from a personality disorder as an adult (Goodyear, 1993).

Categories of personality disorder

The individual disorders outlined in ICD–10 will be described first, and differences, if any, from the DSM–IV scheme mentioned. Descriptions are largely drawn from the detailed account given by Millon (1981). Two categories of personality disorder, borderline and dissocial types, have been given some prominence in this account because subjects with these disorders have a high frequency of contact with medical, psychiatric and forensic services. The boxes that follow use ICD–10 criteria, and any differences from DSM–IV are noted.

Anankastic personality disorder (DSM–IV obsessive–compulsive personality disorder)

The obsessional or anankastic personality was first clearly described by Freud (1908). It is characterised by perfectionism, punctiliousness, indecisiveness, reluctance to take risks, rigidity and orderliness. The anankastic personality has difficulty with uncertainty, yet a great need to be in control. Chance has to be reduced to a minimum, and any unplanned situation is avoided. Such individuals like routine and may have a timetable and a specific menu for each day which is not permitted to vary from week to week. They may be rigid in their views, and in extreme cases insist on others adhering to their views and their timetables as well. As a result their behaviour and expectations impinge upon others and this may lead to disagreements. Preoccupied by order, routine and planning, they lack spontaneity.

Clinically, patients present as neat, stiff and formal individuals, although they are rarely referred for this reason alone since these traits, in a milder form, may be valued by society. Thus minor degrees of obsessionality are not only commonplace but also desirable, leading to reliability and competence, a pattern which should not be classified as personality disorder. The ICD–10 diagnostic criteria are given in Box 18.1, and those for DSM–IV are similar. The personality type may be more common in rural than urban areas (Casey & Tyrer, 1990).

Obsessional personalities may present with any axis I disorder. There is disagreement about whether obsessional personality forms the basis for obsessional symptoms (Rachman & Hodgson, 1980; Reed, 1985), although there does appear to be an association with obsessional neurosis (Tyrer *et al*, 1983).

Hereditary factors may be aetiologically relevant. Clifford *et al* (1984), using the Leyton Obsessional Inventory, showed that obsessional traits and obsessional symptoms had heritability factors of 0.4 and 0.47 respectively, although an earlier and probably less sophisticated study based on the Middlesex Hospital Questionnaire failed to detect any genetic effect (Young & Lader, 1971). The belief that this type of personality is associated with 'endogenous depression' is probably incorrect and stems from the error of assessing personality only when the patient is ill (see also chapter 15).

Paranoid personality

Kretschmer (1918) described a condition he called paranoia sensitiva: an extraordinary sensitivity to rejection by others, and a consequent tendency to resist all social contacts because of difficulty in trusting others and suspiciousness.

Clinically this group of patients is characterised by a constant feeling of threat from others. Individuals are always on the alert for perceived dangers, and even misinterpret common gestures of courtesy as ploys to be used against them. Advice from friends that they are not under siege is not accepted, and they are adamant in their defensive stance. Others describe them as touchy because they take offence easily. Sometimes they may be insensitive to the feelings of others, and fail to trust even those whom they should trust, such as parents or spouses. Not surprisingly they are often disliked by colleagues, and this serves to heighten further their sense of mistrust. A particular fear, which can evoke extreme anxiety, is that of being coerced by a power stronger than they are. It is probably this fear that stops them from seeking help, because they regard doctors and psychiatrists as powerful authority figures.

Because paranoid personalities also have a high degree of anxiety associated with almost any type of attachment, they tend to become isolated

---

Box 18.1 ICD–10 criteria for anankastic personality disorder

1. Feelings of doubt and caution.
2. Preoccupation with details, rules, lists, etc.
3. Perfectionism that interferes with task completion.
4. Excessive conscientiousness, and undue preoccupation with productivity to the exclusion of pleasure and interpersonal relationships.
5. Excessive pedantry and adherence to social conventions.
6. Unreasonable insistence by the patient that others submit exactly to his or her way of doing things; or unreasonable reluctance to allow others to do things.
7. Intrusion of insistent and unwelcome thoughts or impulses.

Three out of seven items required for the diagnosis. DSM–IV describes "obsessive–compulsive personality disorder", and the diagnosis is based on four out of eight items. These include items 1–6 above, but item 7 is excluded. The additional two items in DSM–IV are: a miserly spending style towards both self and others; and an inability to discard worthless objects even when they have no sentimental value.

---

and this leads to a gradual impairment of reality testing. In later stages, there is little difference in their minds between what they have thought and what they have seen. These individuals maintain self-esteem by projecting their malevolence onto others, by denying any personal weakness, and by self-aggrandisement through grandiose and persecutory fantasies. In the face of decompensation they may retreat into fantasy or become depressed. Morbid jealousy of a non-delusional type sometimes occurs. Another rare subtype is the querulous litigant who spends many hours each day trying to sue other people, often over the most trivial issues. An unusual complication in old age is the so-called senile squalor or Diogenes syndrome. These people neglect themselves to a severe extent so that they end up living in extreme squalor. Macmillan & Shaw (1966) found that while half their cases were psychotic, the remainder had lifelong premorbid severe personality traits of being independent, suspicious, unfriendly, obstinate, secretive and quarrelsome, a pattern suggestive of paranoid personality disorder.

ICD–10 criteria are shown in Box 18.2, and DSM–IV criteria show few differences.

Differential diagnosis

Paranoia is a ubiquitous symptom and may be present in schizophrenia (particularly paranoid schizophrenia), organic and affective disorders (both mania and depression). The main differential is from *delusional disorder*, in which the paranoia is of a psychotic type. Schizoid personalities share the aloofness of the paranoid personality, but lack paranoid ideation. Some antisocial personalities are also paranoid, but apart from an occasional outburst, paranoid personalities tend not to commit antisocial acts.

Schizoid personality disorder

Eugene Bleuler (1922) first coined the term "schizoidie" to describe a trait he believed to be present in everyone, varying only in its degree of biological penetrance. In its full-blown form he suggested it led to schizophrenia, but in milder cases it resulted in schizoid personality. These were "people who are shut in, suspicious, incapable of discussion, people who are comfortably dull". Kretschmer (1918) provides an apt literary description of the anaesthetic schizoid:

> We feel we are with something flavourless, boring . . . what is there in the deep under all these masks, perhaps there is nothing, a dark hollow-eyed nothing . . . affective anaemia . . . indifference is a common schizoid variant of affective insensibility. It is an uninterestedness which is ostentatiously manifest. The indifferent notes that he takes absolutely no interest in many things which are important to other people . . . they are devoid of humour, and often serious without exhibiting either sorrowfulness or cheerfulness. Their expression, dullness, denotes their passive lack of feeling, a phlegmatic state which may be distinguished by the lack of warm emotional responsiveness towards mankind.

The modern concept differs little from Kretschmer's, and the core feature is a profound lack of emotion, warmth, or any concept of the normal give-and-take of human relationships. This prevents the patient from making or sustaining any close relationships. Even in a mandatory situation such as

---

Box 18.2   ICD–10 criteria for paranoid personality disorder

1. Excessive sensitivity to setbacks and rebuffs.
2. Tendency to bear grudges.
3. Suspiciousness, misconstrues neutral or friendly actions as hostile.
4. Combative sense of personal rights.
5. Recurrent suspicion without justification of sexual partners.
6. Excess in self-importance, self-referential attitude.
7. Preoccupied with unsubstantiated conspiratorial explanations.

Three out of seven items required for the diagnosis. DSM–IV excludes item 6 and instead has an item "reluctant to confide in others because of unwarranted fear that the information will be used maliciously against him or her".

work, communication tends to be formal or perfunctory. Jobs involving the expenditure of physical or mental energy are generally shunned, and light activities such as reading or watching television are preferred. Schizoid personalities rarely present with symptomatic complaints, and in self-description tend to be rather vague or superficial. This vagueness does not represent any attempt to deny complex feelings, but rather signifies a real impairment in social and emotional processes and the individual's inner world is correspondingly empty. There may be a few residual past memories and emotions, but in general their inner worlds lack the complicated unconscious processes or the intricacies found in other pathological personalities. Introspection about philosophy, science and religion are commonplace and may become the sole concern of the schizoid individual. The ICD–10 definition of schizoid personality disorder is shown in Box 18.3 and shows some minor differences from DSM–IV criteria.

Differential diagnosis

The condition is distinguished from schizophrenia by the absence of psychotic symptoms, although a picture resembling schizoid personality can occur in the prodromal phase of schizophrenia, lasting a few months or years, which may precede the appearance of florid symptoms. The distinction from *simple schizophrenia* is more difficult to make, but simple schizophrenia usually has a later onset (18 or older), the presence of negative symptoms, and the deterioration is rather more severe. *Schizotypal disorder* is associated with a greater degree of eccentric thought and behaviour, but the two disorders are often comorbid. Isolation is also present in *avoidant personalities*, but they are fearful of rejection rather than simply disinterested. A rare differential is chronic *depersonalisation syndrome*. These individuals complain that they relate to the world as if through a wall of glass, but still maintain good human relationships. Asperger's syndrome (also known as a schizoid disorder of childhood) is distinguished by its earlier onset during childhood. Rather than simply being withdrawn, Asperger's subjects show an impairment of social interaction that may be similar to, although milder than, that shown by autistics. They have a range of restrictive and repetitive or stereotyped interests, there are oddities in the way they use language for communication, and their speech is either monotonous, like a mechanical drone, or stacatto. There are abnormalities in non-verbal expression which occur in Asperger's syndrome and are said to distinguish the disorder from schizoid personality disorder (Tantam, 1988). Autistic disorder is a very much more severe disorder and is readily distinguished by the severe language disorder and very early onset. In adult life, some patients with Asperger's syndrome may develop sociopathic traits and commit offences (Wolff & Cull, 1986). The relationship between shy children, Asperger's syndrome, autism and the adult personality disorders is reviewed by Le Couter (1993).

Box 18.3   ICD–10 criteria for schizoid personality disorder

1. Few, if any, activities provide pleasure.
2. Emotional coldness, detachment or flattened activity.
3. Limited capacity to express warmth, tender feelings or anger.
4. Apparent indifference to praise or criticism.
5. Little interest in sexual experience.
6. Preference for solitary activities.
7. Excessive preoccupation with fantasy and introspection.
8. Lack of close friends (or only one).
9. Insensitivity to providing social norms and conventions.

Three criteria required to make the diagnosis; onset in early adulthood or before. DSM–IV stipulates four out of seven similar criteria, but excludes items 7 and 9.

Schizotypal personality disorder

The term *schizotypal* was coined by the analyst Rado (1956) as an abbreviation of the "schizophrenic phenotype". Although Rado's genetic ideas have long since passed into oblivion, more recent adoption and cross-fostering studies have shown a link with schizophrenia, and so schizotypal disorder is included within the schizophrenic spectrum disorders. The DSM–III (and later DSM–IV) criteria for schizotypal personality disorder were based on 14 cases of odd withdrawn personalities who were called the "B3 spectrum disorder cases" among the first-degree relatives of adopted-away schizophrenic probands in the cross-fostering study of Wender (1977). Since then, almost all family studies of schizophrenia have found an excess of both schizophrenia and schizotypal personality disorder among first-degree relatives. The addition of schizotypal personality to the co-twins of schizophrenic probands gives a higher concordance ratio for monozygotic : dizygotic twins than when the diagnosis is restricted to DSM–III schizophrenia alone (Farmer *et al*, 1987). Although the earlier family studies of schizotypal probands found only an excess of schizotypal but not schizophrenic relatives (Baron *et al*, 1983), a more recent study by Battaglia *et al* (1991) based on pure schizotypal probands demonstrated a morbid risk for schizophrenia of around 5%. The earlier studies included probands with borderline as well as schizotypal features, and while this group may be more common, they may be different from the pure schizotypal personalities.

Clinical description

Like schizoid personalities, schizotypal personalities are aloof and isolated but their inner world is not so barren. There may be referential ideas, odd beliefs, magical thinking and suspiciousness, but this is not of delusional intensity. Unlike the schizoid the schizotypal personality has some degree of relatedness to others, and a feeling of being part of the world. Sometimes individuals complain of feelings of estrangement and depersonalisation, and they may socially isolate themselves for long periods. During these phases, there may be inappropriate affect, paranoid ideation, and communication in odd and circumstantial ways. For much of the time they feel out of touch with other people. The DSM–IV criteria are shown in Box 17.4, and in this scheme schizotypal disorder is grouped with the personality disorders, but ICD–10 regards it as a disorder related genetically to schizophrenia, and therefore includes it in the section on schizophrenia.

Dissocial personality disorder (psychopathy, sociopathy, antisocial personality disorder)

History

Pinel (1806) wrote of a condition called "manie sans deliré". Among his cases he described a non-psychotic but ill-tempered French nobleman who, in a fit of rage, pushed a woman down a well. According to Pinel, this disorder consisted of a profound disorder of affective function, blind impulses to commit acts of serious violence (manie) which occurred in the absence of any disorder of perception or intellect. Although Pinel pleaded that his patient suffered from "manie sans deliré", the nobleman was still

---

Box 18.4 DSM–IV criteria for schizotypal personality disorder

1. Ideas of reference (not delusions of reference).
2. Excessive social anxiety.
3. Odd beliefs or magical thinking.
4. Unusual perceptual experiences (e.g. illusions).
5. Odd or eccentric behaviour or appearance.
6. No close friends or confidants (or only one), other than first-degree relatives.
7. Odd speech.
8. Inappropriate or constricted affect (e.g. silly or aloof).
9. Suspiciousness or paranoid ideation.

The disorder should have started in early adulthood, and five out of nine criteria are required for the diagnosis. The symptoms should not be due to schizophrenia or pervasive developmental disorder. In ICD–10, schizotypal disorder is classified together with the schizophrenias rather than with the personality disorders, although the ICD–10 text states that the course resembles that of a personality disorder and the criteria are broadly similar.

Adapted with permission from DSM–IV. Copyright 1994 American Psychiatric Association.

sentenced for life to the Bicetrê, the main asylum in Paris. Pritchard (1835) described a similar condition called "moral insanity" which comprised "a morbid perversion of the natural feelings, tempers, moral dispositions and natural impulses without any defect in intellectual reason and functions or any insane delusions or hallucinations". In France, Trélat (1861) coined the term "folie lucide" to describe "lucid madmen who in spite of their disturbed reason respond to all questions to the point and to the superficial observer looked quite normal", while impulsive behavioural states such as homicidal and suicidal monomanias were held to be cases of "impulsive insanity" in the scheme of Dagonet (1870).

The 19th century French literature was dominated by the concept of degeneration, which, according to Magnan (1886), was a specific inherited physical and mental disorder which became increasingly severe in successive generations, finally resulting in the extirpation of the affected individuals and their families. Lombroso (1887) in Italy also saw a biological link between criminality and moral insanity in his book *L'homme Criminal: Criminal-ne, Fou Moral, Epileptique,* in which he declared "they are born delinquent with the physical stigmata of moral insanity". Lombroso also suggested that an epileptoid state was the main cause of character disorder. Only the earlier German literature defined the abnormal personality of the psychopath in the same way as today, that is in terms of behavioural traits, and the writings of Koch, Schneider and Kretschmer all provide elegant descriptions.

There are many 20th century contributions to this subject. Karpman (1946) described a primary idiopathic psychopathy called anethopathy, to include individuals whose antisocial behaviour occurred as a result of a constitutionally determined failure of personality development. Secondary psychopaths were those whose antisocial behaviour could be explained by other psychopathology. Henderson (1939) described three psychopathic types – aggressive, inadequate and creative – the latter accounting for the high intelligence found among some deviant characters. Cleckley (1976) provided a series of detailed clinical descriptions of psychopathic individuals in his seminal book *The Mask of Sanity,* selecting the title because he felt the individuals were so deranged that they were suffering from a severe, although concealed, mental illness.

Epidemiology

The only category for which there are reliable epidemiological figures is antisocial personality disorder (ASPD). Myers *et al* (1984) reported life-time prevalence rates of 2.1–3.3%. Sociocultural and religious factors may influence the rate. Thus low rates were found in Taiwan, ranging from 0.03% in rural settings to 0.14% in the capital (Hwu *et al*, 1989). No case was found among the Hutterites, a rural religious sect in America (Eaton & Weil, 1955). Around 6.5% of all psychiatric patients have antisocial 'reactions', but higher rates of around 18% are observed among attenders at psychiatric emergency clinics (Robins, 1985). The male:female ratio for the DSM–III definition of ASPD is 6:1, but when the older Schneiderian trait-based criteria are applied it falls to 2.6 in rural Sweden, and 1.25 in Iceland.

Helgason (1964) observed that psychopathy occurred in 16% of men who emigrated from Iceland, while the rate was only 5% in those who remained in Iceland, with a rather smaller difference for women. Robins (1985) has speculated that the higher crime rate observed in the US compared within Europe might be partially explained by selective migration, because the American population is partly made up of successive generations of European immigrants. Higher rates are also found in urban rather than rural settings. An effect for lower social class is doubtful, and if present is likely to be small. Robins (1985) has speculated that the rate for ASPD might be rising, basing her figures on the rising crime rates in Western countries, but it should be noted that many other factors contribute to crime.

Clinical description

These individuals may be charming, brusque, or occasionally belligerent in their manner. There is generally an inner coldness, coupled with insensitivity to the feelings of others, and a lack of empathy. More severe cases are obviously callous, and some will have committed serious crimes. In social or family situations there is a tendency to try to dominate, or at the very least demean, other people. Confrontation on some personal issue may provoke revenge, and among those with poor impulse control this may rapidly escalate into violence.

Dissocial individuals usually have a clear intellectual grasp of the moral values of society, and may even superficially acknowledge that they should change their behaviour. They repeatedly fail to learn from experience, or fail to respond to conventional regimes of punishment. A few, especially the more simple types, may be so grossly insensitive as to be genuinely unaware of the feelings of others. However, most are all too keenly aware of the foibles and weaknesses of other people, and take advantage to prey on them. The defect in affectional responsiveness is serious and permits callous behaviour. There is little capacity to share tender feelings, experience genuine affection, or love. A sham apology, or expression of contrition, may sometimes appear after hurting someone, or following a serious crime, but there is little or no genuine experience of guilt or remorse.

Two psychodynamic mechanisms are commonly employed by sociopaths and these are rationalisation and projection. Aggressive behaviour and unkind actions are rationalised by viewing them as "hard but honest" or saying "the world is a tough place, where dog eats dog". Those with a more vivid imagination resort to lying. Projection and projective identification permits individuals to disown their own malevolent impulses and attribute them to others. Attacks on other people are then justified, as subjects view themselves as the persecuted victim.

Boredom and a low tolerance of frustration are common. These individuals are usually unable to sustain the tedium of a job, or the day-to-day responsibilities of a marriage. They may resort to thrill-seeking behaviours, such as gambling, promiscuity or substance abuse. In spite of their almost total lack of respect for the rights of others, many have a superficial charm and a mask of civility. However, before long the charmer will display his true colours as a con-man or fraudster, and when among other people the urge to demonstrate hostility and vindictiveness soon surfaces.

The more extreme cases may become criminals. One study showed that serious felonies only occurred in around a fifth of those who fulfilled criteria for ASPD. Rather more frequent were problems with aggression, work and promiscuity. Men tended to have more illegal occupations, traffic offences, arrests, and greater promiscuity. Women with ASPD more often deserted or hit their spouses, manifested child-neglect, or failed to work steadily.

Millon (1981) pointed out that there are many more people with milder psychopathic traits who are neither criminal nor sufficiently dysfunctional to satisfy current diagnostic criteria. The ruthless, conniving business man, the brutalising sergeant or the vindictive headmistress all discharge their hostile impulses under the guise of a respectable occupation. Among Cleckley's (1941) case histories were a minister of the church, a lawyer, a physician, and even a psychiatrist!

Diagnosis and differential diagnosis

Equating criminality (a behaviour) with sociopathy (a personality type) has led to much confusion in the past. Most criminals are neither sociopathic nor mentally ill, although some sociopaths may get involved in crime and they commonly become recidivists. In a few cases of chronic schizophrenia, personality deterioration resulting in lack of inhibition may lead to a picture resembling sociopathy. During the early phases of mania, particularly in the paranoid aggressive subtype, there is increased aggression, importuning, rudeness and insensitivity which may be indistinguishable from aggressive sociopathy. DSM–IV specifies that ASPD should not be diagnosed in the presence of mania. Reid (1985) advises caution when applying the label to individuals in late adolescence or early adulthood, particularly among those from disruptive environments. Many such young delinquents lack the inner affectionless core and will later mature out of their antisocial behaviour. The label itself is damaging, and should not be applied unless the pattern has persisted for many years.

Comorbidity

The ECA found no association between ASPD and anxiety, phobic disorder, obsessive–compulsive disorder, depression, mania or schizophrenia. The only disorders which were associated with ASPD were alcoholism and substance abuse, confirming many of the earlier studies. Among women there was an association with somatisation disorder; a correlation was found between the number of antisocial and somatic symptoms for some individuals. These findings echo earlier observations on Briquet's syndrome that personality disorder of the "hysterical" type was linked to antisocial behaviour. The presence of raised rates of depression and anxiety among treated samples has led Robins (1985) to suggest that those with ASPD only seek treatment for their axis I disorder and not for their personality problems. In a special hospital population, Coid (1993) observed much higher rates of comorbidity for affective disorder, as well as for other personality disorders, in particular paranoid disorder in men and borderline disorder among women.

Classification

ICD–10 defines "dissocial personality disorder" as shown in Box 17.5. Subjects usually come to attention because of a growing disparity between behaviour and social norms. The DSM–III definition had quite a different emphasis and described antisocial behaviours rather than abnormal personality traits, and this was continued in DSM–III–R. The DSM–IV definition is now very similar to the ICD–10 definition, differing only in the stipulation that there should be some evidence of conduct disorder before the age of 15.

Other classificatory systems

Cleckley (1941) described a series of 16 traits which he considered to be typical of the psychopath, including cunning, callousness, lack of remorse, shallow affect, impulsivity, irresponsibility, superficial charm, pathological lying, and so on. On the basis of these traits, Hare & McPherson (1984)e devised the "Psychopathic Check List", a scale of 20 items which has been used in neuropsychological investigations of psychopathy. Blackburn (1971) used the MMPI to classify psychopathy and identified four distinct patterns. The first group were highly extroverted, free of guilt, impulsive, and more violent in terms of previous convictions. A second group had more neurotic features, and they were withdrawn, hypochondriacal, suspicious, prone to depression, impulsive with anxious aggression, undersocialised and introverted. A third group were controlled, with a defensive denial of psychological problems, and they also denied experiencing anxiety or other affects, and some were mildly extroverted. The fourth group also showed defensive denial, but were more introverted and suspicious than the third group. Blackburn (1971) argued that the first two MMPI types were aggressive because they *lacked control*, while the latter two groups were *overcontrolled* and became aggressive when their control broke down, according to Megargee's (1966) model of undercontrolled and overcontrolled aggression.

Violent offences

Violent offences committed by dissocial subjects have been compared with violent actions committed by non-dissocial individuals. Dissocial violence tends to be more callous, more aggressive, and more commonly associated with a macho display. Victims are generally male, unknown to the subject, and episodes more often occur in association with alcohol. Violent episodes caused by non-dissocial individuals generally have more understandable motives, and there is usually an affective colouring to the episode (Williamson *et al*, 1987) It is of interest that most of the violent and disruptive prisoners in the English prisons have high scores on Hare's Psychopathic Checklist (Hare & McPherson, 1984).

Legal aspects

Maudsley (1897) was one of the first to suggest that the legal system should not treat such offence-prone individuals in the same way as common criminals: "When such individuals commit an offence, the truest justice would be the admission of a modified responsibility". The category of "moral imbecility" was first included in the 1913 Mental Deficiency Act, and this was changed to "moral defective" in the 1927 Act. The 1959 Mental Health Act included four legal categories for administrative purposes; subnormality, severe subnormality, mental illness and psychopathic disorder, the latter

---

Box 18.5   ICD–10 criteria for dissocial personality disorder

Personality disorder, usually coming to attention because of a gross disparity between behaviour and the prevailing social norms, characterised by:

1. Callous unconcern for the feelings of others.
2. Gross irresponsibility, disregard for social norms, rules and obligations.
3. Incapacity to maintain enduring relationships though no difficulty in establishing them.
4. Low tolerance to frustration; low threshold for discharge of aggression including violence.
5. Incapacity to experience guilt and profit from experience, particularly punishment.
6. Marked proneness to blame others, or offer plausible rationalisations.

DSM–IV criteria are essentially similar, but the individual should be at least 18 years old and have shown evidence of conduct disorder before the age of 15; also the antisocial behaviour should not occur exclusively in the course of schizophrenia or a manic episode.

being defined as "a persistent disorder or disability of the mind (whether or not including subnormality or low intelligence) which results in abnormally aggressive or seriously irresponsible conduct on the part of the individual and requires or is susceptible to medical treatment". Unfortunately, most of these individuals were not susceptible to treatment and the inclusion of the treatability clause proved unworkable, because it required psychiatrists to admit such people to hospital even when little change was possible. In the 1983 Act, although a similar definition was retained, the treatability clause was replaced with the phrase "is likely to alleviate or prevent a deterioration of his condition". This meant that there was less obligation to admit such patients, particularly those for whom treatment would have little or no effect.

Aetiology

This has been more extensively studied than in the other personality disorders. There is evidence for a hereditary contribution, an aggressive temperament, conduct disorder and attention deficit disorder during childhood, as well as an environmental contribution from abuse and deprivation during childhood.

Earlier twin studies of criminality, and the more recent adoption studies of ASPD, all point to a significant hereditary contribution. The pooled results of seven twin studies of adult criminality showed a weighted mean monozygotic (MZ) concordance rate of 51%, but only 22% for dizygotic (DZ) twins. By contrast, delinquency does not appear to be genetically determined: the pooled results for five twin studies of juvenile delinquency found an MZ concordance rate of 87% and a similar high DZ concordance rate of 72%, suggesting that juvenile delinquency may have a strong familial component but that this is not genetic (McGuffin & Gottesman, 1984).

Adoption and cross-fostering studies have the advantage that they can tease out genetic from environmental factors. Crowe (1972) found that the offspring of female felons in Iowa had increased rates of criminality and sociopathy, but not alcoholism or any other psychiatric disorder. Adoption studies also confirm the genetic contribution to antisocial personality (Schulzinger, 1972; Cadoret *et al*, 1985). Hutchings & Mednick (1974) used the interesting approach of cross-fostering in order to attempt to quantify the relative contribution of nature and nurture in the development of antisocial personality. In cases in which neither the biological nor adoptive parents were known to the police, 11% of adoptees had a criminal record, and this was similar to the figure when the adoptive father also had a police record, indicating a familial but non-genetic component. Where only the biological father was known to the police, 21% of the adoptees had a police record, and where both the biological and adoptive parents had police records this figure rose to 36% for the adoptees, suggesting an additive effect. Around 16% of the offspring of sociopathic parents have ASPD, which is similar to the rate found in cross-fostering studies (Robins, 1985). This suggests that environment may play a role, but only if there is a preexisting genetic diathesis. A separate environmental factor, late placement for adoption, also makes an independent contribution to subsequent criminality. Bohman *et al* (1982), in their extensive Swedish cross-fostering studies also showed that the presence of criminality in both biological and adoptive parents independently increased the risk of criminality for adopted children. However, the adopted-away sons of parents who are both alcohol abusers and criminals were only alcohol abusers, suggesting that good parenting might alleviate the antisocial tendency, but had little effect on drinking behaviour. Other environmental factors which were associated with antisocial behaviour identified in these studies were prolonged institutional care, lower socioeconomic status, and for men, multiple temporary placements during childhood.

A question of some interest is whether ASPD has a familial or genetic link with other types of personality disorder and psychiatric illness. A familial association with somatisation disorder was first described by Guze *et al* (1967) and subsequently confirmed by Cloninger & Gottesman (1987). Cadoret (1978) also found a familial association between ASPD and hysteria of the Briquet type, with male family members having ASPD and females showing a Briquet's syndrome. Increased rates of criminality have not been found among first-degree relatives of schizophrenic probands. Evidence to date suggests that the heritable form of criminality has more to do with petty recidivism and property offences, rather than violent crimes against the person.

Biological studies

An earlier observation by Hill & Watterson (1942) that psychopathic subjects had increased theta activity on the electroencephalogram (EEG), suggesting immaturity, has only been partially replicated (Blackburn, 1979). When psychopaths were compared with non-psychopaths, few differences emerged, but a comparison between primary and secondary psychopaths showed that the latter group had a lower level of cortical arousal, fewer spontaneous fluctuations on skin conductance, and more rapid electro-dermal habituation. These changes correlated with trait measures of anxiety and social withdrawal. Howard (1984), in his study of Broadmoor admissions (which included mentally ill and psychopathic subjects), found that those with EEG changes suggestive of cortical under-arousal had more anxiety, and were more likely to have committed offences against strangers.

The trait of impulsivity has also been linked to lowered levels of CSF 5-HIAA because low levels have been found in arsonists (Virkunen *et al*, 1987) and homicidal offenders who had killed a sexual partner, although the levels were normal for other cases of homicide (Lidberg *et al*, 1985). The fenfluramine prolactin challenge test, which measures central serotonergic function, correlates with measures of irritability and aggression in subjects with borderline (BPD) and schizotypal personality disorders (SPD) (Coccaro, 1989). Impulsiveness is a prominent trait among borderline and dissocial personality disorders, but is non-specific and occurs in a variety of psychiatric disorders.

Childhood antecedents

Childhood conduct disorder, attention deficit disorder and constitutional aggression all contribute to ASPD. The association between conduct disorder in childhood and later ASPD is well known, but is very much stronger looking backwards rather than forwards. This is because 4–10% of all 8-year-olds display conduct disorder but only 40% of them will later develop ASPD (Robins, 1985). Risk factors for the development of ASPD include a younger age of onset and a wide variety of childhood conduct disorders, the typical sequence being school problems, fighting and lying among younger school children, followed by vandalism, stealing and drinking in early adolescence. Arrests, exclusion from school, and drug abuse appear *last* in the sequence before ASPD. Follow-up studies by Robins (1966, 1985) demonstrated that all cases of adult ASPD had shown some antisocial behaviour during childhood. It was because of these observations that the DSM–III and DSM–IV diagnostic criteria for ASPD included a history of antisocial behaviour prior to age 15.

Risks are decreased in the presence of protective factors such as a good family background, high intelligence and resilience (Rutter, 1985). Farrington *et al* (1990) found that children from a criminogenic environment who did not later become delinquent were, at the age of 10, rather less daring, more neurotic, more shy, and spent less leisure time with their fathers. Conversely, risk of a poor outcome for childhood conduct disorder was increased in the presence of adverse family circumstances: parental mental illness; marital discord; divorce; inconsistent discipline and family chaos; foster placements; and physical or sexual abuse.

Aggressive behaviour is a key feature of ASPD, and repeated studies have shown that aggression is one of the most stable character traits over time, with only gradual attenuation with increasing age. Aggression at the age of eight correlates highly with aggression at the age of 30, as measured by spouse abuse, self-reported physical aggression and criminality. Among men, an early history of temper tantrums predicts later divorce, ill-tempered parenting behaviours and a poor work record, while women tend to marry men of lower social status (for review see Coid, 1993).

Attention deficit disorder in childhood (formerly known as hyperactivity) occasionally results in ASPD as an adult, but it seems as if this only occurs in cases where conduct disorder is an intervening variable. Attention deficit disorder attentuates with age. In most cases the attention deficit disorder resolves, although a few subjects have persistent poor emotional and impulse control and concentration difficulties in adult life. A rather smaller group develop serious psychiatric or antisocial pathology, sometimes associated with substance abuse and criminal behaviour. A follow-up study of 6–12-year-old subjects with attention deficit disorder showed that 9% were later incarcerated, compared with only 1% among the control group (Mannuzza *et al*, 1989).

Emotionally unstable personality disorder

ICD–10 describes two subtypes of this personality disorder: the impulsive and the borderline types. ICD–10 impulsive type replaces ICD–9 explosive type. DSM–IV does not include this condition as one of the personality disorders, but in its section on "Habit and impulsive disorders" describes a similar condition, intermittent explosive disorder, as discussed later in this chapter, and also on page 1039.

ICD–10 impulsive personality disorder is characterised by a marked tendency to act impulsively with little consideration of the consequences, and behavioural explosions may also occur. The essential component is poor impulse control, a need for immediate reward, an inability to plan ahead, and unpredictability.

Borderline personality disorder

> The borderline of insanity is occupied by many persons who pass their whole life near that line, sometimes on one side, sometimes on the other. Hughes (1884)

The term "borderline" has been used in many different ways: to describe the area between the neuroses and the psychoses; a personality disorder genetically related to schizophrenia (Kety *et al*, 1971; Spitzer *et al*, 1979); a psychoanalytic formulation of a particular type of personality organisation (Kernberg, 1967); and more recently as a specific type of personality disorder in DSM–IV (Box 18.6).

An early description was given by Schneider (1950) in his account of the "labile personality".

> The labile has no chronic moodiness, but is specifically characterised by the abrupt and rapid changes of mood which he undergoes. Sometimes the smallest stimulus is sufficient to arouse a violent reaction. Labile persons present a picture of shiftless social instability . . . as a group the more irritable ones are apt to get into trouble through impulsive violence, and the more inconstant ones have all sorts of chance lapses.

The modern concept of borderline personality disorder (BPD) derives mainly from writings of American analysts of the 1930s and 1940s who were puzzled by those patients who proved refractory to classical psychoanalysis, yet had mainly neurotic symptoms. Stern (1938) was the first to label these patients as comprising "a borderline group of neuroses". Hoch & Polatin (1949), believing that their patients were more seriously ill and nearer to psychoses, applied the term "pseudoneurotic schizophrenia".

Clinical features

The most salient features of this disorder are unstable mood, unstable interpersonal relationships, and a disturbance of identity. Depression is common; the pattern is not one of a continuous depressed mood, but rather of rapid and reactive shifts into depression. The mood is characterised by complaints of boredom, intolerance of being alone, frustration and an unpleasant sense of emptiness. Some analysts, such as Kohut (1971), have written that this state of "affective hunger" is so unpleasant that subjects may resort to impulsive behaviour, such as binge-eating, kleptomania or thrill-seeking behaviour, and take drugs or alcohol to alleviate the dysphoria. Episodes of anxiety, usually lasting no more than a few hours or a day or two at most, occur particularly in the context of separation and abandonment fears. These are the patients who break down when their therapist takes a holiday or their treatment plan is altered. In men, outbursts of anger can result in assaultive behaviour, while among women, anger, dysphoria, and impulsivity are more commonly turned inward, leading to wrist-cutting, self-mutilation and impulsive overdoses. In a large study of non-psychotic subjects who were briefly hospitalised for florid attention-seeking behaviour, four main symptoms were identified: *anger* was the main or only affect, there was a *defect in affectional relationships*; an *absence of self-identity*; and *depressive loneliness* (Grinker *et al*, 1968).

Identity disturbance is an important psychodynamic feature, but this is not the same as low self-esteem, although the two may coexist. Kernberg (1967) originally derived the concept from Erikson's (1956) maturational model. A normal adolescent should negotiate the maturational steps involved in a commitment to *physical intimacy, occupational choice, energetic competition* and *psychosocial self-definition*. Failure to negotiate this maturational phase was termed "identity diffusion" by Erikson (1956), and "identity disturbance" by Kernberg (1967), and the latter term has been retained in DSM–IV. Difficulties in the spheres of work, sexual orientation and self-identity were present in three-quarters of a clinic population of BPD subjects (Clarkin *et al*, 1983).

Impulsive behaviour is frequent, sometimes with recurrent suicidal threats, repeated overdoses, and may occasionally result in an unintended death. Sometimes a very severe state of chaotic impulsivity occurs where subjects respond to every passing whim, behaving like a small child, and these patients often gain admission to hospital. Their pre-admission histories are characterised by wild living, substance abuse, promiscuity, frequent

---

Box 18.6 DSM–IV criteria for borderline personality disorder

A pervasive pattern of instability of interpersonal relationships, self-image and affects, and marked impulsivity beginning by early adulthood and present in a variety of contexts, as indicated by five (or more) of the following:

1. Frantic efforts to avoid real or imagined abandonment. Note: Do not include suicidal or self-mutilating behaviour covered in criterion 5.
2. A pattern of unstable and intense interpersonal relationships characterised by alternating between extremes of idealisation and devaluation.
3. Identity disturbance: markedly and persistently unstable self-image or sense of self.
4. Impulsivity in at least two areas that are potentially self-damaging (e.g. spending, sex, substance abuse, reckless driving, binge-eating). Note: Do not include suicidal or self-mutilating behaviour covered in criterion 5.
5. Recurrent suicidal behaviour, gestures or threats, or self-mutilating behaviour.
6. Affective instability due to a marked reactivity of mood (e.g. intense episodic dysphoria, irritability, or anxiety usually lasting a few hours and only rarely more than a few days).
7. Chronic feelings of emptiness.
8. Inappropriate intense anger or difficulty controlling anger (e.g. frequent displays of temper, constant anger, recurrent physical fights).
9. Transient, stress-related paranoid ideation or severe dissociative symptoms.

Adapted with permission from DSM–IV. Copyright 1994 American Psychiatric Association.

---

outbursts of rage, running away from home and tumultuous relationships. Lacey & Evans (1986) have used the term 'multi-impulsive personality disorder' to describe this very disturbed subgroup.

Borderline subjects enter into ambivalent relationships which are often intense and characterised by a tendency to over-idealise or devalue their partners. Sometimes they make dependent relationships, at the same time provoking the rejection and abandonment they fear so greatly. At other times, manipulative or coercive behaviour is used to humiliate those who care for them. Over the longer term, the picture is one of instability which ameliorates with age.

Reliability and validity of the concept

The DSM–III concept of BPD was rather more popular in the US than in Europe, but studies have shown that the disorder itself is just as common in Europe. For example, Kroll *et al* (1982) found that 8.5% of the in-patients in an admission unit at Fulbourne Hospital, Cambridge, fulfilled criteria for BPD. British psychiatrists preferred to use the terms "histrionic" or "explosive", or simply to diagnose "personality disorder" without specifying the category.

A group of Maudsley psychiatrists thought that the key items for BPD were a pattern of unstable, intense interpersonal relationships, impulsiveness, and self-destructive behaviour (Tarnopolsky & Berelowitz, 1984). These workers also included "stress-related psychotic episodes" or regressions, but this item, originally in Gunderson & Kolb's (1978) definition of BPD, was dropped from the DSM–III–R definition because Spitzer *et al* (1979) suggested that subjects with more eccentric or near-psychotic symptoms should form a separate group (that is, schizotypal personality disorder). It is of interest (although somewhat confusing) that DSM–IV has re-inserted this controversial item once more into the definition of BPD by adding a ninth criterion: "transient stress-related paranoid ideation or severe dissociative symptoms".

The validity of the syndrome has been questioned by Fyer *et al* (1988) who found that, in clinical populations, BPD rarely occurred by itself but was usually associated with some other psychiatric disorder. Of their cases, 91% were comorbid with at least one other psychiatric diagnosis, 30% with two diagnoses, 12% with three other diagnoses, and only 9% had a pure borderline disorder. To explain these findings they suggested that BPD was either an independent diagnostic entity that commonly occurred with other psychiatric disorders, or it represented a rather non-specific dimension of impulsivity and instability that crossed several diagnostic categories. In spite of criticisms of the concept, Fyer *et al* (1988) found that BPD, as presently defined, described a clinically recognisable group of patients, and the diagnosis could be made in around 20% of all hospital admissions.

Relationship to functional psychoses

As defined in DSM–III–R, BPD bears little or no relationship to schizophrenia; for example, Pope *et al* (1983) found no cases of schizophrenia among a group of 33 in-patients with BPD. A 10–15 year follow-up study of around 200 BPD subjects revealed only one who subsequently developed schizophrenia (Stone, 1990). Only long-term follow-up studies can tell if the addition of the item "transient paranoid ideation" in DSM–IV makes any difference to the likelihood of a later schizophrenic denouement.

The association between affective disorder and BPD, at least in clinic populations, is rather stronger. Akiskal *et al* (1983) found that around 50% of BPD subjects had at least one type of affective disorder, and Baxter *et al* (1984) found that 50% of in-patients with unipolar depression had BPD. Such high rates of association may be explained by a tendency for subjects with two or more disorders to be referred to specialist centres, and also because BPD depression is often treatment-resistant, which makes referral more likely. Gunderson & Phillips (1991) suggested that the association may be due to the two disorders being independent but occurring commonly together. BPD is frequently comorbid with other personality disorders, particularly schizotypal, but there is considerable overlap with antisocial, histrionic and narcissistic types.

Aetiology

Although the aetiology is unknown, there is increasing evidence that physical and sexual abuse during childhood is relevant. However, many cases have no history of abuse, and so there is probably a continuum of those who have a strong genetic or constitutional basis to develop BPD, and those in whom a traumatic upbringing is causal, with most cases having a mixture of both elements. A family study of probands with BPD showed that BPD itself was ten times more common among first-degree relatives than among the relatives of schizophrenic probands (Loranger *et al*, 1982). Stone (1990) observed increased rates of affective disorder, alcoholism and BPD, but not schizophrenia, among the parents of borderlines. There is only one twin study by Torgerson (1984) and this failed to find any concordant borderline twins. Early family studies suggested a familial link with affective disorder, but more recent investigations by Pope *et al* (1983) and Androlunis *et al* (1981), which separated pure borderline probands from borderline probands with depression, found increased rates of affective disorder among relatives only in the mixed group, suggesting that BPD is an independent entity rather than a subtype of affective disorder.

Childhood antecedents

There is growing evidence for an association between BPD and sexual abuse during childhood. Thus there is a higher rate of sexual abuse than in depressive controls, and the parents of borderlines also show more mental illness, personality disorder, drug abuse and marital discord (Ogata *et al*, 1990). The early memories of sexually abused borderline subjects may be particularly malevolent and unpleasant (Nigg *et al*, 1991). In an elegant study, Brown & Anderson (1991) examined the histories of childhood abuse of nearly 1000 patients admitted to a US Army Hospital. The prevalence rate of BPD rose with increasing levels of reported abuse: 3% of non-abused patients; 13% with either physical or sexual abuse; and 29% of those with both physical and sexual abuse. BPD accounted for nearly 50% of the personality disorder diagnoses in the abused group. Parental brutality is less common than sexual abuse, and was only present in 6% of Stone's (1990) series, but it may worsen outcome since 12.5% of the BPD subjects who were physically abused later committed suicide. Even witnessing parental violence is thought to be of aetiological significance. Early or multiple separations from the mother, once held to be causal, are probably not in themselves so damaging, but the family context in which such separations occur, whether there is discord, neglect or abuse, appears to be more relevant.

Biological studies

Several, but not all, studies have shown increased rates of dexamethazone suppression among BPD subjects, and one study (Kontaxakis *et al*, 1987) found a similar rate of 50% non-suppression in both borderline patients and depressed controls. Reviewing the findings, Steiner *et al* (1988) concluded that there was no consistent pattern, particularly as in some studies subjects were also comorbid for depression. Abnormalities in the TRH-TSH stimulation test were reported by Sternbach *et al* (1983) but were not replicated in a later study by Korzekwa (1991). One finding of interest that has been replicated is a decrease in rapid eye movement latency similar to the pattern observed in unipolar depressives (Akiskal *et al*, 1983). On this basis, Silk *et al* (1988) suggested that the sleep EEG could be used to diagnose biological depressions among borderline patients. The auditory evoke responses (P300) distinguished BPD from other personality disorders and affective disorders, and it is of note that a similar pattern was only found among schizotypal and schizophrenic subjects.

A more definite biological contribution is present in cases in which there has been some noxious early influence on the brain, particularly in men. Examples include birth injury, damage through infection or trauma during childhood, attention deficit disorder, epilepsy and other neurological conditions. Although each of these categories is rare, Androlunis *et al* (1981) found that 38% of a series of men with BPD had an organic contribution.

Histrionic personality disorder

Histrionic personalities turn to others for protection and the rewards of life. In contrast to the dependent personality, histrionic individuals take the initiative in the quest for nurturance, and this leads to seductive and over-dramatic behaviour. A colourful description that also covers most of the DSM–IV features was given by Kretschmer (1926):

> an over-lively and over-idealistic psychic sexuality, with prudish or rejection of its physical correlate, a rapidly vanishing elan of feelings, enthusiasm for impressive persons, a preference for what is loud and lively, a theatrical pathos, an inclination for brilliant roles, to dream themselves into big purposes in life, the playing with suicide, contrast between enthusiastic self sacrificial abandonment and a naive sultry childish egotism and especially a mixture of the droll and tragic in their way of living . . .

In addition to their social affability, these patients have an overwhelming need for attention and affection. At first meeting, they may impress by the ease and openness with which they discuss their feelings and emotions. They tend to be capricious, easily excited but intolerant of frustration, delay and disappointment. They may be sexually provocative, with shallow expressions of emotion, or manipulative for selfish ends, and craving excitement. There is excessive sensitivity to the moods of others and even inadvertent snubs may be interpreted as rejection. The use of hyperbole in speech is common; women tend to be coquettish while men are overly flattering. Promises are made that are rarely fulfilled and invariably forgotten. Dissatisfaction with single attachments, combined with a constant need for stimulation, results in seductive behaviour to ensure a constant stream of new partners. The ICD–10 features of histrionic personality disorder are shown in Box 18.7.

Histrionic personalities are exclusively "other people directed", and their high degree of exteroceptive vigilance diminishes their capacity for an inner world of thought, memory or emotion. The outside world is everything, introspection is avoided, and so they lack the intrapsychic skills needed for adult modes of thinking and behaving. Earlier life experiences are often repressed and a wealth of inner feelings are therefore unavailable to them, leading to psychic impoverishment and excessive reliability on the fleeting, insubstantial relationships of the moment.

Jung thought these individuals were of an "extraverted intuitive type", while the early analysts stressed fixation at an infantile level, with childlike behaviour and confusion between fantasy and reality (Wittels, 1930). Twin studies based on the Middlesex Hospital Questionnaire showed a modest effect for hysterical traits (Young & Lader, 1971), but Slater & Shields (1969) found no concordant MZ or DZ twin pairs with hysterical disorder suggesting that a hereditary contribution was unlikely, and a study of the hysterical trait in Gottesman's (1963) twin study of normal adolescence showed negligible genetic influences.

Comorbid disorders

Histrionic personalities are prone to anxiety, particularly at times of separation, and generalised anxiety disorder and agoraphobia may occur. It was once thought that conversion symptoms and other dissociative phenomena such as amnesia, fugues and multiple personality disorder were more common among histrionic types, but their frequency is probably no greater than in the other personality disorders (Chodoff & Lyons, 1958). Somatisation is not uncommon, and the combination of multiple somatic complaints and personality disorder known as Briquets syndrome is discussed on page 724. Other personality disorders, particularly borderline and antisocial types, may coexist. Short-lived histrionic features are sometimes observed among young depressed women, but this should not be confused with more long-standing histrionic personality disorder.

Anxious (avoidant) personality disorder

In contrast to the schizoid personality, who lacks any interest in other people, the avoidant personality will actively seek contact, yet at the same time is so hypersensitive to rejection and feelings of humiliation that relationships rarely develop. ICD–10 uses the term "anxious personality", and DSM–IV the term "avoidant", which was introduced by Millon (1969). Earlier this century, Kretschmer (1922) identified two types of schizoid individual: the anaesthetic and hyperaesthetic types. The anaesthetic type corresponds to DSM–IV schizoid personality, and the hyperaesthetic to the avoidant personality:

> . . . here we find the qualities of nervousness, excitability, capriciousness, anxiousness, tenderness and above all sensitive susceptibility. He behaves shyly or timidly or distrustfully or as if he were pushed in on himself. He complains of nerve trouble. He keeps anxiously away from all coarse games and brawls. (Kretschmer, 1922)

Horney (1945) proposed a personality type she called "detached", and in her schema these individuals had an interpersonal style of "moving away from people". She wrote:

> there is an intolerable strain in associating with people and solitude becomes a means of avoiding it, self-sufficiency is maintained consciously, or unconsciously, by restricting one's needs, his goals are negative; he wants *not* to be involved, *not* to need anybody, *not* to allow others to intrude or influence him.

These individuals are habitually self-conscious, persistently in a state of tension and express an overwhelming need for security. There is a tendency to exaggerate the negative aspects of everyday situations. They feel their loneliness and isolated experience very deeply, but also have a strong yet repressed desire to be accepted. Avoidant personalities tend to be

---

Box 18.7 ICD–10 criteria for histrionic personality disorder

1. Self-dramatisation, theatricality, exaggerated expression of emotion.
2. Suggestibility.
3. Shallow and labile affectivity.
4. Continually seeking excitement, being at the centre of attention.
5. Inappropriately seductive in appearance or behaviour.
6. Over-concern with physical attractiveness.

Three out of six items required for the diagnosis. The DSM–IV definition requires four out of eight similar items, the additional items being style of speech that is excessively impressionistic and lacking in detail, and considering relationships to be more intimate than they actually are.

excessively introspective, unsure of their identity and self-worth. The central dynamic is the struggle between affection and mistrust. Their life is restricted and one of great psychic pain. Among the more artistically inclined, the need for affection and closeness may appear in poetry, or else become sublimated into intellectual pursuits such as music or art. The tortured lives of the great musicians bears witness to this. Other people are actively sought out, because to be alone with one's despised self may impose an even greater torment, yet others are also avoided because of feelings of shame and humiliation. They have few friends, although they may wish for more, and because of their obsequiousness are sometimes the butt of taunts and jibes. Relationships are unlikely to be sustained unless the other partner provides a degree of uncritical acceptance.

Comorbid patterns and differential diagnosis

Generalised anxiety disorder is most frequently associated, but depression resulting from the miserable lives these people lead may also occur. *Social phobias* are such a pervasive part of the avoidant pattern that it is difficult to say where the personality disorder ends and the social phobia begins. There are several distinguishing features. Firstly, in the avoidant personality the pattern is much more pervasive, while in social phobia individuals are usually capable of making some normal relationships, at least within the family. Secondly, individuals with social phobia are intensely phobic about meeting people in specific situations, such as going to a restaurant, or meeting a large group at work, but are less likely to be troubled by relationships in general. Thirdly, other personality traits such as low self-esteem or the pathological desire for acceptance are common in the avoidant personality disorder, but unusual in individuals with social phobia.

Some patients present with hypochondriasis, as isolated individuals totally preoccupied with various bodily sensations and constantly seeking medical contact and reassurance. Fatigue, which enables them legitimately to do nothing and hence avoid other people, is a strategy they may use to isolate themselves from others. Conversion symptoms and rituals similar to those seen in obsessive–compulsive disorder also sometimes occur.

Dependent personality disorder

This group is characterised by excessive emotional dependence on others, and individuals have an intense need for social approval and affection and will suppress their own needs to fit in with the wishes of others. They may be self-effacing, ever agreeable, docile or ingratiating, and this may be apparent in their manners and posture. They search for an all-powerful partner who will supply them with the necessary nurturance and affection, and then cling on to them in a dependent relationship. When it breaks down, depression and feelings of isolation may supervene.

Kraepelin (1913) used the term "shiftless" and Schneider (1923) called them "weak willed". Freud described oral dependent characters, but a more detailed description is given by Abraham (1924) who wrote:

> some people are dominated by the belief that there will always be some kind person, a representation of the mother of course, to care for them and give them everything they need. This optimistic belief condemns them to inactivity . . . they make no kind of effort and in some cases they even disdain to undertake a breadwinning occupation.

Dependent personalities perceive themselves as thoughtful, cooperative people, but not ambitious. Beneath their affability they are constantly searching for attention and approval. Self-depreciation is often used as a ploy to obtain reassurance, or at the very least avoid reprimand. Constantly pouring oil on troubled waters, they try to deny their own hostile impulses. Self-esteem is low, and decision-making is difficult. They may make relationships with assertive partners that are ostensibly very close. Many fail to enter long-standing relationships in adult life, but rather stay at home, dependent on their parents until middle-age.

Deutsch (1942) described the "as-if" personality, a variety of the dependent personality, characterised by chameleon-like shifts of attitude and opinion so as to be in conformity with the partner of the moment. ICD–10 also includes self-defeating personality disorder as one of the subtypes of dependent personality disorder. Prevalence is unknown, but the disorder is common and probably more frequent among females. Aetiology is also unknown, but maternal over-protection combined with adverse temperamental factors within the child may contribute. Horney (1945) highlighted pervasive feelings of weakness and helplessness and a "poor little me" feeling. The word "inadequate" has since been used indiscriminately in association with personality disorders, but Sullivan (1947) described an "inadequate type" which corresponds to dependent personality disorder. ICD–9 used the word "asthenic", but the word "dependent" is retained in DSM–IV and ICD–10; features of the latter are shown in Box 18.8.

There is some evidence supporting the validity of dependent personality disorder. A factor analysis of a group of subjects with personality disorders identified submissiveness as a major factor (Presly & Walton, 1973). This factor was composed of the following traits: humility, submissiveness, intropunitiveness, indecisiveness and avoidance of competition. These authors thought such traits were related to dependent personality disorder, although at the time of their study the validity of this category was questioned because it was not included in either the DSM or ICD schemes of that time.

Comorbidity

Dependent personality is most often comorbid with all the anxiety disorders (generalised anxiety and the phobias, particularly agoraphobia and social phobia), although the complete picture of dependent personality disorder is rarely encountered in these anxiety disorders. More severe dependent personality disorders are found among those with the somatoform disorders, particularly somatisation disorder and hypochondriasis. Here there is a lifelong pattern of dependency, with constant reassurance-seeking behaviour in the context of a medical setting. The most commonly associated axis II disorders are histrionic, avoidant and borderline personality disorders. Patients with long-standing psychiatric illness of any type often display a dependent pattern, but in these cases the personality prior to the onset of the axis I disorder was generally normal.

Differential diagnosis

Both histrionic and dependent personalities seek reassurance and affection from their environment, but in the dependent personality this is through submissiveness rather than through dramatic attention-seeking behaviour. Borderline patients may form dependent relationships, but these have a grossly unstable pattern. Individuals with avoidant personality disorder also lead restrictive lives, but the avoidant personality fears the good faith of others and anticipates rejection, while the dependent personality is permanently optimistic and always expects to receive nurturance from all his objects.

Narcissistic personality disorder

People with this disorder have a grandiose sense of self-importance. They may be preoccupied by fantasies of success, power, brilliance or ideal love. They believe it is their right to receive special treatment and there may also be a sense of entitlement. Self-esteem is usually based on a blind naïve assumption of personal worth. Feelings of superiority are fragile, and there may be an exhibitionistic need for constant attention and admiration from others. Depression sometimes arises from the deep feelings of envy for those whom they perceive as being more successful.

These individuals overvalue their personal worth, tend to direct affection towards themselves, and may show interpersonal exploitativeness and lack empathy. Friendships are one-way and only develop if individuals feel the friendship will profit them. In romantic relationships, the other partner is often treated as little more than an object to bolster their self-esteem. Cognitively they tend to be expansive with a pervasive sense of well-being. They have little or no idea that their behaviour may be objectionable, and others may describe them as arrogant. Millon (1981) suggested that the parents of narcissists brought them up to believe they were almost perfect and invariably lovable regardless of their behaviour. Horney (1939) wrote "parents who transfer their own ambitions to the child and regard the boy as an embryonic genius, or the girl as a princess, give the child the feeling

---

Box 18.8 ICD–10 criteria for dependent personality disorder

1. Encouraging or allowing others to make one's important life decisions.
2. Subordination of one's own needs to those of others on whom one is dependent; undue compliance to their wishes.
3. Unwillingness to make even reasonable demands on others.
4. Feeling uncomfortable or helpless when alone, because of exaggerated fears of inability to care for oneself.
5. Preoccupation with fears of being abandoned by person with whom one has a close relationship and of being left to care for oneself.
6. Limited capacity to make everyday decisions without advice from others.

Three out of six items required for diagnosis. DSM–IV requires five out of eight items. Most of the DSM–IV items are similar, but they include three additional items: difficulty in initiating projects on his or her own; volunteers to do things that are unpleasant or demeaning to get others to like him or her; difficulty in expressing disagreement with others because of fear of loss of support or disapproval.

---

that he is loved for imaginary qualities rather than for the true self". Prevalence is unknown and the condition is not included in ICD–10, but diagnostic criteria are given in DSM–IV.

Differential diagnosis

A high degree of egocentricity occurs in most of the other personality disorders, and so this trait is not in itself diagnostic. In ASPD it is associated with a more malevolent feeling towards others, while narcissistic personalities are well-disposed, believing that other people admire them. They are less impulsive and emotional than borderlines, less dramatic than histrionic subjects, and are more cohesive and successful than dependents. However, in practice any of the above disorders may coexist with narcissistic personality disorder.

Passive aggressive personality disorder

Passive aggressive personality disorder is characterised by a pervasive pattern of passive resistance in both the domestic and work situation. People with this disorder resent or oppose demands that may increase their level of functioning. As a result they may not fulfil their promise in the areas of either work or relationships. Their resistance is expressed indirectly through manoeuvres such as procrastination, stubbornness, intentional inefficiency and forgetfulness. There is a tendency for them to become sulky, irritable or argumentative when asked to do something they do not wish to do. Sometimes they are scornful or hypercritical of people making such demands. The name of the disorder is based on the unproven assumption that such people are passively expressing covert aggression.

The clinical picture shows some resemblance to oppositional deficit disorder of childhood and adolescence, and this diagnosis will preempt a diagnosis of passive aggressive personality disorder in those under 18 years of age. Although behaviour consistent with this pattern may be commonly observed in the work place or in general practice settings, it rarely impairs people to such an extent that any clinical intervention is required. The condition was not included in ICD–10, was included in DSM–III–R but in DSM–IV it has been removed from the main section, appearing only in the chapter entitled "Criteria sets and axes provided for further study" indicating a degree of doubt concerning the validity of the disorder.

Depressive personality disorder

This category is not included in ICD–10 or in the main section of DSM–IV, but only in the section entitled "Criteria sets and axes provided for further study". It refers to a lifelong depressive temperament. Individuals have a pervasive pattern of depressive cognitions and behaviour, pessimism and low self-esteem. As well as being critical and derogatory about themselves, they may also be judgemental and hypercritical about others. Although they claim to be realistic, others view them to be unduly pessimistic, humourless and unable to enjoy themselves. They tend to be introverted, quiet individuals.

The condition should not be diagnosed in the presence of major depression because all of the above symptoms may occur in depression. The distinction from dysthymia is much more difficult to make, but in depressive personality disorder most of the changes are held to be cognitive, interpersonal and intrapsychic personality traits rather than depressive symptoms.

DSM–III–R (American Psychiatric Association, 1987) adopted the term "self-defeating personality disorder", which also incorporated the much older psychoanalytic concept of masochistic personality disorder, but the DSM–IV concept is more closely related to the notion of a depressive temperament.

Mixed personality disorders (ICD–10) and personality disorder not otherwise specified (DSM–IV)

Only a minority of patients can be easily placed in one of the specific diagnostic categories outlined in the proceeding sections. The majority of patients with a personality disorder have a series of traits that fulfil criteria for a mixture of two or three personality disorders, and in these cases DSM–IV recommends that two or three separate personality disorders should be recorded, while ICD–10 recommends a diagnosis of "mixed personality disorder". Other cases have insufficient traits to satisfy the criteria for any one type, or are essentially either unclassifiable or very difficult to classify, and for these DSM–IV recommends the category "personality disorder not otherwise specified". It is not surprising that most clinicians prefer to use only a diagnosis of "personality disorder" without specifying the type.

Miscellaneous disorders

The personality disorders usually have their onset in adolescence or early adulthood and there is usually no precipitating event. The implication was that once the personality was formed by late adolescence it could no longer change, regardless of external experiences. It is now recognised that a person's character may change in adulthood as a consequence of stressful events, particularly if the stress was extreme. ICD–10 describes a group of disorders entitled "enduring personality changes", in which the onset of the changed personality can be clearly traced to a particular event or illness. Included in this category are: enduring personality changes following a catastrophic experience; following an episode of severe psychiatric illness which has resolved; chronic pain syndrome; and bereavement. There is no precise equivalent in DSM–IV, but it does include a section on "personality change due to a medical condition" when the medical condition should be specified. A variety of subtypes are described in this category: labile, disinhibited, aggressive, apathetic, paranoid, combined types and others. Personality changes due to organic brain disease are described on page 959.

Enduring personality changes after a catastrophic experience

This follows extreme stress, such that personal vulnerability is not required to explain the effects. Severe stresses include being a concentration camp victim, experiencing torture or a disaster, or prolonged exposure to life-threatening circumstances, such as being a hostage. Personality changes which follow from short-term trauma, such as a car accident, are not included since preexisting vulnerability usually plays a role. The differentiation from a preexisting personality disorder that is unleashed by stress is probably impossible to make, and may be clinically irrelevant.

The clinical picture is usually one of social withdrawal, coupled with a somewhat hostile or mistrustful attitude to the world. Subjects may complain of feelings of hopelessness, estrangement, and a chronic feeling of being on edge, as if constantly threatened. The diagnosis should only be made if the personality changes have lasted more than two years. Although the disorder is differentiated from post-traumatic stress disorder, the latter may sometimes have preceded it.

Enduring personality changes following psychiatric illness

A few individuals find their experience of psychiatric disorder so devastating that it results in a permanent personality change, even after they have fully recovered from their original illness. The clinical picture is mainly one of dependency, a demanding attitude to others, reduced interests and passivity, with persistent claims of being ill associated with illness behaviour, dysphoria, and impaired occupational and social function. Some subjects complain of being changed or stigmatised by their psychiatric illness. The personality change should have been present for at least two years, and there should be no evidence of a preceding personality disorder, although previous vulnerabilities will obviously play a role. The disorder does not appear in DSM–IV and appears for the first time in ICD–10, so little is known about its validity, frequency or cause.

Comorbidity in the personality disorders

A common error in the past (and it still sometimes occurs) has been to try to diagnose *either* mental illness *or* personality disorder, but not both together. This leads to a relative neglect of axis I disorders in these patients, because "the personality disorder explained everything". The diagnosis of an axis I and axis II disorder signifies the presence of two independent psychiatric conditions. However, comorbidity for two axis II disorders (e.g. for borderline and histrionic types) does not signify that there are two separate personalities. It only means that the clinical picture fulfils diagnostic criteria for two personality disorders. The preceding sections highlighted the main axis I and axis II associations for each personality disorder subtype. A rather different picture emerges studying cohorts of patients with a particular axis I disorder.

Comorbidity with schizophrenia

Reviewing five earlier series, from 1912–1972, Cutting (1985) found that 16–26% of patients with schizophrenia appeared to have preexisting schizoid personality disorder. However, in a smaller series of his own, Cutting *et al* (1986) failed to replicate these findings. Using the PAS, Tyrer (1988) found that 45% of a series of 109 patients with schizophrenia were presently comorbid for personality disorder and around 18% were in the schizoid cluster (schizoid or paranoid); a few were in the antisocial group and occasional other types were also encountered. It is uncertain to what extent these cases represent the prodrome of a schizophrenic illness or are independent personality disorders. A premorbid personality disorder in most cases of schizophrenia is unusual; the presence of a behaviour problem suggestive of a personality disorder is usually the result of the psychosis, and may be worse among those with severe schizophrenia. Successful treatment of the underlying psychosis usually abolishes or at least greatly reduces most of the disordered behaviour and antisocial tendencies.

Comorbidity with affective disorder

There is no evidence that premorbid personality disorder makes any contribution to bipolar disorder (Tyrer *et al*, 1988). Cyclothymia, once thought to predispose to bipolar illness, is now classified as an affective disorder and the two disorders may not be easy to distinguish (Akiskal *et al*, 1983). Among patients with depression, particularly in-patients, high rates of borderline personality disorder may be found (Baxter *et al*, 1984), but the two disorders are probably independent and not associated (Gunderson & Phillips, 1991). Life events are associated with depression, and a recent study by McGuffin *et al* (1988) has shown a familial tendency for life events, suggesting their occurrence may be far from random or truly independent. Seivewright (1988) went further, suggesting that personality disorder may be one of the intervening variables that modulate the effect of a life event on the individual. In certain circumstances this may even be the cause of the event, and he speculated that there may be "event-prone personalities".

The neurotic disorders may be more strongly linked with the personality disorders, particularly those in the anxious cluster. In a large general practice-based study, Tyrer *et al* (1988) noted that around half of those presenting with a neurotic disorder (anxiety states, phobias, neurotic depression and hypochondriasis) were comorbid for a personality disorder, usually anankastic, dependent, passive aggressive or histrionic types. No definite association between any one personality type and a specific neurotic disorder was found. Higher rates of personality disorder (particularly explosive type) were observed among those with adjustment disorders (Tyrer *et al*, 1988), but as ICD–10 specifies that adjustment disorder is associated with personal vulnerability, this finding is hardly surprising.

Alcohol dependence and personality disorder

The relationship between alcohol, personality and personality disorder is complex. Premorbid abnormalities of personality (not amounting to a personality disorder) have been observed among those destined to develop alcohol dependence. From 1947–1961, all new students at the University of Minnesota completed the MMPI, and those who later developed alcohol dependence were compared with their classmates. The pre-alcoholic subjects were more impulsive, non-conforming and gregarious, had higher scores on the psychopathic deviate and masculinity/femininity scales, but they were not more maladjusted (Kammeier *et al*, 1973). Women who subsequently became problem drinkers were more often pessimistic, withdrawn, self-defeating, less dependent and less self-satisfied than those who only drank moderately. These findings were echoed in later investigations into the types of personality disorders found among severe female alcoholic in-patients, in whom the borderline–schizotypal constellation is common (Valgum & Valgum, 1989).

Once clinical alcohol dependence has developed, MMPI data tend to show high rates of personality disturbance, but there is no strong association with any one particular category. Tyrer *et al* (1988) found that more than half of a group of alcoholics in the general practice population fulfilled criteria for personality disorder (mainly explosive type).

Assessment

Clinical assessment

Although this is the most common method of assessing personality, it is often quite unreliable. The index of overall agreement between psychiatrists is lower for personality disorder than for any other major class of psychiatric disorder; they are usually able to agree on the presence of a personality disorder, but not on the specific subtype. Test–retest reliability is poor and the diagnosis often changes, usually to one of the neurotic disorders.

There are a number of reasons for this unreliability, particularly when the patient's own account is used to make the diagnosis. Firstly, for some personality disorders items such as over-exaggeration (histrionic disorder) or dishonesty (ASPD) are features of the disorder itself, and so self-assessment will inevitably be biased. Secondly, during an axis I illness self-assessment will be contaminated by the patient's affect, and this will tend to distort the picture in a negative way. Thirdly, traits and symptoms are often confused. For example, a patient who, during an episode of depression, reports anxiety and displays histrionic and dependent behaviour may be wrongly diagnosed as having histrionic personality disorder. Fourthly, it is often wrongly assumed that those with neurotic disorders will inevitably also have personality disorders. This notion stems initially from the work of Alexander (1930) who described the neurotic character, but the assumption persists even in some modern textbooks in which neuroses and personality disorders are often combined in a single, common chapter. Fifthly, there is often the view, now changing, that illness and personality are mutually exclusive. Thus a patient can have either an "illness" or a "personality disorder" but not both. The risks inherent this view are obvious, but it was a commonly held principle before the advent of multiaxial classifications. Finally, value judgements often cloud clinical judgements when assessing personality, and terms such as 'inadequate', 'hysterical' or 'immature' are sometimes applied inappropriately (e.g. for the purpose of rejecting the patient from hospital; Thompson & Goldberg, 1987).

Structured assessment

Older tools

These can be conveniently divided into self-rating instruments and structured interviews. The best known self-rating instrument is the Eysenck Personality Inventory (EPI; Eysenck & Eysenck, 1964). This contains 108 questions relating to the dimensions of neuroticism, extroversion and, controversially, psychoticism, as well as a lie scale. Although widely used in studies of physical as well as psychiatric disorders, it suffers from the problem that current psychiatric disorder will markedly influence the N (neuroticism) scale (Kendell & DiScipio, 1968; Kerr *et al*, 1970). Also, the use of dimensions does not easily fit with clinical practice and the common clinical categories. Most of the scales and interviews require some training, as do some of the longer self-rating questionnaires.

The MMPI was developed to differentiate between the categories of abnormal personality, but it has also been extensively studied in the healthy population. The subject is presented with 550 statements and asked to respond to each with 'true', 'false' or 'cannot say'. Unfortunately the scales have been labelled using the standard nosology of psychiatry (e.g. paranoia, schizophrenia, psychopathy, etc.). Its use to generate the traditional categories of personality disorder is limited, and interpretation by an experienced psychologist is required.

Cattell's 16PF (1965) is a structured interview schedule, more commonly used by occupational psychologists than in the clinical settings. It generates 16 dimensions, e.g. 'tense-relaxed' or 'controlled-uncontrolled', although some of the terms chosen to describe these are rather idiosyncratic, such as 'harria-parmia', 'alexia-protension' and somewhat questionably it includes intelligence as a personality trait.

Newer tools

The Standardised Assessment of Personality (Mann *et al*, 1981) relies on data from an informant, who is required to provide a description of the patient when well. As abnormal traits are revealed, more detailed questioning follows, but the assessment usually takes no more than 15 minutes to complete. The Personality Assessment Schedule (PAS) was developed by Tyrer & Alexander (1979) to generate ICD–9 diagnoses, but has since been updated to provide diagnoses both for ICD–10 and DSM–III–R. The schedule requires either the subject or informant or both to provide information on 24 traits of personality, and during the interview emphasis is placed on the patient's premorbid traits.

The Millon Clinical Multiaxial Inventory (Millon, 1982) is a self-administered questionnaire of 175 items. It takes 25 minutes to complete and analysis is by computer. It provides three sets of results – an individual profile, an interpretive report, and a categorical assessment of personality. The latter, however, is limited to borderline, schizotypal and paranoid types. The main limitation, inherent in all questionnaires, is the failure to distinguish current mental state from personality traits and this may confound the diagnosis. A revised version capable of generating DSM–IV diagnoses is presently being developed.

Structured interviews

The Structured Interview for DSM–III Personality Disorders (SIPD; Pfohl *et al,* 1983) is a comprehensive semistructured interview with 60 items. Data are gathered from the subject and an informant to generate the diagnosis.

The Personality Disorder Examination (Loranger *et al,* 1985) is a lengthy structured interview with 359 items, some traits and some behavioural measures, which also generates both DSM–III–R and ICD–10 diagnoses. It takes around three hours to complete and its size precludes its use except in research settings. The Structured Clinical Interview for DSM–III–R (2) (SCID–2) was developed by Spitzer *et al* (1987) to focus exclusively on axis II diagnosis. Initially, SCID–1 is used to make an axis I diagnosis. This is followed by the Personality Disorder Questionnaire in which the subject is requested to make a series of dichotomous yes/no choices. The SCID–2 interview then focuses on questions to which a positive response has been given, covering all the traits in the DSM–III–R personality disorder section so that the interviewer should be able to make a diagnosis.

Disorder-specific schedules

There are now many schedules that can diagnose and rate the severity of specific categories of abnormal personality. Perhaps the best known is the Diagnostic Interview for Borderlines (Gunderson *et al,* 1981). A less well-established instrument is the Schedule for Interviewing Borderlines developed by Baron (1981). Other schedules include the Structured Interview for Schizotypy (Kendler *et al,* 1989), the Schedule for Interviewing Schizotypal Personalities (Baron *et al,* 1990) and the Diagnostic Interview for Narcissistic Patients (Gunderson *et al,* 1990), and there are many other interviews which focus on one or more DSM–III personality disorders.

Particular traits can also be measured: thus obsessional traits, as well as obsessional symptoms and resistance, can be measured with the Leyton Obsessional Inventory (Cooper, 1970). This 69-item scale uses a card assortment and a post-box technique that is somewhat cumbersome and time-consuming. Hostility is a common feature of some patients with personality disorder, and is both state and trait dependent. In the parasuicide population this trait has received particular attention and the

Hostility–Direction of Hostility Questionnaire (HDHQ; Caine *et al,* 1967) is most commonly used to measure this. As people with a personality disorder have such a profound influence on those around them and may have a serious impairment of social function, it may also be important to assess their social function. A review of the large number of instruments that measure social function is given in Tyrer (1990), which also reviews the many instruments used to assess personality disorder.

There has been a burgeoning interest in cognitive therapy (see chapter 6) particularly with regard to the parasuicide population. In assessing the hopelessness and relative failure to solve personal problems of these patients, cognitive therapists use the "Means–Ends Problem Solving Procedure" (Platt & Spivack, 1975) and the Hopelessness Scale (Beck *et al,* 1974).

Impulse and habit disorders

Both DSM–IV and ICD–10 describe a group of patients with impulsive behaviour and habit disorders, characterised by failure to resist an impulse that is usually ego-syntonic but often harmful. There is an increasing sense of tension prior to committing the impulsive act, with a sense of pleasure or gratification once the act has been committed. These disorders are not personality disorders, and probably represent only a residual category and include five unrelated disorders: intermittent explosive disorder; pathological gambling; trichotillomania (which are described in this chapter); kleptomania and pyromania (both discussed by Chiswick *et al,* 1995).

Intermittent explosive disorder

DSM–IV includes this category as one of the impulse control disorders rather than as a specific personality disorder, although ICD–10 includes impulsive personality disorder as one of the personality disorders. The degree of aggressiveness is out of proportion to any precipitating social stress. Individuals or their relatives usually describe the episodes as spells or attacks. There is some doubt as to whether a pure type of the category really exists, as the vast majority of explosive individuals have either BPD, ASPD, substance abuse, a functional psychosis or organic personality changes.

Pathological gambling

Gambling may be defined as staking something of value, generally money, on a game, or an uncertain event, or some other contingency. Professional gamblers carefully plan their gambling and attempt to decrease the element of risk, for example, by having access to information not available to others. In contrast, pathological gamblers will gamble with repeated and heavy losses, often to a state of financial and social ruin.

DSM–IV defines the essential feature of the disorder as a chronic and progressive failure to resist impulses to gamble, with the behaviour leading to much damage to personal and family life. Efforts to stop or resist gambling generally fail, and the behaviour shows some resemblances to an addiction. Thus there is restlessness and irritability if the person is unable to gamble; an increase in the size and frequency of the stake required to achieve the desired level of excitement; and repeated losses induce a strong urge to return yet again to try to win back the losses. In pathological states the gambling will persist even in the face of mounting debts, marital break-up or other legal problems. Some gamblers steal to maintain their habit and the morbid tendency may only come to light through a court case involving theft or embezzlement. Excessive gambling is a serious health problem and may be associated with other addictions, particularly alcohol and tobacco, but there may also be disturbed eating, sleeping, sexual and relationship problems, as well as impaired function at work. A few subjects present with depression or following an overdose. A comprehensive account of the topic is presented in the review by Legg-England & Gotestam (1991).

Gambling itself is a common pastime and it is estimated that 39% of the British population engage in some form of regular gambling, while in the US a figure of 61% is given (Moran, 1983). Pathological gambling is much less common but is not rare: a survey in Australia gave a prevalence of 0.25% (Dickerson, 1988) while in the US a figure of 0.77% (US Commission on the Review of the National Policy towards Gambling, 1976) was given. Surveys of prison populations show that around 10% of prisoners are pathological gamblers (Royal College of Psychiatrists, 1977). Gambling is probably more common and more obvious among men who indulge in horse and dog racing, with which dramatic losses soon become apparent. Women prefer bingo and football pools in which morbid patterns are less obvious because losses are smaller and spread over longer periods of time.

Aetiology

Experience of risk-taking is generally thrilling and pleasurable, and this is probably the main motivation. The gambling itself is a significant emotional event for those who indulge in it, and large changes in heart rate may occur during gambling. The experience of winning is said to produce a sense of euphoria resembling the effects of amphetamines or opiates. There are also suggestions that gambling will at least temporarily help people switch out of negative internal mood states such as feelings of loneliness, depression or other forms of dysphoria. The obvious self-destructive nature of the behaviour has provoked much analytical speculation, but there is little scientific study on the problem. In his autobiographical novel *The Gambler*, Dostoyevsky described the rewarding sense of power obtained from gambling. Freud (1928), commenting on this book in his paper "Dostoyevsky and parricide", suggested that gambling arose from a need for self-punishment to appease unconscious guilt feelings concerning patricidal urges. After a big loss, Dostoyevsky accomplished his best writing because (according to Freud) he was then freed from the guilt that inhibited his creativity. Greenson (1947) suggested that the gambling served to gratify both oedipal and pre-oedipal wishes. The gambler re-enacts the family drama, in which sometimes fate represents the tyrannical father whom the gambler wished to defeat, while at other times it is the mother whom he wished to woo and whose bounty he longed for (Frosch *et al*, 1985).

Moran (1983) emphasised the presence of social pressures, early exposure to gambling, and having a father who drank or gambled as likely influences upon men, while women who gamble are more likely to have an alcoholic spouse who is often absent. The prevalence of gambling appears to correlate with the number of gamblers in one's social circle (family, friends, work colleagues), and although gambling is initially a social activity, in its later morbid phase the gambling is usually a lone preoccupation. Learning theorists point out that the usual sequence of repeated gambling losses with occasional random wins provides a pattern of intermittent reinforcement, the most potent schedule for conditioning. In this respect a big win is thought to be particularly hazardous, and the financial reinforcement of winning prolongs the habit.

Personality disorder, particularly ASPD, may also contribute, but pathological gambling can arise in the absence of any other disturbance of the personality. Gambling may occur during an episode of depression as a way of obtaining symptomatic relief, similar to secondary drinking or kleptomania. Reckless gambling may sometimes accompany an episode of mania where financial irresponsibility is common. Psychological dependence on gambling is demonstrated by the presence of withdrawal symptoms and craving following cessation of the activity.

Management

There is no specific therapy, although Dickerson (1989) lists 22 uncontrolled studies offering differing treatment approaches, encompassing most known types of psychotherapy. Counselling and support for the family may also be helpful. During history-taking it will often become apparent that help has only been sought to alleviate the consequences of gambling, such as debt, or a distressing marital situation or some other legal problem, with little wish to cease the gambling behaviour. Both psychodynamic psychotherapy and aversive behavioural therapy have been attempted, but neither claim much success. Most gamblers find the notion of complete abstinence abhorrent, but a few may accept the wisdom of a moratorium for a few months, after which more controlled gambling may be permitted.

Among the more severe cases there is usually a disturbed appreciation of the value of money, and in these instances it is wisest for all the family income to be paid into an account over which only the spouse has sole control (Moran, 1983). Gamblers Anonymous, which uses the Alcoholics Anonymous model, allows both the patient and spouse to share information about their struggles with the morbid impulses and provide mutual support: it may be more helpful than the more traditional medical and psychiatric approaches.

Trichotillomania

Francois Hallopeau (1889), a French dermatologist, introduced the term *trichotillomania* to denote an irresistable urge to pull one's hair. This is often done in a specific pattern associated with rituals, such as mouthing the hair afterwards, or even ingesting it (trichophagy). Most subjects report a state of tension before pulling their hair out, and this is included among the diagnostic criteria for DSM–IV. The hair-pulling is not described as painful, but subjects report tingling and pruritis in the affected areas. As well as the scalp, the eyebrows, eyelashes, beard and pubic hair may be involved. Hair-pulling tends to occur during states of relaxation – while sitting down watching television, reading, studying, talking on the telephone, or driving. Most subjects engage in hair-pulling when they are on their own. Hair-pullers commonly also engage in nail-biting, thumb-sucking, head-banging, gnawing and other types of self-mutilation. Greenberg & Sarner (1965) describe the inventiveness some patients have in devising methods to remove their hair. As well as pulling their hair out singly or in tufts, some would rub their scalps with their palms or their pillows until baldness supervened. Others tangle their hair in a comb or brush and then use these instruments to epilate themselves. Bizarre cases were also noted in this series: a patient with schizophrenia who after years of hair-pulling set fire to himself, and a mother and son, with the son inducing the mother to do the hair-pulling for him. Children (usually aged 1–5) who swallow their hair may develop a tracheobezoar and present with epigastric pain, vomiting and palpable mass. The DSM–IV features of trichotillomania are shown in Box 18.9.

The disorder is not uncommon, occurring in around 1% of new psychiatric referrals, and usually presents to dermatological clinics before seeking any psychiatric help. The onset is typically in childhood and adolescence, and there is a marked female preponderance. A study of associated psychiatric comorbidity showed an increased lifetime prevalence for major depression, simple phobia, generalised anxiety disorder, and possibly also for alcohol and substance abuse. There was no association with personality disorder or any particular personality disorder subtype (Christianson *et al*, 1991), and the rate for personality disorder diagnoses was slightly less than in the general psychiatric out-patient sample. It may be more common among individuals with learning impairment, and may also occur in schizophrenia. Depression and substance abuse may lead to exacerbations, but are not thought to be causal.

Box 18.9 DSM–IV criteria for trichotillomania

1. Recurrent pulling out of one's hair resulting in noticeable hair-loss.
2. Increasing sense of tension prior to hair-pulling.
3. Pleasure, gratification or sense of relief when pulling out the hair.
4. Not due to another mental disorder, or a general medical condition (e.g. a dermatological condition).
5. Causes significant distress or impairment in social or occupational functioning.

Adapted with permission from DSM–IV. Copyright 1994 American Psychiatric Association.

The differential diagnosis is mainly with alopecia areata. Both disorders present with bald patches, but in trichotillomania the short broken strands of hair will appear alongside normal hairs, while in alopecia all the hairs are short. In addition, when the hair regrows there is no change in pigmentation in trichotillomania, which can occur in alopecia. Among the more difficult cases, or those in which the habit of hair-pulling is denied, a scalp biopsy will demonstrate the traumatic nature of the disorder with categen hairs, absence of inflammation and scarring, and dilated follicula infundibula. Hair follicle changes known as tricomalacia are said to be characteristic and differentiate the disorder from other forms of alopecia.

Management

The disorder often starts in childhood, has a prolonged course, and behavioural strategies appear to be the most useful. These include self-monitoring, covert desensitisation and habit reversal. The latter technique involves asking the patient to practice some alternative motor response such as grasping or clenching the hands for three minutes, which competes with the urge to pull hair. The behavioural regime relies on identifying situations where the habit takes place, commonly while reading or watching television, and response prevention is attempted in these situations. Relaxation therapy is sometimes also helpful. Another component of the behavioural regime is "overcorrection" or positive attention, requiring the subject to brush or comb their hair or repair eye make-up (for eyelash pullers) after each episode of hair-pulling. Arzin *et al* (1980) reported a successful outcome for 34 hair-pullers, and also provided a detailed account of the behavioural methods they used. Facial screening by covering the subject's scalp with a soft cloth is sometimes helpful. Patients will often deliberately cover affected areas out of feelings of shame, but also to protect these areas from further damage. Drug treatments may also help. Swedo *et al* (1989) conducted a cross-over trial of desipramine and clomipramine in non-depressed women with trichotillomania. Both drugs were helpful, but there was some advantage for clomipramine suggesting a possible link with obsessive–compulsive disorder, and interestingly there have been some promising reports for fluoxetine. While both behaviour therapy and drug treatment may offer some relief in the short-term, little is known about relapse rates or long-term outcome.

References

Abraham, K. (1925) Psychoanalytische Studien zur Characterbildung Internationale Psychoanalytische Bibliothek XVI. Leipzig Internationaler Psychoanalytischer Verlag, p. 1–64.

Adler, A. (1964) *Problems of Neurosis*. New York: Harper.

Akiskal, H. S., Hirschfield, R. M. A. & Yerevanian, B. I. (1983) The relationship of personality to affective disorders: a critical review. *Archives of General Psychiatry*, **40**, 801–810.

Alexander, F. (1930). The neurotic character. *International Journal of Psychoanalysis*, **11**, 291–311.

Alnaes, R. & Torgersen, S. (1988) DSM–III symptom disorders (axis I) and personality disorders (axis II) in an out-patient population. *Acta Psychiatrica Scandinavica*, **78**, 348–455.

American Psychiatric Association (1980) *Diagnostic and Statistical Manual of Mental Disorders* (3rd edn) (DSM–III). Washington, DC: APA.

—— (1987) *Diagnostic and Statistical Manual of Mental Disorders* (3rd edn, revised) (DSM–III–R). Washington, DC: APA.

—— (1994) *Diagnostic and Statistical Manual of Mental Disorders* (4th edn) (DSM–IV). Washington, DC: APA.

Androlunis, P. A., Gluech, B. C., Stroebel, C. F., *et al* (1981) Organic brain dysfunction and borderline personality disorder. *Psychiatric Clinics of North America*, **4**, 61–66.

Arzin, N. H., Nunn, R. G. & Frantz, S. E. (1980) Treatment of hair pulling (Tricotillomania): A comparative study of habit reversal and negative practice training. *Journal of Behaviour Therapy and Experimental Psychiatry*, **11**, 13–20.

Baron, M. (1981) *Schedule for Interviewing Borderlines*. New York: New York State Psychiatric Institute.

——, Gruen, R., Asnis, L., *et al* (1983) Familial relatedness of schizophrenic and schizotypal states. *American Journal of Psychiatry*, **140**, 1437–1442.

——, Asnis, L. & Gruen, R. (1990) Schedule for interviewing schizotypal personalities: a diagnostic interview for schizotypal features. *Psychiatry Research*, **4**, 213–228.

Battaglia, M., Gasperini, M., Sciuto, G., *et al* (1991) Psychiatric disorders in the families of schizotypal subjects. *Schizophrenia Bulletin*, **17**, 659–665.

Baxter, L., Edell, W., Gerner, R., *et al* (1984) Dexamethazone suppression test and axis I diagnosis of inpatients with DSM–III borderline disorder. *Journal of Clinical Psychiatry*, **45**, 150–153.

Beck, A. T., Weissman, A., Lester, D., *et al* (1974) The measurement of pessimism: the hopelessness scale. *Journal of Consulting and Clinical Psychology*, **42**, 861–865.

Blackburn, R. (1971) Personality types among abnormal homicides. *British Journal of Criminology*, **11**, 14–31.

—— (1979) Cortical and autonomic arousal in primary and secondary psychopaths. *Psychophysiology*, **16**, 143–150.

—— (1988) On moral judgments and personality disorder. The myth of psychopathic disorder revisited. *British Journal of Psychiatry*, **153**, 505–512.

Bland, R. C., Newman, S. C., Dyck, R. J., *et al* (1990) Prevalence of psychiatric disorders in a prison population. *Canadian Journal of Psychiatry*, **35**, 407–413.

Bleuler, E. (1922) Die probleme der Schizoidie und der Syntonie. *Zeitschrift fuer die gesamte Neurologie und Psychiatrie*, **78**, 373–388.

Bohman, M., Cloinger, R., Sigvardsson, S., *et al* (1982) Predisposition to petty criminality in Swedish adoptees: genetic and enviromental heterogenecity. *Archives of General Psychiatry*, **39**, 339–341.

Bowlby, J. (1977) The making and breaking of affectional bonds. II. Some principles of psychotherapy. *British Journal of Psychiatry*, **130**, 421–431.

Brown, G. R. & Anderson, B. (1991) Psychiatric morbidity in adult inpatients with childhood histories of sexual and physical abuse. *American Journal of Psychiatry*, **148**, 55–61.

Cadoret, R. J. (1978) Psychopathology in adopted-away offspring of biological parents with antisocial behaviour. *Archives of General Psychiatry*, **35**, 176–184.

——, O'Gorman, T. W., Troughton, E., *et al* (1985) Alcoholism and antisocial personality – interrelationships, genetics and environmental factors. *Archives of General Psychiatry*, **42**, 161–167.

Caine, T. M., Foulds, G. A. & Hope, K. (1967) *Manual of the Hostility–Direction of Hostility Questionnaire*. London: University of London Press.

Casey, P. R. (1989) Personality disorder and suicide intent. *Acta Psychiatrica Scandinavica*, **79**, 290–295.

——, Dillon, S. & Tyrer, P. J. (1984) The diagnostic status of patients with conspicuous psychiatric morbidity in primary care. *Psychological Medicine*, **14**, 673–681.

—— & Tyrer, P. J. (1986) Personality, functioning and symptomatology. *Journal of Psychiatric Research*, **20**, 363–374.

—— & —— (1990) Personality disorder and psychiatric illness in general practice. *British Journal of Psychiatry*, **156**, 261–265.

Cattell, R. B. (1965) The Scientific Analysis of Personality. Harmondsworth: Penguin.

Chodoff, P. & Lyons, H. (1958) Hysteria, the hysterical personality and "hysterical" conversion. *American Journal of Psychiatry*, **114**, 734–740.

Christianson, G. A., McKenzie, T. B. & Mitchell, J. E. (1991) Characteristics of 60 adult chronic hair pullers. *American Journal of Psychiatry*, **148**, 365–370.

Clarkin, J. F., Widiger, T. A., Frances, A., *et al* (1983) Prototypic typology and the borderline personality disorder. *Journal of Abnormal Psychology*, **92**, 263–275.

Cleckley, H. (1941) *The Mask of Sanity* (5th edn). St. Louis, MO: Mosby.

Clifford, C. A., Murray, R. M. & Fulker, D. W. (1984) Genetic and environmental influences on obsessional traits and symptoms. *Psychological Medicine*, **14**, 791–800.

Cloninger, C. R. (1987) A systematic method for clinical description and classification of personality variants. *Archives of General Psychiatry*, **44**, 573–588.

—— & Gottesman, I. I. (1987) Genetic and environmental factors in antisocial behaviour disorders. In *Cases of Crime: New Biological Approaches* (eds S. A. Mednick, T. E. Moffitt & S. A. Stack). Cambridge: Cambridge University Press.

Coccaro, E. F. (1989) Central serotonin and impulsive aggression. *British Journal of Psychiatry*, **155** (suppl. 8), 52–62.

Coid, J. (1993) Current concepts and classification of psychopathic disorder. In *Personality Disorders Reviewed* (eds P. Tyrer & G. S. Stein), pp. 113–164. London: Gaskell.

Cooper, J. (1970) The Leyton obsessional inventory. *Psychological Medicine*, **1**, 48–64.

Cote, G. & Hodgins, S. (1990) Co-occurring mental disorders among criminal offenders. *Bulletin of the American Academy of Psychiatry and Law*, **18**, 271–281.

Crowe, R. R. (1972) The adopted offspring of women criminal offenders – a study of their arrest records. *Archives of General Psychiatry*, **27**, 600–603.

Cutting, J. (1985) *The Psychology of Schizophrenia*. Edinburgh: Churchill Livingstone.

——, Cowen, P. J., Mann, A. H., *et al* (1986) Personality and psychosis: use of the Standardized Assessment of Personality. *Acta Psychiatrica Scandinavica*, **73**, 87–92.

Dagonet, H. (1870) Des impulsions dans la folie et de la folie impulsive. *Annales Medico-Psychologique*, **4**, 5–32, 215–259.

Department of Health and Social Security (1985) *Mental Illness Hospitals and Units in England. Results from the Mental Health Enquiry*. Statistical Bulletin, Government Statistical Service. London: HMSO.

Deutsch, H. (1942) Some forms of emotional disturbance and their relationship to schizophrenia. *Psycho-analytic Quarterly*, **11**, 301–321.

Dickerson, M. G. (1988) The prevalence of excessive and pathological gambling in Australia. *Journal of Gambling Behaviour*, **4**, 125–151.

—— (1989) Gambling; dependence without a drug. *International Review of Psychiatry*, **1**, 157–172.

Dilling, H. & Weyerer, S. (1989) Incidence and prevalence of treated mental disorders. Health care planning in a small-town rural region of upper Bavaria. *Acta Psychiatrica Scandinavica*, **61**, 209–222.

Eaton, J. W. & Weil, R. J. (1955) *Culture and Mental Disorder*. Glencoe, IL: Free Press.

Ennis, J., Barnes, R. A., Kennedy, S., *et al* (1989) Depression in self-harm patients. *British Journal of Psychiatry*, **154**, 41–47.

Erikson, E. H. (1956) The problem of ego identity. *Journal of the American Psychoanalytical Association*, **4**, 56–121.

Essen-Moller, E. (1956) Individual traits and morbidity in a Swedish rural population. *Acta Psychiatrica Scandinavica* (suppl. 2), 100.

Eysenck, H. J. (1979) The conditioning model of neurosis. *Behavioural and Brain Sciences*, **2**, 155–166.

—— & Eysenck, S. B. G. (1964) *Manual of the Eysenck Personality Inventory (EPQ)*. London: University of London Press.

—— & —— (1979) The Structure and Measurement of Personality. London: Routledge & Kegan Paul.

Farmer, A. E., McGuffin, P. & Gottesman, I. I. (1987) Twin concordance for DSM–III schizophrenia. Scrutinising the validity of the definition. *Archives of General Psychiatry*, **44**, 634–641.

Farrington, D., Loeber, R. & Van Kammen, W. B. (1990) Long-term criminal outcomes of hyperactivity-impulsivity-attention deficit and conduct problems in childhood. In *Straight and Devious Pathways from Childhood to Adulthood* (eds L. N. Robins & M. Rutter). Cambridge: Cambridge University Press.

Feighner, J. P., Robins, E., Guze, S.B., *et al* (1972) Diagnostic criteria for use in psychiatric research. *Archives of General Psychiatry*, **26**, 57–63.

Freud, S. (1908) Character and anal eroticism. In *Collected Papers* (English translation, 1929). Vol. 2. London: Hogarth.

Freud, S. (1928) Dostoyevsky and parricide. In *The Complete Works of Sigmund Freud* (standard edn, 1961) (ed. J. Strachey), Vol. 21, p. 177. London: Hogarth Press.

Frosch, W. A., Frosch, J. P. & Frosch, J. (1985) The impulse disorders. In *Psychiatry 1* (eds R. Michels & J. O. Cavenar). Philadelphia: J.B. Lippincott.

Fyer, M. R., Frances, A., Sullivan, T., *et al* (1988) Comorbidity of borderline personality disorder. *Archives of General Psychiatry*, **45**, 348–352.

Goodyear, I.(1993) Continuities and discontinuities from childhood to adult life. In *Seminars in Child and Adolescent Psychiatry* (eds D. Black & D. Cottrell), pp. 276–290. London: Gaskell.

Gottesman, I. I. (1963) Heritability of personality: a demonstration. *Psychological Monograph*, **77**, 1–21.

Greenberg, H. R. & Sarner, C. A. (1965) Trichotillomania: symptoms and syndrome. *Archives of General Psychiatry*, **12**, 482–489.

Greenson, R. (1947) On gambling. *American Imago*, **4**, 61.

Grinker, R. R., Werble, B. & Drye, R. C. (1968) *The Borderline Syndrome*. New York: Basic Books.

Gunderson, J. G. & Kolb, J. E. (1978) Discriminating features of borderline patients. *American Journal of Psychiatry*, **135**, 792–796.

——, —— & Austin, V. (1981) The diagnostic interview for borderline patients. *American Journal of Psychiatry*, **138**, 896–903.

——, Ronningstam, E. & Bodkin, A. (1990) The diagnostic interview for narcissistic patients. *Archives of General Psychiatry*, **47**, 676–680.

—— & Phillips, K. A. (1991) A current view of the interface between borderline personality disorder and depression. *American Journal of Psychiatry*, **148**, 967–975.

Gunn, J. (1988) Personality Disorder: a clinical suggestion. In *Personality Disorders. Diagnosis, Management and Course* (ed. P. Tyrer), pp. 33–42. London: Wright.

Guze, S. B., Wolfgran, E. D., McKinnery, J. K., *et al* (1967) Psychiatric illness in the families of convicted criminals. A study of 519 first-degree relatives. *Disease of the Nervous System*, **28**, 651–659.

Hallopeau, F. (1889) Alopecie par grattage: trichomanie on trichotillomanie. *Annales de Dermatologie et de Syphiligraphie*, **10**, 440–441.

Hanson, W. & Wang, A. G. (1984) Suicide attempts in a Danish region. *Social Psychiatry*, **19**, 197–201.

Hare, R. D. (1983) Diagnosis of antisocial personality disorder in two prison populations. *American Journal of Psychiatry*, **140**, 887–890.

—— & McPherson, L. M. (1984) Violent and aggressive behaviour by criminal psychopaths. *International Journal of Law and Psychiatry*, **7**, 35–50.

Helgason, T. (1964) *Epidemiology of Mental Disorders in Iceland*. Copenhagen: Munksgaard.

Henderson, D. K. (1939) *Psychopathic States*. London: Chapman & Hall.

Herzog, D. B., Keller, M. B., Lavori, P. W., *et al* (1992) The prevalence of personality disorders in 210 women with eating disorders. *Journal of Clinical Psychiatry*, **53**, 147–152.

Hill, D. & Watterson, D. (1942) Electroencephalographic studies of psychopathic personalities. *Journal of Neurology and Psychiatry*, **5**, 47–52.

Hoch, P. H. & Polatin, P. (1949) Pseudoneurotic form of schizophrenia. *Psychiatric Quarterly*, **23**, 248–276.

Horney, K. (1939) *New Ways in Psychoanalysis*. New York: W. W. Norton.

—— (1945) *Our Inner Conflicts*. New York: Norton.

Howard, R. C. (1984) The clinical EEG and personality in mentally abnormal offenders. *Psychological Medicine*, **14**, 569–580.

Hughes, C. H. (1884) Moral (affective) insanity: psycho-sensory insanity. *Alienist and Neurologist*, **5**, 296–315.

Hutchings, B. & Mednick, S. A. (1974) Registered criminality in the adopted and biological parents of registered male adoptees. In *Genetics, Environment and Psychopathology* (eds S. A. Mednick, F. Schulzinger, J. Higgins, *et al*), pp. 215–230. Amsterdam: Elsevier.

Hwu, H. F., Yeh, E. K. & Chang, L. Y. (1989) Prevalence of psychiatric disorders in Taiwan defined by the Chinese Diagnostic Interview Schedule. *Acta Psychiatrica Scandinavica*, **79**, 136–147.

Jackson, H. J., Whiteside, H. L., Bates, G. W., *et al* (1991) Diagnosing personality disorders in psychiatric inpatients. *Acta Psychiatrica Scandinavica*, **83**, 206–213.

James, W. (1890) *The Principles of Psychology*. New York: Holt.

Jung, C. G. (1921) *Psychologische Typen*. Zurich: Rascher.

Kammeier, M. L., Hoffman, H. & Lopes, R. G. (1973) Personality characteristics of alcoholics as freshmen and at the time of treatment. *Quarterly Journal of Studies on Alcohol*, **34**, 390–399.

Karpman, B. (1946) Psychopathy in the scheme of human typology. *Journal of Nervous and Mental Disease*, **103**, 276–288.

Kass, F., Skodol, A. E., Charles, E., *et al* (1985) Scaled ratings of DSM–III personality disorders. *American Journal of Psychiatry*, **142**, 627–630.

Kendell, R. E. & DiScipio, W. J. (1968) Eysenck Personality Inventory scores of patients with depressive illness. *British Journal of Psychiatry*, **114**, 767–770.

Kendler, K., Lieberman, J. A. & Walsh, D. (1989) The structured interview for schizotypy (SIS): a preliminary report. *Schizophrenia Bulletin*, **15**, 559–571.

Kernberg, O. F. (1967) Borderline personality organisation. *Journal of the American Psychoanalytical Association*, **15**, 641–685.

Kerr, T. A., Shapiro, K., Roth, M., *et al* (1970) The relationship between the Maudsley Personality Inventory and the course of affective disorder. *British Journal of Psychiatry*, **116**, 11–19.

Kessel, N. (1960) Psychiatric morbidity in a London general practice. *British Journal of Preventive and Social Medicine*, **14**, 16–22.

Kety, S. S., Rosenthal, D., Wender, P. H., *et al* (1971) Mental illness in the biological and adoptive families of adopted schizophrenics. *American Journal of Psychiatry*, **128**, 302–306.

Kohut, H. (1971) *The Analysis of the Self*. New York: International University Press.

Kontaxakis, V., Markionis, M., Vaslamtsis, J., *et al* (1987) Multiple neuroendocrinological responses in borderline personality disorder patients. *Acta Psychiatrica Scandinavica*, **76**, 593–597.

Korzekwa, M. I. (1991) Biological markers in borderline personality disorders. Proceedings of the Conference on Borderline Personality Disorder, Hamilton, Ontario, January 1991.

Kraepelin, E. (1913) *Psychiatrie: Ein Lehrbuch* (8th edn), Vol. 3. Leipzig: Barth.

Kretschmer, E. (1918) *Der sensitive Beziehungswahn*. Berlin: Springer.

—— (1922) *Korperbau und Charakter*. Berlin: Springer Verlag.

—— (1926) *Hysteria* (English translation). New York: Nervous and Mental Disease.

Kroll, J., Carey, K., Lloyd, S., *et al* (1982) Are there borderlines in Britain? A cross validation of US findings. *Archives of General Psychiatry*, **39**, 60–63.

Lacey, J. H. & Evans, C. D. H. (1986) The impulsivist: a multi-impulsive personality disorder. *British Journal of Addiction*, **81**, 641–649.

LeCouter, A. (1993) Clinical syndromes in early childhood. In *Seminars in Child and Adolescent Psychiatry* (eds D. Black & D. Cottrell), pp. 95–123. London: Gaskell.

Legg-England, S. & Gotestam, K. G. (1991) The nature and treatment of excessive gambling. *Acta Psychiatrica Scandinavica*, **84**, 113–120.

Leighton, D. C., Harding, J. S., Macklin, D. B., *et al* (1963) Psychiatric findings of the Stirling County Study. *American Journal of Psychiatry*, **143**, 718–722.

Lewis, G. & Appleby, L. (1988) Personality disorder: the patients psychiatrists dislike. *British Journal of Psychiatry*, **153**, 44–49.

Lidberg, L., Tuck, J. R., Asberg, M., *et al* (1985) Homicide, suicide and CSF 5HIAA. *Acta Psychiatrica Scandinavica*, **71**, 230–236.

Lombroso, C. (1887) *L'Homme Criminal: Criminal-ne, Fou Moral, Epileptique*. Paris: Alcan.

Loranger, A. W. (1990) The impact of DSM–III on diagnostic practice in a University Hospital. *Archives of General Psychiatry*, **47**, 672–675.

——, Oldham, J. M. & Tulis, E. H. (1982) Familial transmission of DSM–III borderline personality disorder. *Archives of General Psychiatry*, **39**, 795–799.

——, Susman, V. L., Oldham, J. M., *et al* (1985) *Personality Disorder Examination (PDE). A Structured Interview for DSM–III–R and ICD–9 Personality Disorders. WHO/ADAMHA Pilot Version*. White Plains, NY: New York Hospital, Cornell Medical Centre.

Macmillan, D. & Shaw, P. (1966) Senile breakdown in standards of personal and environmental cleanliness. *British Medical Journal*, **2**, 1032–1037.

Magnan, V. (1886)Lecous Clinique sur les maladies mentales. Paris: Battaille.

Maier, W., Lichtermann, D., Klingler, T., *et al* (1992) Prevalence of personality disorders (DSM–III–R) in the community. *Journal of Personality Disorder*, **6**, 187–196.

Mann, A. H., Jenkins, R., Cutting, J. C., *et al* (1981) The development and use of a standardised assessment of abnormal personality. *Psychological Medicine*, **11**, 839–847.

Mannuzza, S., Gittleman Klein, R., Horowitz Kongi, P., *et al* (1989) Hyperactive boys almost grown up: IV. Criminality and its relationship to psychiatric status. *Archives of General Psychiatry*, **46**, 1073–1079.

Maudsley, H. (1897) Responsibility in Mental Disease. New York: Appleton & Co.

McGuffin, P. & Gottesman, I. I. (1984) Genetic influences on normal and abnormal development. In *Child Psychiatry: Modern Approaches* (2nd edn) (eds M. Rutter & L. Hersov). London: Blackwell.

——, Katz, R., Aldrich, J., *et al* (1988) The Camberwell Collaboration Depression Study 2. Investigation of family members. *British Journal of Psychiatry*, **152**, 766–775.

Megargee, E. I. (1966) Undercontrolled and overcontrolled personality types in extreme antisocial aggression. *Psychological Monographs*, **80**, No. 611.

Millon, T. (1969) *Modern Psychopathology: A Bisocial Approach to Maladaptive Learning and Functioning*. Philadelphia: W. B. Saunders.

—— (1981) *Disorders of Personality, DSM–III: Axis II*. New York: John Wiley.

—— (1982) *Millon Clinical Multiaxial Inventory Interpretative Scoring System* (2nd edn). Minneapolis.

Mischel, W. (1968) *Personality and Assessment*. New York: John Wiley.

Moran, E. (1983) Gambling. In *Handbook of Psychiatry, 4. The Neurosis and Personality Disorders* (eds G. F. M. Russell & L. A. Hersov), pp. 385–390. Cambridge: Cambridge University Press.

Morgan, H. G., Burns-Cox, C. J., Pocock, H., *et al* (1975) Deliberate self-harm: clinical and socio-economic characteristics of 368 patients. *British Journal of Psychiatry*, **127**, 564–574.

Myers, J. K., Weissman, M. M., Tischler, G. L., *et al* (1984) Six month prevalence of psychiatric disorders in three communities, 1980–1982. *Archives of General Psychiatry*, **41**, 959–967.

Nigg, J. T., Silk, K. R., Western, D., *et al* (1991) Object representations in the early memories of sexually abused borderline patients. *American Journal of Psychiatry*, **148**, 864–869.

Ogata, S. N., Silk, K. R. & Goodrich, S. *et al* (1990) Childhood sexual and physical abuse in adult patients with borderline personality disorder. *American Journal of Psychiatry*, **147**, 1008–1013.

Ovenstone, I. K. (1973) Spectrum of suicidal behaviours in Edinburgh. *British Journal of Preventive and Social Medicine*, **27**, 27–35.

Pfohl, B., Stangl, D. & Zimmerman, M. (1983) *Structured Interview for DSM–III Personality (SIDP)*. Iowa City: University of Iowa.

——, —— & —— (1986) The implication of DSM–III personality disorders for patients with major depression. *Journal of Affective Disorders*, **7**, 309–318.

Pinel, P. H. (1806) *A Treatise on Insanity* (transl. D. Davis, 1962). New York: Hafner Publishing.

Piran, N., Lerner, P., Garfield, P.E., *et al* (1988) Personality disorders in an anorexic patient. *International Journal of Eating Disorders*, **7**, 589–599.

Platt, J. & Spivack, G. (1975) *Manual for the Means-Ends Problem-Solving Procedure. A Measure of Interpersonal Cognitive Problem-Solving Skill*. Philadelphia: Hahnemann Medical College and Hospital.

Pope, H. G., Jonas, J. M., Hudson, J. I., *et al* (1983) The validity of DSM–III borderline personality disorder. *Archives of General Psychiatry*, **40**, 23–30.

Presly, A. J. & Walton, H. J. (1973) Dimensions of abnormal personality. *British Journal of Psychiatry*, **122**, 269–276.

Pritchard, J. C. (1835) *Treatise on Insanity*. London: Gilbert & Piper.

Rachman, S. J. & Hodgson, R. (1980) *Obsessions and Compulsions*. Englewood Cliffs, NJ: Prentice-Hall.

Rado, S. (1956) Schizotypal organization: Preliminary report on a clinical study of schizophrenia. In *Changing Concepts of Psychoanalytic Medicine* (eds S. Rado & G. E. Daniels), pp. 225–236. New York: Grune & Stratton.

Reed, G. F. (1985) *Obsessional Experience and Compulsive Behaviour: a Cognitive–Structural Approach*. London: Academic Press.

Reich, W. (1933) *Charakteranalyse*. Leipzig: Sexpol Verlag.

Reich, J., Yates, W. & Nduaguba, M. (1989) Prevalence of DSM–III personality disorders in the community. *Social Psychiatry and Psychiatric Epidemiology*, **24**, 12–16.

Reid, W. H. (1985) Antisocial personality disorder. In *Psychiatry 1* (eds R. Michels, J. D. Cavender, H. K. H. Brodie, *et al*), pp. 1–11. Philadelphia: J. B. Lippincott.

Ribot, T. (1890) *Psychologie des Sentiments*. Paris: Delahaye & Lecrosnier.

Robins, L. (1966) *Deviant Children Grown Up*. Baltimore: Williams & Wilkins.

—— (1985) Epidemiology of anti-social personality disorder. In *Psychiatry 3* (eds R. Michels, J. O. Cavenar, H. K. Brodie, *et al*), pp. 1–14. Philadelphia: J. B. Lippincott.

Royal College of Psychiatrists (1977) *Submission of Evidence to the Royal Commission on Gambling*. London: Royal College of Psychiatrists.

Rutter, M. (1985) Resilience in the face of adversity: Protective factors and resistance to psychiatric disorder. *British Journal of Psychiatry*, **147**, 598–611.

— (1987) Temperament, personality and personality disorder. *British Journal of Psychiatry*, **150**, 443–458.

Schneider, K. (1923) *Die psychopathischen Personlichkeiten*. Vienna: Deuticke.

— (1950) *Psychopathic Personalities* (9th ed., English transl.). London: Cassell.

Schulzinger, F. (1972) Psychopathy, heredity and environment. *International Journal of Mental Health*, **1**, 190–206.

Seivewright, N. (1988) Personality disorder, life events and onset of mental illness. In *Personality Disorders. Diagnosis, Management and Course* (ed. P. Tyrer). London: Wright.

Sheldon, W. H. (1940) *The Varieties of Human Physique: An Introduction to Constitutional Psychology*. New York: Harper.

Shepherd, M., Cooper, B., Brown, A. C., *et al* (1966) *Psychiatric Illness in General Practice*. Oxford: Oxford University Press.

Silk, K. R., Lohr, E., Shipley, E., *et al* (1988) Sleep EEG and DST in borderlines with depression. Proceedings and summary, 141st Annual Meeting, American Psychiatric Association, p. 206. Washington, DC: APA.

Skodol, A. E., Oldham, J. M., Hyler, S. E., *et al* (1993) Comorbidity of DSM–III–R eating disorders and personality disorders. *International Journal of Eating Disorders*, **14**, 403–416.

Slater, E. & Shields, J. (1969) Genetic aspects of anxiety. In *Studies of Anxiety* (ed. M. H. Lader). *British Journal of Psychiatry* Special Publication No. 3. Ashford: Headley Brothers.

Spitzer, R. L., Endicott, J. & Robins, E. (1978) Research Diagnostic Criteria: rationale and reliability. Archives of General Psychiatry, *35*, 773–782.

—, — & Gibbon, M. (1979) Crossing the border into borderline personality and borderline schizophrenia. *Archives of General Psychiatry*, **36**, 17–34.

—, Williams, J. & Gibbon, M. (1987) *Structured Clinical Interview for DSM–III–R (SCID–II)*. New York: Biometrics Research, New York State Psychiatric Institute.

Srole, L., Langer, T., Michael, S., *et al* (1962) *Mental Health in the Metropolis*. New York: McGraw Hill.

Steiner, M., Links, P. & Korzekwa, M. I. (1988) Biological markers in border personality disorders. An overview. *Canadian Journal of Psychiatry*, **33**, 350–354.

Stern, A. (1938) Psychoanalytic investigation of and therapy in the borderline group of neuroses. *Psychoanalytic Quarterly*, **7**, 467–489.

Sternbach, H. A., Fleming, J. & Extein, J. (1983) The dexamethazone suppression test and thyrotrophin releasing tests in depressed borderline patients. *Psychoneuroendocrinology*, **8**, 459–462.

Stone, M. H. (1990) Treatment of borderline patients: a pragmatic approach. *Psychiatric Clinics of North America*, **13**, 265–286.

— (1993) *Abnormalities of Personality. Within and Beyond the Realm of Treatment*. New York: W. W. Norton.

Sullivan, H. S. (1947) *Conceptions of Modern Psychiatry*. New York: Norton.

Swedo, S. E., Leonard, H. L. & Rapoport, J. L. (1989) A double blind comparison of clomipramine and desipramine in the treatment of trichotillomania (hair pulling). *New England Journal of Medicine*, **321**, 497–501.

Tantam, D. (1988) Lifelong eccentricity and social isolation: II. Asperger's syndrome or schizoid personality disorder. *British Journal of Psychiatry*, **153**, 777–782.

Tarnopolsky, A. & Berelowitz, M. (1984) "Borderline personality": Diagnostic attitudes at the Maudsley Hospital. *British Journal of Psychiatry*, **144**, 364–369.

Thomas, A. & Chess, S. (1982) Temperament and follow up to adulthood. In *Temperamental Differences in Infants and Young Children* (eds R. Porter & G. M. Collins). Ciba Symposium 89, pp. 168–172. London: Pitman.

Thompson, D. J. & Goldberg, D. (1987) Hysterical personality disorder. The process of diagnosis in clinical and experimental settings. *British Journal of Psychiatry*, **150**, 241–245.

Torgersen, S. (1984) Genetic and nosological aspects of schizotypal and borderline personality disorders. *Archives of General Psychiatry*, **41**, 546–554.

Trélat, U. (1861) *La Folie Lucide*. Paris: Delahaye.

Tyrer, P. (1988) *Personality Disorders. Diagnosis, Management and Course*. London: Wright.

—— (1989) General neurotic syndrome and mixed anxiety-depressive disorders. In *Classification of Neurosis*, pp. 153–160. Chichester: John Wiley.

—— (1990) Personality disorder and social functioning. In *Measuring Human Problems* (eds D. F. Peck & C. M. Shapiro), pp. 119–142. Chichester: John Wiley.

—— & Alexander, J. (1979) Classification of personality disorder. *British Journal of Psychiatry*, **135**, 163–167.

——, Casey, P. & Gall, J. (1983) The relationship between neurosis and personality disorder. *British Journal of Psychiatry*, **142**, 404–408.

——, —— & Ferguson, B. (1988) Personality disorder and mental illness. In *Personality Disorders: Diagnosis Management and Course* (ed. P. Tyrer), pp. 93–104. London: Wright.

Urwin, P. & Gibbons, J. L. (1979) Psychiatric diagnosis in self-poisoning patients. *Psychological Medicine*, **9**, 501–507.

US Commission on the Review of the National Policy Towards Gambling (1976) *Gambling in America: Final Report*. Washington, DC: US Government Printing Office.

Vaillant, G. E. (1977) *Adaptation for Life*. Boston: Little, Brown & Co.

Valgum, S. & Valgum, P. (1989) Co-morbidity for borderline and schizotypal personality disorders. A study of alcoholic women. Progress in neuropsychopharmacology and biological psychiatry. *Journal of Nervous and Mental Disease*, **177**, 279–284.

Virkunen, M., Nuutila, M. & Goodwin, F. K. (1987) Cerebrospinal fluid. Monoamine metabolite levels in male arsonists. *Archives of General Psychiatry*, **44**, 241–247.

Waller, G. (1993) Association of sexual abuse and borderline personality disorder in eating disordered women. *International Journal of Eating Disorders*, **13**, 259–263.

Weissman, M. M., Myers, J. K. & Harding, P. S. (1978) Psychiatric disorders in a US urban community: 1975–1976. *American Journal of Psychiatry*, **135**, 459–462.

Wender, P. H. (1977) The scope and the validity of the schizophrenic spectrum concept. In *Psychiatric Diagnosis* (eds V. M. Rakoff, H. C. Stancer & H. B. Kedward). New York: Brunner/Mazel.

Williamson, S., Hare, R. D. & Wong, S. (1987) Violence: criminal psychopaths and their victims. *Canadian Journal of Behavioural Science*, **19**, 454–462.

Wittels, F. (1930) The hysterical character. *Medical Review of Reviews*, **36**, 186–190.

Wolff, S. & Cull, A. (1986) 'Schizoid' personality and anti-social conduct: a retrospective case note study. *Psychological Medicine*, **16**, 677–687.

World Health Organization (1992) *International Classification of Diseases and Related Health Problems (ICD–10)*. Geneva: WHO.

Young, J. P. R. & Lader, M. H. (1971) The inheritance of neurotic traits: a twin study of the Middlesex Hospital Questionnaire. *British Journal of Psychiatry*, **119**, 393–398.

19 Treatment and outcome of the personality disorders

Michael Stone, Patricia Casey & George Stein

Psychotherapy • Eccentric disorders • Dramatic disorders • Anxious disorders • Lowered self-esteem • Countertransference • Group therapy • Other treatment approaches • Social and prison programmes • Drug treatments • Long-term outcome

---

It would be wrong to talk of a cure in connection with the personality disorders, but a generation ago a diagnosis of personality disorder was generally equated with untreatability. Advances in the fields of diagnosis, psychotherapy and psychopharmacology have now provided clinicians with a useful range of treatment options – even if the quest for a cure remains elusive. Many patients still remain beyond the reach of any therapy, either because they are too severely affected or are too contemptuous. Certain general principles are common to the management of the personality disorders. These derive mainly from the writings of a few psychoanalysts with a special interest in the area, but the same principles equally apply to treatment in general psychiatric settings as well. In this chapter the principles of psychotherapy will be outlined first, followed by a consideration of the more medical interventions.

Psychotherapy

The word "enduring" is included in the ICD–10 definition of personality disorders. This implies long-lasting although not totally immoveable features. Personality is in effect a most stable mechanism. It represents the sum of a huge number of programmes, each with a high survival value, for example, for getting along with parents, attracting sexual partners, rearing one's children or coping with bosses. Costa & McCrae (1986) pointed out that personality is resistant to change, whether or not it is normal and in harmony (and therefore in no particular need for change), or highly disagreeable to others, making it self-defeating, and therefore greatly in need of change. Personality disorders call out for some sort of therapeutic intervention because they have the capacity to spoil patients' lives and the lives of others.

Maladaptive traits are difficult to change, and in most cases strenuous efforts and prolonged treatment are required. Therapists must content themselves with small improvements and a relatively slow advance, extending over a period of years rather than weeks or months. Waldinger

& Gunderson (1984), in their survey of psychotherapists with an interest in borderline personality disorder (BPD), found that the treatment duration was between two and seven years, with an average of four years for most cases. A general psychiatrist using supportive measures and medication may also find the duration of the therapeutic contact extends for some 3–6 years.

In the more prolonged analytical treatments of severe personality disorders, three phases are recognised: firstly, a holding or containing phase in which the therapist serves almost as a transitional object; secondly, a gradual weaning phase when previously tolerated regression is increasingly questioned and during which there is a gradual process of optimal disillusionment; and thirdly, a separation phase when autonomy and self-worth are encouraged. For those treating the personality disorders there is no quick fix; if the maladaptive traits disappear after a few sessions or a brief course of medication, then the original diagnosis of personality disorder, at least as the cause of the presenting behaviour rather than as a coincidental diagnosis, should be questioned.

Many different methods of psychotherapy have been tried in the treatment of disorders of personality. These include supportive therapy, classical psychoanalysis, psychodynamically orientated psychotherapy, cognitive–behavioural psychotherapy (Linehan, 1993; Beck & Freeman, 1990), and a host of eclectic pragmatic approaches. With each method most authorities agree that the emphasis should be on the "here and now" rather than the "distant past" because the aim is to change present behaviour patterns and current modes of relating. For the analytically-based therapist this means greater emphasis on interpreting the transference, while cognitive therapists will explore current distortions of reality. Regardless of the theoretical orientation of the therapist, the cognitive style of the patient needs to be taken into account during treatment. Therapists should also guard against too facile formulations or simplistic interpretations that view the different personality disorders as defences against this or that conflict. Alexander (1957) suggested that the treatment of personality disorders entailed providing a "corrective emotional experience". Fromm-Reichmann (1950) put the case even more strongly and wrote "what these patients need is an experience, not an explanation". This holds true whether treatment takes the form of five times weekly psychoanalysis or an admission to a general psychiatric unit.

Unlike most axis I disorders, many subjects with personality disorders do not complain of symptoms. Their problems bother other people rather than themselves. A very self-centred person might see himself as "tough yet reasonable", while others would perceive him as a narcissist. The term 'ego-syntonic' has been used to describe this, *syntonic* signifying comfort with themselves, as opposed to *dystonic* suggesting disharmony with themselves or their environment. Some maladaptive traits such as being moody, shy, or absentminded, even if they are ego-syntonic, impinge only lightly on friends and intimates. However, other ego-syntonic traits such as being wilful, impulsive or callous have a much more damaging effect and are therefore of clinical importance. Some subjects with personality disorders are ego-dystonic and regret their maladaptive traits, and their distress provides some motivation for therapeutic change. The degree of syntonicity has important implications with regard to the initiation and ultimate success of treatment. A second feature common to almost all personality disorders is the self-defeating nature of the maladaptive traits. These patients are adept at making matters worse for themselves. Subjects with a paranoid personality will suspect and alienate even their closest friends; histrionic personalities will spare no effort to become involved with the most inappropriate person; obsessional personalities stifle all pleasure for themselves and their families; and for almost all there will be attempts to destroy or subvert those who seek to treat them or change their ways.

Treatment goals among those with personality disorders should be limited. A wholesale change of character is unlikely to occur, but limited change may be possible. A patient with a schizoid personality will never become the life and soul of the party, but there is progress if he begins to meet a friend once a week. A borderline personality will continue to make emotionally intense relationships, but if there is only sadness rather than self-mutilation when the relationship ends, her reactions will be within the normal range. For some chronically suicidal adolescents the aim is quite modest – simply the preservation of life and prevention of suicide. Even this basic goal may require a generous allocation of psychotherapeutic time, hospital admissions, medication and nursing support. The goals for the three DSM–IV personality disorder clusters are quite different: for the *dramatic* cluster (borderline, histrionic, sociopathy), it is to curb impulsivity and overheated emotionality; for the *eccentric* cluster (paranoid and schizotypal) to undo the cognitive distortions; for the *anxiety* cluster to alleviate the excessive inhibitedness.

It should be noted that both psychoanalysis and psychotherapy rest on the assumption that a patient's maladaptive traits and behaviour are born out of conflicts, and that resolution of these conflicts will help the patient. The method may be of relatively little use if the main difficulty is one of temperament (e.g. extreme intensity, irritability, emotional insensitivity) because temperament is largely innate or genetic (Buss & Plomin, 1984) and less likely to change in the long-term as a result of purely psychological intervention.

A key goal in treating subjects with a personality disorder is the amelioration of their maladaptive traits. If rudeness and stinginess are maladaptive and to be extinguished, then their opposites (politeness and generosity) represent the ideal and should be fostered. By aiming to train patients out of their more maladaptive habits and behaviours, the therapist will instinctively find himself behaving in a manner opposite to the prevailing pathological trend in the patient's personality. For example, when treating an avoidant person the therapist will find himself being more affable and outgoing than is usual for himself, and so demonstrate that the world is not such a hostile place. For the chaotic patient, sticking to the rules, insisting on punctuality and starting and finishing sessions on time is essential; while for the clingingly dependent individual, almost by instinct the therapist avoids over-long stays in hospital, frequent extra individual sessions or out-of-hours telephone calls. Table 19.1 shows the therapeutic counterforces that apply to the various DSM–IV personality disorders. The use of the technique of counterforces requires some care, particularly in the presence of an axis I disorder. Thus the dependent personality with depression may try to remain in hospital because of depressive feelings rather than because of dependency needs, and the clinical distinction is often fine and rarely easy to make.

Therapy with these subjects is hard work: a successful outcome depends on the presence of a certain glue which binds the patient and therapist together. What is the nature of this glue? Woolcott (1985) emphasised that the most important component is the quality of *likeableness*. It is this that motivates the therapist to work assiduously on the patient's behalf. Likeableness is difficult to define, but is probably a composite of several traits including flexibility, forgiveness, respectfulness, consideration and perseverence. Unfortunately the medical model, with its emphasis on disease types and negative traits, pays insufficient attention to the patient's strengths and positive traits, which may be of critical importance in determining outcome. Positive qualities, such as high intelligence, artistic sensitivity or talent, and strong moral fibre may also help to motivate therapists.

Table 19.1 Prevailing traits and corresponding countermeasures

Personality disorder	Prevailing trait(s)	Countermeasures
Schizoid	Aloofness	Affability
Schizotypal	Eccentricity	Conventionality
Paranoid	Mistrustfulness	Candour, honesty
Borderline	Unreasonableness, seductiveness, impulsivity	Compassionate neutrality, strict boundaries
Histrionic	Over-emotionality	Orderliness, logical approach, modulated responses
Narcissistic	Grandiosity, condescension	Sympathy, humility, not taking offence
Antisocial	Contempt for rules	Strict adherence to rules
Obsessive–compulsive	Constricted affect	Emotional vividness
Passive aggressive	Argumentativeness	Non-defensiveness
Avoidant	Timorousness	Encouragement
Dependent	Clinginess	Kind but distant
Depressive	Pessimistic	Optimism, enthusiasm
Irritable	Angry	Calmness

When both patient and therapist have some degree of mutual respect, each participant is minimally anxious and therefore best able to engage in harmonious dialogue. Therapists are unable to like everybody, and in the presence of even a mild degree of dislike, anxiety and defensiveness will soon paralyse any form of self-expression, while in the presence of mutual dislike, therapy will soon come to an end. The paradox is that those with the most disabling disorders who are in the greatest need of change are usually quite unlikeable. They alienate their relatives, employers, co-workers and, however well-meaning or well-trained, their therapists as well.

For those at the milder end of the spectrum with more likeable characteristics, psychotherapy serves as a useful catalyst for change; for those with severe disorders who are grossly unlikeable, therapy rarely takes off at all. If they have entered therapy (which is usually at someone else's request) they soon quit. To some extent, likeability is also socially determined, thus the private therapist will soon come to dislike the patient who skips a few sessions and fails to pay his bills. By contrast, therapists working in a forensic setting would hardly be troubled by such behaviour and might find they are able to "click" quite well with certain "likeable rogues". Even so, there are some severely dystonic individuals with, for example, sadistic or sociopathic personalities who are so grossly contemptuous of almost all other people (including therapists) that they would not be amenable to this form of treatment.

A final point concerns the qualities of the therapist. Just as there are some doctors who dislike almost any psychiatric patient, there are some psychiatrists who dislike or cannot effectively cope with these most taxing and devious individuals. Gunderson (1984) suggested that psychotherapists who treat BPD subjects should have qualities that include "a comfort with aggression, sensitivity to separation experience, a sense of adventurousness and clarity of conceptual organisation". Supervision is essential for novices, and often helpful even for those with experience. Working in a unit that specialises in the treatment of the personality disorders may be helpful in familiarising trainees with the more common problems as well as acquiring some basic skills. However, the more intensive and longer-term therapies are perhaps best left to those who are temperamentally suited to such work.

Eccentric disorders

Schizotypal personality disorder is characterised by eccentric ideas, and the area of concern for the therapist includes the cognitive distortions. Rapport is often difficult to establish, and few subjects will be able to tolerate or understand a classical transference-based type of interpretation. It is best for the main thrust of the therapy to focus around candid discussions of practical everyday or real issues. This should be done in conventional, simple language, discouraging strange speech on the part of the patient, with the therapist also taking care to avoid jargon. The therapist should try to help the patient to remain in tune with others at work or at home, rather than be solely at the mercy of his strange ideas. In this function the therapist will serve almost as an "auxiliary ego" and has a psycho-educative role in teaching the patient how the world works. Schizotypal personalities are often poor at applying what is learned in one situation to new situations; repeated gentle challenges to their cognitive distortions over a lengthy period may sometimes be required.

Schizoid patients seldom come spontaneously for treatment and psychotherapy has little effect because motivation is so poor. They keep their distance and are content to live that way. Group therapy occasionally offers some form of contact because they learn that they are not alone in harbouring strange ideas, and may find it easier to relate to peers rather than an authority figure.

Paranoid personalities

Patients with paranoid personalities require extraordinarily deft handling, particularly during the early phases of therapy when only the paranoia is manifest. Outwardly paranoid subjects may be sure and self-confident although at the same time dogmatic and suspicious, but inwardly they are generally insecure, fearing a sleight at every turn. Beneath the surface there may be extreme degrees of jealousy; sometimes even classical morbid jealousy may be present. Confronting or even asking questions about their distorted views of the world may be interpreted as an attack.

Rapport is often difficult to establish in the first place. A paranoid patient might say at the first meeting, "I don't know if I can trust you, doctor, you are a man, and my father was a man, and he beat the living daylights out of me and put me down. I just don't trust men." To become defensive, or even reassuring, or throw the question back, or seek more information about the patient's distressing circumstance, would probably only serve to heighten tension. Far better to accept some truth in the patient's assertion and reply "How could you possibly trust me? You have only just met me. You have no way of knowing whether all those diplomas on the wall are really mine or whether I am genuine or a charlatan. If I were in your shoes I would tread very carefully as well."

Such a reply conveys an understanding of what it must be like to be that person and see the world through the patient's eyes. If the doctor really was a charlatan he would be unlikely to be so candid. Such a high degree of open honesty may go some way to mitigating the patient's suspiciousness.

Once treatment has been established and trust has developed, the paranoid patient can be seen to be struggling with intense feelings of rejection, humiliation and impotence. Therapy will soon lead into a world of earlier conflicts where there are feelings of humiliation, of being put down or subjected to withering criticism, often by the same sex parent (Frosch, 1983). Older Freudian notions that the paranoid feelings represent repressed homosexuality are now largely discounted, as it is recognised that most subjects have a heterosexual orientation, and the high frequency of sexual jealousy tends to confirm this. However, paranoid personalities are extremely touchy about the idea of homosexuality, possibly because this has become a symbol for not being able to perform adequately with a partner, and the idea is associated with a more widespread sense of failure and impotence. Empathic, rather than confrontational, interventions that accept the patient's position appear to be most helpful.

Dramatic disorders

Patients in the dramatic cluster present with obvious distress or attention-seeking behaviour that, by implication, almost demands therapeutic intervention. Similar psychotherapeutic principles govern the treatment of these disorders, and fundamental to them is Kernberg's (1967) concept of borderline personality organisation. An organisation, or pathological organisation, refers to the relative structures of impulses, anxieties and defences. Its purpose is to protect the individual from the chaos of earlier developmental stages. It is therefore a somewhat rigid structure that has the disadvantage of depriving the individual of more advanced modes of functioning (Higgit & Fonagy, 1993). Kernberg's borderline personality organisation consists of four elements:

(1) ego weakness, which includes a poor ability to tolerate anxiety, control impulses, or develop socially acceptable ways that can channel energy;
(2) a tendency to shift towards irrational dream-like thinking patterns in the context of generally intact reality testing (there is no psychosis);
(3) the dominance of developmentally less mature psychological defences, such as splitting, projection and projective identification;
(4) identity diffusion, so that mental representations of important other people are fragmented or strongly charged as either good or bad.

This formulation has been very influential in the psychoanalytic literature on personality disorder, and is thought to be common to borderline, narcissistic, histrionic and "as if" personalities, and to a certain extent also the antisocial disorders. It may be present in up to 10% of the population, but does not represent a clinical psychiatric disorder.

Therapeutic techniques

Acting as a container

Borderline subjects lead a chaotic existance and are prey to intolerable affects. Kohut (1971) used the term "disintegrative anxiety", while Bion

(1959) wrote of a "nameless dread". The phrase a "holding environment" is attributed to Winnicott (1965). It is a description of the mother's primary and almost exclusive concern for her infant's welfare. During analysis, "holding" refers to the therapist's ability to create a milieu in which many different powerful affects can be both experienced and explored in safety. Winnicott believed that the quality of reliability was at least as important as the therapist's interpretation in these cases. Bion also used the term "container", which Gunderson (1984) specifically applied to borderline subjects and suggested that the therapist should serve as a container for all the patient's powerful affects. Sometimes patients need a bigger and stronger container than a single therapist, and in these cases admission to hospital may be invaluable.

Limit-setting

Limit-setting techniques will usually be necessary for almost every borderline patient, particularly at the beginning of treatment. Firmness will be needed concerning the timing and duration of sessions, and any conditions which warrant an extra session. Sometimes written contracts help to convey the notion that the therapist is neither omnipotent nor able to cope with every chaotic or deviant action in which the patient indulges. The express delineation of what is, and what is not, acceptable during therapy helps to place at least some responsibility on the patient. It should be noted that therapists working in a one-to-one out-patient setting have little power to set limits, and are only really able to rely on their own persuasiveness. Among out-patients with suicidal tendencies, a contract may sometimes stipulate that the patient is to telephone the doctor or report to a casualty department rather than act directly on any impulses. If a contract results in a delay in impulsive gratification, it has been helpful. A manoeuvre that prevents acting-out is of value because it brings to the surface the complex underlying emotions, which can then be scrutinised. Unfortunately, many patients are unable to stop acting-out by merely promising not to do so.

For those with severe dyscontrol, admission is often required. Therapeutic contracts for in-patients should be written with caution. A common error is to stipulate discharge (which may be unsafe) if the patient breaks the contract. Adler (1977) wrote of the need for empathic, non-confrontational limit-setting in the hospital situation. A rejecting response is commonly found among hospital staff, representing no more than a manifestation of hate in the counter-transference. The more obvious confrontational elements in contracts should be removed and a more gentle terminology applied. Adler wrote that limit-setting is "a way of defining how staff and patients can work together".

Splitting and its management

One of the key features of patients with a borderline personality is to view everything somewhat unrealistically in black and white terms of good and bad. Ambivalent feelings towards themselves or other people are avoided at all costs. Beneath this avoidance is a deep fear that if good and bad feelings are brought together, the bad feelings will inevitably overwhelm and destroy the good feelings and annihilate any sense of loving or being loved. Defences such as projection, externalisation and splitting are kept in operation to enforce rigid compartmentalisation. An important aim for therapy is to help to resolve the defensive need for splitting, which is characterised by persistent division within the mind of impressions about self and others into extreme opposites of 'good' and 'bad'. This is mainly accomplished through interpreting the transference and the "holding" function of the therapist, allowing a patient gradually to explore new ways of relating to others. In a hospital, a borderline patient has more than one individual caring for them and may find it easier to find good and bad objects, and so externalise the splitting within themselves. They usually make determined attempts to split or polarise by constantly attacking the links between others, and in doing so tend to create disharmony among those who care for them.

Kernberg (1975) described the need to help patients to knit back together the various split images of the self. One way of doing this is to read back to the patient the many contradictory statements made in therapy concerning their key interpersonal relationships. A patient may begin by describing her mother as "perfect and saintly", but in a later session speak of some earlier memory of the mother having whipped her mercilessly for some childhood trifle. Discrepancies of this sort give the therapist a chance to suggest "Well, isn't it possible that your mother is a more complex figure than you make her out to be . . . that she could shift between kindness and cruelty?"

Similarly, the self-image may be equally unintegrated. A borderline patient who has been a victim of incest may, because of the early overstimulation, later become promiscuous. At one moment she may see herself as an innocent victim and at another as a whore, and therefore alternates between self-pitying and self-loathing. An important facet of therapy is to help patients to achieve a more unified and realistic picture of their personal world.

Aggression and hostile feelings

Kernberg (1967) believed that the primary problem of borderline patients is their innate aggression (which may have a constitutional basis). This results in distortions of the mental picture of the self and others. A similar view is expressed by Kleinian analysts who also believe that the seeds of later human psychopathology arise from innate destructiveness. During treatment, hostility towards the therapist will sooner or later appear in the form of some abuse of the therapeutic situation. This may be mild, such as being late or missing sessions, or more severe in the direct expression of criticism and hostility or by acting-out. These negative transference reactions should be interpreted early on in therapy, and, if necessary, repeatedly in a neutral and non-critical atmosphere. Failure to bring the issue of aggression to the fore, or being either too supportive or overly critical, would foster the feeling in the patient that the therapist cannot cope with the patient's main problem – aggression and hostility. By withstanding the patient's repeated onslaughts, the therapist gradually enables the patient to become less fearful of his destructive impulses, and a degree of integration to the personality becomes possible (Higgit & Fonagy, 1992).

Kohut (1971) provided a contrasting causal model and method for treating BDP. In his view, the disorder arises as a consequence of insufficient parental attention and lack of empathy, which results in an inadequately developed sense of the self. In essence, this is a deficiency theory that results in "developmental arrest". Anger is the result of narcissistic injury and deprivation, rather than due to innate aggression. In Kohut's scheme, the therapist's role is to provide a soothing or mirroring function that gradually leads to a restoration of the self.

A useful example of how the two different approaches might operate in practice is given by Horowitz (1987). During a session, a patient complains bitterly of feeling severe loneliness at the weekend. Kernberg's approach relies on a direct confrontation of the patient's negative transference feelings, and a classic drive/defence transference interpretation might be "You are angry with me and perceive me as cold and uncaring since I was not available for you at the weekend. You would like me to be available at all times and without limitation." Explicitly or implicitly, the therapist tells the patient that his wishes or drives are both unrealistic and insatiable.

A Kohutian interpretation of this common therapeutic situation might be "You are angry at me for not being available during the weekend, when you were feeling alone, and this is quite understandable in terms of your early experience of your mother rarely being around when you needed her". The latter interpretation emphasises *empathic understanding* of an insatiable emotional wish, instead of focusing upon the wish *per se*. In both approaches the ultimate aim is to help the patient to tame the wish, which is clearly unreasonable. In the classical model, the drive will eventually be tamed by the patient's increasing awareness of the negative consequences of his reactions. In the Kohutian model, the benign parental imago comforts, soothes and supports, so that it ultimately becomes internalised. In practice, which approach is selected will be determined mainly by the characteristics of the patient. Some sensitive or paranoid individuals might find even the second empathic type of interpretation overly critical, while for others the more direct approach might be more appropriate.

Vengeance, manipulation and self-mutilation

Many of the difficulties that BPD patients experience or impose on others stem from the poor modulation of their affects; they overreact, behave impulsively or unreasonably, and coerce by suicidal threats or other forms of blackmail. Kernberg (1975) suggested that suicidal behaviour in BPD subjects often coincides with intense attacks of rage on the object.

Brobyn *et al* (1987) described a severe borderline patient who as a child had been beaten for many years by her father. One day she was found with a knife under her sleeve waiting for her father to come home. When asked whether she intended to kill her father, she replied "God, no, I was going to kill myself in front of him". The only overt manifestation of the patient's vengeful impulses is the wish to punish her father by making him watch her death, and her own murderous impulses are at least overtly denied. Ego boundaries are broken down; he is she, (she will be killed instead of him) and she is he (the perpetrator of the violence). Such a degree of fusion of this type may assume a terrifying and destructive quality (Giovacchini, 1982).

A common situation occurs when a relationship ends, and a borderline patient cuts her wrists with the intention of coercing her partner back into the relationship, or at the very least provoking guilt feelings. The vengeful element in these situations is usually obvious. Sometimes during treatment, as the therapeutic relationship deepens, an episode of self-mutilation or other acting-out may occur as a means of expressing guilt or fear of the growing closeness, and this signifies a negative therapeutic reaction. Following episodes of self-mutilation there is sometimes (but not always) a feeling of well-being. The patient has a sense of triumph at her victory over pain and death, while family and therapists are reduced to a state of bewildering impotence.

Although innate aggression was once thought to be the main cause of such behaviour, recent studies have suggested that parental abuse of various types in childhood may be a more important factor. These aggressive and manipulative behaviours should, as Gunderson & Szabo (1993) point out, be understood in the light of adaptations made in response to past traumas and be interpreted as "unfortunate survival techniques" that result from mistreatment. In the case mentioned above (Brobyn *et al*, 1987), the patient's mother had discovered that suicidal threats seemed to diminish the harshness of the beatings the father meted out to the children. Not surprisingly, her daughter learnt to use suicidal threats when dealing with her father and later authority figures. Much of the aggressiveness and manipulativeness found among borderline subjects amounts to vengefulness directed at the parents or other key figures. The therapist's task is to help the patient slowly to unravel the pattern, and see the uselessness and ultimate self-destructiveness of vengefulness, for example, in demolishing current ongoing relationships.

Dealing with vengeance

Among subjects who have experienced severe maltreatment by a parent, later relationships may be clouded by high levels of vengeance and a tendency to go to extremes. Pain-seeking behaviour becomes the norm, showing itself as some point on the spectrum of sadomasochism. At the extreme masochistic end are individuals who mutilate themselves, or select partners who inflict physical or psychological pain and so earn their title of 'martyr'. At the other extreme are individuals who are pure sadists, who rarely present themselves for treatment but are determined to inflict as much or more suffering than they received when young. Pure types are uncommon, and most borderline patients will oscillate wildly between adoration of their partners followed by threats to self-mutilate, or walk out in the face of some minor unpleasantness. In their behaviour they alternate between being kind and compassionate, and being cruel and humiliating like the abusing parent. Once therapists become aware that a patient is locked into a cycle of this sort, any initial sympathy and compassion may rapidly wane. The therapist will need to alternate between compassion and firmness, with the ultimate therapeutic goal of trying to help the patient to see the futility of wreaking vengeance.

In cases when the partner appears normal, well-meaning and not cruel, the patient needs to be taught *not* to overreact to minor problems in the relationship; not to react impulsively or spitefully; and above all not to treat the partner as a whipping boy or transference symbol of a cruel or sexually molesting parent. In other patients where the current relationship appears to be a re-enactment of the previous childhood trauma, it may be best to try to support the subjects in their efforts to leave the relationship. While some patients are able to use the therapists' interpretations and attempts to link the present sadomasochistic pattern to the previous traumatisation, it should be remembered that subjects with borderline personalities are less adaptive in handling their childhood abuse than many others who may have been equally abused.

A particular difficulty arises among those with a pronounced sadistic streak. Here almost any intervention (but most of all remarking on the patient's own unkind or cruel behaviour) is interpreted as a 'put down'. The patient might turn vengefully on the therapist and say "you hate me" or "you think I'm a bad person". An interpretation which offers some explanation might be tried, such as: "Look, when you locked yourself in the bathroom and cut your wrist with the razor, after your husband said he did not want to go to the movies, your reaction may have been a bit extreme for that situation, and besides, you weren't getting back at him so much as at your father." This might restore some calm, but among patients who are severely vengeful, sadistic or hypersensitive, such a remark may be taken as criticism and these patients often quit therapy.

In subjects who experienced real parental maltreatment, the therapist will often feel compassion for what the patient suffered, enabling him to empathise with the patient and then gently help to pry the patient loose from the maladaptive vengeance-motivated behaviour patterns. If there was no real mistreatment, and where the patient misperceived the parents as bad owing to his irritability and inordinate demands, the therapist's task will be to help the patient to develop a more realistic picture concerning the patient's own irritability and the effect this may have had on the parents.

Counselling for borderline personalities who were sexually abused

Many borderline patients report sexual molestation by persons within or outside the family, and have valid histories of traumatic backgrounds including incest, physical or other types of abuse. Even witnessing cruelty or physical abuse being meted out to a sibling or a parent may have a traumatising effect. Flashbacks , nightmares, episodes of panic or intense anxiety, irritability, and other manifestations of post-traumatic stress disorder are commonly found among BPD patients who are admitted to hospital (Putnam & Trickett, 1993). There is evidence that women who were traumatised, particularly under the age of 14, tend to resort to self-mutilation, substance misuse, suicidal gestures or acts in the context of interpersonal stress, and it is their life-threatening behaviour that results in hospitalisation. An example highlighting possible therapeutic interventions is described below.

> *Case example*
> A woman of 28, married with two small children, was in twice-weekly therapy because of depression, irritability and tendencies to mutilate herself and strike out at her children. Due to her irritability, the husband's parents had temporarily taken over the care of the children. Overdoses and episodes of self-mutilation had resulted in four brief admissions to hospital over the previous year.
> She had married at the age of 17 in order to escape an abusive home. Between the ages of 8 and 11 she was fondled genitally and sometimes penetrated by her father. At the age of 12 she was molested by a stranger who poked an object into her vagina. Her mother was both hypercritical and physically abusive, often punching her in the face and occasionally causing nosebleeds for trivial or non-existent offences. At age 11 her alcoholic father abandoned the family, leading her mother to make a suicide attempt requiring hospitalisation. Three years later the father returned and resumed fondling her. At age 15 she began abusing alcohol and cutting her wrists.
> The relationship with her husband, a pathologically jealous man, was sadomasochistic, alternating between his cursing her for her alleged infidelities and then making up by having sex three or four times a day. The only time she felt calm was during sex; immediately afterwards she would cry copiously "not wanting the good feeling to end", and descending once more into depression. Her husband was extremely jealous and intolerant of her telephoning or meeting her female friends. Her social life became increasingly constricted so that she felt like a "caged animal".
> A variety of drug treatments produced little benefit, and in recent months a problem had arisen in therapy in that she noticed herself

becoming inordinately attracted to her psychiatrist. She idolised him as the only consistently kind person in her life, could not bear to leave the sessions, and became disconsolate on the days between them. This, combined with her perception that her life seemed to be spiralling downwards, led her to seek a consultation with another psychiatrist who adopted a more multifaceted approach to treatment and made the following recommendations:

(1) As the marriage was vital to the patient's well-being (psychologically as well as economically), joint marital therapy was given the highest priority. Within a few months there was an improvement in the husband's ability to control his temper, he became more compassionate towards his wife's difficulties and needs, and was able to "loosen up" on his exaggerated need to control her every movement. This helped to lessen her sense of desperation and the feeling that the only safe person in her environment was her doctor.

(2) A different psychopharmacological regime, including fluoxetine (60 mg daily) and sodium valproate, helped to reduce her impulsivity, and a small dose of pimozide helped to decrease the erotomanic preoccupation with the first therapist.

(3) With the second therapist the patient was eager to "get it all out" by exposing and reliving the earlier scenes of sexual abuse, as if she was in a hurry to put her illness behind her. Previously she had revealed almost nothing of her traumatic past during the sessions. The second therapist encouraged her to pursue a middle course, and to reveal and recount the old experiences of trauma, but at a pace that was compatible with her need to stay out of hospital and remain with her family. Too rapid an immersion in the old trauma might prove too overwhelming and lead to a recrudescence of her self-destructive behaviour.

It was also important for her to work through her intense feelings of love and adoration towards the therapist, but this needed to be done at a similar slow pace. The twice-weekly regime seemed appropriate: a week's absence was too long and could not be tolerated, while increasing the frequency beyond twice-weekly might overstimulate feelings that were already too intense and result in a kind of transference drowning.

In this case the correct dynamic interpretations alone would not have sufficed unless something was done to change the husband's abusive and over-controlling behaviour, hence the need for marital therapy. To some extent even this represented her own psychopathology, as the husband was provoked into behaviour which duplicated the trauma of the past, and this constellation is not uncommon among subjects with borderline personality disorder (Van Der Kolk, 1989). Medication may also be helpful (but not always) in controlling impulsive behaviour (see 'Drug treatments', below).

Poor self-esteem

Damage to self-esteem in borderline subjects is generally profound as a consequence of repeated childhood trauma, and interpretative work is usually insufficient. The patients' social, intimate and occupational lives, besides being meagre, are usually well below what might have been expected under more favourable circumstances. This impoverishment serves as a perpetual proof of their "worthlessness" and both corroborates and perpetuates their low self-esteem. They therefore need to see themselves function on a higher plane in at least one major sphere of activity. In the above case, couple therapy led to an improvement in the marriage, which helped to negate the global feelings of worthlessness, but any suitable intervention such as occupational therapy or vocational counselling that improves functioning may be equally helpful. Attending a day hospital, or a group such as Alcoholics Anonymous may be useful in raising self-esteem. Also, any social or pharmacological measure that helps to decrease impulsivity will also tend to improve self-esteem, because without adequate self-control, self-esteem will inevitably remain low, leaving the patient vulnerable to depression and other dysfunctional behaviours.

Subjects who have experienced sexual abuse as children may display a range of abnormal sexual behaviour in adulthood. Some become prematurely erotised and have heightened sexual cravings, in the sense that they focus on sex as an antidote for all their tensions, whether sexual or not, such as feelings of loneliness, marital conflict or anxiety. Others who become hypererotised may later became promiscuous. But in some cases, revulsion towards the victimising relation outweighs both the love (as towards a father or older brother) and any physical pleasure that may have accompanied the incest. In these instances there may be a total rejection of sex throughout adult life, sometimes expressed as a preference for homosexual attachments. This is because an incestuous relationship results in heightened ambivalence, at first towards the original offender, and then to later sexual partners.

Ambivalent sadomasochistic relationships are characteristic during adult life (Stone, 1988) unless therapy succeeds in interrupting the pattern. There may be an endless succession of ugly scenes and fights followed by passionate reconciliations. In later life, as the passion declines, there may be rather less in the way of passion and reconciliation, with only a chronic abusive relationship remaining.

Loneliness and fears of abandonment

Earlier commentators on borderline conditions (Masterson, 1981; Rinsley, 1982) put much weight on the theme of fears of abandonment as the central issue in borderline patients. More recent findings have stressed the importance of sexual and physical abuse as causative factors, and simple separations in non-distressing circumstances do not appear to be causal. Still, fears of being alone or being abandoned are commonplace among borderline subjects, even if there were no unusual separations in childhood. Innate factors, such as separation anxieties, may contribute in some cases. In others, parental seductiveness or overdependency upon a particular child may in turn produce excessive dependency on the parent, and thus rob the child of experiences such as the development of hobbies, or having a wide circle of childhood friends that would help to build self-sufficiency. The task of the psychotherapist is to work out with the patient the probable causes of the inability to be alone. Even so, knowing the relevant psychodynamics will rarely remedy the problem, because the patient is now *in the habit* of being unable to handle separations with ease. Up to a point, the presence of the therapist is helpful, with the possibility of telephone access. However, eventually some sort of behavioural intervention is required, such as encouraging hobbies or other interests, as well as a gradual weaning from the supportive presence of the therapist.

Narcissistic personality disorder

Narcissistic personalities are preoccupied with being a success, whether famous, beautiful or wealthy. They have a sense of entitlement, and are contemptuous of others or display envy. Narcissistic traits are commonly found in other personality disorders, particularly the borderline and antisocial types. Sometimes the narcissistic character arises from being spoiled or drowned in empty praise as a child. These subjects rarely present themselves for treatment, or if they do only remain in therapy for a very brief period. More commonly there is a diet of parental neglect and humiliation, and here the grandiosity is no more than a compensatory mechanism for obscuring thinly veiled feelings of worthlessness, unattractiveness, low self-esteem and unloveability. These patients alienate others through their sarcasm and disdain, or sometimes even through jealousy and clingingness, but these distortions should be viewed as desperate measures of the inferior yet "true self".

Only the latter group are prepared to engage in therapy, which aims at the delineation of these mechanisms and the enhancement of self-esteem in a genuine way, by the achievement of success through work or through the patient's own efforts, rather than through entitlement. In relationships, narcissistic personalities should be encouraged to make durable friendships by being more compassionate and less contemptuous of others. If they reach this more mature state, with improved relationships, the older pathological narcissistic defences can be dropped. Some of these patients are so hypersensitive they may only be able to recognise trust in the form of positive feedback. This does not necessarily help them, because it tends to evoke the original trauma and resultant anger at not being valued for themselves (Patrick, 1985). Narcissistic personalities are not as decompensated as borderline personalities, and so limit-setting, or providing a holding environment, need not apply unless borderline features are also present.

As for *envy*, one of the most corrosive of human emotions, psychodynamic exploration of its childhood antecedents is often ineffective. However, greater success in life may be helpful for the subject, rendering it inoperative, although it does not eradicate the tendency.

> *Case example*
> A narcissistic young surgeon complained to his therapist that no one appreciated his brilliant operating skills, and he was contemptuous of his boss, an idiot who only promoted other ignorant doctors. During therapy he was encouraged to distinguish himself, and in due course discovered a small modification for a thyroid operation. He wrote papers and gave lectures on the subject, and was then invited to become the senior man at another hospital – and became the envy of others.

Histrionic disorders

The DMS–IV concept of histrionic personality disorders encompasses some patients at the milder end of the spectrum of what was previously known as hysterical personality disorder, as well as those who lie at the more severe end of the spectrum who also manifest narcissistic and borderline features. A short-lived exaggeration of previous histrionic traits can sometimes occur in depression, in which case standard antidepressive treatment may be helpful.

In the milder hysterical personalities, there is intense repression that serves as a defence against hidden sexual striving, usually relating to an incestuous relationship, and this is accompanied by a tendency to sexualise other non-sexual relationships, such as the doctor–patient relationship. Patients often act out conflicts, and there is greater reliance on fantasy than on logic and reality. Here the aim of psychotherapy is the lifting of an abnormal inhibition. Classical psychoanalysis or psychoanalytically oriented psychotherapy, with free association and dream analysis, was originally devised for this group. Therapy is directed at undoing the repression and exposing the hidden sexual strivings. These usually focus on incestuous choices, for example, the daughter who wished for her father in the absence of any actual experiences with the taboo object. Resolution of the oedipal conflict leads to a better integration of sexuality into the fabric of the personality, with less need to seek those with an "aura of forbiddenness" or unsuitable sexual partners, and eventually there is a more appropriate selection of partners. Therapy in these cases involves eliminating repression and fostering a more normal sexuality.

Among the more severely affected, disinhibition rather than repression or inhibition is the main problem. These patients, who manifest repeated and strident demands for praise and attention, have overlapping narcissistic and borderline features and they function at a more infantile or borderline level (Kernberg, 1967). Among borderline in-patients with prominent histrionic traits, a history of incest or molestation is common (Stone, 1989; Zanarini & Gunderson, 1990). Non-molested hysterical personalities need to realise that, while potential sexual partners may symbolise one or other parent, they are not really forbidden. Those who have suffered molestation need to learn during therapy that not all partners are as exploitative and unworthy as the individuals who once misused them.

In all instances, the origins of the hysterical and dramatic behaviour need to be sympathetically explored, but at the same time the therapist should help to educate or train the patient to overcome these maladaptive tendencies. Instead of encouraging profuse apologies for being late, punctuality should be encouraged; rather than agree that the bank manager is avaricious and demanding, the patient should be encouraged to adopt a more disciplined approach to personal finances. The patient should learn to rely less on emotional appeal, and more on a rational solution, and so become less childlike and dependent and more self-sufficient.

Hospitalisation for borderline patients

> This syndrome is difficult to treat and tends to create massive problems of management. (Main, 1957)

Main (1957) treated 12 borderline subjects in a psychoanalytically-oriented in-patient unit, and some years later interviewed the nursing staff involved who recounted how deeply distressed, almost to the point of illness, they had become while caring for these patients. Borderline subjects are often admitted to hospital, usually for treatment of an associated axis I disorder. There are two areas of concern for this group: regression and splitting. A few patients seem to worsen after admission, with more frequent episodes of self-mutilation, and this apparently retrograde step is termed regression. Some therapists, while not condoning the deviant behaviour, view the regressed state as providing a greater opportunity for therapy and for inducing changes.

The hospital milieu may be an ideal place for mapping out the various elements in the patient's "splitting" since the different members of staff may each be the recipient of a different attitude or behaviour from the patient. The feared therapist, the adored head nurse, the despised ward clerk, and so on, may each answer to an abusive father, a fondly loved mother, and an irritating older sister. In other cases the splitting may repesent one ambivalently regarded parent, who at different times inspired all these contradictory feelings. By meeting frequently, the staff can build a more integrated picture of the patient, so that those who interact directly with the patient, especially the therapist, can now help the patient to knit together these compartmentalised patterns into a more unified and adaptive personality.

Among more severe cases the splitting may assume a more destructive quality, and with it the tendency characteristic of borderline patients to divide hospital staff, play one off against another, extract special favours, and convert staff into friends or even lovers: in short, to *actualise transference themes* rather than to think about them. These patients try to manipulate the environment rather than conform to it. As a counterforce to these antitherapeutic tendencies, it is best if staff maintain a united front, share a common philosophy about the optimal treatment plan, and communicate frequently in ward rounds, supervision and team meetings. Once decisions are made, staff should support one another and resist any temptation to cross professional boundaries or become overfamiliar with the patient, even in the face of intense pressure or subtle seductive behaviour on the part of the patient.

Borderline patients will often provoke crises. The therapist and the hospital staff will have to become flexible in "rolling with the punches", shifting seamlessly from one type of intervention to another in accordance with the needs of the moment. No matter what the therapist's major orientation, a healthy degree of pragmatism is essential.

A second controversial area relates to the duration of stay: whether it should be brief or prolonged. Because of the dangers of regression, and the requirement for most general psychiatric units to care for psychotic patients who may be even more regressed, most psychiatric units will only tolerate the briefest possible stay for borderline subjects. These brief admissions may be helpful, and Kernberg (1984) provided three indications: (1) brief psychotic episodes; (2) suicidal concerns; and (3) clarification of diagnosis, mainly the exclusion of major functional psychosis, particularly if the patient is unknown to the treatment unit.

Longer-term hospitalisation may also be helpful, but with the current reduction in hospital beds this is becoming a less viable proposition. Kernberg (1984) suggested that long-term hospitalisation is indicated when the patient has: (1) low motivation; (2) poor object relations; or (3) severe ego weakness with a poor tolerance of anxiety and decreased impulse control. Fenton & McGlashan (1990) add a further group: chronically suicidal adolescents and young adults who come from destructive homes. Discharge for such patients might involve the return to a home where abuse would continue with more despair and suicidal attempts, and in these instances the hospital serves as an asylum.

In hospital, borderline patients tend to be envious of others who function at a higher level, but often disparage or may even be cruel to other patients, such as those with schizophrenia who function at a lower level, indicating the merit in segregating borderline patients in specialised units. These have the advantage that staff become more experienced at managing acting-out behaviours, and can be both sympathetic yet firm in the face of manipulative behaviour, rather than only rejecting. Specialised facilities function as therapeutic communities, with a treatment programme consisting of individual therapy, ward groups and active participation by patients in the life of the unit (Jackson & Pines, 1986; Fenton & McGlashan, 1990).

Anxious disorders

Patients in the anxious cluster struggle with inhibitions against normal assertiveness and enjoyment to which they would be entitled. They retreat from what belongs to them, in contrast to those in the dramatic cluster who reach out for what does not belong to them. Rather than place external limits, treatment should focus on the removal of internal limits or inhibitions that impair normal interactions. The patients are dominated by fear, such as sexual fears, social fears, or fears of voicing an opinion. DSM–IV includes obsessive–compulsive, dependent and avoidant personalities in this group, but some of the other non-official categories such as passive aggressive, masochistic, self defeating, the "as if" personality and depressive personality types show similar inhibitions and require a similar approach. The typical background features, inner scripts and coping strategies of these patients are shown in Table 19.2.

Many of these individuals are well-integrated and function at much higher levels than borderline subjects, and will respond to out-patient treatment. Techniques differ little from those employed for individuals with neurotic disorders, and may include classical techniques such as free association and the analysis of dreams as well as psychodynamic psychotherapy. Occasionally, a few patients in the anxious cluster will only respond to 3–5 times weekly psychoanalysis focusing largely on dreams. This applies particularly to severe compulsive or passive aggressive men who are (1) remarkably out of touch with their emotions, or (2) grossly contemptuous of psychiatry and its treatment methods, but who may in spite of their scepticism accept evidence from more objective sources such as dreams.

Lowered self-esteem

Lowered self-esteem is common among subjects with personality disorders of any type. Even narcissistic personalities, beneath their facade of grandiosity, may be struggling with feelings of worthlessness, while among depressive personalities pessimism and low self-esteem are almost universal.

Low self-esteem in borderline patients may partly relate to their innate tendency to depression, but also to abuse and rejection by parents. Incest victims who become borderline often blame themselves for seducing their offending relative, who may have compounded the issue by calling the victim a "whore" or a "tramp" at the time of the incest.

Table 19.2 Personality disorders dominated by anxiety

	Background	Inner script	Strategy
Obsessive–compulsive	Undue parental concern with obedience	Respect is more important than love	Conform, be neat, perfect, logical and contained
Dependent	Parent was dependent or fostered dependency	I can't manage; others can take care of me	Be compliant, submissive; cling for dear life
Avoidant	Being shamed into feeling socially unacceptable	I'm no good; others are out to hurt me	Better safe than sorry
Passive aggressive	Being intruded on and bullied by parents	I have to get even in a way I don't get hurt	Procrastinate, frustrate, sabotage, do the minimum
Depressive	Disappointment, privation, loss, abuse, shaming	My life is tragic; pessimism is justified	If I cry, others might just come to my rescue
Masochistic	Love interspersed with undeserved punishment	Martyrs can sit at the right hand of God	If I suffer enough, I can buy a little love

Patients often cling to their low self-image, almost with the tenacity of a delusion, and it may be helpful to elucidate the dynamic reasons behind this. A beautiful woman who had been molested as a child may have an underlying fear of men's predatoriness, especially if she were to acknowledge her attractiveness, and because of this might feel safer to maintain she was ugly. An intelligent student who feared the envy of other children or his siblings during childhood, if he were to acknowledge his intelligence, sustains a belief that he is stupid, almost as a defence.

Unfortunately, unearthing the real reasons or providing appropriate interpretations concerning the dynamics underlying the low self-esteem rarely brings anything more than minor relief. Psychotherapy alone is unlikely to be sufficient, and the appropriate interpretations should be understood as just preliminary steps in a process that requires real life experience. The interpretations and the presence of the therapist serve to embolden the patient to test the world more forcefully. The intelligent student learns that a top-grade mark does not provoke a backlash of murderous envy, while the beautiful woman should learn that, in encounters with men, most are trustworthy and very few are carbon copies of the truly predatory and untrustworthy figures from earlier life. To acknowledge being attractive need not come at such a high price.

The curative process for lowered self-esteem is thus interactive, and similar to overcoming a phobia by behavioural means as suggested by Marks & Marks (1990). At this point a cognitive–behavioural intervention is often useful, and the therapist may try to urge the patient to take some small steps into the forbidden zone (e.g. by calling someone for a date, or trying for a non-stressful job). Anxieties that have hitherto remained dormant now rise to the surface and can be discussed and alleviated. The strength of the therapeutic bond serves to embolden the patient to test the reality of his fears. Eventually the need for the low self-image is diminished, and with that the self-esteem rises to a more realistic level.

In persons whose low self-esteem stemmed largely from withering criticism and rejection from parents, there is usually the additional problem of intense ambivalence toward the parent(s); the difficulty arises from the loyalty to the cruel parent, and from the pain involved in gradually realising that the parent was deeply at fault, perhaps even malicious. Patients often fight against the recognition of the truth, when their parents have actually been monstrous, because the parents were the only straw to which the patients could cling when they were small and helpless. Such patients prefer to blame themselves for being "bad", as though they deserved their maltreatment, since this may be the easier notion to entertain. Perhaps in this situation psychotherapy by itself can be effective in bringing about the necessary reversal of images; that the patient is not such a bad sort after all, and that the parents were pretty grim. The therapist, first hearing the accounts from the patient's childhood, and then offering a more realistic appraisal of how the offending (or rejecting) parent would be viewed by ordinary people, can in many instances overturn the patient's incorrect and self-damaging appraisals.

Countertransference

Pines (1978) described how the therapist finds himself being "dragged unwillingly but inevitably as if by a great force into the pattern imposed by the patient so that we begin to feel provoked, hostile, persecuted and to behave exactly as the patient needs us to, becoming rejecting, hostile". Borderline patients are extremely sensitive to dyadic relationships and may have an eerie understanding of the weaknesses of other people, so that it is almost inevitable that therapists develop stronger reactions to their borderline patients than to their other patients (Higgit & Fonagy, 1993). Lorand (1955) pointed out that the analyst must be constantly aware of his countertransference, whether the feelings are friendly or antagonistic, and there is a danger to treatment from unrecognised countertransference attitudes. In a famous paper concerning the treatment of antisocial personalities, Winnicott (1949) wrote, "The therapist must be so thoroughly aware of his counter-transference that he can sort out and study his projective reactions to the patient. These will include *hate.*"Common countertransference reactions to different personality disorders are shown in Table 19.3.

Provided the countertransference feelings can be understood they may serve as a useful tool in therapy.

Case example
Searles (1979) described how a young trainee presented a session with a female borderline subject in which the patient talked non-stop, extolling the virtues of her boyfriend, without letting the trainee get a word in edgeways. The young doctor was perplexed by the meaning of the session and Searles commented "Well, if I were in your shoes I'd feel mighty jealous – having to listen to her praise someone else while sitting there with me in the room. Maybe she wished to alert you to her own hidden struggle with the emotion of jealousy by causing you to experience that very emotion." In a later session and at an appropriate moment the trainee enquired whether jealousy played any role in the patient's life, and she described an unbearable jealousy of her older sister whom she felt had always been greatly favoured by her parents.

Therapists are usually nudged into making mistakes, and Dawson (1988) provided a comprehensive list of these errors. Therapists may become "all-knowing and all-understanding" and so apparently become the only competent one in the therapeutic dyad. In these situations, it may be better to admit ignorance or even a failure to understand. Therapeutic neutrality is easily dislodged by being over-emotional or responsive to affective displays by the patient. Sometimes therapists become the vehicle for the patient's intolerable self-critical part, and so are driven into the role of confronter and accuser; they then reject the patient completely and so repeat the patient's previous pattern. In the face of sexual seductiveness, therapists may defend themself by becoming harsh, rejecting or over-critical; but occasionally rescue fantasies may develop with romantic involvement, and these may be a serious hazard to therapists' own professional career. Rescue fantasies are a particular hazard for those dealing with young borderline patients in whom the "pathetic child victim" elicits strong parental feelings in the therapist, who may as a result try to usurp the real parents.

Sometimes a more neurotic countertransference occurs, with the patient coming to symbolise an important character for the therapist, such as a detested sibling or a former sweetheart. Unless these feelings are brought to light they may undermine psychotherapy altogether, because the therapist may become excessively fond of or needlessly dislike the patient. In these cases therapists should discuss the matter during supervision, or even return briefly to therapy themselves.

Table 19.3 Common countertransference reactions to personality types

Disorder	Countertransference reaction(s)
Schizoid	Boredom; lack of sympathy
Schizotypal	Disdain at the patient's "weirdness"
Paranoid	Fear at being menaced; impatience at the patient's misreading of social situations
Borderline	Feeling put-upon; aroused; overwhelmed; rescue fantasies
Narcissistic	Offence at patient's contempt or grandiosity
Antisocial	Contempt, fear, indignation, envy (at patient's "freedom" to do as he pleases)
Histrionic	Charmed, aroused; swamped by patient's emotionality
Obs.–compuls.	Boredom (at excessive, dry details)
Avoidant	Impatience, disdain (at patient's lack of courage)
Dependent	Annoyance (at the clinginess); powerful (at being needed)
Pass. aggr.	Annoyance, impatience (at the covert hostility)
Depressive	Impotence, despair (at being unable to help)
Hypomanic	Charm, envy, irked (at the overfamiliarity)
Irritable	Outrage
Masochistic	Impatience (at patient's continued bad choices)
Sadistic	Hatred, outrage, contempt, fear

Group therapy

Groups may sometimes have a civilising influence on individuals, but there are some patients with very severe degrees of narcissism or disruptive behaviour who cannot fit into a group. For patients who can tolerate group therapy, other group members are able to provide a form of reality orientation therapy, and so give useful insights into a patient's maladaptive traits. Sometimes this is highly effective and can be accomplished by the other group members in a language that a therapist could not afford to use in individual therapy. In a study of Yalom's therapeutic factors, altruism and self-understanding were most highly rated as being important by borderline subjects (Macaskill, 1982). Empathic interpretation by the therapist in connection with feelings of narcissistic injury were also found to be helpful. Provided there is some degree of cohesiveness, groups appear to have a comforting and containing role for the borderline individual without resulting in any damage to other members. However, one group composed exclusively of borderline subjects failed, as it plunged into emotional chaos and a degree of mutual destructiveness (Kutter, 1982). On the other hand, groups which specialise in dealing with patients with histories of incest and sexual molestation (common among BPD subjects) may be successful, as they help to decrease the sense of isolation and shame. Among BPD subjects with impulsive behaviours such as binge-eating, drinking and gambling, the group methods of the appropriate 'anonymous' group may be helpful. Higgit & Fonagy (1992) and others recommend that group therapy can be a useful addition to individual therapy, but in order to avoid splitting and countertransference difficulties, it is better for the same therapist to be involved in both group and individual treatments.

Other treatment approaches

Beck *et al* (1990) described a cognitive approach to the treatment of the personality disorders. Cognitive therapy relies on the inner scripts of patients (see Table 18.3), which are thought to underpin the abnormal behaviours, and certain traits appear to be amenable to a cognitive approach, particularly anger, dependency, lack of assertiveness, and low self-esteem.

Anger is a common and serious problem for patients with BPD and ASPD. The basis for the cognitive approach to management is identification of the triggers that provoke anger. Role-play and videotape feedback are used to assist the patient in the emotional recall of previous angry outbursts, and this is then used to help identify the most likely triggers. The significance of these triggers is explored and the therapist models a more appropriate response to such situations, usually in the form of a verbal expression of the underlying hostile feelings, or simply control of the anger. With practice the patient is taught to achieve better self-control.

For the trait of *dependency*, Trukatt & Carlson (1984) recommended a hierarchical exposure to situations that require the subject to make their own decisions. Because decision-making in dependent subjects may result in heightened anxiety, anxiety management techniques form an important component of the treatment. Patients with dependent, anxious, or passive aggressive personality disorders have difficulties in saying "no" to others, cannot set limits on the behaviour of other people, and are therefore readily exploited. In such cases, assertiveness training and teaching patients how to say "no" in specific situations may be helpful. This can be done using the standard techniques of role-play, modelling and videotape feedback.

Beard *et al* (1990) described a combined cognitive–analytic approach. In the first few sessions, the patient and therapist together write a description of the patient's history and this is linked to the patient's present maladaptive behaviour. Then the therapist asks the patient to monitor and record whenever they use such maladaptive mechanisms. The therapist introduces diagrams to help the patient to see how different frames of mind can lead to different behaviours. The patient is encouraged to recognise them, discuss them with the therapist, and in due course the maladaptive behaviours hopefully diminish. Many subjects (not only those with personality disorders) have difficulties in expressing their feelings verbally, but find it rather easier to describe their interpersonal problems with diagrams, which may form a useful starting point for therapy. Lansky (1988) described a more directly educational programme, even providing patients and their relatives with a tape which described the features and difficulties posed by "self-control disorder".

Social and prison programmes

Certain prisons specialise in the psychotherapeutic treatment of severely dissocial people, and have developed their own psychotherapeutic programmes based on the principles of a therapeutic community. Programmes vary widely and are usually specific to particular prisons, with a mixture of group and individual methods being used (Dolan & Coid, 1993). Group methods are more helpful in enabling subjects to see how destructive some of their behaviour can be, while individual therapy serves to increase an individual's capacity to experience a more normal range of affects, fantasies, and to develop trust. In some regimens there is hierarchical progress through the prison, with the possibility of early parole serving as an incentive for some inmates. The high security offered in prison means that these regimes are probably not applicable to ambulant patients or even those with ASPD in the hospital setting.

A novel approach to the treatment of young offenders in the US is the wilderness programmes, which include an 'outward-bound' type experience. In the first phase of these programmes the offenders are taught the elements of camping and techniques required for surviving in a wilderness. In the second phase, the offenders and counsellors spend two weeks in the wilderness together and during this period attempt to achieve a complex physical goal, such as climbing a mountain together. During the final phase, offenders are sent off on a wilderness trip on their own, with the counsellors being available but only at some distance. High success rates in terms of reduced recidivism are reported (Reid & Matthews, 1980), but the programme has not been attempted in the UK, possibly because of the distinct lack of wilderness.

It should be noted that the DSM–IV definition of antisocial personality disorder is largely based on behavioural disturbances, and there are many individuals, particularly those from a traumatic background, who are not necessarily amoral, and who with guidance or therapy may outgrow such tendencies. The same cannot be said for the psychopath as defined by Cleckley (1972) or by Hare's Psychopathic Check-List (Hare *et al*, 1990), because subjects with marked psychopathic traits are by definition contemptuous of authority, and this usually includes the psychiatric profession. Traits such as severe callousness or the absence of any sense of remorse or shame places the more extreme psychopathic cases beyond the realms of treatment. Hare (1993) commented on the untreatability of psychopaths: "The term implies that there is something to treat . . . but as far as we can determine psychopaths are perfectly happy with themselves and they see no need for treatment."

Drug treatments

The beneficial effects of medication in patients with a personality disorder are generally quite modest, and far less impressive than when the same drugs are given for treatment of affective disorder or schizophrenia. Drugs may be helpful in cases of behavioural dyscontrol, self-mutilation, suicidal behaviour and psychotic episodes, particularly during the more severe phases requiring hospital admission. Only borderline and schizotypal personality disorders show any benefit from medication. Except when there is an associated axis I disorder, the other categories, such as dissocial, narcissistic, schizoid, anankastic or avoidant types, generally do poorly with medication.

Neuroleptics

Soon after the introduction of chlorpromazine for treating schizophrenia, a few adventurous psychoanalysts in the US tried it with their more difficult borderline patients. The analysts observed decreased anxiety, improved reality testing, less frequent acting-out, and an increased ability to tolerate the therapeutic situation, and in some cases improved relationships as well (Winkleman, 1955; Kernberg, 1967). Brinkley *et al* (1979) reported on five treatment-resistant borderline patients who responded well to small doses of neuroleptics (perphenazine 10 mg, thioridazine 25 mg) while an open trial of low-dose pimozide (2 mg daily) demonstrated improvement in mental symptoms and behaviour among a group of subjects with DSM–III personality disorders, particularly if the drug was taken for three or more months (Collard, 1976).

Placebo-controlled trials have now established a more definite role for small doses of neuroleptic medication among subjects with BPD. In a group of in-patients and out-patients with BPD, SPD or both, haloperidol (7 mg daily) resulted in significant improvements in behavioural dyscontrol, psychoticism and paranoid ideation, as well as in many neurotic symptoms, especially anxiety, hostility and depression, and was significantly superior to both placebo and amitriptyline (Soloff *et al*, 1986*a*). In a community sample of subjects with BPD and SPD, thiothixene was shown to be superior to placebo for a variety of psychotic symptoms as well as for hostility, phobias, anxiety and obsessive–compulsive symptoms. There were only small drug/placebo differences for the symptoms of somatisation, depersonalisation, derealisation and suspiciousness. There were no drug/placebo differences for sensitivity to interpersonal rejection or depressive hostility, and so for these symptoms a psychotherapeutic approach may be more helpful (Goldberg *et al*, 1986).

A more recent trial by Soloff *et al* (1993) questioned many of the earlier findings. Using a rather lower dose of haloperidol (4 mg daily) among a group of mainly out-patients with BPD, there were few drug/placebo differences for most symptoms. Haloperidol was superior to placebo only for anger and depression, as well as for objective measures of behavioural dyscontrol. Possibly the drugs were less effective among out-patients because compliance was lower.

Suicidality (for example, by taking repeated overdoses) is common in BPD. Montgomery & Montgomery (1982) demonstrated that flupenthixol (20 mg fortnightly) was superior to placebo in diminishing the frequency of such behaviour, while in the same study, mianserin (30 mg daily) had no beneficial effect. Depot preparations may be a better way of achieving symptom control than oral preparations among subjects who are paranoid, irritable, prone to take overdoses or act out in other ways. Cowdrey & Gardner (1988) found that trifluoperazine (8 mg daily) also diminished suicidality, but many patients stopped this drug because of postural hypotension and extrapyramidal side-effects.

There are suggestions that small doses of neuroleptics, for example, trifluoperazine (2–4 mg daily) or thioridazine (25 mg daily), taken over a long period may be beneficial and may be compatible with psychotherapy, although most psychotherapists prefer to treat patients drug-free whenever this is possible. Subjects with personality disorders seem to benefit from much lower doses of antipsychotic medication than when the same drugs are used in schizophrenia. They are generally less tolerant of side-effects, and dose titration is a critical aspect of therapy. Apart from the well-known neuroleptic side-effects, a few patients become increasingly agitated, depersonalised, paranoid and even mildly psychotic on these drugs. This worsening has been called "behavioural toxicity" and is rare and unexplained, but may be due to a type of akathisia without motor effects, or an atropine-like psychosis. It generally resolves upon drug withdrawal (Steiner *et al*, 1979).

Antidepressants

Patients with personality disorders do not respond as well to standard antidepressant drugs as patients with uncomplicated depressions. In one of the earliest open trials of imipramine, Klein & Fink (1962) observed that subjects with histrionic and manipulative features did less well, while Kiloh *et al* (1962), in a discriminant function analysis, also confirmed that self-pity, irritability and hysterical features were associated with a poor response to imipramine. In a later study it was noted that young depressive patients with personality disorders did less well than patients with psychotic depression (Paykel, 1972). A large retrospective case note sample showed that 64% of subjects with pure depression responded well to tricyclics, but only 27% of those with both personality disorder and depression responded (Black *et al*, 1988). The response to monoamine oxidase inhibitors (MAOIs) is also worse among subjects who have depression and personality disorder; for example, 70% of a group of phenelzine non-responders were found to have a personality disorder (Shawcross & Tyrer, 1985).

Can antidepressants help the personality disorder itself? Clinicians often prescribe antidepressants to patients with personality disorders in the hope that alleviation of their misery will somehow result in an improvement in character. The only group to evaluate this notion systematically were Akiskal *et al* (1980), who prescribed antidepressants to patients with what they termed "characterological depressions", who had had mild depressive symptoms for more than five years, yet were not suffering from major depression. (Today many of these subjects would be diagnosed as having dysthymia, which is now classed as an affective disorder.) Approximately a third responded well to therapeutic doses (150–200 mg) of either desipramine or clomipramine. Responsiveness was associated with female sex, a previous history of major depression, hypersomnia and a mild degree of elation following tricyclic medication. Non-responders were more often male, had a history of substance abuse, and had a more unstable personality.

Although the tricyclics have been available for more than 35 years and have been prescribed to many patients with personality disorders, there is only one placebo-controlled study of a tricyclic (amitriptyline) in patients with BPD (Soloff *et al*, 1986*b*). Around half the subjects improved, but among the remainder there was a marked deterioration, with more impulsive behaviour and paranoid ideation, indicating that for some BPD subjects tricyclics could have paradoxical effects similar to those described for benzodiazepines (Soloff *et al*, 1986*b*).

Monoamine oxidase inhibitors (MAOIs)

Early studies suggested that MAOIs had beneficial effects in BPD. In a recent study, tranylcypromine was shown to be superior to placebo, alprazolam, carbamazepine and trifluoperazine for a variety of affective and behavioural symptoms in a group of BPD subjects (Cowdrey & Gardner, 1988). The only predictor of a positive response to tranylcypromine was a history of childhood hyperactivity. As a result it is unclear whether the beneficial effect of the MAOI was due to antidepressive effects or its psychostimulant properties. MAOIs are relatively contraindicated among those with the personality disorders because of risks associated with alcohol and overdose. The new generation of reversible MAOIs such as moclobemide lack the 'cheese effect' (are less likely to trigger hypertensive crises), and so their role as antidepressants in BPD merits further exploration.

Selective serotonin reuptake inhibitors (SSRIs)

Serotonergic dynfunction has been implicated in a number of key borderline symptoms, particularly depression, impulsivity and obsessive–compulsive phenomena. Three recent open trials have reported beneficial effects for fluoxetine in cases of BPD. Norden (1989) treated 12 patients with BPD with fluoxetine in doses of up to 40 mg daily, and rating scales showed 75% improvement, particularly for the symptoms of depression and impulsivity. In a group of 22 treatment-resistant patients who had been ill for an average of 18 years, most subjects improved with fluoxetine and there was a dramatic decrease in the rate of self-mutilation (Markovitz *et al*, 1991). Cornelius *et al* (1991) successfully treated five refractory BPD subjects with doses of 40–80 mg fluoxetine who had previously failed on phenelzine, neuroleptics and tricyclics. While these early reports on SSRIs appear promising, there is an urgent need for placebo-controlled trials before more specific recommendations can be made.

Lithium

In the US in the 1970s, studies on chronically assaultive prisoners showed a beneficial effect with lithium. Such studies would probably fail to obtain ethical approval today, and so are unlikely to be repeated. Tupin *et al* (1973), in an uncontrolled trial, showed a beneficial effect in 56% of 27 male convicts who had a pattern of easily triggered violence, but 11% became more aggressive. Among those who benefited, lithium levels tended to be at the upper end of the therapeutic range, and the drug appeared to induce a state of reflective delay. Sheard *et al* (1976) conducted a much larger placebo-controlled trial in a group of chronically assaultive prisoners with a variety of personality disorders. After three months the rate of serious assaults dropped to zero among the lithium-treated group, but remained unchanged in the group taking placebo. When the lithium was stopped, violent episodes escalated to their previous rate within one month.

A placebo-controlled study of lithium among a group of turbulent adolescent females with brief spontaneous mood swings of depression, anger, elation and over-talkativeness, showed a modest response to lithium (Rifkin *et al*, 1972). The long-term follow-up study of borderline subjects of Stone (1990) found a few cases (around 8%) who later developed bipolar II disorder, and these subjects did well on lithium. In general, most subjects with aggressive or borderline personality disorders do not respond to lithium, and selecting the few responders is rather like looking for a needle in a haystack. The presence of anger, affective features (particularly bipolar II disorder), a family history of affective disorder, alcoholism and a family history of alcoholism are all possible but unproven pointers. Some patients with "episodic dyscontrol syndromes" may also empirically respond to lithium. Among in-patients with serious problems of depression or aggression, a two-month trial of lithium may help clarify the issue. Lithium may also benefit around 70% of those with self-mutilation and learning difficulties (Wickham & Read, 1987).

Benzodiazepines

These drugs are generally contraindicated in patients with personality disorders. The first descriptions of benzodiazepine-induced rage reactions were among subjects with personality disorders (Tobin *et al*, 1960). A systematic evaluation of alprazolam in BPD found that episodes of self-mutilation were more frequent and more severe than when the same subjects took placebo (Cowdrey & Gardner, 1988). Although benzodiazepines are now the focus of many adverse reports, some earlier studies described benefits in certain specific situations; for example, diazepam is a proven antiepileptic, and may also have a calming effect in aggression and the inter-ictal personality disturbance found in some epileptic patients (Goddard & Lokare, 1970). It may be useful in some subjects with destructive attacks of rage or outbursts of temper (Lion, 1979). Intramuscular lorazepam can help both psychotic and non-psychotic aggression (Bick & Hannah, 1986). Although neuroleptic drugs should be the first choice, for those who develop severe extrapyramidal side-effects or hypotension, benzodiazepines may be an alternative. There are also descriptions of patients being able to abort episodes of self-mutilation when prodromal symptoms appear by taking lorazepam or triazolam (Griffiths, 1985).

Episodic dyscontrol has been defined by Monroe (1982) as "an abrupt onset of intense mixed dysphoric effects". This recurrent maladaptive behaviour interferes with the life flow of the individual, and is probably not a unitary phenomenon. It has been likened to epilepsy, and patients and their relatives often refer to such episodes as "spells" or "attacks", but although there may be prodromal symptoms reminiscent of an aura, the patient does not lose consciousness and the electroencephalogram (EEG) is normal. Earlier trials with antiepileptics such as diphenylhydantoin were disappointing, but more recently carbamazepine has been shown to be effective in some cases. It reduces the frequency and severity of aggressive episodes in schizophrenia, and there has been one trial demonstrating a beneficial effect in BPD (Cowdrey & Gardner, 1988). Mattes (1984) also found that carbamazepine reduced the frequency of aggressive episodes in a group of patients with heterogeneous psychiatric diagnoses, an effect which was independent of investigations such as neuropsychological tests or the EEG.

Just occasionally a few patients, particularly those with a history of childhood hyperactivity or previous amphetamine responsiveness in childhood, will respond well to D-amphetamine (15–30 mg daily). Needless to say, amphetamines must only be used with extreme caution, but among patients who respond there is no tendency to increase the dose, in contrast to the drug-misusing population who will soon seek to raise the dose. Eliciting an earlier history of attention deficit disorder in cases of adult personality disorder is important, because some of these patients will respond to other drugs such as MAOIs, neuroleptics or lithium.

Prescribing for borderline patients is an art in itself, as the medication itself is often used as yet another medium for acting-out, for example, by taking overdoses. It is often extremely difficult to obtain an honest appraisal of whether a drug has been helpful or not because some subjects, such as patients with a histrionic personality, may wildly exaggerate any benefits, while many borderline patients will seek to devalue almost anything their doctor tries to do. Sweeney (1987) recommended that prescribing should always be done in the context of a 'therapeutic trial' in order to obtain maximal participation by the patient, and to avoid any risk of the doctor appearing to be too authoritarian.

In patients with suicidal tendencies, drugs that are rather more lethal in overdose, such as the tricyclics, MAOIs and lithium, should be avoided if possible, while the relative safety of benzodiazepines, neuroleptics and SSRIs in overdose should be noted.

Although there may be valid theoretical reasons why psychotherapy should not be combined with medication, a psychiatrist who treats subjects with severe personality disorders will inevitably have to use admission, medication *and* psychotherapy. There is somewhat more controversy over the use of small doses of neuroleptics among ambulant patients. Drugs may have some benefits for mood and other symptoms, but the majority of psychotherapists prefer their patients to be drug-free if at all possible. Selecting the optimum drug for cases of BPD is not easy, especially as there are no useful clinical predictors of drug responsiveness. One interesting finding in the sequential trial of Cowdrey & Gardner (1988) was that when patients were offered a sequence of four separate drugs, even though the response rate for any individual drug was low, a majority of the patients were able to respond to at least one of them. Thus a pragmatic approach may be most helpful, with patients being offered two or three drugs in succession so that the most suitable one can be selected.

Electroconvulsive therapy (ECT)

Patients who are comorbid for personality disorder and depression may show a good initial response to ECT, but there is often an early relapse. Kramer (1982) reported on five subjects with BPD and depression. One had a good response with an early relapse, two had an equivocal response with rapid relapse, and two showed no response. Zimmerman *et al* (1986) confirmed these findings and found a higher readmission rate after ECT for patients with personality disorders and depression compared with those who only had depression. In a large retrospective case note study, Black *et al* (1988) showed that 68% of patients with pure depression responded well, but only 40% of those with concomitant personality disorders. Against this, Casey & Butler (1995) failed to detect any difference in either the short-term or one-year outcome between these groups, and Black *et al* (1988) also demonstrated an 80% response rate in both groups.

The prescription of ECT among subjects with personality disorders raises problems. In spite of evidence that the outcome may be less successful, ECT should not be withheld. In some cases a severe depression may be concealed; thus frequent self-mutilation may lead to intensive nursing involvement, which may itself trigger further manipulative behaviour on the part of the patient, and so confuse the diagnosis. The high doses of phenothiazines used for sedation may mask the more diagnostic biological symptoms of depression, and ECT may be helpful in such cases. In addition, there are some patients who may be suffering from a drug-responsive depression, but whose behaviour is so chaotic, immature or wilful that they are unable to comply with a simple course of antidepressants, let alone discuss their difficulties with a psychotherapist. Even so, these patients are just as keen to be free of their depression, and ECT may be the only type of antidepressive remedy that they can use. Therapeutic pessimism may lead to a failure to prescribe either ECT or other drug treatments among personality disordered subjects, and this in itself has been shown to affect outcome (Black *et al*, 1988). Remembering the tendency of these patients to act-out dangerously, it may be all the more important to pursue standard physical treatments among subjects who are depressed and who also have a comorbid personality disorder.

Long-term outcome

Follow-up studies provide information on how well a group of subjects with a particular diagnosis will do over time, and whether the diagnosis itself has long-term stability and hence meaning. For chronic disorders such as a personality disorders, short-term follow-up may provide some indication about the effect of any intervention, but only long-term studies will give a picture of the lifetime course. However, long-term studies are fraught with the problem of diagnostic validity, because diagnostic criteria may change from the outset of the study to the time when outcome is examined. For example, does the old diagnosis of 'pseudoneurotic schizophrenia' identify the same group of patients as DSM–III–R BPD?. Because the older diagnosis included brief psychotic experiences among the criteria, up to 20% of such cases (who confusingly were also sometimes called borderline) later developed schizophrenia. DSM–III–R criteria for BPD excluded brief psychotic episodes, and so the development of schizophrenia in these patients was unusual. On the other hand, the new criteria in DSM–IV have reintroduced the criterion of "brief paranoid episodes", making it more likely that some DSM–IV BPD subjects may develop schizophrenia as a late outcome.

There are further difficulties; few subjects have a pure syndrome. In Fyer *et al*'s (1988) group of BPD subjects, only 9% had uncomplicated BPD. Secondly, only those with the more extreme disorders are hospitalised and are therefore diagnosed with enough documentation to serve as a starting point for follow-up studies. Finally, some traits such as being antisocial may themselves lead to significant later events being expressly concealed from investigators.

Mortality and suicide

Zilber *et al* (1989) studied the five-year standardised mortality ratio (SMR) of all the patients admitted to psychiatric hospitals in Israel in 1978 (*n* = 16 147). The SMR for all types of personality disorder in the 20–39 year age group was 6.9, which was similar to that found for schizophrenia (SMR = 6.3) but slightly lower than that for affective disorders (SMR = 8.5). Around half the deaths of those with personality disorder were due to natural causes, mainly infections (SMR = 3.2). Certain complications dramatically increased mortality, such as alcohol abuse (SMR = 27) or substance abuse (SMR = 21), mainly as the result of natural causes, usually infections. The risk for suicide was higher among subjects with a personality disorder (SMR = 2.6) although this was considerably lower than that for affective disorder (SMR = 6.1), but in the same range as that for schizophrenia (SMR = 3.2).

The mortality of subjects with antisocial personality disorders is high, and although DSM–III–R stated "they sometimes have a violent end", reliable mortality data relating specifically to ASPD are lacking. Follow-up studies by Robins (1985) indicated that excess mortality in this group was mainly due to homicide, accidents, and the complications of alcohol or substance abuse.

Among those who have been incarcerated, there is more clear-cut evidence of increased mortality. Robertson (1987) followed up a population of 1347 mentally disordered offenders (all diagnoses) in the UK, and 23 years later found that 21% had died; a quarter of the deaths were by violent or unnatural means (suicide, homicide and accidents). Offenders with non-psychotic disorders (mainly personality disorders) met a violent death in 29% of cases during the follow-up period. A similar but rather smaller study in the US showed that 7 (5.9%) out of 118 delinquents who were incarcerated had met a violent end, giving them a 76-fold higher risk of having a violent death compared with a similar age and sex-matched group in the general population (Yaeger & Lewis, 1990). Those with personality disorders who end up in prison are generally at the more severe end of the spectrum, and so these alarming figures probably do not apply to community samples.

Suicide is an appreciable risk for BPD, and rates of around 8% (Paris *et al*, 1987; Stone, 1990) are given, although McGlashan's (1986) series (from the expensive and exclusive Chestnut Lodge Hospital) gave a figure of only 3%. Factors associated with suicide in Stone's (1990) series were a previous or family history of affective disorder, alcoholism, a history of incest or parental brutality. Although numbers were small, a very high suicide rate of around 40% was found for women who had all eight of the DSM–III–R criteria, those with schizoaffective features, or those who were comorbid for alcoholism and major affective disorder as well as BPD. For the milder disorders mortality rates are unknown, but even a high neuroticism score may be associated with an SMR of 2 (Allebeck *et al*, 1988).

Outcome of borderline personality disorder

Disorders which impinge more on clinicians have a greater likelihood of becoming the focus of a detailed outcome investigation. Two large series of BPD patients by Fenton & McGlashan (1986) (*n* = 87) and Stone (1990) (*n* = 196) confirmed that two-thirds of the patients had a good outcome when traced 10–15 years after the index admission. In Stone's larger series, a better outcome was associated with high intelligence (IQ more than 130), obsessional features, artistic talent, attractiveness (among women) and attendance at AA (among alcoholics). A worse than average outcome was associated with parental physical cruelty, a history of transgenerational incest, schizotypal features, extreme impulsivity leading to a chaotic lifestyle, and antisocial traits.

The DSM–III–R criterion "inordinate anger" worsened outcome. Since this item is not included in the criteria for Kernberg's borderline personality organisation, the latter condition has a rather more benign outcome than DSM–III–R BPD. The diagnosis of BPD tended to be stable over time, although by the fourth or fifth decade only a quarter of the subjects still had sufficient features to justify such a diagnosis. A small number, around 11%, switched diagnosis to affective disorder (Stone, 1990), but schizophrenia only developed in one out of 196 cases in Stone's series. A recurrence of borderline symptoms was sometimes observed among subjects in their mid-40s following widowhood or divorce (sometimes the result of the patient's irascibility) when patients presented once again for treatment (McGlashan, 1986).

Although at the time of the initial index admission BPD appeared to be just as severe as a schizophrenic illness, follow-up studies indicate a better outcome. Readmission rates were lower (28% v. 77%) and more borderline patients had a job (66% v. 18%). However, in comparison with the general population the marriage and fertility rates were significantly lower (Stone, 1990).

Dissocial personality disorder

Robins (1985) pointed out that sociopathy is a life-long disorder, possibly marked by three distinct phases, but it can abort at any time. In early childhood there may be arguments, tantrums and stubbornness with oppositional behaviour. In middle childhood there is aggression and conduct disorder, while in adolescence there is truancy and stealing. Around 40% of conduct-disordered boys and 20% of conduct-disordered girls go on to develop adult ASPD, which is most prominent in young adulthood.

The disorder tends to attenuate with age, and in later life there is a dramatic decline in the rates of aggression and theft, the hallmarks of ASPD. Many explanations are offered for the high rate of termination of the criminal lifestyle that occurs in the mid-40s, including increasing maturity, the development of more satisfying relationships, commitment to legitimate employment, less self-absorption, and less rebelliousness or pleasure-seeking behaviour. The decline in physical and emotional energy may result in criminal burnout, while fear of further incarceration may also play a role (Coid, 1993), although there are a few individuals who fail to make any adjustment in mid-life.

It should be noted that criminal burnout does not necessarily imply maturity in a psychopathic personality. Reid (1986) suggested that many ageing psychopathic subjects are still antisocial, but just less successful, lacking the physical strength and emotional stamina needed to continue in the criminal world, so they can no longer compete with younger psychopathic personalities.

Reliable figures for the outcome of ASPD are almost impossible to find, for, as Dilalla & Gottesman (1990) pointed out, there are many young people from abysmal environments who pass through a delinquent phase and later mature out of it, and the inclusion of such cases in any series would paint an unduly optimistic picture. On the other hand, confining a follow-up study to hardened criminals from a prison setting would give too pessimistic a picture. The presence of ASPD worsens the outlook for those with alcohol and substance misuse, and even for convicted criminals; recidivism rates rise for criminals who also have ASPD. For example, the four-year reconviction rate for discharged rapists was higher if they were also comorbid for ASPD (Rice *et al*, 1990).

Schizoid and schizotypal disorders

There is considerable interest in the long-term outcome of schizotypal subjects, in particular to see whether subjects develop schizophrenia and to determine if there are any predictors of such an outcome. Chick *et al* (1979) examined 22 children with schizoid disorders between the ages of 5 and 14 and showed that the disorder was essentially stable over time, but by age 22, two subjects (9%) had developed schizophrenia. Fenton & McGlashan (1989) followed up 105 subjects with schizotypal personality disorder (STP), of whom 75 were comorbid for BPD and 30 had mainly pure STP. Around 15 years later, 16% developed schizophrenia, and the items which more strongly predicted a schizophrenic outcome were those specific to STP (that is, magical thinking, suspiciousness, paranoid ideation and social isolation) whereas the borderline features were not associated with later schizophrenia. Additional predictive factors included transient delusional experiences, lower IQ, and a poorer premorbid quality of work. These findings tend to confirm the earlier observations of Spitzer & Gibbon (1979) that STP, but not BPD, belong within the schizophrenia spectrum of disorders. The presence of features of STP appears to worsen the outlook for obsessional disorder (Minichiello *et al*, 1987), the combined BPD–STP syndrome has a poorer outlook than BPD alone (Stone, 1990), and among women is associated with higher rates of alcoholism (Valgum & Valgum, 1989).

Milder disorders

There is little long-term follow-up information on the milder personality disorders, particularly those in the anxious group, or on the outcome of individual traits. Tyrer *et al* (1993) observed a negative correlation of traits with age, suggesting a gradual improvement over time. He suggested that there were two groups of personality disorders: the *mature*, which changed little with the passage of time, and the *immature*, which attenuated with increasing age. The mature group included mainly those in the eccentric and anxious groups; the anankastic, paranoid, schizoid and anxious. The immature group included those in the dramatic cluster, the antisocial, borderline and histrionic types, as well as the dependent and narcissistic types.

This suggestion is supported by two studies that assessed the presence of personality traits with age (Tyrer & Seiverwright, 1988; Reich *et al*, 1988). Both studies showed that traits associated with antisocial, borderline and explosive character disorders become less frequent with older age, while increasing age had little effect on the schizoid, compulsive, anxious or hypochondrial traits. Fogel & Westlake (1990) found that 15.8% of a large cohort of subjects with major depression also had a diagnosis of personality disorder. Borderline personality disorder was not diagnosed in anyone aged 45 or over. Histrionic and dependent personality disorders were less frequent with increasing age, while compulsive personality disorder increased with age (3% at 25–44 years, up to 5% for those aged over 69) (Fogel & Westlake, 1990).

Additional information can be obtained from psychogeriatric studies using older samples, adopting a retrospective view of the patient's life. Bergmann (1991) examined a group of elderly subjects in the community and tried to correlate an earlier history of interpersonal difficulties and abnormal personality traits with psychiatric symptomatology in old age. He identified four main groups of subjects. Firstly, those who in younger life were prone to anxiety, in late life manifested hypochondriasis and affective symptoms, particularly depression. A second group were those who in earlier life had been "insecure or rigid", had poor relationships with their parents and sometimes psychiatric disorders in childhood, and in later life experienced loneliness, obsessional and affective symptoms. A third group were designated "paranoid and hostile types" in old age, and when younger had many features of ASPD such as poor relationships with parents, "neurotic disorders" in childhood, marital disharmony, and poor work records. Finally, those with dependent features and apparently inadequate in their younger years seemed to fit in rather better later, particularly in middle age when they assumed submissive roles and their compliance was perceived as more of an asset than a liability, although in late life these subjects also had a tendency towards depression.

Conclusions

The high morbidity and mortality of subjects with the personality disorders, as well as the suffering caused to others, means that treatment issues cannot be ignored. The notion that at least some subjects with the personality disorders may be amenable to treatment is relatively new to psychiatry, although it remains uncertain whether treatment has any influence over the longer-term trajectory. For some patients, particularly those in the severe psychopathic group, it may be best for psychiatry to leave well alone, as the protection of society and forensic issues take precedence over any marginal improvement that psychotherapy may bring about in a severely dangerous individual. There are, however, many other patients, perhaps with milder or less contemptuous character disorders, who may have a need to change, a modicum of insight and some degree of motivation. A variety of psychotherapies ranging from the psychodynamic through to the cognitive–behavioural may offer some hope for amelioration. The discovery of genetic and other associations with the functional disorders has provided some theoretical justification for psychopharmacological intervention, which, particularly if combined with psychotherapy, may be beneficial. All methods of treatment aim at the same goal: the gradual conquest of preexisting habits by new, more adaptive habits of thought and behaviour.

References

Adler, G. (1977) Hospital management of borderline patients and its relation to psychotherapy. In *Borderline Personality Disorders* (ed. P. Hartocollis), pp. 307–323. New York: International Universities Press.

Akiskal, H. S., Rosenthal, T. L., Haykal, R. F., *et al* (1980) Clinical and sleep EEG findings separating "subaffective dysthymias" from "character spectrum disorders". *Archives of General Psychiatry*, **37**, 777–793.

Alexander, F. (1957) *Psychoanalysis and Psychotherapy*. London: George Allen.

Allebeck, P., Allgulander, G. & Fisher, L. D. (1988) Predictors of completed suicide in a cohort of 50 465 young men: role of personality and deviant behaviour. *British Medical Journal*, **297**, 176–178.

Beard, H., Marlowe, M. & Ryle, A. (1990) Management and treatment of personality disordered patients. The use of sequential diagrammatic reformulation. *British Journal of Psychiatry*, **156**, 541–545.

Beck, A. T. & Freeman, A. (1990) *Cognitive Therapy of Personality Disorders*. New York: Guilford Press.

Bergmann, K. (1991) The psychiatric aspects of personality in older patients. In *Psychiatry in the Elderly* (eds R. Jacoby & E. Oppenheimer), pp. 852–871. Oxford: Oxford University Press.

Bick, P. A. and Hannah, A. L. (1986) Intramuscular lorazepam to restrain violent patients. *Lancet*, *i*, 206.

Bion, W. R. (1959) Attacks on linking. *International Journal of Psychoanalysis*, **40**, 307–315.

Black, D. W., Bell, S., Hulbert, J., *et al* (1988) The importance of axis II in patients with major depression. *Journal of Affective Disorders*, **14**, 115–122.

Brinkley, J. R., Beitman, B. D. & Friedel, R. O. (1979) Low dose neuroleptic regimes in the treatment of borderline patients. *Archives of General Psychiatry*, **36**, 319–326.

Brobyn, L. L., Goren, S. & Lego, S. (1987) The borderline patient: Systemic versus psychoanalytic approach. *Archives of Psychiatric Nursing*, **1**, 172–182.

Buss, A. H. & Plomin, R. (1984) *Temperament: Early Developing Personality Traits*. Hillsdale, NJ: Lawrence Erlbaum.

Casey, P. R. & Butler, E. (1995) The effects of personality in response to ECT in major depression. *Journal of Personality Disorders*, **9**, 134–142.

Cleckley, H. (1972) *The Mask of Insanity*. St Louis: Mosby.

Coid, J. (1993) Current concepts and classifications of psychopathic disorder. In *Personality Disorder Reviewed* (eds P. Tyrer & G. Stein), pp. 113–164. London: Gaskell.

Collard, J. (1976) Pimozide in the treatment of some "social maladjustments" in "personality disorders". *Acta Belgica Psychiatrica*, **79**, 686–703.

Cornelius, J. R., Soloff, P. H., Peril, J. M., *et al* (1991) A preliminary trial of fluoxetine in refractory borderline patients. *Journal of Clinical Psychopharmacology*, **11**, 116–120.

Costa, P. T. Jr & McCrae, R. R. (1986) Personality stability and its implications for clinical psychology. *Clinical Psychology Review*, **6**, 407–423.

Cowdrey, R. & Gardner, D. L. (1988) Pharmacotherapy of borderline personality disorder. *Archives of General Psychiatry*, **45**, 111–119.

Dawson, D. F. (1988) Treatment of the borderline patient: relationship management. *Canadian Journal of Psychiatry*, **33**, 370–378.

Dilalla, L. F. & Gottesman, I. I. (1990) Heterogeneity of causes of delinquency and criminality: lifespan perspectives. *Development and Psychopathology*, **1**, 339–349.

Dolan, B. & Coid, J. (1993) *Psychopathic and Antisocial Personality Disorders*. London: Gaskell.

Fenton, W. S. & McGlashan, T. H. (1990) Longterm residential care: treatment of choice for refractory character disorders. *Psychiatric Annals*, **20**, 44–49.

Fogel, B. S. & Westlake, R. (1990) Personality disorder diagnosis and age: inpatients with major depression. *Journal of Clinical Psychiatry*, **51**, 232–235.

Fromm-Reichmann, F. (1950) Principles of Intensive Psychotherapy. Chicago: University of Chicago Press.

Frosch, J. (1983) *The Psychotic Process*. New York: International Universities Press.

Fyer, M. R., Frances, A. J., Sullivan, T., *et al* (1988) Comorbidity of borderline personality disorders. *Archives of General Psychiatry*, **45**, 348–352.

Giovacchini, P. L. (1982) Structural progression and vicissitudes in the treatment of severely disturbed patients. In *Technical Factors in the Treatment of the Severely Disturbed Patient* (eds P. Giovacchini & L. Bryceboyer), pp. 3–64. New York: Aronson.

Goddard, P. & Lokare, V. G. (1970) Diazepam in the management of epilepsy. *British Journal of Psychiatry*, **117**, 213–214.

Goldberg, S. C., Schulz, S. C., Schulz, P. M., *et al* (1986) Borderline and schizotypal personality disorders treated with low-dose thiothixene vs placebo. *Archives of General Psychiatry*, **43**, 680–686.

Griffiths, J. L. (1985) Treatment of episodic behavioural disorders with rapidly acting benzodiazepines. *Journal of Nervous and Mental Disease*, **173**, 312–315.

Gunderson, J. G. (1984) *Borderline Personality Disorder*. Washington, DC: American Psychiatric Press.

—— & Szabo, A. N. (1993) Treatment of borderline personality disorder: A critical review. In *Borderline Personality Disorder: Etiology and Treatment* (ed. J. Paris), pp. 385–406. Washington, DC: American Psychiatric Press.

Hare, R. D., Harpur, T. J., Hakstian, A. R., *et al* (1990) The revised Psychopathy Checklist. *Psychological Assessment*, **2**, 338–341.

Higgit, A. & Fonagy, P. (1992) Psychotherapy in borderline and narcissistic personality disorder. *British Journal of Psychiatry*, **161**, 23–43.

—— & —— (1993) Psychotherapy for personality disorder. In *Personality Disorder Reviewed* (eds P. Tyrer & G. S. Stein), pp. 225–261. London: Gaskell.

Horowitz, L. (1987) Indications for group psychotherapy with borderline and narcissistic patients. *Bulletin of the Menninger Clinic*, **51**, 248–260.

Jackson, M. & Pines, M. (1986) Inpatient treatment of borderline personality. *Neurologia et Psychiatrica*, **9**, 54–87.

Kernberg, O. F. (1967) Borderline personality organisation. *Journal of the American Psychoanalytic Association*, **15**, 642–685.

—— (1975) *Borderline Conditions and Pathological Narcissism*. New York: Aronson.

—— (1984) *Seven Personality Disorders: Psychotherapeutic Strategies*. Yale: New Haven.

Kiloh, L. G., Ball, J. R. B. & Garside, R. F. (1962) Prognostic factors in treatment of depressive states with imipramine. *British Medical Journal*, i, 1225–1227.

Klein, D. F. & Fink, M. (1962) Psychiatric reaction patterns to imipramine. *American Journal of Psychiatry*, **119**, 432–438.

Kohut, H. (1971) *The Analysis of the Self*. New York: International Universities Press.

Kramer, B. A. (1982) Poor response to ECT in patients with a combined diagnosis of major depression and personality disorder. *Lancet*, i, 1048.

Kutter, P. (1982) *Basic Aspects of Psychoanalytic Group Therapy*. London: Routledge & Kegan Paul.

Lansky, M. (1988) The subacute hospital treatment of the borderline patient – I: an educational component. *Hillside Journal of Clinical Psychiatry*, **10**, 24–37.

Linehan, M. M. (1993) *Cognitive–behavioural Treatment of Borderline Personality Disorder*. New York: Guilford.

Lion, J. R. (1979) Benzodiazepines in the treatment of aggressive patients. *Journal of Clinical Psychiatry*, **40**, 70–71.

Lorand, S. (1955) The teaching of psychotherapeutic techniques to residents in psychiatry. *Acta Psychother. Psychosom. orthopaedag*, **suppl. 3**, 218–224.

Macaskill, N. D. (1982) Therapeutic factors in group therapy with borderline patients. *International Journal of Group Psychotherapy*, **32**, 61–74.

Main, T.(1957) The ailment. *British Journal of Medical Psychology*, **30**, 129–145.

Markovitz, P. J., Calabrese, J. R., Schulz, S. C., *et al* (1991) Fluoxetine in borderline and schizotypal personality disorders. *American Journal of Psychiatry*, **148**, 1064–1067.

Marks, I. & Marks, J. (1990) Exposure treatment of agoraphobia/panic. In *Handbook of Anxiety, vol. 4. The Treatment of Anxiety* (eds R. Noyes, Jr, M. Roth & G. D. Burrows), pp. 298–310. Oxford: Elsevier.

Masterson, J. F. (1981) *The Narcissistic and Borderline Disorders*. New York: Brunner/Mazel.

Mattes, J. A. (1984) Carbamazepine for uncontrolled rage outbursts. *Lancet, ii*, 1164–1165.

McGlashan, T. H. (1986) The Chestnut Lodge follow-up study: III. Long term outcome of borderline personalities. *Archives of General Psychiatry*, **43**, 20–30.

Minichiello, W. E., Baer, L. & Jenike, M. A. (1987) Schizotypal personality disorder: a poor prognostic indicator for behaviour therapy in the treatment of obsessive–compulsive disorder. *Journal of Anxiety Disorder*, **1**, 273–276.

Monroe, R. R. (1982) DSM–III style diagnosis for the episodic disorders. *Journal of Nervous Mental Diseases*, **170**, 664–669.

Montgomery, S. A. & Montgomery, D. (1982) Pharmacological prevention of suicidal behaviour. *Journal of Affective Disorders*, **4**, 291–298.

Norden, M. J. (1989) Fluoxetine in borderline personality disorder. Progress in neuropsychopharmacology. *Biological Psychiatry*, **13**, 885–893.

Paris, J., Brown, R. & Nowlis, D. (1987) Long term follow up of borderline patients in a general hospital. *Comprehensive Psychiatry*, **28**, 530–536.

Patrick, J. (1985) Therapeutic ambience in the treatment of severely disturbed narcissistic personality disorders. *American Journal of Psychoanalysis*, **45**, 258–267.

Paykel, E. S. (1972) Depressive typologies and response to amitriptyline. *British Journal of Psychiatry*, **120**, 147–156.

Pines, M. (1978) Group analytic psychotherapy of the borderline patient. *Group Analysis*, **11**, 115–126.

Putnam, F. W. & Trickett, P. K. (1993) Child sexual abuse: a model of chronic trauma. *Psychiatry*, **56**, 82–95.

Reich, J., Nduaguba, M. & Yates, W. (1988) Age and sex discrimination of DSM–III personality cluster traits in a community population. *Comprehensive Psychiatry*, **29**, 298–303.

Reid, W. H. (1986) Antisocial personality. In *Psychiatry 1* (eds R. O. Michels, J. O. Cavenar *et al*), pp. 1–11. Philadelphia: J. B. Lippincott.

Reid, W. H. & Matthews, W. M. (1980) A wilderness experience treatment program for antisocial offenders. *International Journal of Offender Therapy and Comparative Criminology*, **24**, 171–176.

Rice, M. E., Harris, G. T. & Quinsey, V. L. (1990) A follow up of rapists assessed in a maximum-security psychiatric facility. *Journal of Interpersonal Violence*, **5**, 435–448.

Rifkin, A., Quitkin, F., Carrillo, C., *et al* (1972) Lithium carbonate in emotionally unstable character disorders. *Archives of General Psychiatry*, **27**, 519–523.

Rinsley, D. (1982) *Borderline and Other Self Disorders*. New York: Aronson.

Robertson, G. (1987) Mentally abnormal offenders; manner of death. *British Medical Journal*, **295**, 632–634.

Robins, L. N. (1985) Epidemiology of antisocial personality disorder. In *Psychiatry 3* (eds R. O. Mithels & J. O. Cavenar). Philadelphia: J. B. Lippincott.

Searles, H. F. (1979) *Countertransference*. Madison, CT: International Universities Press.

Shawcross, C. R. & Tyrer, P. (1985) The influence of personality on response to monoamine oxidase inhibitors and tricyclic antidepressants. *Journal of Psychiatric Research*, **19**, 557–562.

Sheard, M., Marini, J. L., Bridges, C. I., *et al* (1976) The effect of lithium on unipolar aggressive behaviour in man. *American Journal of Psychiatry*, **133**, 1409–1413.

Soloff, P. H., George, A., Nathan, R. S., *et al* (1986*a*) Progress in pharmacotherapy of borderline disorders: a double-blind study of amitriptyline, haloperidol and placebo. *Archives of General Psychiatry*, **43**, 691–697.

——, Anselm, M. G., Nathan, S., *et al* (1986*b*) Paradoxical effects of amitriptyline on borderline patients. *American Journal of Psychiatry*, **143**, 1603–1605.

——, Cornelius, J., George, A., *et al* (1993) Efficacy of phenelzine and haloperidol in borderline personality disorder. *Archives of General Psychiatry*, **50**, 337–385.

Spitzer, R. L. & Gibbon, M. (1979) Crossing the border into borderline personality and borderline schizophrenia. *Archives of General Psychiatry*, **36**, 17–24.

Steiner, M., Elizur, A. & Davidson, S. (1979) Behavioural toxicity: neuroleptic induced paradoxical behavioural toxicity in young borderline schizophrenics. *Confinia Psychiatrica*, **2**, 226–233.

Stone, M. H. (1988) The borderline domain: the "inner script" and other common psychodynamics. In *Modern Perspectives in Psychiatry, vol. II* (ed. J. Howells), pp. 200–230. New York: Brunner/Mazel.

—— (1989) Individual psychotherapy with victims of incest. *Psychiatric Clinics of North America*, **12**, 237–256.

—— (1990) *The Fate of Borderline Patients*. New York: Guilford Press.

Sweeney, D. R. (1987) Treatment of outpatients with borderline personality. *Journal of Clinical Psychiatry*, **48** (suppl. 8), 32–35.

Tobin, J. M., Bird, I. F. & Boyle, D. F. (1960) Preliminary evaluation of librium in the treatment of anxiety reactions. *Diseases of the Nervous System*, **21** (suppl.), 11–19.

Trukatt, I. D. & Carlson, C. R. (1984) Database versus symptomatic formulation of treatment: the case of dependent personality. *Journal of Behaviour Therapy and Experimental Psychology*, **15**, 153–160.

Tupin, J. P., Smith, D. B., Clanon, T. L., *et al* (1973) The long term use of lithium in aggressive prisoners. *Comprehensive Psychiatry*, **14**, 311–317.

Tyrer, P. & Sieverwright, H. (1988) In studies of outcome. In *Personality Disorders: Diagnosis, Management and Course* (ed. P. Tyrer), pp. 119–136. London: Wright.

——, Casey, P. & Ferguson, B. (1993) Personality disorder in perspective. In *Personality Disorder Reviewed* (eds P. Tyrer & G. Stein), pp. 1–16. London: Gaskell.

Valgum, S. & Valgum, P. (1989) Co-morbidity for borderline and schizotypal personality disorders. A study of alcoholic women. Progress in neuro-psychopharmacology and biological psychiatry. *Journal of Nervous and Mental Disease*, **177**, 279–284.

Van Der Kolk, B. A. (1989) Compulsion to repeat the trauma. Re-enactment, revictimisation and masochism. *Psychiatric Clinics of North America*, **12**, 389–402.

Waldinger, R. J. & Gunderson, J. G. (1984) Completed psychotherapies with borderline patients. *American Journal of Psychotherapy*, **38**, 190–202.

Wickham, E. A. & Read, J. V. (1987) Lithium in the control of aggression and self-mutilating behaviour. *International Clinical Psychopharmacology*, **2**, 181–190.

Winkleman, N. W. (1955) Chlorpromazine in the treatment of neuropsychiatric disorders. *Journal of the American Medical Association*, **155**, 18–21.

Winnicott, D. W. (1949) Hate in the countertransference. *International Journal of Psychoanalysis*, **30**, 69–75.

—— (1965) *The Maturational Processes and the Facilitating Environment*. New York: International Universities Press.

Woolcott, P. Jr. (1985) Prognostic indicators in the psychotherapy of borderline patients. *American Journal of Psychotherapy*, **39**, 17–29.

Yaeger, C. A. & Lewis, D. O. (1990) Mortality in a group of formerly incarcerated juvenile delinquents. *American Journal of Psychiatry*, **147**, 612–614.

Zanarini, M. & Gunderson, J. G. (1990) Childhood experiences of borderline patients. *Comprehensive Psychiatry*, **30**, 18–25.

Zilber, N., Schufman, N. & Lerner, Y. (1989) Mortality among psychiatric patients, the groups at risk. *Acta Psychiatrica Scandinavica*, **79**, 248–256.

Zimmerman, M., Coryell, W., Pfohl, B., *et al* (1986) ECT response in depressed patients with and without a DSM–III personality disorder. *American Journal of Psychiatry*, **143**, 1030–1032.

20 Anorexia nervosa and bulimia nervosa

Janet Treasure

---

*Clinical description • Measurement • Epidemiology • Aetiology •
Medical complications • Assessment • Treatment • Outcome •
Bulimia nervosa*

Historical accounts of young women who eat very little are plentiful, but the causes and meaning ascribed to such behaviour have varied. The religious interpretation was that extreme piety led to this asceticism. Bell (1985) in his book *Holy Anorexia* described the practices of Italian holy women from the 13th century, and questioned whether there are similarities with anorexia nervosa. Once scientific thinking began to hold sway, "miraculous maids" such as the tragic Welsh fasting girl, Sarah Jacob, were a curiosity as they appeared to defy the laws of nature. Doctors and nurses from Guy's Hospital set up a watch committee to provide rigorous proof as to whether Sarah Jacob could indeed survive without food or drink (Fowler, 1871). She died after six days in 1869, one year after Gull brought the condition, which he initially termed apepsia hysterica, to medical attention.

Richard Morton (1694) is usually credited with the first medical descriptions of patients with anorexia nervosa. In his book on wasting illnesses *Phthisiologica, or a Treatise of Consumptions*, he described two patients whose illness appeared to be due to voluntary food restriction. One was an 18-year-old girl who

> "fell into a total suppression of her Monthly Courses from a multitude of Cares and passions . . . From which time her appetite began to abate . . . she was wont by her studying and continuing pouring upon Books to expose herself both day and night . . . she was like a Skeleton only clad with skin."

This girl unfortunately died, but the second patient, a 16-year-old schoolboy, who "fell gradually into a total want of appetite, occasioned by studying too hard and the Passions of the Mind . . ." was cured by advice which was to "abandon his studies, to go into the country Air, and to use Riding and a milk diet".

Unequivocal descriptions of anorexia nervosa appeared in the 19th century. Marcé, a young French psychiatrist, wrote (1860) of

> "young girls who at the period of puberty become subject to inappetancy carried to the utmost limits . . . these patients arrive at

the delirious conviction that they cannot or ought not to eat ... All attempts made to constrain them to adopt a sufficient regimen are opposed with infinite strategies and unconquerable resistance."

Sir William Gull (a physician at Guy's Hospital) and Charles Lasegue (a French psychiatrist) brought the illness to the attention of the medical community between 1868 and 1888 with articles and case presentations. Lasegue's (1873) account is particularly vivid and well observed:

" ... gradually she reduces her food further and further, and furnishes pretexts for so doing ... the abstinence tends to increase the aptitude for movement."

He describes the lack of insight into the dangerousness of the weight loss and gives a typical ripost when confronted: "I do not suffer and therefore must be well."

Attempts to classify the illness reflect some of the uncertainties that remain today:

"the want of appetite is, I believe, due to a morbid mental state." (Gull, 1873)
" ... the cases were not strictly insane; there was however something wrong in the nervous equilibrium, and usually something queer in the family history." (Ryle, 1936)

The name given to the disorder has changed over time reflecting beliefs about both aetiology and psychopathology. Marcé used the expression 'hypochondriacal delirium', probably because many of his patients explained their reluctance to eat in terms of abdominal discomfort and he considered that the lack of appetite and abdominal complaints were hysterical phenomena. Lasegue did not refer to Marcé and used the term 'anorexia hysteric'. The current French term is 'anorexie mentale'. Although Gull (1868) initially called the syndrome 'apepsia hysterica', four years later he replaced 'apepsia' with 'anorexia', as he observed that food, if taken, was digested, indicating that the stomach was not at fault. He later argued that because men could be afflicted and the deficit was central rather than peripheral, 'nervosa' was a better term than 'hysterica'. In recent years many have questioned whether 'anorexia' is appropriate. There are physiological, psychological and behavioural features characteristic of starvation that lead to the premise that appetite should be present, and therefore there is a block at some level between the perception of hunger and the motivation to eat. In the West, explanations of the reluctance to eat now focus on dissatisfaction with weight and shape rather than on abdominal discomfort. It is interesting that the German name for the condition describes more accurately the current content of the psychopathology, thinness addiction or 'Magersucht'.

Treatment recommendations were remarkably similar from all sources, and centred upon removal of the patient from her family and home surroundings.

"The hypochondriacal delirium, then, cannot be advantageously encountered so long as the subjects remain in the midst of their own family and their habitual circle: the obstinate resistance that they offer, the sufferings of the stomach, which they enumerate with incessant lamentation, produce too vivid an emotion to admit of the physician acting with full liberty and obtaining the necessary moral ascendancy. It is therefore indispensable to change the habitation and the surrounding circumstances and to entrust the patients to the care of strangers." (Marcé, 1860)

"the patient should be fed at regular intervals and surrounded by persons who would have most control over them . . . the inclination of the patient must be in no way consulted . . . "(Lasegue, 1873)

Clinical description

The historical clinical descriptions are still relevant to current clinical practice. The onset of the illness commonly occurs within a few years of the menarche, with a median age of 17, but cases as young as 8 and as old as 60 have been described. The female to male ratio is 10:1. The onset is insidious, and the gradual weight loss is frequently unnoticed by the family or even commended as an adoption of a healthy lifestyle. Nutritional knowledge and dietary fashion have changed eating behaviour over time. The carbohydrate avoidance of the 1960s and 1970s has been replaced by the exclusion of fat. Parents often do not react until the weight loss has been considerable. The family may even protest that their daughter eats large amounts, if her plate is piled with large quantities of vegetables or salads or other low-calorie foods. As observed by Morton (1694), the contrast between the degree of emaciation and the level of mental and physical activity is striking. Often the first indication that something is amiss is that menstruation ceases. Parents may describe a change in temperament, where their previously "good girl" has become "difficult", emotional and excessively conscientious. It is usually held that anorexia nervosa is more common within the upper social classes. However, this may reflect a referral bias since case registers do not confirm the association, but suggest a relationship with educational achievement.

In the majority of cases it is easy to make the diagnosis of anorexia nervosa. The following is a vignette of a typical case.

Case example

Susan was a 21-year-old undergraduate at Oxford reading philosophy. Her eating became erratic after difficulties in a relationship in her first year. Her weight fell from 63 kg to 42 kg (body mass index (weight/ height^2) 14 kg/m^2) and amenorrhoea developed. She was sent home from college as she could not cope with her studies, her tutors noted that her academic performance had deteriorated, and her friends were concerned about her misery. She refused to accept that she had anorexia nervosa, stating that she was a fraud, wasting medical time. Her parents insisted that she eat, but she described feeling "gross" and contemplated suicide: "Nothing could be worse than having to eat". Even low-calorie foods were threatening. She could not finish anything she ate, not even a tomato or a slice of cucumber or pot of yogurt; it was "too excessive and greedy to do so". She weighed herself five or six times a day and would feel her thighs for excess flesh with disgust. The only time she felt happy was when she lost weight, and conversely she became despondent and despairing when she failed to do so, or if she lost control in any way.

She became obsessed with food and would go for long walks that included frequent visits to supermarkets where she handled many items but bought nothing. She became preoccupied by a new interest in preparing food for others and even dreamed about force-feeding and woke up terrified. Her interest turned from philosophy to diet magazines, recipe books and cooking. She was driven to be always on the go, and even in bed she would furtively clench and stretch her muscles.

Mental state

The clinical features of anorexia nervosa are entwined with those of starvation. It is useful to digress slightly to highlight which features are secondary to weight loss and which will therefore be ameliorated by nutritional rehabilitation. Keys *et al* (1950) outlined the profound effects that starvation has on physiology and psychology. They reported the Minnesota Experiment, in which a series of 32 male conscientious objectors were semistarved for six months to 76% of their premorbid weight, and followed-up during 12 weeks rehabilitation. The men started to toy with the food and increase the use of spices and salt, and to dawdle for two hours over a meal. Food became the principal topic of conversations and dreams, and their attention to food-related items increased. The men became emotionally unstable, irritable and aggressive. Social activity decreased; it was "too much trouble", "too tiring". Sexual interest also dwindled, one man ruefully observing: "I have no more sexual feeling than a sick oyster". We can conclude from this study that much of the food-related behaviour, psychological distress and social isolation seen in anorexia nervosa is a weight-related phenomenon.

It is often difficult to pinpoint the core primary features of anorexia nervosa, the characteristic psychopathology. The explanations given for the refusal to eat vary over time and place. Currently the control of weight or shape are central. Fatness epitomises moral degradation and is equated with sloth, gluttony and selfishness. These strongly-held views and overvalued ideas constitute what has been described as a morbid fear of fatness, and is present in both ICD–10 and DSM–IV descriptions. However, Crisp (1980) believed that the key component is a phobia of normal weight. In addition to the global attitudes about fatness or weight, there may be a sensitivity to a particular part of the body. This feature has been termed a disturbance of body image. It is not always present, and it has been difficult to measure experimentally as it may be a metaphor for more abstract discontent. ICD–10 (World Health Organization, 1992) differs from DSM–III–R (American Psychiatric Association, 1987) in that, because of this controversy, it no longer includes a perceptual aspect of body image in the definition (Hsu & Sobkiewicz, 1991). The diagnostic criteria for anorexia nervosa in ICD–10 and DSM–IV (American Psychiatric Association, 1994) are given in Box 20.1. The sufferer may acknowledge that she is thin, but will explain that she needs a margin of safety to ensure that her body does not become too fat. In order to elicit this feature, the patient should be asked to volunteer her "ideal weight", which will be well below her premorbid weight.

This preoccupation with weight and shape is a contemporary phenomenon and was not present in the classical descriptions of the illness, and is frequently absent in males. In non-Western cultures, for example in Hong Kong, the explanations are in terms of internal physical discomfort. Others explain that eating impairs their academic performance. Changes in the content of the psychopathology (pathoplasticity) over time and across cultures resemble those seen in other psychiatric illnesses, such as hysteria.

In contrast to externally imposed starvation, which produces mental and physical inertia, anorexia nervosa is associated with heightened activity until over 30% of weight is lost. Excessive exercise to "burn off" calories occurs. In others the activity is driven by a compulsion for tidiness or cleanliness. Academic work is pursued with excessive zeal.

Physical state

A typical patient with anorexia nervosa will have gaunt facial features, with the rest of the body hidden under layers of bulky clothes. The hands, feet and nose are pinched, blue and cold. Skin and hair are dry and downy, and lanugo hair may be present on the cheeks, nape of the neck, forearms and legs. In severe cases a proximal myopathy will be present, as may a petechial rash. The pulse rate is slow (60/minute) and blood pressure low (90/60 mm Hg).

Additional psychiatric disorders

Over 80% of subjects with anorexia nervosa have additional psychiatric morbidity during the course of their lives. Depression and obsessive–compulsive disorder are the most frequent. These syndromes are also common among first-degree relatives (Halmi *et al*, 1991).

Box 20.1 Diagnostic criteria for anorexia nervosa given in ICD–10 and DSM–IV

ICD–10 anorexia nervosa
1. Significant weight loss (BMI<17.5 kg/m^2) or failure of weight gain or growth
2. Self-induced weight loss
   (a) avoid fattening foods
   (b) vomiting
   (c) purging
   (d) excessive exercise
   (e) appetite suppressants
   (f) diuretics
3. Psychopathology
   (a) fear of fatness
   (b) low weight-threshold
4. Widespread endocrine disorder
   (a) amenorrhoea
   (b) raised growth hormone
   (c) raised cortisol
   (d) reduced T3

(Quetelet's body-mass index (BMI) = weight (kg)/height (m)^2)

DSM–IV anorexia nervosa
1. Refusal to maintain normal minimal weight (15% below expected)
2. Fear of weight gain or fatness even though underweight
3. Abnormal perception of weight, size or shape
4. Amenorrhoea (minimum 3 cycles)

Adapted with permission from DSM–IV. Copyright 1994 American Psychiatric Association.

Low mood, anhedonia, lack of concentration, pessimism and sleep disturbance (see page 1216) often occur. However, these symptoms also developed in the subjects in Keys *et al*'s (1950) starvation study. Therefore they are not specific to anorexia nervosa, but are a more general consequence of starvation; the symptoms usually disappear with weight gain. It is difficult, if not impossible, to distinguish these depressive features from those of an affective disorder. Specific characteristics of anorexia nervosa such as a preoccupation with food may help, although when the weight loss is severe, hunger itself will diminish. Active suicidal ideation is rare. Patients with anorexia nervosa will usually state that they do not want to die, they will vigorously deny that their behaviour is putting their life in danger, and reject the idea that they are undertaking a slow passive form of suicide. Once the illness becomes chronic and the quality of their life diminishes, more active suicidal ideation occurs and accounts for over half of the mortality in this group.

Although it has been argued, because of the frequent history of affective disorders within the families, that anorexia nervosa is a variant of an affective disorder (Cantwell *et al*, 1977), the clinical features, epidemiology and course of the two conditions suggest they are distinct (Halmi, 1985; Strober & Katz, 1987). In addition, there is no reciprocal increased risk of an eating disorder among affective disorder families (Strober *et al*, 1990). Symptomatic treatment with antidepressants is usually ineffective at low weight.

Obsessional symptoms, particularly centred around food and eating, are present in approximately a third of cases. For example, there are often rituals about which plate a patient can use and who can wash it. Any disturbance to the routine, such as an unexpected visitor, leads to refusal to eat. Often the rituals are associated with calorie-counting; for example, one patient noted with despair how she would drive ten miles out of her way to buy a wheat cereal product from a large supermarket, as this brand had 10 fewer calories per serving than other brands. More general cleaning or checking rituals can also arise. In most cases the obsessional behaviour diminishes with weight restoration. Starvation produces rituals and obsessive behaviour around food, as documented in Solzhenitsyn's *One Day in the Life of Ivan Denisovich* (1963):

> "picking up Shuhov's bread ration he handed it to him . . . though he was in a hurry he sucked the sugar from his bread with his lips, licked it under his tongue . . . he broke his ration in two, one half he stuck into his bosom into a little pocket he had specially sewn into his jacket . . . he considered eating the other half but food gulped down is no food at all; its wasted; it gives you no feeling of fullness . . . so he crawled barefoot up to his bunk, widened a little hole in his mattress and there amid the sawdust, concealed his half ration . . . Meanwhile the sugar in his mouth had melted . . . "

The ritualised meal is regarded as a reward to be earned and is associated with great pleasure that compensates for the hassles and discomforts of everyday life. Again this is clearly described by Sozhenitsyn:

> "Shukov with his two bowls . . . And now they had nothing more to say to one another – the sacred moment had come . . . He set to. First he only drank the liquid, drank and drank. As it went down filling his whole body with warmth, all his guts began to flutter inside him at that meeting with that skilly. Gooo-ood! There it comes, that brief moment for which a zek lives. And now Shukov complained about nothing . . . This was all he thought about now . . . "

Approximately a third of women who present with obsessive–compulsive disorder later in life have a past history of anorexia nervosa (Kasvikis *et al*, 1986). Anxiety and panic disorder are less common. Personality disorders, particularly in the avoidant, anankastic and emotionally unstable domains, are present in approximately half of those referred for psychiatric treatment (see also page 765). Patients with a mixed pattern of anorexia nervosa and bulimia may show borderline features and impulsively harm themselves, steal or misuse alcohol. Even though patients could qualify for an axis II diagnosis when ill during their anorexic phase, these features frequently disappear on recovery. Other personality traits such as poor self-esteem and little confidence in their academic abilities or their attractiveness are more persistent. Perfectionist traits are usual; flawed work may be destroyed and repeated, or personal belongings strictly ordered.

Measurement

A structured interview, the Eating Disorder Examination, that assesses the relevant psychopathology has been developed (Cooper & Fairburn, 1987). Several self-report questionnaires are also in common use. The Eating Attitudes Test (EAT) is a self-report questionnaire which has been validated in clinical samples but has poor sensitivity and specificity when used in the community (Garner & Garfinkel, 1979). The same group (Garner *et al*, 1983) later produced another self-report questionnaire, the Eating Disorders Inventory, which incorporates factors from the EAT as well as personality dimensions.

Epidemiology

Anorexia nervosa can present to a variety of medical specialities under several diagnostic guises. Therefore it is not sufficient to calculate the incidence from psychiatric case registers. The ascertainment of missed or misdiagnosed cases was meticulously undertaken in the Mayo Clinic study (Lucas *et al*, 1991) in which the average incidence in the general population was estimated to be 7 per 100 000. This is comparable to European figures (4/100 000: Szmukler *et al*, 1986; 5/100 000: Hoek, 1991). Anorexia nervosa has increased in case registers over the last two decades (Szmukler *et al*, 1986; Willi *et al*, 1990), but this may represent better recognition of the condition since no such trend was found at the Mayo Clinic over the period 1930–1980, although an increase in young women was found in the first five years of the 1980s.

Establishing the prevalence of anorexia nervosa is fraught with difficulties, as large populations need to be screened and all studies so far have found that "cases" actively avoid participation. A Swedish study avoided these difficulties by carrying out a survey of a group at high risk for the condition, 15-year-old school children (Rastam *et al*, 1989). The prevalence was 700 per 100 000, and 90 per 100 000 school boys. The estimated prevalence in Rochester, US, is 200 per 100 000 females.

Certain groups in whom weight and appearance are at a premium are at high risk. Ballet dancers and models have a prevalence rate of between 4–6%. Dieticians also may have increased rates.

There have been many case reports of anorexia nervosa from Asia and Africa. Although definitive epidemiological studies in non-Western cultures have not been performed, it is thought that anorexia nervosa is less prevalent in non-Western cultures. However, it has been argued that cases of anorexia nervosa can be seen in non-Western societies if the "fear of fatness" criterion (a culture-bound symptom) is removed (Lee, 1991; Littlewood, 1992).

Aetiology

Speculations about the aetiology of anorexia nervosa range from the biological to the sociological. None of the theories so far proposed can account fully for the epidemiological and clinical findings.

It has been argued that anorexia nervosa may have increased in prevalence during the time of the flappers in the 1920s, and in the 1960s at the time of the model Twiggy. Feminists conceptualise anorexia nervosa as a form of hunger strike undertaken to resolve the conflict between the expectations of a traditional female role and those of the modern woman (Orbach, 1986). The assumption that the incidence of eating disorders has risen is a central argument in such sociocultural models of aetiology (Brumberg, 1988). The evidence for an increase in anorexia nervosa is controversial (see above), but it is less so for bulimia nervosa, even though there is little hard evidence (the disorder was not classified until the mid-1980s).

Another influential theory is that maladaptive patterns of family interaction give rise to the disorder. One of the first controversies in the literature on anorexia nervosa concerned the question of whether it was possible to treat a patient with anorexia nervosa without isolation from the family (Myrtle, 1988; Playfair, 1988). Rigidity (resistance to change), enmeshment (overclose involvement between a child and parent so that each is poorly differentiated), conflict avoidance and overprotection were described as characteristic features of the family of a child with anorexia nervosa (Minuchin *et al*, 1978). One family model is that the child with anorexia nervosa provides a joint focus for parents who themselves have problems sustaining a relationship. The girl is stuck with this role in the family and has difficulties establishing autonomy. Many of these so-called "psychosomatic" family patterns may be no more than the normal parental response towards a sick child. A more plausible explanation is that the family members are not causal but are ineffective in the face of the illness, and so fail to arrest its progression. Crisp (1980) described the family in anorexia nervosa as one in which there are difficulties adjusting to adolescence and the increasing autonomy of the children.

Many theories have been developed to account for individual vulnerability; Bruch (1974) suggested that early parenting experiences contributed to later difficulties, leading to a poor sense of identity, uncertainty about the relevance and meaning of internal states, and an overwhelming sense of ineffectiveness. Slade (1982) also had a theoretical model focused around the individual. He suggested that personality traits such as low self-esteem and perfectionism provide the background against which anorexia nervosa develops in response to specific triggers. The control and self-discipline of anorexia nervosa compensate for an underlying sense of inadequacy, which might explain the preponderance of eating disorders in those who opt for prolonged education.

Another theory is that anorexia nervosa develops because of conflict relating to sexual maturity. The physiological and social regression of anorexia nervosa enables avoidance of the conflict (Crisp, 1980). Difficulties with sexuality may arise from earlier traumatic experiences, as approximately a third of cases of anorexia nervosa have been victims of sexual abuse in childhood, but it is unlikely that there is a specific link between childhood sexual abuse and eating disorders (Palmer *et al*, 1990).

Feeding and reproductive functions are integrated within the same areas of the hypothalamus. Bhanji & Mattingly (1985) described a few subjects with hypothalamic brain tumours who had an anorexic-like picture. A recent hypothesis suggests that anorexia nervosa results from stress with the consequent release of corticotrophin-releasing hormone, which in turn suppresses appetite (Morley & Blundell, 1988). Also, 5-hydroxytryptamine has been implicated in pathophysiological studies and is a reasonable candidate in view of its spectrum of action, which involves the suppression of eating and sexual activity (Curzon, 1992; Treasure & Campbell, 1994). Further support for a biological vulnerability trait comes from twin studies (Treasure & Holland, 1993, 1995). The concordance rate for anorexia nervosa between monozygotic twins (55%) is significantly greater than that between dizygotic twins (24%) (Holland *et al*, 1988), and approximately 5–7% of first-degree relatives are affected.

Medical complications

Medical problems often arise in anorexia nervosa and it is not possible to give a comprehensive account here. (For a more complete review see Treasure & Szmukler, 1995.) Box 20.2 displays the questions that are useful to ask. Boxes 20.3 and 20.4 outline common problems related to weight loss and weight control measures, and Box 20.5 outlines the investigations that are of value.

Endocrine system

The endocrine dysfunction reflects both the acute and the chronic nutritional disturbance. Amenorrhoea is one of the diagnostic criteria for anorexia nervosa, but it may be masked by withdrawal bleeds from the oral

---

**Box 20.2 Questions for the assessment of the medical
sequelae of eating disorders**

1. When was your last period?
2. Do you feel the cold badly? How does it affect your peripheral circulation?
3. Have you noticed any changes in your body hair, head hair, skin or nails?
4. Have you noticed any weakness in your muscles? What about climbing stairs or brushing your hair?
5. Are you troubled by aches in your bones or have you had fractures?
6. What is your sleep like? Do you have to wake to go to the toilet?
7. Have you fainted or had dizzy spells?
8. Have you noticed palpitations?
9. Have you had any pain or trouble with your teeth? What about temperature sensitivity? Do you attend to mouth hygiene after you have vomited?
10. Have you vomited blood or lost blood from your back passage?
11. Do you suffer from bloating or abdominal pain?
12. Have you noticed if the glands on your face have become swollen?

---

contraceptive pill. The hypothalamic–pituitary–gonadal axis regresses to a prepubertal state. Luteinising hormone (LH) and follicle stimulating hormone (FSH) are reduced, oestrogen and progesterone levels are undetectable, and pelvic ultrasonography reveals ovaries diminished in size but with a multifollicular appearance, and a small uterus.

All of the hormonal components of the hypothalamic pituitary adrenal axis are increased; this is thought to reflect increased hypothalamic secretion of corticotrophin-releasing hormone (CRH), and there is an impaired response to the dexamethasone suppression test. Thyroxine and T3 are reduced, and reverse T3 is increased. The thyroid stimulating hormone (TSH) response to thyroid releasing hormone (TRH) is delayed (Goodwin, 1990). Growth hormone levels are increased, probably as a consequence of poor nutrition, but somatomedin levels are decreased. These endocrine abnormalities disappear with weight recovery.

Metabolism

Fatal hypoglycaemia can supervene rapidly and without warning, especially in the context of exercise in severe cases. Asymptomatic hypoglycaemia is often found on routine testing of in-patients, and does not require active management other than the usual refeeding regime. Raised liver function tests settle on refeeding. Ironically, in view of the low-fat diet of these

---

Box 20.3 Medical consequences of starvation

1. Reproductive function
   (Loss of menstruation, fertility and pregnancy difficulties)
2. Musculoskeletal
   (Myopathy – particularly of the limb girdle muscles. Pathological fractures.teeth)
3. Cardiovascular
   (Palpitations and syncope)
4. Renal
   (Nocturia. Renal stones)
5. Skin and hair
   (Loss of head hair, increase in body hair, dry skin, acrocyanosis, chilblains)
6. Metabolic
   (Hypoglycaemia. Liver dysfunction, high cholesterol, hypothermia)
7. Gastrointestinal
   (Delayed gastric emptying, constipation)
8. Central nervous system
   (Poor concentration, difficulty in undertaking complex thought)
9. Psychological symptoms
   (Depression, obsessive–compulsive behaviour)

Box 20.4 Medical consequences of weight control methods used by patients with eating disorders

1. Gastrointestinal tract
   (Teeth, salivary gland hypertrophy, upper and lower gastro-intestinal tract bleeding, abdominal distension, constipation)
2. Renal
   (Oedema, dehydration, stones, failure)
3. Cardiovascular
   (Dysrhythmias, postural hypotension)
4. Central nervous system
   (Tetany, fits)
5. Metabolic
   (Dehydration, hypokalaemia, hyponatraemia)
6. Drug effects
   (Caffeine, slimming tablets such as diethyl proprion, amphetamine and ecstasy can be abused. Toxicity leads to nervousness and overt psychotic features)

A more detailed account is given by Bhanji & Mattingly (1985)

Box 20.5 Useful investigations

1. *Physical examination*
   Skin for petechial rash/lanugo hair/ Raynaud's/chilblains/
   callous on hand/self-mutilation
   Mouth and teeth for caps/loss of enamel/abrasions
   Lying and standing blood pressure for dehydration
   Abdomen for constipation
   Ability to rise from a squat for proximal
   myopathy

2. *Blood count*
   Anaemia (Hb 9–12 g/l) (usually normocytic normochromic)
   White-cell count between 2000–4000
   Platelet deficiency (rare)
   ESR normal

3. *Blood chemistry*
   (Urea and electrolytes are usually sufficient unless there are
   other indications)
   Urea usually low in restricting anorexia nervosa, but can be
   increased with vomiting and laxative misuse
   Potassium <3.5 mM/l (vomiting or laxative misuse)
   Bicarbonate >30 mM/l (vomiting): <18 mM/l (laxative misuse)
   Aspartate transaminase, alkaline phosphatase, gamma
   glutamyl transaminase may all be increased
   Cholesterol >6.5 mM/l
   Amylase (salivary isoenzyme) increased (bulimia vomiting)
   Phosphate levels decreased
   Carotene increased
   Protein usually normal

4. *Blood hormones*
   (These are of no use diagnostically and do not need to be
   performed routinely)
   LH, FSH decreased
   Oestrogen decreased
   T4 decreased, with increase in reverse T3
   Growth hormone increased
   Cortisol increased
   Prolactin normal
   Basal TSH normal (delay response to TRH)
   Basal ACTH normal (decrease reponse CRH)
   Basal insulin reduced (increased sensitivity to insulin)

patients, a high cholesterol level is often present. This may be caused by altered oestrogen and thyroid hormone metabolism.

Salt and electrolyte balance

Electrolyte abnormalities are frequent in the underweight subgroup who vomit and abuse laxatives. Plasma potassium levels occasionally fall below 3 mM/l. The electrocardiogram may show prolonged QT intervals and U waves. Fatal arrhythmias can occur without warning. Sodium, magnesium and phosphate are also sometimes reduced. Too rapid correction of these abnormalities can tip the patient into an acute confusional state. Although the electrolyte abnormalities are profound, they develop slowly and there is a degree of metabolic adaptation. Supervision to prevent vomiting and oral potassium supplements are the first line of management for hypokalaemia. Intravenous potassium is rarely required and should only be administered under the care of physicians. Oedema may result from the rehydration after stopping laxative abuse and vomiting: so-called "refeeding oedema". Patients may gain as much as 15 kg in a week.

Haematology

Marrow suppression with haemoglobin levels reduced to 9 g/100 ml and white-cell counts of less than 4000 are common. Platelet suppression is rare, but is a sign of dangerous weight loss. The erythrocyte sedimentation rate (ESR) is low and usefully distinguishes the anaemia and weight loss of anorexia nervosa from that of inflammatory bowel disease. Surprisingly, subjects with an eating disorder are often free of the common viral infections, but tuberculosis and other chronic infections occur sporadically.

Gastrointestinal system

Gastric emptying is delayed and leads to distension and discomfort once refeeding is instituted. In the most extreme cases, acute gastric distension may occur which can be fatal. It is therefore common practice to start refeeding gradually with "half portions" (approximately 1000–1500 kcal). Cisapride or metoclopramide, which increase gastric motility, can occasionally be used for symptomatic benefit. Constipation is common and may become intractable in cases of laxative misuse.

Central nervous system

Concentration is impaired and the capacity for complex thought diminished. Cerebral atrophy associated with ventricular dilatation and widened sulci may be related to vomiting or raised cortisol, and resolves in most cases following weight gain.

Long-term health problems

The detrimental medical consequences in both the short and long-term can be used to help motivation and obtain compliance. It is usual to find one item on the health checklist that is of personal concern to the individual. For example, some patients are extremely concerned about the loss of their periods and the implications this will have for their future fertility. The use of pelvic ultrasonography to image the ovaries and uterus may be particularly motivating for such women. Others may be concerned about the risk of osteoporosis, which becomes more severe with the length and severity of the illness and weight loss. Pathological fractures may appear after ten years of amenorrhoea. Further details of the long-term effects on reproduction and the skeleton are given in Treasure (1995).

Assessment

The diagnosis of anorexia nervosa rarely poses difficulties, but the crucial step at the first assessment interview is to engage the patient in treatment. Ambivalence about treatment is usual, and often patients are unforthcoming and angry at being coerced into seeing a doctor by concerned relatives and friends. Even if the patient has been brought for assessment by the family, it is important to establish an individual relationship with the sufferer initially. A structured style of interviewing that questions how the disorder has affected her physical health and psychological well-being, career and social life can often help to overcome this resistance, reassuring the patient that her problems can be understood. Avoid any comments which could be interpreted as critical or hostile, as patients will be acutely sensitive to these.

A weight and diet history is necessary to establish whether there is any degree of stability and control. Both the rate of change of weight as well as the absolute weight are markers of dangerousness (see Table 20.1). Patients with the restricting form of illness usually maintain a regular meal pattern, while those who are in the prodrome of the bulimic form will have prolonged periods of abstinence.

It is important to establish whether symptoms associated with bulimia nervosa are present, because these may terrify the patient and reinforce her need to have rigid control over her diet. Direct questioning may lead to denial. It is better to normalise the behaviour with probes such as:

"It is a common occurrence when people are as underweight as you that they have episodes when their eating seems excessive or out of control. Has this ever happened to you?"

"At times like this people experience discomfort and may even vomit. Has this happened to you? Have you ever had to make yourself sick to give you some relief?"

Table 20.1 A chart of weight thresholds for women for use in anorexia nervosa

Height	5'0"	5'2"	5'4"	5'6"	5'8"
Normal weight range (kg) (body-mass index (BMI) 20–25 kg/m^2)	45–56	48–60	51–64	54–68	58–72
Weight threshold for anorexia nervosa (BMI 17.5 kg/m^2)	39	42	45	48	51
Medical danger (BMI<13.5 kg/m^2)	30	33	34	37	39

"Often people who are underweight suffer badly from constipation. Has this ever happened to you? Have you had to take something to help?"
"Sometimes people with this illness are driven to be very active. Does this apply to you?"
"Many people with this problem use other methods to control their weight, such as health-shop preparations or street drugs. Perhaps you have had to do this?"

The weight history establishes the relationship between eating and life circumstances and context. A weight, physical and psychiatric history of all the other family members is also required, and may provide material that can be used in later psychotherapeutic sessions.

The formulation should detail the constitutional risk factors, patterns of interaction and behaviour, precipitating events and factors (which often lie within the family) that perpetuate the illness. A physical examination paying particular attention to the cardiovascular system, with lying and standing blood pressure, tests of proximal muscle strength, examination of the skin, and a screen for haematological and electrolyte abnormalities, is required. The patient should be told that she has anorexia nervosa and also given a brief reformulation that highlights the difficulties which have arisen following the illness, and encapsulates the relevant antecedant factors. It is useful to encourage the patient to read widely about the illness so that she can work in partnership with the therapist to overcome the problem.

Treatment

The classical treatment advocated by Gull was to remove the sufferer from her home environment to a nursing home, where "moral management" would be applied. There has been a marked change away from this approach over the last 20 years, during which new specific psychotherapeutic treatments have been developed. A recent study produced the remarkable finding that specialist out-patient treatment, in selected cases, can lead to an outcome that is as good as, if not better than, in-patient treatment, and with improved compliance (Crisp *et al*, 1991). This replicates the findings from Bristol (Morgan *et al*, 1983) where early out-patient intervention was effective.

A stepped care approach towards treatment should be followed (see Table 20.2).

Stage 1

Early or mild cases can be treated within the community by suitably trained general practitioners or community psychiatric nurses, with additional support from self-help associations.

Weight gain should be a focus of treatment for two reasons. Firstly, starvation leads to a cascade of secondary disabilities (medical, psychological and social) and these perpetuate the disorder. Secondly, it is a widely-held clinical impression that the disease runs a chronic course

Table 20.2 A stepped care approach to anorexia nervosa

Phase of illness	Treatment	Care provider
Excessive dieting	Education (nutritional, weight, clinical) Weight monitoring	General practitioner, community psychiatric nurse, school counsellor Specialised voluntary organisations
Clinical anorexia nervosa	Specific psychotherapy (educational, behavioural, cognitive, problem-solving)	General or child psychiatrist Clinical psychologist
Anorexia nervosa > 1 year duration	Specific out-patient psychotherapy (family or cognitive analytical)	Specialised eating disorder unit
Anorexia nervosa with life-threatening complications or treatment-resistant to out-patient care	In-patient or day patient treatment	Specialised eating disorder unit

unless weight is restored to a healthy level. Weight should be graphed at regular intervals. A target range of weight (see Table 20.1) should be set that encompasses the premorbid weight. For those who were obese premorbidly, a range of body–mass index (BMI) between 22–24 kg/m² is appropriate. It is useful to establish a regular routine for weighing. The therapist may wish to set a pattern by weighing the client at the beginning of each session. Whatever the weight change, it is important not to appear judgemental but to ask whether the weight was as expected, and how this made the client feel.

Although weight gain in the long-term will lead to tangible benefits, in the short-term it can lead to severe distress. Anxiety and despair are common, and the struggle between accepting the weight gain and continuing to diet becomes harder. It is helpful to warn patients and relatives about this in advance, and inform them that "anorexic attitudes about weight, shape and eating may persist for several years, even after apparent recovery of weight and menstrual function".

(a) *The therapeutic alliance*

At all stages the therapeutic relationship should be collaborative, with a kind, firm and consistent approach used to tackle the anorexic behaviour. The therapist should be knowledgable about eating disorders and nutrition. The first phase of treatment is to engender motivation to recover from the illness. The goal of treatment is to produce a balanced eating pattern. The issues of power, control and trust within the therapeutic relationship need to be recognised, as they can lead to coercion, frustration or collusion. Mutual trust is essential since it is futile for the therapist or carers to insist on goals that are unattainable. Women with anorexia nervosa may try to placate the therapist by lying about vomiting, laxative misuse or food intake. On the other hand, a failure to set goals and discuss the expectations of therapy can lead to a collusive relationship and a persistent illness. A focus on low self-esteem, lack of appropriate assertiveness and the binds of perfectionism and over-control is required; alternative ways to cope with stress other than weight loss should be developed. Hilda Bruch (1985), a psychoanalyst with wide experience in the treatment of eating disorders, advised against traditional psychoanalytical therapy for eating disorders. She described how sufferers may experience interpretations made by the therapist as a repetition of a pattern in which they have been told what to think and feel by significant others. A style of therapy with active participation in homework tasks such as reading, diary-keeping and problem-solving is often successful.

It is probably useful to set a limit on therapy (a minimum of 12 sessions over a year), although follow-up "booster" sessions are recommended for up to five years, as the trust and support engendered by treatment need to be continued.

(b) *Education*

Education about the consequences of the disorder and its treatment, and correction of mistaken assumptions (particularly about aetiology) is crucial. Women with anorexia nervosa consistently state that there is nothing wrong with them, and they consider themselves to be "frauds, wasting medical time". It is important to counter these arguments by providing information about the condition, for example, to warn that without treatment less than half of patients may make a full recovery, and that severe life-threatening physical problems may arise. The best recovery possible can only be obtained by joint work.

The patient needs to be aware of how much she will need to eat to gain weight. A supplement of approximately 7000 kcal is required to gain 1 kg, so a calorie intake of 3000 kcal per day is necessary to gain weight at a rate of 1 kg per week. In-patient treatment has to balance the difficulties of rapid weight-gain with the dangers of institutionalisation. This dilemma is not present with out-patient treatment, and weight gain can proceed more slowly, although goals should be clear. Overactivity at low weight can be dangerous and this should be discouraged.

Information about the medical consequences of anorexia nervosia are an important component of treatment. A screen of haematology, urea and electrolytes, liver function tests and cholesterol is useful for those who are severely underweight. Pelvic ultrasonography and bone-density measurement may be relevant.

Bulimia nervosa follows anorexia nervosa in a quarter of cases, and fear of this complication is often present. It is helpful to discuss the topic and develop strategies to minimise its occurrence. Useful strategies include adopting a regular pattern of eating with a mixed diet, and avoiding the seductive dangers of vomiting or laxative misuse. Hunger frequently increases when the dietary restrictions are lifted, and combined with the difficulty in monitoring fullness this can lead to terrifying feelings of lack of control. The therapist should reassure the patient that this is a normal and transient phase.

(c) *Support*

It is useful to engage the family or other carers in treatment, although active control over eating is less appropriate or successful for older patients. However, relatives need to be clear about the goals of treatment. They can get information and support from the self-help organisation, the Eating Disorders Association. These and other specialist centres often run groups for parents and carers.

(d) *Problem-solving*

Once an atmosphere of trust has been established, it is possible to focus on the difficulties that were blocked off once the anorexia nervosa developed.

This might include looking at difficulties in developing an adult relationship with the parents, or some deeply-held attitudes and beliefs such as the need to be perfect or to be in control.

Stage 2

Family approaches

In the 1970s there were enthusiastic reports about the efficacy of family therapy in the treatment of anorexia nervosa. Unfortunately, in inexperienced hands family therapy can be perceived as an indication that the family is somehow at fault, and some families have found it aversive.

A randomised control trial that compared family therapy with individual treatment indicated that family therapy was more effective in preventing relapse following in-patient treatment in the subgroup whose illness had begun before the age of 18 and was of short duration (Russell *et al,* 1987). Individual therapy was more effective than family therapy in older patients. These research findings support clinical pragmatism in that it is helpful to involve the family of a young adolescent who lives at home. It remains unclear which specific components of family therapy are of value, although recent research suggests that parental counselling combined with individual treatment may be more effective and more acceptable than a more formal family therapy approach. It often comes as a surprise to many parents that they need to set firm limits on eating. Family therapists encourage both parents to work together as a team on this problem. If one parent takes sole responsibility for the illness, a collusive relationship can develop. At times it may be necessary to refer one or both parents for counselling or support, since caring for their daughter can be exhausting.

As in individual therapy, education is an important component of treatment. The family should learn about the medical, psychological and social ramifications of anorexia nervosa. It is helpful to dispel mistaken beliefs about aetiology, for example, that it is caused by stubbornness or naughtiness on the part of the sufferer or that the behaviour of the family is responsible. Such mistaken attitudes will perpetuate guilt, recrimination and criticism and make treatment difficult. Family therapists help parents to find ways in which they can encourage their daughter to eat, such as direct supervision of meals with firm limit-setting. Parents can start to take control over their daughter's health and welfare, which requires them to negotiate a consistent plan of management.

> #### Case example
> Rose was 18 years old and had developed anorexia nervosa with additional obsessional symptoms one year earlier. She was seen individually, but her parents were also seen by her therapist and the dietician. Rose and her parents were given verbal and written information about anorexia nervosa and encouraged to find out more

by joining the Eating Disorders Association. During the initial six months of treatment, the parents adopted a structured approach to their daughter's eating. Family members would sit with Rose for meals and ensure that she ate them. Rose gained 4 kg in weight. After six months of treatment the mother admitted that she had been under a great deal of stress, as this approach often led to arguments. Rose considered that she had made some improvement and resented her parents being so intrusive. It was therefore decided that Rose should take total charge of her food. She would buy and prepare it herself and her parents would make a determined effort not to interfere. A few joint meetings were needed to establish the new rules and to reassure the parents that progress was continuing by weighing Rose at the clinic. Nine months later the family appeared wreathed in smiles. Rose had begun to menstruate and now had a boyfriend. Her mother recounted the joy she felt when for the first time in three years she heard her daughter laugh.

There are possible contraindications to family therapy. If the parents are divorced or separated, the act of including the parental couple in therapy together may fuel the fantasy of the family reuniting. It is also inappropriate to entrust treatment to parents with severe psychopathology, or to those who have physically or sexually abused their child, which will apply to approximately a third of cases and may be difficult to detect. Another contraindication is a previous attempt at family therapy that failed, leaving parents hostile and angry. In such cases, parent support groups can be of help.

Stage 3

Day patient treatment

Several specialised centres within the UK now offer day patient treatment for anorexia nervosa. This allows a greater degree of personal autonomy than an in-patient unit. The programmes that have been devised use a multidisciplinary team approach and many of the components outlined above. At least one or two meals a day are supervised, and patients usually attend five days a week for 2–4 months. In addition to nutritional treatment and education, programmes also provide therapeutic groups, family therapy and social support. Research shows that patients gain weight and are able to maintain this over the subsequent six months. A detailed account of this treatment approach can be found in Piran *et al* (1990).

In-patient treatment

In-patient treatment is required if the patient's physical or mental state is dangerous or there are contraindications to out-patient treatment. An outline of some of the complications that signal the need for urgent treatment is given in Box 20.6. In-patient treatment should not be seen as a cure for anorexia nervosa, but as a means of alleviating the physical and psychological distress that starvation produces. Intensive treatment after discharge is required to prevent later relapse.

A common approach in specialised in-patient units is for the nurses to take the control of eating away from the patient in the initial stages. Food portions are gradually increased to obtain a steady rate of weight gain, with snacks and drinks between meals. The daily caloric content of meals starts at about 1000 calories and gradually increases to 3000 calories. Strict behavioural regimens in which all privileges are taken away and total bed-rest is prescribed are no more effective than lenient regimes, and may increase the risk of developing bulimia nervosa. It is important that clear limits are set and that there is effective anticipation of the patient's needs and difficulties. The advantage of the specialist unit is that patients can be treated in a group, which means that there are sufficient resources to ensure that nursing care is given during the meal.

The nursing care delivered during and around meal times varies between units. One model is to have a nurse present during the meals, which are shared with other patients with anorexia nervosa. The nurse aims to facilitate mutual support among the group, which might involve a patient towards the end of treatment reassuring and empathising with the novice, but on other occasions the aim will be to remove the focus from food. The expectation is that patients will finish their food and it is the group's task to ensure that this is done. If meal times are prolonged, high calorie drinks may be substituted for some of the food. The countertransference can be intense and the nurse should be sensitive to this. It is necessary to continue supervision after meals to prevent habitual vomiting. Similarly, it is necessary

---

Box 20.6 Clinical and psychiatric grounds for admission

A. *Medical indications*
   1. BMI below 13.5 kg/m² (or a rapid rate of fall)
   2. Syncope
   3. Proximal myopathy
   4. Hypoglycaemia
   5. Electrolyte imbalance
   6. Petechial rash and platelet suppression.

B. *Psychiatric indications*
   1. Risk of suicide
   2. Chronicity >5 years
   3. Comorbidity with impulsive behaviour
   4. Intolerable family situation
   5. Extreme social isolation
   6. Failure of out-patient treatment

to guard against the use of other methods of weight control, such as laxative misuse and furtive exercising. Ambivalence about treatment makes the nurse's role difficult. Overvalued ideas about weight, shape and eating are impossible to shift by logical discussion. It is probably more reassuring for the patients to hear that the nurse understands but remains firm in her resolve to help the patients to gain weight.

Nurses managing patients with eating disorders have to work as a team, anticipate splitting, set limits without excessive coercion, and cope with the intense countertransference. Such nursing skills are more effective than any drug treatment so far tried, but they can lead to exhaustion and so the medical staff and senior nursing staff need to provide a lot of support. Families should be involved in in-patient care so that they are aware of the treatment goals and are prepared for the difficulties of the post-discharge phase. A more detailed account of in-patient treatment is given in Treasure *et al* (1995).

Difficulties in management

Occasionally a patient will lose insight into the dangerousness of her condition and staff need to implement the treatment order of the Mental Health Act to ensure that her health and safety are safeguarded. This measure should only be used after there have been several interviews with the patient and her family. Although parents are often concerned that if they take this step their daughter will never forgive them, it is our experience that patients later come to recognise the need for this step and are grateful that their lives were saved. A recent decision in the English Court of Appeal recognised that anorexia nervosa sometimes destroys the ability of the sufferer to make rational decisions regarding her medical treatment (Roberts, 1992). Compulsory admission should probably only be used as a last resort, but this does not signify that it should be rarely used (Goldner *et al*, 1991).

> *Case example*
> Clarissa rapidly lost weight after starting a diet for fun. Her parents were divorced and she lived with her father. It was several months before her mother became so worried about her weight that she arranged to have the family doctor call when she was visiting her daughter at home. Clarissa was admitted to a local psychiatric unit where she was offered the freedom to eat as she wished. She later recounted "They didn't make me eat, so I didn't". She collapsed on the third day with a cardiac arrest. She was successfully resuscitated but required ventilation on an intensive care unit for several days. Her parents were warned about the nature and danger of her illness and agreed to put their daughter on a treatment order of the Mental Health Act. She was transferred to a specialised unit where she refused to eat and drink for two days, despite the nurses sitting

with her for several hours after meals and encouragement from fellow sufferers. The nurses told her that they were not going to let her die, but they understood how difficult it was for her to eat and they would help by assisting her more actively. Two nurses gently but firmly ensured that several spoons of porridge were eaten. This did not need to be repeated. She gained weight and left the hospital after 14 weeks. She was seen intensively as an out-patient and managed to maintain her weight.

On rare occasions such as that of Clarissa, assisted feeding has to be used. This has far fewer complications than tube or intravenous feeding, but does require skilled nursing. It is important that this is discussed with the patient before starting, using the clear explanations given above. Two nurses are needed. One nurse spoon-feeds the patient while the other gently restrains and comforts her. The nurses should explain that they have to take over control as the anorexia is putting the patient's life at grave risk, and that they have an ethical duty to safeguard her life as her own judgement has become so clouded by the illness that she fails to recognise the danger she is in. It is usual for the patient to eat herself when she has experienced the firm resolution of the staff. In adult patients there is time for this gradated nursing strategy, but for children who have fewer reserves, more acute measures such as nasogastric feeding may be necessary. This should be time-limited and needs to be carefully supervised. Intravenous feeding may be required, particularly if life-threatening medical emergencies are present, but the nursing in this case would be provided on a medical ward.

Medication

There are two basic reasons for adopting a pharmacological approach in the management of eating disorders. The first is that a drug may correct the basic biochemical deficit underlying the condition. The second is that a drug may produce symptomatic benefit. In the early half of the century hormonal extracts such as thyroid hormone and oestrogen were given. Later, insulin treatment, sometimes in combination with chlorpromazine (Dally & Sargant, 1960), was used.

A small number of controlled trials have been undertaken to investigate whether pharmacotherapy can facilitate weight gain. Most of these have been conducted in an in-patient setting and it is possible that any beneficial effect is obscured by a "ceiling" phenomenon resulting from the therapeutic in-patient milieu. Cyproheptidine, an antiserotoninergic drug, was found to be marginally superior in terms of weight gain compared with standard in-patient management, particularly in the group with restricting anorexia nervosa (Vigersky & Loriaux, 1977; Goldberg *et al*, 1979; Halmi *et al*, 1986), while clomipramine, amitriptyline and pimozide had little additional benefit (Lacey & Crisp, 1980; Vandereycken & Pierloot, 1983; Biederman *et al*, 1985; Crisp *et al*, 1987).

Despite the general ineffectiveness of drug treatment in terms of weight gain (see Szmukler, 1982; Russell, 1985) they may have some role in alleviating symptoms of anxiety and depression. The depressive symptoms that accompany anorexia nervosa occasionally do not improve or may even worsen during weight gain. In such cases, treatment with a tricyclic antidepressant may result in recovery from the depressive symptoms. Another atypical subgroup who may benefit are middle-aged women who, in the course of a major depressive illness, lose a great deal of weight, not simply from a depressive want of appetite, but because they develop typical anorexic attitudes of food avoidance and over-concern with weight. Merely administering an antidepressant often fails to remedy their depression and their weight loss. On the other hand, combining the antidepressant with a weight-gain programme is most likely to restore such patients to their former health. Chlorpromazine has been used in small doses to reduce anxiety and guilt.

Overall, for restricting anorexia nervosa the benefits of drug treatment are small, and need to be balanced by the finding that a significant proportion of the mortality found in anorexia nervosa is a result of an overdose of antidepressant medication (Patton, 1988). In practice, compliance with medication is usually poor, perhaps because this represents sacrificing control. Alternatively the patient may discover from her own research that weight gain is a side-effect of such medication.

Outcome

Russell (1977) stated that anorexia nervosa is an illness that must run its course and has cycles of recovery and relapse, and a reliable expectation of outcome can only be made after four years have elapsed. Even when the outcome is favourable, the illness usually lasts 2–3 years. Follow-up studies have found that, on average, up to half of the patients recover fully with a return to normal weight and menstruation: weight is restored in 60%, menstrual functioning resumes in 55%, and normal eating behaviour in 40%. Psychosocial adaptation is often impaired. Two-thirds are in employment or in a normal educational career, very few are married, and approximately a third have a negative attitude to sexuality (there is wide variation between studies).

Often with the glamorisation of eating disorders by the press, the ominous course taken in a third of cases gets forgotten. A summary of important outcome studies is given in Table 20.3. These studies were chosen as they provide information from different age cohorts, the numbers were large and the follow-up complete enough to have confidence in the findings. It is clear that patient selection affects outcome. The outcome of those referred for psychiatric care is generally worse than for those presenting to a general hospital. There is a trend for the outcome of more recent studies to be better, but this conclusion may be confounded by the length of time for follow-up. During the initial phase of the illness the standardised mortality ratio is increased six-fold, and the mortality rate rises to 20% after 20 years of illness (Theander, 1970; Patton, 1988). Suicide accounts for half of the deaths. There is a suggestion in the literature that the mortality rate may decline where specialised treatment is given (Crisp *et al*, 1992).

Normal weight bulimia nervosa develops in approximately a quarter of cases of anorexia nervosa. Affective disorders and obsessional disorders are less common and are more usually present in those who have failed to recover.

The prognostic factors found from many studies are shown in Box 20.7. For age of onset there is some evidence to suggest that there is a bimodal relationship, with both very early (premenarchal) and later onset (>20 years) associated with a poor outcome. Dally (1969) suggested that the chances of recovery were poor if the illness had lasted for over seven years, but a more recent study extended this to 15 years (Ratnasuriya *et al*, 1991). For a more detailed account of outcome studies, see Steinhausen *et al* (1991).

Bulimia nervosa

History

Bulimia derived from the Greek *bous*, meaning ox, and *limos* (hunger), indicating a state of pathological voracity that has been described for centuries. However, in many accounts the bulimia was a symptom of a physical disorder. Four of the 14 historical examples described by Parry Jones & Parry Jones (1991) were infested with parasitic worms. The symptoms in the remaining cases resembled those seen in pyloric stenosis. Other historical accounts describe a fluctuating course rather similar to the Kleine Levin syndrome. Binge-eating in association with obesity was described by Stunkard (1959), and Bruch (1974) used the term "thin fat

---

Box 20.7 Poor prognostic factors for anorexia nervosa

A. *Illness-related*
 1. Long duration, resistant to treatment
 2. Lower minimum weight
 3. Age of onset (lower gives better outcome)

B. *Premorbid adjustment*
 4. Personality difficulties
 5. Poor relationship with family
 6. Social difficulties

Table 20.3 Chronic outcome of anorexia nervosa

Study	Cohort year	Minimum follow-up (yrs)	Maximum follow-up (yrs)	n	Mortality	Suicide	Poor outcome	Mortality and morbidity
Theander (1985)	1931–1960	25	54	94	17 (18%)	5 (5%)	5 (5%)	22 (23%)
Ratnasuriya et al (1991)	1959–1966	20	27	41	7 (17%)	3 (7%)	8 (19%)	15 (36%)
Tolstrup et al (1985)	1960–1976	8	25	151	9 (6%)	6 (4%)	29 (19%)	38 (25%)
Hsu et al (1979)	1968–1973	4	20	105	2 (2%)	0 (0%)	20 (20%)	22 (21%)
Morgan et al (1983)	1973–1978	4	8	78	1 (1%)	1 (1%)	19 (24%)	20 (26%)

people" to describe ex-obese subjects who regurgitated food after indulging in large meals.

Russell (1979) described a similar pattern of behaviour developing after an episode of anorexia nervosa. He used the term 'bulimia nervosa' to describe the syndrome in which bulimia was associated with purging and a morbid fear of fatness. It took Russell six years to collect 30 cases, but today the condition is very common, indicating that the prevalence has increased rapidly over the last three decades.

Definition

A variety of systems for classifying binge-eating disorders has evolved. Broad criteria were used for "bulimia" in DSM–III (American Psychiatric Association, 1980). They differed from Russell's criteria for bulimia nervosa in that purging, a morbid fear of fatness and a past history of anorexia nervosa were not considered necessary. In DSM–III–R the criteria were tightened, the preoccupation with weight and shape was included, and frequency cut-off points were introduced. The ICD–10 criteria for bulimia nervosa (Box 20.8) differ from those of DSM–IV in that frequency criteria (a minimum of two binges a week over three months) are not present, and the link with anorexia nervosa remains although it is not essential.

Clinical description

The median age of onset of bulimia nervosa is 18 (slightly later than that of anorexia nervosa), females predominate (M:F ratio = 1:10) and all social classes are affected. Patients are usually of a normal body weight. It is more common in groups where weight and shape issues are important, such as ballet dancers, models and actresses. A recent study in the UK suggests that British Asian girls may be particularly at risk (Mumford *et al*, 1991). Approximately a third of patients have a past history of anorexia nervosa and another third a history of obesity.

A characteristic set of attitudes to shape and weight is a key feature resembling the overvalued ideas that are commonly present in anorexia nervosa, and have been termed "a morbid fear of fatness". Preoccupation with weight and shape concerns is the driving force behind the abnormal eating behaviours and can interfere with concentration and social life.

A history of weight loss preceding onset is typical and there is usually an attempt to follow a strict diet with protracted periods of fasting. Binging has not been clearly defined but there is a move to use operational criteria such as objective overeating (1000 kcal or more) accompanied by a sense of loss of control, followed by feelings of shame and disgust. The content of binges varies from an array of "forbidden" palatable foods, to foodstuffs that would normally be regarded with disgust (leftovers, or food from the dustbin). The usual precipitants for binges are transgressions of self-imposed

---

Box 20.8 Criteria for a diagnosis of bulimia nervosa

DSM–IV
1. Recurrent episodes of binge-eating
2. Feeling of lack of control of eating during binge
3. Regular use of methods of weight control
   (a) vomiting
   (b) laxatives
   (c) diuretics
   (d) fasting/strict diet
   (e) vigorous exercise
4. Minimum average of two binges a week over three months
5. Persistent overconcern with shape or weight

ICD–10
1. Episodes of overeating
2. Methods to counteract weight gain
   (a) vomiting
   (b) laxatives
   (c) fasting
   (d) appetite suppressants
   (e) metabolic stimulants
   (f) diuretics
3. Morbid fear of fatness with a sharply defined weight threshold
4. Often a history of anorexia nervosa

Adapted with permission from DSM–IV. Copyright 1994 American Psychiatric Association.

---

dietary rules, or feelings of depression, anxiety, loneliness and boredom. Swollen parotid glands can give the face a rounded appearance; the teeth may be capped or smooth and shiny, and a callous may be present on the dorsum of the hand (Russell's sign).

Extreme attempts to control weight and shape are used and are notable for both their ingenuity and for the tenacity with which patients pursue them in the face of dangers to their health. The most common method is self-induced vomiting. The capacity to induce vomiting varies; some need to conjure up an image, while others have to stimulate their fauces. Tolerance to laxatives develops, and ever larger amounts are taken, which occasionally produces vomiting. Dehydration and severe electrolyte abnormalities can develop. Some of the most dangerous methods of weight loss are used by women with coexistent medical problems. Patients with diabetes mellitus omit their insulin and run their blood glucose at high levels, leading to coma and severe complications such as retinopathy and neuropathy (Steele, 1989). Patients with Crohn's disease fail to comply with steroid treatment, and those with thyroid disease take thyroxine to excess.

Case example
Charlotte grew up in a rural community. Her father used physical and sexual violence to control the family. She left home at the age of 16, and with little money for food she lost weight. She began to binge-eat, and self-induced vomiting and laxative misuse rapidly ensued. She binged several times a day on a gruel that she made from flour and water. Her laxative consumption gradually increased so that in the mornings, after taking a full bottle of laxatives, she vomited and was unable to walk without feeling faint. She described her body with loathing and spent over an hour each morning finding suitable clothes from her wardrobe (size range 10–16). She lost many friends because she often phoned to cancel an arrangement at the last minute if she felt too fat to go out. Her first job was in a bakers, which she quickly lost as she was caught stealing food. She was unable to maintain any job for longer than a few months as her concentration was poor and she had many days off sick. Her debt gradually increased and was a source of grave concern. She had a series of short relationships, usually with men who abused her in a variety of ways. She tried a variety of medications to control her weight. Initially she obtained diet pills from private slimming clinics, but then bought amphetamines or ecstasy. Over the years, excessive alcohol consumption became a regular part of her life, and she described being less concerned about her weight when drunk. She was regularly admitted to hospital after episodes of self-harm, which usually involved cutting herself or overdoses.

Measurement

The interviews and schedules described for anorexia nervosa also apply for bulimia nervosa. The Bulimia Investigatory Test, Edinburgh (BITE; Henderson & Freeman, 1987) is a widely used self-report questionnaire.

Differential diagnosis

As discussed in the historical section, binge-eating can accompany a variety of medical conditions. A tendency to gluttony has been described in frontal lobe dementia (Erb *et al*, 1989). Prader Willi syndrome is also associated with gross episodes of overeating, as is the Kleine-Levine syndrome.

Comorbidity

Additional psychiatric features are common; depressive and anxiety symptoms predominate. These patients often have disorders of impulse control: self-mutilation (10%), suicide attempts (30%), promiscuity (10%), and shoplifting (20%). Alcohol abuse occurs in 10–15%, and conversely, approximately a third of female alcoholic patients have a history of an eating disorder (Lacey & Moureli, 1986; Peveler & Fairburn, 1990). Patients often fulfil the criteria for borderline personality disorder, but binge-eating is one of the criteria for borderline personality disorder and so the argument is circular. Surveys using structured interviews have found that approximately 20% of cases have abnormal personalities within the dramatic cluster, and 13% have borderline personality disorder (Levine *et al*, 1986). The association between eating disorders and personality disorders is also discussed on page 765.

Epidemiology

There are few studies on the incidence of bulimia nervosa, as it has only recently been added to psychiatric case registers. A study from Holland found that the incidence of cases presenting for medical care is 11.4 per 100 000 population per year (Hoek, 1991). Estimates of the prevalence have varied as the definition has altered. Studies over the last five years have consistently found a point prevalence of 1–2% among young women (Johnson-Sabine *et al*, 1988; Bushnell *et al*, 1990). Bulimia nervosa is therefore 5–10 times more common than anorexia nervosa.

Aetiology

The aetiology of bulimia nervosa is often subsumed under the broader category of "eating disorders". This followed Russell's original observation that bulimia nervosa was a variant of anorexia nervosa. Russell (1985) later argued that bulimia nervosa was probably an example of pathoplasticity within psychiatry. He suggested that bulimia nervosa is one of the contemporary modes of presentation of a neurosis or personality disorder. However, there are antecedents and predisposing conditions which are unique to bulimia nervosa.

A history of weight loss is always present, and a third to a half of patients have a history of anorexia nervosa. Dieting increases the risk of developing bulimia nervosa eightfold (Patton *et al*, 1990; Marchi & Cohen, 1990; Tuschl, 1990). The predisposition to overeat in response to weight loss is probably a normal homeostatic response, and is seen in famines or following experimental food restriction such as the famous Minnesota starvation studies. A psychological explanation of binge-eating has been termed counter-regulation. This followed from the observation that subjects with rigid dietary rules over-ate if they broke any of the rules. One physiological explanation is that weight loss alters central 5-HT function, which in turn weakens the normal satiety response. No consistent pathophysiological features have been found. Interest has focused on cholecystokinin, noradrenaline, 5-HT, YY and neuropeptide Y (Morley & Blundell, 1988; Geracioti & Liddle, 1988; Kaye *et al*, 1990).

However, although dieting may be a necessary condition it is not sufficient. The nervosa stem of the title is also relevant. The background of patients with bulimia nervosa is similar to that of patients with other neurotic conditions. Affective disorders, alcoholism and eating disorders occur frequently in other family members (Kissett *et al*, 1989; Kendler *et al*, 1991). Family function is often disturbed, with multiple family arrangements, a lack of warmth, high levels of control and often physical and sexual abuse (Schmidt *et al*, 1991).

Assessment

As with all psychiatric conditions, treatment should only take place after a comprehensive evaluation. Eating pathology and the methods of weight control used need to be fully assessed. A physical examination and a screen for electrolyte abnormalities is required if potentially damaging weight control measures are employed. The combination of vomiting and laxative misuse can lead to an unusual combination of low potassium and acidosis. The presence of comorbidity should be established. Anxiety and depression (Laessle *et al*, 1987), personality disorder (Yates *et al*, 1989), and drug and alcohol abuse (Russell, 1979), which are common in patients with bulimia nervosa, may lead to treatment difficulties.

Social difficulties and current life stresses should be sought as they may play a role in maintaining the illness. The formulation will often encompass trauma during childhood and persisting difficulties and stresses. Patients with bulimia nervosa are initially less ambivalent about treatment than patients with anorexia nervosa. However, when they later realise that treatment may entail a sacrifice of their control over their weight and eating, the situation may reverse, leading to poor compliance. The initial assessment should focus on a patient's reasons for "giving up bulimia" because when she starts treatment the therapist can use these reasons to encourage her to persevere.

Treatment

Psychological treatment is regarded as the treatment of choice for bulimia nervosa, since numerous studies have confirmed its effectiveness in research trials. A recent meta-analysis of psychotherapy for bulimia nervosa revealed no clear advantage of one type of therapy over another, or of group over individual treatment (Hartmann *et al*, 1992).

Cognitive-behavioural therapy was introduced for the treatment of bulimia nervosa by Fairburn (1981). It is now the "gold standard" in view of its good performance when given either individually or in a group (Fairburn, 1985; Garner *et al*, 1986; Freeman *et al*, 1988), but it is costly in terms of therapist time and training. The amount of therapy time was 60 hours or more for the group in Minnesota, spread over several evenings a week (Mitchell *et al*, 1990); in the Edinburgh programme, standard cognitive–behavioural treatment was given in 16–20 sessions starting with twice-weekly meetings (Lacey, 1983).

Group approaches are cost-effective and the format and content has varied. Some are educational/behavioural/psychodynamic (for example Lacey, 1983), others emphasise a cognitive–behavioural approach (Freeman *et al*, 1988), while a third group are more psychoeducational (Olmsted *et al*, 1991). However, the organisational problems involved in forming a cohesive group suitable for each member's needs can be formidable (Freeman, 1991).

Although effective treatments for bulimia nervosa are available, we need to know more about how to apply them judiciously, matching treatment to need. Many of the therapies that have been evaluated are costly and are only available in specialised units. The next stage is to design programmes which can provide effective care within community settings, taking into account the constraints on resources. Early intervention may prevent a symptom pattern from becoming established. A stepped care approach to treatment, in which additional elements are added as patients fail to respond or only show partial improvement, is a rational development that can satisfy the service requirements (Garner *et al*, 1986; Fairburn, 1991). An outline of the approach which is being developed at the Maudsley Hospital follows (see Table 20.4).

A stepped care approach developed at the Maudsley Hospital

A stepped care approach to the treatment of bulimia nervosa allows the development of a pragmatic management plan. It is emphasised to the patient that she is an active collaborator in her own treatment and that she will be required to take responsibility for her actions. Therapists acknowledge that it will always be possible for patients to deceive them if that is what they wish, but that this behaviour is self-defeating. The therapist's role is not to act as a policeman or to "cure" a passive patient.

Step 1

Minimal interventions, particularly those which educate and empower the sufferer, can benefit those with mild or early-onset illness. The advantages for the healthcare provider are that they are cost-effective, and for the patient they avoid the possible stigmatisation associated with psychiatric referral, and can increase her sense of mastery and foster independent coping strategies.

Education and specific behavioural interventions are an integral component of the therapy. These can be given effectively in the form of a self-treatment book (Schmidt & Treasure, 1993), which can produce symptomatic improvement in a fifth of cases (Treasure *et al*, 1994). The patient is introduced to the idea that physiological and psychological factors underpin binge-eating. The concept of weight homeostasis is presented, together with the theory that overeating counterbalances weight loss.

Table 20.4 Stepped care approach to the management of bulimia nervosa

Phase of illness	Treatment	Care provider
Subclinical disorder, binge-eating disorder, or early onset bulimia nervosa with no previous treatment	Education (nutritional, weight regulation and clinical consequences of bulimia nervosa)	Self-administered, general practitioner or community psychiatric nurse
Established bulimia nervosa	Cognitive–behavioural (group or individual), possible adjunctive antidepressants	General psychiatrist Clinical psychologist
Severe disorder or significant comorbidity	Cognitive analytical or interpersonal therapy Adjunctive antidepressants Day patient care In-patient care	Specialised eating disorder unit

Similarly, compensatory overeating occurs if intervals between meals are prolonged or if food is not absorbed because of vomiting. The notion that this pattern of behaviour is circular is gradually introduced.

Instruction on the medical consequences of vomiting, laxative misuse or other weight control measures is needed. It is helpful to warn patients that laxatives do not significantly impair calorie absorption, and vomiting becomes less and less successful as a weight control measure the longer it is used.

Patients are instructed to refrain from dieting and to eat regular meals. The concept of self-monitoring in the form of a diary is introduced. Patients should be advised to read about their condition and encouraged to join a self-help organisation such as the Eating Disorders Association, which produces a newsletter and a reading list.

Step 2

Patients who fail to respond to education alone will need a more complex therapeutic approach. Motivation difficulties and self-defeating attitudes or patterns of thinking may block change. Cognitive–behavioural therapy (CBT) can tackle these difficulties. CBT can be administered as a group therapy, but in order to minimise attrition groups should have fewer than ten patients and follow a well-structured format. Homework assignments should be individualised for each patient in the group.

The mainstay of the behavioural treatment is a food diary. The patient enters into the diary eating and purging behaviour and their emotional and practical antecedents and consequences as they occur. The ultimate goal is to eat three meals with one or two small snacks regularly throughout the day, but this should be approached gradually. The therapist should be alert to the ramifications of the therapeutic alliance. On the one hand there may be a tendency to dissimulate in order to please the therapist; alternatively there may be a stubborn resistance to "play the game" and homework assignments will be jettisoned. The therapist should anticipate these two responses and explore their origin and meaning with the patient.

A variety of stimulus control techniques can help stop the urge to overeat, such as distraction, detachment, imagery and alternative behaviours including relaxation. Meals should be carefully structured in place, timing and performance. Eating should take place away from the site of food preparation. Binge triggers such as left-overs and "dangerous foods" should be controlled. Shopping should take place on a full stomach and with a list of items to buy.

A programme to minimise vomiting and laxative misuse should be implemented. One of the first stages in treatment will be to plan to eat a meal, however small, which should not be followed by vomiting. An alternative is to increase gradually the interval between a binge and vomiting. A variety of techniques (similar to those used to arrest binging) can be tried to prevent the urge to vomit. Laxative consumption should either be gradually decreased or the number of laxative-free days each week increased. Tolerance to the effects of laxatives leads to distension, discomfort and constipation during withdrawal. Soluble fibre such as that in fruit and vegetables will alleviate some of these symptoms, while insoluble fibres such as bran can exacerbate them. Any reduction in vomiting or laxative misuse may lead to weight gain due to rebound fluid retention, but this settles within two weeks.

Cognitions are usually tackled in tandem with the behavioural component, as irrational assumptions about shape and weight can be elicited using the diary as a focus. Typical dysfunctional thoughts are "eating a chocolate Easter egg will increase your weight by a stone" or "2 lbs weight increase is the forerunner of inevitable rapid weight gain". The disparagement of body image is often linked to low self-esteem. If feelings of self-worth are linked to external factors such as weight or shape or academic performance and combined with perfectionist traits, this results in unrealistic goals and assumptions. The inevitable failure to achieve the goals further diminishes self-worth. Interpersonal relationships are often characterised by the need to please others. Patients need to learn to recognise self-defeating patterns of behaviour and to use alternative strategies. Techniques such as problem-solving and assertiveness training should be taught, and the patient should consider changes in lifestyle. Relapses should be seen as inevitable, and preparation to limit the extent of a relapse is essential. When a relapse occurs it should give the patient a chance to practise behavioural strategies she has learnt.

Step 3

Patients with a severe concurrent depression or those who fail to respond to CBT, perhaps because they are unwilling to accept the treatment rationale, may be considered for pharmacological treatment. Drug treatment alone compares unfavourably with the "gold standard" psychotherapy. Even the most ardent enthusiasts for the traditional antidepressant treatment acknowledge that careful titration and rotation of antidepressants is required to prevent relapse. Also, adverse side-effects are common in this clinical setting (severe electrolyte imbalance is a contraindication to medication), and symptoms are only controlled while the treatment is maintained. Compliance is often poor. However, the combination of pharmacotherapy and psychotherapy may be of value (Agras *et al*, 1992).

The choice is between a 5-HT reuptake inhibitor such as fluvoxamine or fluoxetine (Fluoxetine Bulimia Nervosa Collaborative Study Group, 1992), or a tricyclic antidepressant such as imipramine. This decision may be based on the patient's tolerance of side-effects. Fluoxetine, although more expensive, may be of advantage in the overweight patient as it appears less likely to cause weight gain. It should probably be prescribed in a dose of 60 mg/day, while tricyclics should be prescribed in standard antidepressant doses. The optimum duration of treatment is unknown, but six months is generally regarded as appropriate (Walsh *et al*, 1991).

In view of the tendency for patients with bulimia nervosa to act impulsively, the potential risk of self-harm by overdose should be remembered. Medication should not be given to patients who are unlikely to comply with follow-up or monitoring of side-effects, or those with a history of repeated overdoses, unless indicated for the treatment of depression in which case admission may be necessary.

Step 4

It is increasingly recognised that CBT is less effective in a proportion of patients, usually those with coexistent personality difficulties. In such cases binge-eating arises as a response to dysphoric mood, rather than as a simple consequence of dietary restraint. This affective change arises as a result of low self-esteem and underlying interpersonal problems. Patients in whom CBT has failed should be referred for specialist treatment. Different approaches such as cognitive analytical therapy (Ryle, 1990), or cognitive therapy adapted for personality disorders (Beck & Freeman, 1990) or interpersonal therapy (Klerman *et al*, 1984) have been successfully used by Fairburn *et al* (1991) in bulimia nervosa. All these therapies share techniques derived from psychodynamically orientated therapies to focus on the patient's current relationships and circumstances.

Step 5

Patients with severe symptoms and comorbidity may require brief periods of hospitalisation at times of crisis or for treatment of associated conditions, for example, depression or alcohol misuse. Such an admission may serve as a break in the pathological eating pattern, but improvements are unlikely to generalise to the outside environment without additional treatment. Patients with severe electrolyte disturbances or physical illness may benefit from day patient care prior to out-patient CBT, to enable them to control their vomiting and to regularise their electrolyte imbalance. If patients fail to respond to the intensive out-patient treatment package detailed above, in-patient treatment may need to be considered. First, the patient's history and cooperation with treatment should be reviewed. Have important maintaining factors not been addressed in the therapy? Did the patient comply with treatment, completing homework assessment and self-monitoring? Have important transference issues leading to resistance been appropriately addressed? Day patient treatment is probably the treatment of choice (Piran & Kaplan, 1990), allowing the patient to remain in contact with the everyday situations that precipitate binge-eating while having an intensive therapeutic contact.

The aim of day patient treatment is not to develop new approaches to treatment, but to provide an intensive course of closely supervised therapy. Day patient care relies on a multidisciplinary approach and the peer support given by fellow patients, with the skilled nurse as the main care-provider. The patient eats on the ward, and nurses are available to help her to practise behavioural strategies to prevent vomiting or to cope with the urge to binge. Relatives and friends are encouraged to learn ways to help patients to cope with their eating, and family meetings are regarded as an important component of therapy. Participation in ward groups (such as projective art, relaxation, assertiveness training and psychodrama) is required, and an occupational therapy programme is tailored to the needs of each individual. Body-orientated exercises can help patients to address the interoceptive disturbances that are characteristic of the illness. Sessions with the dietician allow evaluation of their nutritional knowledge and help to prevent the development of a limited repertoire of safe foods. Peer group support encourages patients to be more realistic in their self-appraisal, and group discussions enable them to consider their attitudes to shape and weight in the light of societal pressures. Medication, if considered appropriate, can be safely taken under supervision, and physical complications can be monitored.

Treatment pitfalls

It is not uncommon for patients to come for sessions without doing their homework and then to blame their therapist for their lack of progress. It should be gently but firmly explained to the patient that the only person who can control her eating is herself, and that the therapist is there to help and guide her on the path to recovery. Therapists should acknowledge their own frustrations to the patient, and try to help her see the self-defeating nature of her behaviour. The patient's reasons for entering into treatment should be reviewed and used to increase her motivation. If this fails, therapists can offer a dynamic understanding of the patient's resistance. In some cases it may be necessary to suggest to the patient that she stops treatment to consider her motivation and commitment to therapy.

Patients may lie or keep secrets from the therapist, and it should be explained to the patient early on in treatment that the therapist knows the temptation to lie may be so strong at times that the patient will give into it. The therapist aims to maintain an accepting stance, giving the suspicious and defensive patient a rare opportunity to establish a trusting relationship.

Among the most serious therapeutic problems are threats or attempts at self-harm. The therapist should try to examine the context of each suicide threat, including timing. Is it related to an underlying depressive illness, to issues in the therapy or transference, or is it related to a situation in the patient's emotional life? It may be necessary to admit patients for a brief period if it is felt that they are at genuine risk of suicide.

Relapses should be expected and patients encouraged to view each relapse as a learning experience. The relapse prevention model proposed for other addictive problems (Marlett & Gordon, 1985; Wanigaratne *et al*, 1990) can be usefully applied in the context of eating disorders.

Outcome

Conflicting reports of the course of bulimia nervosa within the community have been recorded; little improvement was found in one study (King, 1991), while approximately 40% improvement was found in other studies (Yager *et al*, 1987; Patton *et al*, 1990; Fichter *et al*, 1992). In clinical populations the illness runs a relapsing and remitting course, with a recovery rate of between 50–70% after 2–5 years of illness (see Table 20.5).

Prognostic factors

The following factors are associated with a poorer outcome:

(1) psychiatric comorbidity;
(2) mixed anorexia and bulimia nervosa;
(3) severe symptoms;
(4) poor social support.

Table 20.5 Outcome studies of bulimia nervosa

Study	Year of cohort	Follow-up interval (yrs)	n	Good outcome	Poor outcome
Patton (1988)	1971–81	6–15	96	–	3[1] died
Lacey (1983)	1980–82	2	30	–	26%
Fallon *et al* (1991)	1980–87	2–9	52	39%	41%
Hsu & Sobkiewicz (1989)	1983–88	4–6	35	57%	20% 1[2] death
Herzog *et al* (1991)	1987–90	3	30	69%	21%
Fichter *et al* (1992)	1985–88	2–3	196	41%	40%

1. Two from road traffic accidents, one from malnutrition.
2. Death from hypertensive crisis treatment phenelzine.

Conclusion

In spite of the vast amount of research done since the condition was first described just over ten years ago (Russell, 1979), the treatment of bulimia nervosa remains a therapeutic challenge. The stepped care approach allows the pragmatic application of current techniques within a structured framework and should ensure that each patient receives the best possible care, given our current knowledge.

References

Agras, W. S., Rossiter, E. M., Arnow, B., *et al* (1992) Pharmacological and cognitive–behavioural treatment for bulimia nervosa: A controlled comparison. *American Journal of Psychiatry*, **149**, 82–87.

American Psychiatric Association (1987) *Diagnostic and Statistical Manual of Mental Disorders* (3rd edn, revised) (DSM–III–R). Washington, DC: APA.

—— (1994) *Diagnostic and Statistical Manual of Mental Disorders* (4th edn) (DSM–IV). Washington, DC: APA.

Beck, A. T. & Freeman, A. (1990) *Cognitive Therapy of Personality Disorders*. New York: Guilford.

Bell, R. M. (1985) *Holy Anorexia*. Chicago: University of Chicago Press.

Bhanji, S. & Mattingly, J. L. (1985) *Medical Aspects of Anorexia Nervosa*. London: Wright.

Biederman, J., Herzog, D. B., Rivinus, T.M., *et al* (1985) Amitriptyline in the treatment of anorexia nervosa: a double-blind, placebo-controlled study. *Journal of Clinical Psychopharmacology*, **5**, 10–16.

Bruch, H. (1974) *Eating Disorders: Obesity, Anorexia Nervosa and the Person Within*. London: Routledge Kegan Paul.

—— (1985) Four decades of eating disorders. In *Handbook of Psychotherapy for Anorexia Nervosa and Bulimia* (eds O. M. Garner & P. E. Garfinkel), pp 7–18. New York: Guilford.

Brumberg, J. J. (1988) *Fasting Girls: The Emergence of Anorexia Nervosa as a Modern Disease.* Cambridge, MA: Harvard University Press.

Bushnell, J. A., Wells, E., Hornblow, A. R., *et al* (1990) Prevalence of three bulimia syndromes in the general population. *Psychological Medicine*, **20**, 671–680.

Cantwell, D. P., Sturzenburger, S., Burroughs, J., *et al* (1977) Anorexia nervosa: an affective disorder? *Archives of General Psychiatry*, **34**, 1087–1090.

Cooper, Z. & Fairburn, C. G. (1987) The Eating Disorder Examination. A semi-structured interview for the assessment of the specific psychopathology of eating disorders. *International Journal of Eating Disorders*, **6**, 1–8.

Crisp, A. H. (1980) *Anorexia Nervosa: Let Me Be.* London: Plenum.

——, Lacey, J. H. & Crutchfield, M. (1987) Clomipramine and 'drive' in people with anorexia nervosa: an inpatient study. *British Journal of Psychiatry*, **150**, 355–358.

——, Norton, K., Gowers, S., *et al* (1991) A controlled study of the effect of therapies aimed at adolescent and family psychopathology in anorexia nervosa. *British Journal of Psychiatry*, **159**, 325–333.

——, Callender, J. S., Halek, C., *et al* (1992) Long term mortality in anorexia nervosa. A 20-year follow-up of the St George's and Aberdeen Cohorts. *British Journal of Psychiatry*, **161**, 104–107.

Curzon, G. (1992) Serotonin and eating disorders: pharmacological relationships. *International Academy of Biomedical Drug Research*, **1**, 112–128.

Dally, P. J. (1969) *Anorexia Nervosa.* London: Heinemann.

—— & Sargant, W. (1960) A new treatment of anorexia nervosa. *British Medical Journal*, **2**, 793–796.

Erb, J. L., Gwirtsman, H. E., Fuster, J. M., *et al* (1989) Bulimia associated with frontal lobe lesions. *International Journal of Eating Disorders*, **8**, 117–121.

Fairburn, C. G. (1981) A cognitive behavioural approach to the management of bulimia. *Psychological Medicine*, **11**, 707–711.

—— (1985) A cognitive–behavioural treatment of bulimia nervosa. In Handbook of Psychotherapy for Anorexia and Bulimia (eds O. M. Garner & P. E. Garfinkel). New York: Guilford.

—— (1991) The heterogeneity of bulimia nervosa and its implications for treatment. *Journal of Psychosomatic Research*, **35**, 3–9.

——, Jones, R., Peveler, R. C., *et al* (1991) Three psychological treatments for bulimia nervosa: a comparative trial. *Archives of General Psychiatry*, **48**, 463–469.

Fallon, B. A., Walsh, B. T., Sadik, C., *et al* (1991) Outcome and clinical course in inpatient bulimic women: A 2- to 9- year follow-up study. *Journal of Clinical Psychiatry*, **52**, 272–278.

Fichter, M. M., Quadflieg, N. & Reif, W. (1992) The course of eating disorders. In *The Course of Eating Disorders* (eds W. Herzog, H. C. Deter & W. Vandereycken), pp. 133–149. Heidelberg: Springer.

Fluoxetine Bulimia Nervosa Collaborative Study Group (1992) Fluoxetine in the treatment of bulimia nervosa: a multicenter, placebo-controlled double-blind trial. *Archives of General Psychiatry*, **49**, 139–147.

Fowler, R. (1871) *A Complete History of the Case of the Welsh Fasting Girl (Sarah Jacob).* London: Henry Renshaw.

Freeman, C. P. (1991) A practical guide to the treatment of bulimia nervosa. *Journal of Psychosomatic Research*, **35** (suppl. 1), 41–47.

——, Barry, F., Dunkeld-Turnbull, J., *et al* (1988) Controlled trial of psychotherapy for bulimia nervosa. *British Medical Journal*, **296**, 521–525.

Garner, D. M. & Garfinkel, P. E. (1979) The Eating Attitudes Test: An index of the symptoms of anorexia nervosa. *Psychological Medicine*, 9, 273–279.

——, Olmsed, M. P. & Polivy, J. (1983) Development and validation of a multidimensional eating disorder inventory for anorexia nervosa and bulimia. *International Journal of Eating Disorders*, 2, 15–34.

——, Garfinkel, P. E. & Irvine, M. J. (1986) Integration and sequencing of treatment approaches for eating disorders. *Psychotherapy and Psychosomatics*, 46, 67–75.

Geracioti, T. D. & Liddle, R. A. (1988) Impaired cholecystokinin secretion in bulimia nervosa. *New England Journal of Medicine*, 319, 683–688.

Goldberg, S. C., Halmi, K. A., Eckert, R. C., *et al* (1979) Cyproheptidine in anorexia nervosa. *British Journal of Psychiatry*, 134, 67–70.

Goldner, E. M., McKenzie, J. M. & Kline S. A. (1991) The ethics of forced feeding in anorexia nervosa. *Journal of the Canadian Medical Association*, 144, 1205.

Goodwin, G. M. (1990) Neuroendocrine function and the biology of the eating disorders. *Human Psychopharmacology*, 5, 249–253.

Gull, W. W. (1868) The address in medicine to the Annual Meeting of the British Medical Association at Oxford. *Lancet*, Aug. 8, 171–176.

—— (1873) Proceedings of the Clinical Society of London. *British Medical Journal*, 1, 527–529.

Halmi, K. A. (1985) Relationship of the eating disorders to depression: biological similarities and differences. *International Journal of Eating Disorders*, 4, 667–680.

——, Eckert, E. & Cohen, J. (1986) Anorexia nervosa: treatment efficacy of cyproheptidine and amitriptyline. *Archives of General Psychiatry*, 43, 177–181.

——, ——, Marchi, P., *et al* (1991) Comorbidity of psychiatric diagnosis in anorexia nervosa. *Archives of General Psychiatry*, 48, 718.

Hartmann, A., Herzog, T. & Drinkman, A. (1992) Psychotherapy of bulimia nervosa: what is effective? A meta-analysis. *Journal of Psychosomatics*, 36, 159–167.

Henderson, M. & Freeman, C. L. (1987) A self-rating scale for bulimia. The BITE. *British Journal of Psychiatry*, 150, 168–174.

Herzog, T., Hartman, A., Sandholz, Z., *et al* (1991) Prognostic factors in outpatient psychotherapy of bulimia. *Psychotherapy and Psychosomatics*, 54, 48–55.

Hoek, H. W. (1991) The incidence and prevalence of anorexia nervosa and bulimia nervosa in primary care. *Psychological Medicine*, 21, 455–460.

Holland, A. J., Sicotte, N. & Treasure, J. L. (1988) Anorexia nervosa: evidence for a genetic basis. *Journal of Psychosomatic Research*, 32, 561–571.

Hsu, L. K. G., Crisp, A. H. & Harding, B. (1979) Outcome of anorexia nervosa. *Lancet*, i, 62–65.

—— & Sobkiewicz, T. A. (1989) Bulimia nervosa: a four-to-six year follow-up study. *Psychological Medicine*, 19, 1035–1038.

—— & —— (1991) Body image disturbance: time to abandon the concept for eating disorders. *International Journal of Eating Disorders*, 10, 15–30.

Johnson Sabine, E., Wood, K., Patton, G., *et al* (1988) Abnormal eating attitudes in London school-girls – a prospective epidemiological study: factors associated with abnormal response on screening questionnaires. *Psychological Medicine*, 18, 615–622.

Kasvikis, Y. G., Tsakiris, F., Marks, I. M., *et al* (1986) Past history of anorexia nervosa in women with obsessive–compulsive disorder. *International Journal of Eating Disorders*, 5, 1069–1075.

Kaye, W. H., Berrettini, W., Gwirtsman, H., *et al* (1990) Altered cerebrospinal fluid neuropeptide Y and peptide YY immunoreactivity in anorexia and bulimia nervosa. *Archives of General Psychiatry*, **47**, 548–556.

Kendler, K. S., MacLean, C., Neal, M., *et al* (1991) The genetic epidemiology of bulimia nervosa. *American Journal of Psychiatry*, **148**, 1627–1637.

Keys, A., Brozak, J., Henshall, A., *et al* (1950) *The Biology of Human Starvation*, Vol II, 850–857. Minneapolis: University of Minnesota Press.

King, M. B. (1991) The natural history of eating pathology in attenders to primary medical care. *International Journal of Eating Disorders*, **10**, 379–387.

Kissett, J. A., Gershon, E. S., Maxwell, M. E., *et al* (1989) Psychiatric disorders in first degree relatives of probands with bulimia nervosa. *American Journal of Psychiatry*, **146**, 1468–1471.

Klerman, G. L., Weissman, M. M., Rounsaville, B. J., *et al* (1984) *Interpersonal Therapy*. New York: Basic Books.

Lacey, J. H. (1983) Bulimia nervosa, binge eating and psychogenic vomiting: a controlled treatment study and long term outcome. *British Medical Journal*, **286**, 1609–1613.

—— & Crisp, A. H. (1980) Hunger, food intake and weight: the impact of clomipramine on a refeeding anorexia nervosa population. *Postgraduate Medical Journal*, **56**, 79–85.

—— & Moureli, E. (1986) Bulimic alcoholics: some features of a clinical subgroup. *British Journal of Addiction*, **81**, 389–393.

Laessle, R. G., Zoettl, C. & Pirke, K. (1987) Meta-analysis of treatment studies for bulimia. *International Journal of Eating Disorders*, **6**, 97–110.

Lasegue, E. C. (1873) On hysterical anorexia. *Medical Times Gazette*, **2**, 265–269.

Lee, S. (1991) Anorexia nervosa in Hong Kong: a Chinese perspective. *Psychological Medicine*, **21**, 703–712.

Levin, A. P. & Hyler, S. E. (1986) DSM–III personality diagnosis in bulimia. Comprehensive Psychiatry, 27, 47–53.

Littlewood, R. (1992) DSM–IV and culture: is the classification internationally valid? *Psychiatric Bulletin*, **16**, 257–261.

Lucas, A. R., Beard, M. C., O'Fallon, M. W., *et al* (1991) 50-year trends in the incidence of anorexia nervosa in Rochester, Minn.: a population-based study. *American Journal of Psychiatry*, **148**, 917–922.

Marcé, L. A. (1860) On a form of hypochondriacal delirium occurring consecutive to dyspepsia and characterized by refusal of food. *Journal of Psychological Medicine and Mental Pathology*, **13**, 204–206.

Marchi, M. & Cohen, P. (1990) Early childhood eating behaviours and adolescent eating disorders. *Journal of the American Academy of Child and Adolescent Psychiatry*, **29**, 112–117.

Marlett, G. A. & Gordon, J, R. (1985) *Relapse Prevention: Maintenance Strategies in the Treatment of Addictive Behaviours.*

Minuchin, S., Rosman, B. L., Liebman, R., *et al* (1978) *Psychosomatic Families: Anorexia Nervosa in Context.* Harvard, MA: Harvard University Press.

Mitchell, J. E., Pyle, R. L., Eckert, E. D., *et al* (1990) A comparison study of antidepressants and structured intensive group psychotherapy in the treatment of bulimia nervosa. *Archives of General Psychiatry*, **47**, 149–157.

Morgan, H. G., Purgold, J. & Welbourne, J. (1983) Management and outcome in anorexia nervosa: A standardised prognosis study. *British Journal of Psychiatry*, **143**, 282–287.

Morley, J. E. & Blundell, J. E. (1988) The neurobiological basis of eating disorders: some formulations. *Biological Psychiatry*, **23**, 53–78.

Morton, R. (1694) *Phthisiologia: Or, a Treatise of Consumptions*. London: Smith & Walford.

Mumford, D. B., Whitehouse, A. M. & Platts, M. (1991) Eating disorders among Asian schoolgirls in Bradford: socio-cultural correlates. *British Journal of Psychiatry*, **158**, 222–228.

Myrtle, A. S. (1888) Letters to the Editor. *Lancet*, 1, 899.

Olmsted, P. M., Davis, R., Rockert, W., *et al* (1991) Efficacy of a brief group psychoeducational intervention for bulimia nervosa. *Behavioural Research Therapy*, **29**, 71–83.

Orbach, S. (1986) *Hunger Strike*. Harmondsworth: Penguin.

Palmer, R. L., Oppenheimer, R., Dignon, A., *et al* (1990) Childhood sexual experiences with adults reported by women with eating disorders: an extended series. *British Journal of Psychiatry*, **156**, 699–703.

Parry-Jones, B. & Parry-Jones, W. Ll. (1990) Bulimia: an archival review of its history. *Psychosomatic Medicine*, **10**, 129–143.

Patton, G. (1988) Mortality and eating disorders. *Psychological Medicine*, **18**, 947–951.

—, Johnson-Sabine, E., Wood, K., *et al* (1990) Abnormal eating attitudes in London schoolgirls: a prospective epidemiological study. Outcome at twelve month follow up. *Psychological Medicine*, **20**, 383–394.

Peveler, R. & Fairburn, C. (1990) Eating disorders in women who abuse alcohol. *British Journal of Addiction*, **85**, 1633–1638.

Piran, N. & Kaplan, A. (eds) (1990) *A Day Hospital Group Treatment Program for Anorexia Nervosa and Bulimia Nervosa*. New York: Brunner/Mazel.

—, —, Kerr, A., *et al* (1990) A day hospital program for anorexia nervosa and bulimia. *International Journal of Eating Disorders*, **8**, 511–521.

Playfair, W. S. (1888) Note on the so-called anorexia nervosa. *Lancet*, 1, 817.

Rastam, M., Gillberg, C. & Garton, M. (1989) Anorexia nervosa in a Swedish urban region: a population-based study. *British Journal of Psychiatry*, **155**, 642–646.

Ratnasuriya, R. H., Eisler, I., Szmuckler, G. I., *et al* (1991) Anorexia nervosa: outcome and prognostic factors after 20 years. *British Journal of Psychiatry*, **158**, 495–502.

Roberts, A. (1992) Judges explain why anorexia must be treated. *The Times*, 11 July.

Russell, G. F. M. (1977) Editorial: The present status of anorexia nervosa. *Psychological Medicine*, **1**, 363–367.

— (1979) Bulimia nervosa: an ominous variant of anorexia nervosa. *Psychological Medicine*, **9**, 429–488.

— (1985) Premenarchal anorexia nervosa and its sequelae. *Journal of Psychiatric Research*, **19**, 363–369.

—, Szmukler, G. I., Dare, C., *et al* (1987) An evaluation of family therapy in anorexia nervosa and bulimia nervosa. *Archives of General Psychiatry*, **44**, 1047–1056.

Ryle, A. (1990) *Cognitive-Analytic Therapy: Active Participation in Change. A New Integration in Brief Psychotherapy*. Chichester: John Wiley.

Ryle, J. A. (1936) Anorexia nervosa. *Lancet*, ii, 893–899.

Schmidt, U., Tiller, J. M. & Treasure, J. L. (1991) Psychosocial factors in the origins of bulimia nervosa. *International Review of Psychiatry*, **5**, 51–60.

— & Treasure, J. (1993) *Getting Better Bit(e) by Bit(e)*. London: Lawrence Erlbaum.

Slade, P. D. (1982) Towards a functional analysis of anorexia nervosa and bulimia nervosa. *British Journal of Clinical Psychology*, 21, 167–179.

Solzhenitsyn, A. (1963) *One Day in the Life of Ivan Denisovitch*. Harmondsworth: Penguin.

Steinhausen, H. C., Rauss-Mason, C. & Seidel, R. (1991) Follow-up studies of anorexia nervosa: a review of four decades of outcome research. *Psychological Medicine*, 21, 447–454.

Strober, M. & Katz, J. L. (1987) Do eating disorders and affective disorders share a common etiology? A dissenting opinion. *International Journal of Eating Disorders*, 6, 171–180.

Strober, M., Lampert, C., Morrell, W., *et al* (1990) A controlled family study of anorexia nervosa: evidence of familial aggregation and lack of shared transmission with affective disorders. International *Journal of Eating Disorders*, 9, 239–254.

Stunkard, A. J. (1959) Eating patterns and obesity. *Psychiatric Quality*, 33, 284–292.

Szmukler, G. I. (1982) Drug treatment of anorexic states. In *Drugs and Appetite* (ed. J. T. Silverstone), pp. 159–181. London: Academic Press.

——, McCance, C. & McCrone, L. (1986) Anorexia nervosa: a psychiatric case register study from Aberdeen. *Psychological Medicine*, 16, 49–58.

Theander, S. (1970) Anorexia nervosa: a psychiatric investigation of 94 female patients. *Acta Psychiatrica Scandinavica*, suppl. 214, 5–194.

—— (1985) Outcome and prognosis in anorexia nervosa and bulimia: some results of previous investigations compared with those of a Swedish long-term study. *Journal of Psychiatric Research*, 19, 492–508.

Tolstrup, K., Brinch, M., Isager, T., *et al* (1985) Long-term outcome of 151 cases of anorexia nervosa. *Acta Psychiatrica Scandinavica*, 71, 380–387.

Treasure, J. L. (1995) Eating disorders. In *Handbook* (ed. W. Studd). London: Royal College of Obstetrics and Gynaecology.

—— & Holland, A. J. (1993) What can discordant twins tell us about the aetiology of anorexia nervosa? In *Advances in the Neurosciences Vol. 90. Primary and Secondary Eating Disorders: A Psychoneuroendocrine and Metabolic Approach* (eds E. Ferrari, F. Brambilla & S. B. Solerte), pp. 113–122. Oxford: Pergamon Press.

—— & Campbell, I. (1994) The case for biology in the aetiology of anorexia nervosa. *Psychological Medicine*, 21, 3–8.

——, Schmidt, U., Troop, N., *et al* (1994) The first step in the management of bulimia nervosa. A controlled trial of a therapeutic manual. *British Medical Journal*, 308, 686–689.

—— & Szmukler, G. I. (1995) Medical and surgical complications of chronic anorexia nervosa. In *Handbook of Eating Disorders: Theory, Treatment and Research* (eds G. Szmukler, C. Dare & J. L. Treasure), p. 197–220. Chichester: Wiley.

——, Todd, G. & Szmukler, G. (1995) The inpatient treatment of anorexia nervosa. In *Handbook of Eating Disorders: Theory, Treatment and Research* (eds G. Szmukler, C. Dare & J. L. Treasure), pp. 275–292. Chichester: Wiley.

Tuschl, R. J. (1990) From dietary restraint to binge eating: some theoretical considerations. *Appetite*, 14, 105–109.

Vandereycken, W. & Pierloot, R. (1983) Combining drugs and behaviour therapy in anorexia nervosa: a double blind placebo/pimozide study. In *Anorexia Nervosa: Recent Developments in Research* (eds P. L. Darby, P. E. Garfinkel, D. M. Garner, *et al*), pp. 365–376. New York: Alan Liss.

Vigersky, R. A. & Loriaux, D. L. (1977) The effect of cyproheptidine in anorexia nervosa: A double blind trial. In *Anorexia Nervosa* (ed. R. Vigersky), pp. 349–356. New York: Raven Press.

Walsh, T. B., Hadigan, C. M., Devlin, M. J., *et al* (1991) Long-term outcome of antidepressant treatment for bulimia nervosa. *American Journal of Psychiatry*, **148**, 1206–1212.

Wanigaratne, S., Wallace, W., Pullin, J., *et al* (1990) *Relapse Prevention for Addictive Disorders*. Oxford: Blackwell.

Willi, J., Giacometti, G. & Limacher, B. (1990) Update on the epidemiology of anorexia nervosa in a defined region of Switzerland. *American Journal of Psychiatry*, **147**, 1514–1517.

World Health Organization (1992) *The Tenth International Classification of Diseases and Related Health Problems*. Geneva: WHO.

Yager, J., Landsverk, J. & Edelstein, C. K. (1987) A 20-month follow-up study of 628 women with eating disorders. 1: course and severity. *American Journal of Psychiatry*, **144**, 1172–1177.

Yates, W. R., Seileni, B., Reich, J., *et al* (1989) Co-morbidity of bulimia nervosa and personality disorder. *Journal of Clinical Psychiatry*, **50**, 57–59.

21 Postpartum and related disorders

George Stein

Puerperal psychoses ● Non-psychotic postnatal depression ●
Maternity blues ● Measurement ● Pregnancy ● Cross-cultural aspects
● Still birth ● Miscarriage ● Termination of pregnancy ●
Premenstrual syndrome ● The menopause

The first recorded clinical description of postpartum mental illness was written in the 4th century BC by Hippocrates (Hamilton, 1962). He cited the case of the wife of Epicrates who gave birth to twins, then developed severe insomnia and became restless on the sixth day, was delirious on the 11th day and died on the 17th day. Hippocrates offered two explanations: firstly, that the lochia had been suppressed and redirected to the brain and this caused mania; and secondly, that there was an influx of blood into the breasts. Bleeding from the nipple after delivery was regarded as a particularly ominous sign. Esquirol (1845) quoting earlier authors wrote that milk deposits were formed in the brain, and this caused insanity by compressing the brain, or by distending its fibres.

It was not until the early part of the 19th century that a firm distinction was made between the puerperal mania caused by sepsis and the mania caused by insanity. Gooch (1829), a lecturer in midwifery at St Bartholomew's Hospital, divided puerperal mania into two types, the one fatal and the other not.

> "Women who are out of their senses attended with fever-like paraphrenitis will, in all probability, die: but when without fever it is not fatal. I have several private patients where a great number of stimulating medicines and blisters have been applied, but they have gone on talking nonsense till the disease has gone off and they have become sensible." (Gooch, 1829)

Meanwhile in France, Esquirol (1845) published his textbook *Des Maladies Mentale*, which included a lengthy chapter entitled "Mental alienation of those recently confined and of nursing women". Esquirol's brilliant pupil Marcé (1858) went on to make the most substantive contribution to the 19th century literature, publishing a whole book on the topic, which included over 310 cases, of which 79 were his own. Nine per cent began during pregnancy, 58% had a "puerperal" psychosis because the illness started during the first six weeks after childbirth, and a further 33% had a "lactational psychosis" because the illness started more than six weeks after childbirth. Marcé described these illnesses in

903

detail, highlighting the ways in which they both resembled and differed from non-puerperal mental disorder. The question as to whether puerperal disorders are a separate group of illnesses, or are merely psychoses that have been triggered by childbirth, has been a recurring theme both in the 19th century and more recently.

During the second half of the 19th century and the early 20th century, interest in the topic grew and psychiatric textbooks of this period such as that by Savage (1875) often described the puerperal and lactational psychoses. The puerperal psychoses continued to have an appreciable mortality of around 10%, mainly due to infection, debility and suicide, but the introduction of electroconvulsive therapy (ECT) led to a dramatic fall in the mortality of the illness. Today the prognosis is generally held to be good, although there are still occasional suicides.

Finally, the earlier policy of separating a mother from her infant during a postnatal illness was called into question when Main (1958) arranged the first joint admission for a mother and her baby to the Cassell Hospital, and so ushered in the modern practice of joint admissions for mothers and babies to psychiatric hospitals.

Puerperal psychoses

The illness commonly starts on the fourth or fifth day, with mood changes, some confusion or even delirium. In some cases there is a symptom-free latent interval during the first two to three days. Not all cases start on the fourth or fifth day, but Brockington *et al* (1982) estimated that most will have started during the first two weeks.

Savage (1875) likened puerperal delirium to alcohol withdrawal states:

> ". . . a condition hardly to be distinguished from delirium tremens in which there are hallucinations of the senses, such as the seeing of vermin and the smelling of foul odours and the same creamy tongue tending to dryness and the same restless tremulousness; refusal of food is a common symptom."

The sleep disorder was described as "miserable sleeplessness". Karnosh & Hope (1937) described puerperal delirium as:

> "panic, sudden aversion and mistrust of relatives, misidentification, hallucinosis, singsong chat, and disintegration of poor affect together with a rapid pulse and a fever ranging from 99°–102°F. This delirium usually abates but mania, depression, schizophrenia, occasionally normality and rarely even death may ensue."

Today puerperal delirium may still be associated with a mild fever, but this is rarely due to infection. Martin (1958) noted that 2.6% of her cases with puerperal psychosis had a toxic confusional picture associated with an infective cause.

Affective disorders

Puerperal mania is among the most florid conditions encountered in psychiatric practice, and the motor symptoms of mania, hyperactivity and distractibility are marked. The onset may be abrupt, but more often there is increasing irritability or elation, with severe blues around the fourth or fifth day postpartum. Sleep is invariably severely disturbed, with patients waking in the early hours and then displaying manic behaviour. Some women have a pleasant or humorous grandiosity, but many are paranoid or querulous, believing themselves to be totally competent mothers and fiercely resenting any suggestion otherwise. A degree of sexual disinhibition is common. One patient, after trying to throw herself through a closed window pane, arrived in hospital wearing pink high-heeled shoes, sprayed herself heavily with perfume, and told the ward staff she had come to a party. Savage (1875) wrote "patients are often seized with an erotic tendency, I have several times judged a case of insanity to be puerperal from the mincing gait and lascivious looks of the patient". Patients with puerperal manias tend to have more confusion, disorganised communications, are less competent and require more in the way of task supervision than patients with non-puerperal mania (Brockington *et al*, 1982). Some episodes of puerperal mania switch into depression, which may persist over the next few months, but others may settle into euthymia without passing through a depressive phase. Occasionally mixed affective states are encountered postpartum, and these are particularly dangerous because they combine the boundless energy of the manic with the suicidal urges of the depressive.

Depressive disorders

Around half of the women admitted for puerperal psychoses are suffering from a depressive disorder, usually psychotic depression, and these illnesses follow around one in a thousand deliveries (Kendell *et al*, 1987). Savage (1875) provides a good description:

> ". . . the melancholy patients are generally pale and sallow, averse to tasting food from some other hallucination of hearing or other cause. They suffer from constipation and often from uneasy feelings about the epigastrium, and according to Marcé they may have analgesia at the nape of the neck, the forearm or the epigastrium. As in mania we have to be on our guard against infanticide. Suicide is, however, the chief danger. This is often attempted under the delusion that the patient is deserted, ruined or cursed. Some attempt it jumping out of the window, others fancying themselves watched, others fancying they are ordered by God to do it, others that they may save their souls or their honour; but the most anxious cases are those that are impulsively suicidal. These patients exhibit no delusions but never miss a chance of self-destruction."

Hospitalisation for depression usually occurs at the request of relatives, nursing staff on the postnatal wards, or other referring agencies who are fearful for the life of either the mother or the baby. The main indications are stupor, not eating and drinking, severe depressive delusions, suicidal thoughts with intent, infanticidal urges, severe rejection of the infant or when the infant is thought to be at serious risk. Delusional beliefs that the baby would be better off dead or adopted or should be in another family are common. Some women harbour very active suicidal thoughts, but others just wish they would never wake up. Patients with puerperal depression tend to have more in the way of delusions and are more often treated with ECT than patients with non-puerperal depression (Katona, 1982). A small number of single women with milder depressions, but more severe associated personality disorder and social problems, may also gain admission to psychiatric mother and baby units.

Puerperal schizophrenia

Puerperal schizophrenia is rare, and figures of 4–16% of cases of puerperal psychoses are given in most UK series (Davidson & Robertson, 1985; Kendell *et al*, 1987). Higher rates are reported from some non-Western countries, such as 22–34% in India (Shah *et al*, 1971; Agrawal *et al*, 1990), even when modern diagnostic criteria are used. Most cases of puerperal schizophrenia are the result of pregnancies occurring in women with previous schizophrenia, although in some instances the schizophrenia may start for the first time after childbirth. Although rare, the prognosis is much worse than for puerperal affective disorder, and the ability to care for the new-born infant is often severely impaired.

As with the other puerperal psychoses, schizophrenia may have a delirious onset and this may progress through both manic and melancholic phases before the full picture of "dementia" emerges (Savage, 1875), and the disorder is then indistinguishable from non-puerperal schizophrenia. Delusions and hallucinations often focus around the baby; thus one woman with previous paranoid delusions believed her baby to be a cat. Another, with catatonic features and marked echolalia, began to scream loudly every time her baby cried. Most authorities do not believe that puerperal schizophrenia comprises a separate schizophrenic subgroup. Hays (1978) suggested there may be a special subgroup of patients with schizophrenia with a greater predilection to puerperal relapses.

Schizoaffective disorder

Schizoaffective cases occur in between 7% (Kendell *et al*, 1987) and 25% of cases (Klompenhouwer & Van Hulst, 1991). The distinction from schizophrenia is not always easy, as the delusions are often similar.

Case example 1

Jane became confused almost immediately after delivery, gradually become more depressed and was admitted at five days postpartum. She expressed a delusional belief that her husband was an imposter, and also feared that her baby would be sexually abused by a child molester, and asked her doctor to teach her baby not to talk to strangers. She was unable to cope with the day-to-day management of her baby because she said opposing forces were inserting clicks into her mind. After a four-month admission with little improvement, the addition of lithium to her phenothiazines led to a rapid resolution of her illness, and her diagnosis was changed from schizophrenia to schizoaffective disorder.

Distinguishing schizoaffective disorder from schizophrenia is important because the prognosis with regard to infant care is generally excellent in schizoaffective cases, but sometimes poor in schizophrenia.

Mixed pictures

Many cases of puerperal psychoses present with a mixture of schizophreniform, affective and organic features, particularly confusion. Brockington *et al* (1982) has likened these atypical illnesses to cycloid psychoses (see page 494). In some studies this category of puerperal psychosis is classified under the group "psychotic disorders not otherwise specified", and the variable use of the term in different series has contributed greatly to the diagnostic confusion. Thus a recent UK study found only 10% of cases fitted this group (Kendell *et al*, 1987), while a Dutch study found 30% (Klompenhouwer & Van Hulst, 1991) and in India as many as 47% had mixed pictures of this type (Agrawal *et al*, 1990). It should also be noted that a small number of patients may only be ill for a few days or a week or two; these subjects are not always admitted to hospital and are best classified as having "brief psychosis".

Epidemiology

Puerperal psychosis is an uncommon disorder, and the original estimate of 2.2 per 1000 deliveries by Marcé (1858) has stood the test of time. Similar figures have recently been reported from Scotland (Kendell *et al*, 1987) and England (Meltzer & Kumar, 1985), but published figures range from between 2.2 to 6.8 per 1000 (Janssen, 1964), the latter including 2/1000 cases admitted to a mental hospital and 4.8/1000 being admitted to a university hospital where perhaps the illnesses were rather less severe. The condition is described in most countries where psychiatric services exist, but there are few thorough population-based epidemiological studies that examine all cases drawn from a defined geographical area.

Paffenbarger (1964) examined all the case notes of women aged between 15 and 44 who were admitted to either public or private hospitals in Hamilton County, Ohio, during the years 1940–1958. He identified 314 patients with first episodes of mental illnesses associated with childbirth. Seventy-two had their onset during pregnancy (between 7–9 per month) which was lower than in non-childbearing women; 242 occurred during the first six months postpartum, but the most dramatic rise was in the first month when 164 women became ill. A puerperal psychosis was associated with increased age and a perinatal death, but only with one obstetric complication, cervical dystocia (failure of cervical dilation). Contrary to expectation, there was no increased risk for single parenthood or lower social class.

In a Scottish study, information from the Edinburgh psychiatric case register was matched with data from the Scottish maternity discharge computer for all women who had delivered in Edinburgh for the years 1970–1978 (Kendell *et al*, 1987). As in Paffenbarger's study there was a dramatic rise in the admission rate during the first month after delivery, but the admission rate remained high for up to two years after childbirth.

Pregnancy was also found to be a time of decreased psychiatric morbidity, and the relative risk of admission during pregnancy was 0.65. The relative risk for admission for the first two postpartum years was elevated at 3.8. Even if the high-risk period of the first 90 days was excluded, the risk of admission still remained raised at 2.1. Risks were greatest for the first month, when the relative risk for admission for psychosis was 22. If only primigravid women are considered this relative risk rises to 35. Risk factors of this magnitude are unusual in medicine and otherwise almost unheard of in psychiatry, and are presumably due to some biological factor, the nature of which presently remains elusive.

Aetiology

Heredity

"It is a fact," wrote Savage (1875) "that the neuroses of pregnancy and childbirth are often associated with a hereditary tendency." Thuwe (1974), pooling the data of ten series published between 1911 and 1973, found that 40% of 614 cases had a positive family history of mental illness. Illnesses in the relatives were not confined to the psychoses, but rather there was a mixture of depression, manic–depression, psychopathy, alcoholism and suicide. Thuwe also found that around 10% of the children of patients with puerperal psychosis developed an acute psychotic illness later in life, and this was a six-fold increase over the rate in the control groups. In a large family study, Protheroe (1969) reported that for female probands with a puerperal affective disorder, the risk for any affective disorder for siblings was 10% and for parents 14.7%, and these figures were similar to those reported for probands with non-puerperal affective disorder. Very few of the affective episodes in the relatives were associated with childbirth, and Protheroe (1969) concluded that while the tendency for affective disorder might run in families, there was little evidence that puerperal psychosis itself was familial. Also, around 10% of the first-degree relatives had a psychiatric disorder, and in all except one case this was schizophrenia (Protheroe, 1969). Similarly, probands with puerperal mania had fewer affected first-degree relatives than probands with non-puerperal mania, suggesting that there is less genetic loading in cases of puerperal mania (Kadramas *et al*, 1980). Childbirth may be a more potent trigger, so that even those with low genetic loading can be precipitated into developing mania following delivery (Kendell *et al*, 1987).

Previous constitution

Most series highlight the importance of the previous psychiatric history. Janssen (1964) found around a third of his patients with puerperal psychosis had previously been admitted to hospital, which is similar to the rate found in the non-puerperal control psychiatric patients but much higher than the 0.7% found among normal controls. Previous affective disorder appears to be more common than a previous history of schizophrenia, thus Kendell *et al* (1987) found that 21% of those with a previous affective illness but only 3.4% with a schizophrenic illness later developed a puerperal psychosis. Even the latter rate is much higher than the population base-rate of 0.2%. A manic–depressive diathesis appears to be the main constitutional as well as heritable component in puerperal psychosis.

Social factors

Savage (1875) thought that psychosocial factors were of little relevance for this disorder and wrote:

> "I have been much struck at seeing how few cases could be traced to fright, grief, losses, etc. No doubt my cases being nearly all taken from respectable married women do not include those in whom shame and grief play the chief part in causation. It is in the lower orders and after illegitimate births that we should find most instances of that kind."

These early observations have been confirmed in two recent studies that showed that life events are not associated with severe postpartum depressive psychoses (Brockington *et al*, 1990; Dowlatschahi & Paykel, 1990). Social class is also unrelated, although there is an increased rate of admission for single women. Increased rates of psychoses are found for caesarian section, perinatal death and in single mothers, all of which might be considered to be stressful situations, although the size of the effect is uncertain (Kendell *et al*, 1987). Hormonal and biochemical hypotheses are discussed below.

The problem of classification

Are puerperal illnesses schizophrenic episodes, organic psychoses, affective disorders, or a completely separate category on their own? The latter position has never been generally accepted, and so ICD–10 does not accord them a separate category, but there has been some move in this direction in DSM–IV. Although obstetric conditions have greatly improved, puerperal psychosis itself has changed little over the last 150 years, but as diagnostic fashions have come and gone, so the manner in which the puerperal psychoses have been classified has shown considerable variation. Thus the phenomenology of the illness itself as measured by the frequency of individual symptoms has changed little over the last 100 years, because when modern diagnostic criteria were applied to a group of 19th century cases, Rehmann *et al* (1990) found a similar frequency for individual symptoms as well as an equally high rate for affective disorder as is found today. Also, in most series there is a sizeable number of mixed or atypical cases (which could be placed in almost any category) and this tends to confuse the nosology. Most 19th century writers, such as Esquirol (1845), considered that these illnesses were either mania, depression or monomania (a type of delusional disorder), with a few cases of "schizophrenia". By the turn of the century, following the discovery of bacteria, there was renewed interest in organic causes. High rates of delirium were reported; in one series 34% of the cases had delirium with infection being suspected as a possible cause (Strecker & Ebaugh, 1926). During the 1950s, the steep fall in mortality following the introduction of ECT and antibiotics led to greater prominence being given to the role of functional psychoses, and in some American series schizophrenia comprised more than 50% of the cases (Pugh *et al*, 1963). More recently, the introduction of lithium and antidepressants has led to a further reappraisal, and the modern view is once more similar to that of the Victorian era, that most puerperal illnesses are affective in origin (Kendell *et al*, 1987).

Present classification in ICD–10 and DSM–IV

ICD–10 (World Health Organization, 1992) states that most postpartum illnesses are affective in origin and should be classified in their respective affective category, such as depression, mania, and so on. In order to code these disorders, the relevant psychiatric code from the affective disorders section is used. To show that onset was associated with childbirth, a code in the obstetric section (099.3) of ICD–10, "Mental diseases and diseases of the nervous system complicating the puerperium", is then added. ICD–10 also includes a short section on puerperal disorders which are not classified elsewhere. These should have commenced within six weeks of delivery and are entitled "Mental and behavioural disorders associated with the puerperium not classified elsewhere". Three groups are recognised: mild, which includes postnatal depression; severe, which includes those cases of puerperal psychoses that cannot be classified elsewhere; and other puerperal disorders. In addition there is a category called "puerperal mental disorder, unspecified" for other disorders with an onset soon after childbirth that are difficult to classify.

Classification in DSM–IV (American Psychiatric Association, 1994) is rather different, and in one respect represents an advance on both DSM–III–R and ICD–10. Although there is no separate category for puerperal disorders, and the text recognises that most of these disorders are affective, it is possible to add a *postpartum onset specifier* to any affective episode which starts within four weeks of childbirth. This means that the vast majority of puerperal illnesses (which are affective) can be separately coded, which was not possible with the previous systems. The postpartum onset specifier can be applied to the current or most recent episode of major depression, mania, or mixed episodes in major depressive disorder, bipolar I, bipolar II disorder or brief psychotic disorder.

Treatment

"Tonics and a change of scene are useful" wrote Savage (1875), and today admission to hospital, occasionally under Section, for rest and appropriate drug treatment remains the mainstay of therapy. If possible the baby should also be admitted. The mother should be closely observed to assess her degree of maternal competence and the risks of harm and neglect to her baby, to determine the subsequent level of nursing supervision.

The pharmacological treatment of the psychoses that occur after childbirth is essentially similar to their treatments at other times, although there may be one or two minor differences in strategy. Manic syndromes require sedation with combinations of phenothiazines and lithium, and for very severe manic states, short-term use of a potent benzodiazepine, lorazepam, may also be helpful because it is not associated with dyskinesias. The combination of haloperidol with lithium can result in unpleasant dyskinesias, difficulties in swallowing, and occasionally even the neuroleptic malignant syndrome. As puerperal mania is often associated with a profound disturbance of sleep, restoration of normal sleep is essential and the combination of chlorpromazine with a benzodiazepine hypnotic is often helpful, while the night nursing staff should always care for the baby during the night. A few women with very severe mania may fail to eat and drink properly or neglect their personal hygiene, and therefore may be more prone to infection; as a wise precaution the patient's pulse and temperature should be observed. Occasionally ECT may be required in unresponsive mania or where the patient is unable to take oral medication. Severe puerperal depression also responds well to ECT, but there is a high early relapse rate. Martin (1958) gave ECT to 28 patients (27 depressive, 1 manic), all of whom had an excellent initial response, but ten women relapsed within 17 days and required a further course of ECT. A tricyclic antidepressant or lithium should be given after a course of ECT to prevent this early relapse, but even with modern drugs a second course of ECT may be helpful.

In spite of its proven efficacy, ECT is unpopular with patients and most prefer treatment with medication. The response rate to tricyclics in the severe puerperal depressions is low and probably worse than in non-puerperal depressives (Dean & Kendell, 1981). However, the addition of lithium to tricyclic antidepressants in resistant puerperal depressions is often helpful. There is only one uncontrolled study on the use of lithium specifically in the puerperal disorders, and this suggests that lithium may be effective for confusional, depressive and schizoaffective syndromes as well as for its more usual indication, mania (Silbermann *et al.* 1975). Patients presenting with a mixed affective and schizophreniform picture often respond well to a combination of tricyclics, chlorpromazine and lithium, and it may therefore be best to hold ECT in reserve for those women who fail to respond to the various drug regimes.

Schizophrenic illnesses are often coloured by affective syndromes during the early months after delivery, and so manic and depressive episodes may require separate treatment. Although the puerperal affective disorders usually improve within a few weeks, schizophrenic illnesses may take several months to resolve and so decisions about the longer-term care of infants should, if possible, be delayed. Pharmacological aspects of managing schizophrenia are also discussed on page 413. A later schizophrenic relapse, for example, occurring during the second or third postpartum year may be very dangerous for both mother and infant, and depot maintenance therapy should be used if possible. As well as reducing the risk of non-compliance, there may be advance warning of an imminent relapse when a patient fails to appear for her injection. Most women with a severe psychotic illness are either too chaotic or unwilling to breastfeed. A few women with milder illness continue to breastfeed successfully, and in these cases lithium is contraindicated because of risks of neonatal lithium toxicity, although the *British National Formulary* (BNF) does not give an absolute contraindication. The effect of psychotropic drugs on breast milk and neonates as described in the BNF is given in Box 21.1. More detailed information on individual drugs is given by Briggs *et al* (1990).

Hormones have little place in the management of acute psychotic illnesses, except in a few instances in which there is a premenstrual exacerbation of a puerperal disorder, particularly depression. These exacerbations are usually a sign that the illness is resolving, and they may sometimes be abolished by increasing the antidepressants or prescribing progesterone suppositories for the two weeks prior to menstruation. This premenstrual exacerbation tends to subside over the next 6–12 months, and only rarely indicates the onset of a more prolonged premenstrual syndrome.

Mother and baby units

Before the introduction of joint admissions, infants had to be separated from their mothers, and the prolonged separation was thought to weaken the mother–infant bond. Mothers often felt guilty about their absence, especially once they resumed responsibilities for infant care (Glaser, 1962). In other cases, overzealous social workers or other family members failed to return the baby to the mother once her illness had resolved. Earlier fears that babies might come to harm in mother and baby units, either at the hands of the mother, or from other patients, or as a result of ward infections, have proved unfounded (Margison & Brockington, 1982).

A mother and baby unit is critically dependent on the quality and flexibility of its nursing staff who fulfil a variety of different roles, quite apart from their traditional role as psychiatric nurses caring for patients with mania, depression or other mental disorders. For the more severely ill women, who may have to be briefly separated from their babies, the nurse may have to substitute for the mother in practical matters such as feeding and changing the infant. Primigravid women suffer from the dual handicap of being psychotic as well as being inexperienced with new-born babies, and during a psychosis new learning is difficult. A common error is to try to make incompetent primigravid women care for their infants when they are too ill to do so. It is more sensible to wait until the psychosis has subsided before attempting to teach basic mothering skills, as the mother will be rather more receptive at this stage. A third more subtle role sometimes fulfilled by older nurses who have had children themselves is to provide a more "maternal" type of support as the women begin to form a relationship with their newborn baby. Finally, nursing staff should be able to assess the quality of the mother–infant relationship, monitor progress, and provide information for the longer-term decisions (e.g. where the more serious illnesses fail to resolve and long-term fostering or adoption is being considered).

Margison (1982) recommends that assessment of the mother–baby interaction should cover four areas, usually taking about two weeks:

(1) the practical competence of the mother in feeding, bathing, and changing the baby;
(2) untoward incidents such as handling the baby roughly or leaving the baby unattended, or verbal or physical attacks on the baby;
(3) what mothers say about the babies, particularly if they are deluded or hallucinated;
(4) a mother's overall affective response to her baby.

Box 21.1 Psychotropic drugs and breastfeeding

Tricyclics (including mianserin and trazodone)	Small amounts are secreted in breast milk but too small to be harmful. Low doses of amitriptyline appear safe.
Doxepin	Accumulation of a doxepin metabolite may cause sedation or respiratory depression. Avoid. One near-fatal case reported.
Fluoxetine	Only small amounts in breast milk, but it may accumulate in the infant. Avoid.
Paroxetine, sertraline	No information (less than 1% of daily dose excreted in breast milk).
Fluovoxamine	Little risk. One case report showed only 0.5% of daily maternal dose in the infant.
Moclobemide	Amounts too small to be harmful, but patient leaflet advises avoid.
Lithium	Risks of adverse side-effects (neonatal lithium toxic ity increased by continuous ingestion). Intercurrent illness in the baby (e.g. diarrhoea) is a danger. 40% of maternal serum lithium concentration excreted into the breast milk. Infant serum and maternal milk levels are approximately equal. BNF advises close monitoring of maternal and infant serum lithium if breastfeeding is undertaken (other authorities say avoid).
Antipsychotics	Only small amounts excreted in the milk. Possible adverse effects in the developing nervous system. Therefore best avoid.
Chlorpromazine	Drowsiness and lethargy in infants, particularly with higher doses.
Sulpiride	Excreted in significant amounts in breast milk. Avoid.
Benzodiazepines	Avoid. Repeated doses cause lethargy, and weight loss may occur in the infant.
Zopiclone	Contraindicated. Excreted in appreciable amounts in breast milk (15–50% maternal levels).

Box 21.1 cont.

Thioxanthenes	Safe at low doses. Higher doses of flupenthixol and zuclopenthixol can produce drowsiness.
Clozapine	Avoid in breastfeeding. Risk of sedation and agranulocytosis.
Risperidone	Avoid.
Carbamazepine	Amounts too small to be harmful. Accumulation does not occur. Considered safe in monotherapy.
Valproate	Use with caution at high doses.
Phenytoin	Clinically safe.
Phenobarbitone	Drowsiness in the infant. Also one case each of methaemoglobinaemia with phenobarbitone and phenytoin reported. Use with caution.
Opiates, diamorphine, morphine	Therapeutic doses unlikely to affect infant; withdrawal symptoms in infants of dependent mothers. Breastfeeding no longer considered the best method of treating dependence in offspring and should be stopped.
Amphetamines	Significant amounts in breast milk. Avoid.
Beta-blockers	Infants should be monitored, possible toxicity due to beta blockade but the amount in breast milk is usually too small to affect the infant. Acebutolol, atenolol, nadolol and sotalol are excreted in higher amounts than other beta-blockers.
Progesterones	High doses may suppress lactation.

Effects of psychiatric disorder on mothering abilities

Severely depressed mothers with psychomotor retardation, difficulties in concentration, and feelings of exhaustion may have insufficient energy to complete the practical tasks required for infant care. Depressed, irritable women, or those with hostile, infanticidal or suicidal thoughts, may require especially close observation. Occasionally psychotically depressed women try to smother their babies with a pillow or drown them in the bath. This can occur even after admission to hospital, and those with severe psychotic depression may require a nurse to be present with them at all times.

Manic patients are also unsafe, particularly during their overactive phase. Their distraction makes them either forget to complete a feed or change their baby, or walk away during changing and leave the baby unattended on a nappy-changing table. Others may wake their babies up from sleep to cuddle them in a sentimental fashion, or give unnecessary feeds or feed inappropriately, for example, with solids. Their irrational anger is usually directed at their husband or the nurses, but may occasionally be directed towards the baby. Grandiosity, disinhibition and general lack of sensitivity may all diminish the quality of infant care, and sometimes the mother hands the baby round the ward for anyone, however unsuitable, to look after. Infant care is generally poor until the mother's distractability has resolved and she has a reasonable degree of concentration. During phases of severe mania or catatonic excitement, mothers must be separated from their infants, and nurseries where babies sleep should be locked to prevent access. In a few cases it may be advisable to remove the baby from the ward while a severe psychotic phase is being treated.

In women with schizophrenia, thought disorder may result in major defects in practical competence, while negative symptoms such as apathy and emotional blunting can grossly impair the sensitivity required for good infant care. The presence of negative symptoms, which may be long-lasting, is a poor prognostic sign. Delusions may preoccupy a subject's mind to such an extent that the infant is excluded or neglected. Delusions and hallucinations that focus around the baby may be particularly dangerous, as patients with schizophrenia sometimes act on the basis of their delusions. Dangerous mistakes such as bathing the baby in cold water, giving the baby feeds that are boiling hot, substituting sterilising fluid for milk, or other bizarre practical errors may occur. One patient, in a distracted state, repeatedly let her baby's face slip under water while bathing her so that nursing staff always had to be present at bathing time to rescue the infant from drowning. Another patient soon after discharge threw her baby into a local swimming pool in a dangerous fashion, yet afterwards was quite unable to explain why she had done so. The long-term prognosis for mothers with schizophrenia and their babies is often poor. In a 5–10 year follow-up study of 17 subjects with puerperal schizophrenia, two women committed suicide, and six made further serious attempts on their lives, while many of the others were involved in episodes of child abuse or neglect to such an extent that only one of the 17 mothers was still caring for her infant and was symptom-free (Da Silva & Johnstone, 1981). Some cases of puerperal schizophrenia may respond well to medication after a period of months; in other cases the child is brought up by relatives (usually the father or the infant's grandparents). Where the social support is poor and the illness fails to respond to medication, the social services may have to remove the baby for fostering or adoption.

The law

Under certain circumstances it may be necessary to prevent a disturbed mother from removing her baby from hospital. In these cases, any person, but usually a social worker may make an application to the magistrate for an Emergency Protection Order (Section 44 of the 1989 Children Act). This replaces the old Place of Safety Order of the 1969 Act. Except in cases of emergency, the applicant should give notice to the parents who have the right to appeal in the first 72 hours. This order lasts for seven days and is extendable once only for a further seven days to a maximum of 14 days, with provision for a medical examination. When more prolonged intervention is required, an interim care order (Section 37) that lasts for eight weeks should be instituted. This can be repeatedly renewed for further four-week periods, but eventually a full care order (Section 31) may be necessary.

Once the social services are involved in looking after an infant of a mother with mental illness, they are required to hold a child protection conference (Section 47). To do this they may require the assistance of other authorities, such as the health authority, and the Children Act uses the phrase "*shall* comply with the request" (Section 27) to indicate a fairly high degree of obligation to attend these case conferences. At these conferences usually only the psychiatrist has any specialised knowledge of puerperal mental disorder, and so his role at the conference is often educational as well as clinical. Commonly, conference members are unduly pessimistic, believing the abnormal mental state found in puerperal depression or mania will last for ever, or at best recur frequently. In other cases, the rather longer-term risks associated with schizophrenia may not be recognised. Even though decisions on the level of risk and future management are made on a consensus basis, the psychiatrist's view of the long-term prognosis of the mother's illness is often a crucial determining factor in deciding whether the infant should stay with the natural mother.

Outcome and risks of recurrence

The natural history, as described by the 19th century authors, was of a rather lengthy illness. Savage (1875) reported on 84 cases of puerperal mania, finding that only a third were better after six months. In 54 cases of melancholia, 50% were better after six months, and 85% by one year, but 8% had died. Writing nearly a century later, Janssen (1964) gave the following figures: 75% of cases of puerperal psychoses had admissions of less than six weeks duration, 15% were ill for 6–12 weeks, 3% for more than six months, and there were no deaths.

There is an increased risk of further psychotic breakdown following a subsequent pregnancy. Relapses tend to have a similar time of onset and duration and are of the same diagnostic category. Thus, if the initial illness commenced during late pregnancy, subsequent relapses would also start in late pregnancy. Summarising information from several different series, Brockington *et al* (1982) calculated the recurrence rate to be around one in five for subsequent pregnancies, and one in three women experience a further puerperal illness sometime during their life. There is a suggestion that the relapse rate may be higher among women with more severe illnesses. Among women with previous puerperal schizophrenia, relapse rates of 45% (Yarden *et al*, 1966) and 47% (Protheroe, 1969) are given. Similarly, women with bipolar disorder who have had both puerperal as well as previous non-puerperal episodes have a 50% chance of a relapse, while the risk is only 36% for those with a previous postpartum illness (Dean *et al*, 1989). Garvey *et al* (1983) gave a much higher figure for their cases of affective disorder: 85% for bipolar, and 67% for unipolar depressions. Pregnancy itself does not appear to have a long-term deleterious effect on schizophrenia, and a controlled study also showed no difference in subsequent hospitalisation rates between patients with schizophrenia who became pregnant, and a matched control group (Yarden *et al*, 1966). On the other hand, pregnancy may have some long-term influence on rates for affective disorder, because the raised admission rates found for women with unipolar affective disorder are confined to parous women, and rates for nulliparous women are the same as those found for men (Gater *et al*, 1989).

Suicide

There has been a steady decline in the suicide rate of pregnant women. Thus for the years 1900–1947, 12.6% of all women of child-bearing age who committed suicide were pregnant at the time of the suicide, and this figure had fallen to 1.8% for the years 1943–1980 (Kleiner & Greston, 1984). The UK suicide statistics of 1973–1984 suggest a standardised mortality ratio for suicide of 0.17 (as compared with the general population of a similar age) during the postnatal period and only 0.05 during pregnancy (Appleby, 1991). This reduction may be attributed to changes in social attitudes, particularly the loss of stigma associated with having children out of wedlock, more readily available contraception and abortion. Appleby (1991) also suggested that motherhood may confer some protection against suicide, but his study still identified certain high-risk groups: pregnant teenagers, single mothers, and those with stillbirths. Many of the suicides appear to occur in the first few weeks after childbirth, often by violent means, suggesting that mental illness was probably at least a factor in these cases. The rate for parasuicide may also be reduced, although not so dramatically, and the relative risk is around 0.43 for the first postpartum year (Appleby, 1991).

Infanticide

Infanticide, in law, refers to the killing of a child under the age of 12 months by its mother, under circumstances that would otherwise amount to murder. The balance of the mother's mind is thought to be disturbed at the time, and it is classed as a type of manslaughter and dealt with leniently by the court, for example, by probation order. D'Orban (1979) examined 89 women charged with infanticide and found that only 27% had a psychotic illness or were seriously mentally ill at the time. Rather more frequent were battering mothers (40%), mainly individuals with personality disorders who had repeatedly battered their infants. There was a small group of women (12%) who were not mentally ill, usually single mothers who killed their baby on the first or second day and this is called neonaticide. A few (8%) killed in the context of the Medea complex (when the baby reminded them of a hated partner and these were revenge killings), a few women killed their infants because they were unwanted, and there was one case of a mercy killing. Reactive depression, and minor ailments in the babies, generally infections, were common at the time of the killing. Infanticide is associated with attempted suicides in over half the cases in one series (Gibson & Klein, 1961), although these are generally unsuccessful. Even though infanticide itself is rare, women with severe puerperal depression and infanticidal ideation will sometimes describe repeated, apparently serious, attempts to take their infant's life, which somehow they fail to carry through to completion. Apnoeic episodes caused by the mother smothering the baby, which can be distinguished from apnoea due to medical causes, are most commonly the result of personality disorder in the mothers (Samuels *et al*, 1992).

Prophylaxis

Some women who have had a puerperal psychosis after their first child wish to have more children, and therefore seek advice on the risks of a recurrence and the possibility of prevention of psychosis. Hamilton (1982) gave a mixture of oestrogen and testosterone in oil by injection to 40 women soon after delivery and noted that none had a recurrence. Dalton (1985) suggested that progesterone may be helpful for cases of previous non-psychotic depressions, but her claims have not been adequately substantiated. As most puerperal illnesses are thought to be affective, Stewart *et al* (1991) administered lithium to 25 women with previous manic or schizomanic illnesses and only two relapsed, although a few women developed mild attenuated illnesses, suggesting that the relapse had been suppressed or was partially treated rather than being prevented.

When women seek prophylactic advice, a careful history of the previous episode should be obtained because puerperal relapses are remarkably similar to the original illness. Critical information includes: the time of onset; duration; the diagnostic category as indicated in the case notes; and which treatments appeared to work. It is then relatively easy to select medications that are most likely to be beneficial, decide when they should start, and how long they should be taken for.

Women who were previously admitted are usually quite anxious to prevent any possibility of recurrence and therefore keen to take any medication the doctor might suggest, while women with previous milder depressions are more reticent about taking prophylactic psychotropic medication. It is best to explain the risks of recurrence, as well as the pros and cons associated with each drug: for example, "lithium is the best prophylactic agent for depression or mania, but breastfeeding will not be possible". Then agree with the patient on the most suitable regime for her particular case. It is also essential to ensure there is psychiatric contact at around the expected time of onset of the illness, and again one or two weeks later. This is because some patients experience recurrences that are mild attenuated illnesses, and these can sometimes be successfully dealt with on an out-patient basis when previously there had been an admission.

The following regimes are offered, and they should all start on the first day after delivery:

For previous mania or schizomania, lithium. A hypnotic may be added because it is essential to ensure that women with a history of previous mania have good and unbroken sleep during the early puerperium.

For milder depressions, amitriptyline 20–30 mg at night (the higher doses are poorly tolerated).

For more severe depressions, lithium with amitriptyline can be given. It should be noted that breastfeeding is not possible with this regime, but is safe with amitriptyline alone.

Hormonal therapy in the form of progesterone is commonly requested, and may be given with or without any of the above psychotropic drugs. This is popular among patients because it is thought of as a "natural hormone" and its use has been much publicised by Dalton (1985), in spite of any proper scientific study of its merits. If it is used, progesterone cannot be taken by mouth and should be given by injection (100 mg l-M b.d. for a few days) followed by progesterone 400 mg b.d. as suppositories. If suppositories are started too early there is a small risk of infection.

It should be noted, however, that there are no controlled trials for any of the above regimes.

Non-psychotic postnatal depression

Postnatal depression in the community is a much more common illness than puerperal psychosis; around 10% of women become depressed in the first few months after delivery. Depression sufficiently severe to present to an out-patient clinic occurs in around 16 per 1000 cases (Oates, 1988) and the account given below refers more to out-patient cases than those found in the community, who probably have milder disorders. Postnatal depression, although severe, lacks the life-threatening quality of the hospitalised cases. The illness usually presents in the first few weeks or months after delivery, with low mood, depressive thoughts and feelings of inadequacy. Weeping is ubiquitous, and the frequency and intensity of crying spells may give an indication of the severity of the illness. Daily crying spells occur at the onset of the illness, but these gradually diminish in frequency to only occasional tearful episodes as the illness resolves. Anhedonia is an almost universal complaint, which usually presents as a failure to derive any pleasure from caring for the new-born baby. A normal mother may describe a degree of lability, but unless she is also suffering from depression she will usually gain much pleasure from caring for her baby.

Pitt (1968), in his classic description of postnatal depression, highlighted the strong association with anxiety, which may be focused on the baby's health, feeding, sleeping and other bodily functions or any other minor ailments. Such a high degree of anxiety is rarely justified by the baby's health, which is generally excellent. In some cases there may also be panic attacks with dizziness, palpitations, shakiness, sweating and feelings of terror usually qualifying for a diagnosis of DSM–IV panic disorder (more than two panics in four weeks). Emotional lability is also common, and any additional stress may trigger a crisis. Rather more troublesome symptoms are the increased irritability, aggression and hostility. In some women there may be angry outbursts, marital rows become more frequent or prolonged, and are even complicated by actual violence. For those women who become ill after their second or third pregnancy, this hostility may be directed at older children who have their own difficulties in adjusting to the new arrival.

Feelings of exhaustion, poor concentration, psychomotor retardation and confusion are also common, resulting in difficulties achieving any task requiring effort, particularly the practical tasks of mothering. These women sometimes also complain of feeling confused about the advice that different health professions offer them. Housework becomes an impossible chore, adding to their sense of guilt. In the more severe cases, in which there is severe psychomotor retardation or hypersomnia, mothers may take to their beds while domestic work and child care are left to other relatives.

Morbid thoughts in postnatal depressed women are of four types: depressive, obsessional, suicidal and infanticidal. Simple depressive morbid thoughts, such as low self-esteem, worthlessness and guilt are common. Obsessional phenomena often include an element of harming the baby: for example, one patient had recurrent thoughts of putting her baby in the oven. Another had recurrent visual obsessions of knifing her baby, while a third had obsessions of throwing her baby downstairs each time she reached the landing at the top of the stairs. They are not always harmless; one woman had a curious obsession about wasting water, and as a consequence refused to cool the baby's feed down with running cold water and gave the baby overheated feeds. However, the baby is not always the focus of obsessional thoughts; one woman was persistently troubled by the thought of everyone falling off the edge of the world.

Suicide is rare, but suicidal thoughts are more common as some patients express the wish that they could go to sleep forever, usually to escape from their depression. Infanticidal thoughts often accompany suicidal thoughts, and because of this the presence of such thoughts or half-hearted infanticidal attempts should alert the clinician to the risk of suicide, which is very much more common than infanticide. As with obsessional thoughts, the infanticidal thoughts also share themes of harming the baby, but they tend to have a more realistic quality than obsessional thoughts, are less repetitive and more often have elements of planning exactly how the baby would be killed, generally by suffocation or drowning. In a severe depression these thoughts may become overwhelming, and in a state of impulsive anger lead to action.

Depressive sleep disorder with difficulty getting off to sleep, early morning wakening and sometimes nightmares should be distinguished from the sleeplessness resulting from the demands of the infant. Diurnal mood variation is sometimes present, but Pitt (1968) wrote that many patients were worse in the evening. Weight loss is difficult to assess because the extra weight gained during pregnancy is lost during the first three months after delivery, and a degree of weight loss is therefore normal. Most breastfeeding women usually maintain a good appetite, but once lactation ceases anorexia may appear, and occasionally a mild anorexia nervosa-like state is encountered. A decrease in sexual feelings is common after childbirth, but during a postnatal depression loss of libido is almost universal. The return of normal sexual feelings is commonly delayed until well after the resolution of any underlying depression, and may be further delayed by the use of antidepressant drugs.

A variety of psychiatric symptoms may be exacerbated or appear for the first time after childbirth, usually in the presence of a postnatal depression. As Savage (1875) wrote, "dypsomania, kleptomania and other morbid tendencies may be present, but all I would say of them is that they are more curable with puerperal conditions than with others". Agoraphobia may start for the first time, or a preexisting agoraphobic disorder may become worse. Acute depersonalisation can also start after childbirth, and is not only very distressing but can persist for very much longer than the original postnatal depression. Alcoholism may start, particularly among those with a previous or family history of alcoholism.

A premenstrual exacerbation of almost any postpartum symptom is common, particularly towards the end of the first postpartum year and during the second year. Any acting-out episodes such as an overdose, a severe marital dispute or violence tend to occur during the premenstrual phase. Curiously, as the postnatal depression resolves the premenstrual tension seems to become more distressing because the sudden switch from euthymia to acute depression is less well tolerated than a more continuous depression.

Aetiology

Postnatal depression in the community is similar to the illness presenting to the out-patient department, although the illness is probably milder with fewer morbid thoughts. One study found that most women in the community with depression had neurotic depression, but there were also a few cases of obsessional disorder, agoraphobia and alcoholism (Watson *et al*, 1984). At three months postpartum the point prevalence rate for depression is around 10% (Pitt, 1968; Kumar & Robson, 1984) and the one-year prevalence rate for episodes of depression is around 25% (Watson *et al*, 1984), but these rates are similar to those found among non-puerperal women of similar age studied in community surveys (Surtees *et al*, 1983). It is only in the first three months following delivery that the rates are actually increased (Cooper *et al*, 1988), and a recent study has suggested there is a three-fold increase in inception rate (Cox *et al*, 1993) in this period. Associated factors include a constitutional predisposition as shown by a previous history of depression, particularly postnatal depression, more severe maternity blues, and elation during pregnancy (Dalton, 1971). Parity and the complications of labour are not associated, with the possible exception of caesarian section (Hannah *et al*, 1992; Edwards *et al*, 1994).

Social factors such as recent life events are important, and some, but not all, of Brown's vulnerability factors (lack of a close confiding relationship, early maternal loss, three or more children under 14 years of age, and lower social class) are associated with postnatal depression. Lack of a close confiding relationship, a poor marriage, life events, and early maternal loss are associated, but the illness does not appear to have any predilection for women with many children, nor does it spare the upper classes. Paykel *et al* (1980) found 20% of their sample of women were depressed six weeks following delivery, and recent life events were the most powerful predictor; a poor marriage acted as a vulnerability factor only in the presence of stressful life events. Other associations noted in this study included a previous depression, maternity blues, a younger age and housing problems. J. L. Cox (1988) argued that childbirth itself is an important life event and results in depression as a consequence of the associated psychosocial stress. It is of interest that there are also descriptions in the earlier literature of women who became psychotic after they had adopted a baby (Tetlow, 1955).

Marriage and postnatal illness

Most studies on postnatal depression report an association between marital disharmony and postnatal depression (Kumar & Robson, 1984; Watson *et al*, 1984). The reasons for this are complex. A few women begin their pregnancy in the context of an unstable or unsupportive relationship, but most couples describe a deterioration in the quality of their marriage coincident in time with the illness. Loss of libido is frequent in postnatal depression and this may result in a weakening of the affectionate bond. Psychoanalysts point to the change from a two-person to a three-person situation that follows the birth of a first child, and highlight the potential for destructive envy resulting from the altered situation. A study of the spouses of women who had been admitted for a puerperal psychosis showed that 42% became sufficiently disturbed to qualify for a DSM–III diagnosis, generally an anxiety state or major depression, compared with only 4% in the control group (Harvey & McGrath, 1988). However, psychiatric case registers show an increase in the morbidity only for women and not for their husbands during the first two years after delivery. Marital disturbance does not always resolve as the depression lifts, and occasionally a resentful husband who has apparently cared well for his wife during her depression leaves once she is recovered. Conversely, a woman may cease to regard her husband as a sexual partner during her depression, and when sexual feelings return she may have an extra-marital affair. The clinician should take note of any marital deterioration, and offer separate supportive interviews for both the husband and wife rather than attempt conjoint marital therapy, at least while one or both partners remains disturbed. It is not uncommon for a marriage to break either during an episode of postnatal depression or shortly afterwards. Such an outcome, even if the depression resolves, is not usually in the best interests of the mother, father or child. Depression is probably only one of several contributory factors in such cases, but because it is so preeminently treatable the psychiatrist should make every effort to treat the disorder vigorously, and so shorten its duration and at the same time involve the husband in the treatment programme in an attempt to reduce harmful social sequelae.

Male reactions

Men occasionally become psychiatrically ill during their wives' pregnancies, and this has been termed the Couvade syndrome (French *couver* = to hatch). Anthropologists have long been interested in couvade rituals, for example, men taking to their beds, fasting or developing abdominal pains, that have been described in different parts of the world. A controlled study (Trethowan & Conlon, 1965) showed that around 1 in 9 men develop symptoms associated with their wives' pregnancies. These were most commonly gastrointestinal – loss of appetite, toothache, nausea, vomiting, early morning sickness, ill-defined abdominal pains and constipation. Anxiety was the most common mental symptom, but depression, tension, irritability, insomnia, nervousness, weakness and headaches were also described. Occasional patients somatise all their anxiety (Enoch & Trethowan, 1979). Symptoms generally start in the third month of their wife's pregnancy and abate soon after parturition. Reik (1931) suggested that the underlying psychopathology comprised an ambivalent identification with the pregnant wife. The identification is obvious, but the ambivalence includes negative feelings, particularly anger because of the unconscious sexual taboo, but also envy related to the woman's creativity which the man does not have.

Infant development

Mothers with postnatal depression are thought to be slightly less responsive to infant cues, being either more withdrawn with flatness of affect, or else more intrusive and hostile (Murray *et al*, 1991). Their infants are thought to be more withdrawn from maternal contact and may be more discontented. Stein *et al* (1991), in a study of 19-month-old infants, found that postnatally depressed mothers helped their children less during play, and their infants behaved more negatively towards their mothers than controls. More behavioural problems and difficulties in expressive language have been observed in toddlers (Cox, 1988), while among 4-year-olds a minor degree of cognitive deficit and some behavioural difficulties can still be detected, even when the effects of current depression, marital disharmony, and paternal psychiatric history are taken into account (Coghill *et al*, 1986). In spite of these observable changes, the balance of opinion seems to suggest that uncomplicated postnatal depression does not result in serious behavioural difficulties in children (Murray *et al*, 1991).

Treatment

Psychotherapy

The initial consultation is often the most critical and provides many useful opportunities for psychotherapy. Patients usually present with numerous complaints, such as depressive symptoms, disappointment in motherhood, and shame associated with morbid thoughts, particularly infanticidal or obsessive thoughts of harm. The act of sharing such thoughts with a professional person may provide immediate cathartic relief. Other symptoms, such as panic attacks, depersonalisation and agoraphobia appearing for the first time may puzzle the patient and an explanation is, in itself, reassuring.

Some illnesses are obviously dangerous, and so a frank recognition and discussion of the risk of suicide and infanticide at an early stage is often helpful, with dangerousness being viewed as a quite separate dimension to severity. During the initial interview the strengths and weaknesses of a patient's current and previous family set-up should be discussed to give the therapist some idea of the direction of future management. Towards the end of the initial consultation, if there is a clear-cut depressive illness the patient should be told that she has a definite illness, which should be named as "postnatal depression". The act of naming the illness by someone in authority, such as the doctor, appears to have a beneficial effect for many women, possibly because the blame is shifted from themselves on to some definite medical cause.

Psychotherapy should be mainly supportive and can be conducted by a variety of different health professionals, but a degree of specialisation in postnatal depression is helpful. Allowance should be made for real practical difficulties, such as illnesses in babies and caring for other children in the family, but at the same time the therapist should also be able to recognise some of the more alarming situations. Women with the more severe depressions usually only wish to talk about their symptoms, permitting little time or space for reviewing relationships with either their babies or families. In these cases, sympathetic listening, permission to talk expansively on symptomatic distress and a cognitive approach may be helpful. Feelings of rejection or hostility directed at the spouse and other children are commonplace, and as the depression lightens the more traditional psychotherapeutic themes of relationships with parents and other family members begin to emerge. The motivation to remain in psychotherapy usually lasts for the duration of the depression, but once the depression lifts many women cease contact.

Group therapy in the form of peer-group support is often helpful for women with postnatal depression. Such support groups, which are often led by community psychiatric nurses or psychologists, work well with relatively small numbers. Previously well-integrated individuals appear to derive most benefit, and patients often strike up close friendships with each other. However, many women cannot tolerate group therapy and so this should never be a substitute for individual treatment.

Drug therapy

Many women, particularly those with brief or mild episodes of postnatal depression, neither wish for nor require pharmacotherapy. However, most of those referred to specialist services are usually suffering from major depression, panic disorder or other affective disorders that may benefit from antidepressant therapy, and this is described in Chapter 4. A few points deserve special mention. Most patients respond well to standard tricyclic antidepressants, but two common tricyclic side-effects are particularly abhorred by postnatal women: sleepiness, because of the obvious risks of being drowsy while caring for the baby; and dizziness, for fear of dropping the baby. It is therefore best to start with small doses of tricyclics such as amitriptyline (10 mg at night) and then slowly titrate the dose upwards. Most patients will respond in the 30–75 mg range, which does not seem to interfere with breastfeeding, while only a minority require higher doses in the 100–200 mg range. The patient's main presenting complaint may offer some guide as to the initial choice of antidepressant. Those with obsessional thoughts and panic disorder may benefit from clomipramine. If sleep disturbance is prominent, trimipramine may be helpful. For those with morbid thoughts, the addition of a non-sedating phenothiazine such as trifluoperazine to the tricyclic medication may be helpful. However, among out-patients who have to care for their babies the more sedating neuroleptics such as chlorpromazine and thioridazine should be avoided.

The selective serotonin reuptake inhibitors (SSRIs) are relatively new and appear to be helpful, but their role in postnatal depression has yet to be evaluated. They may be useful for women who are fearful of side-effects such as weight gain, and may be indicated for those with obsessional features. Breastfeeding is safe on low doses of tricyclics, but is not recommended for patients on SSRIs.

Although Pitt (1968) used the term "atypical" to describe postnatal depression, many cases are quite typical major depressions and therefore there are no special reasons why MAOIs should be offered as the initial antidepressant (Kendell, 1985). In the few women who fail to respond to a single antidepressant, lithium augmentation is probably the most useful strategy, but if lithium is used patients must *always* be actively forewarned about possible teratogenic risks during further pregnancies, because a few women will be thinking of embarking on further pregnancies at this time.

Once the patient is better, drug therapy should continue for 3–6 months and then the tricyclic dosage should be cautiously reduced, possibly at the rate of 25 mg per month. Evidence from case register studies (Kendell *et al*, 1981) suggests that psychiatric morbidity remains high during the second postpartum year. This later morbidity presumably includes recurrences of an earlier postnatal depression, a few new cases of depression and the tail end of some prolonged episodes. For example, Cox *et al* (1982) found that 6% of all women were still depressed at the end of the first year, and Pitt (1968) found that only a half of his cases had resolved at one year. Either way, many patients require supervision well into their second postpartum year, and they should not be discharged from the out-patient clinic until they are not only drug-free, but also symptom-free for at least three months as well. This is because there are a small number of patients who have a chronic relapsing/remitting course following a puerperal onset, and these patients may need to take antidepressants on a long-term basis. Recurrence risks after a subsequent pregnancy for postnatal depression may be higher than those found for puerperal psychoses: Dalton (1985) gave a figure of 64%.

More problematic cases

Although most women do well with conventional psychotherapy and drug treatment, a variety of different approaches may be required for those who fail to respond. A few women with severe illnesses complicated by suicidal or infanticidal thoughts cannot be hospitalised, or admission itself has failed to provide any relief. They require intensive therapy with higher doses of tricyclics, earlier lithium augmentation and a high psychotherapeutic profile, with community psychiatric nurses visiting very frequently. Among cases in which there appear to be risks to the baby or other children in the family, a social worker should be involved to monitor safety, and to consider short-term fostering during a crisis, help from another family member, or the placement of older children in day nurseries. The involvement of a social worker and regular case conferences also ensures that there is a proper structure to coordinate the efforts of all the professionals involved.

In contrast to these severe illnesses, which may be of relatively brief duration, there are prolonged, milder depressions that fail to respond to any treatment. Occasionally there is an associated medical problem, such as thyroid or pituitary disorder, hypertension or the use of anti-hypertensive drugs. Supportive interviews on a fortnightly or monthly basis may be helpful for these longer illnesses, and should continue for two or three years until a spontaneous resolution occurs.

A third problematic group are mothers with personality disorders, some with preexisting borderline features that become much more prominent after delivery. The main problems include a poor response to all the antidepressants, impulsive behaviour in the form of overdoses, occasional child abuse, poor compliance with therapy, and an overdemanding, abusive relationship with both spouses and therapists. For some of these women the stress of looking after their baby seems to provoke hostility and depression, and so an early return to work may prove beneficial. These women often do poorly with medication and require a high psychotherapeutic input, often from two or more therapists. They enter into repeated emotional and social crises, which the team should anticipate in their care plan.

A few women turn to alcohol during a postnatal depression, and this can make them too sleepy, irritable or insensitive to care properly for their infants. These women sometimes come to medical attention, having been arrested and charged by the police for being "drunk in charge of a child under the age of seven" (Section 21 of the 1902 Licensing Act). For some the fear of losing their babies may be sufficient to curb drinking, but among others for safety it may be best to remove the child.

Women with medically ill babies are naturally highly anxious, but do not have a raised rate of postnatal depression. If they become depressed, large fluctuations of mood may follow all the ups and downs of their infant's illness, but antidepressants and support can help dampen the severity of these swings. Women with handicapped babies often have overpowering feelings of hurt and anger ("Why me? Why my baby?"), and even in the presence of depression regard a psychiatric referral as yet another blow to their self-esteem, dismissing both drug and psychological support.

Finally, for those women with agoraphobia, obsessional disorder, depersonalisation or kleptomania (usually presenting as shoplifting), it is usually only necessary to treat the underlying depression, as these symptoms will then often resolve spontaneously.

Maternity blues

Transient mild depression and crying spells after childbirth are frequent and have been called the baby blues, third day blues, the maternity blues and the transitory syndrome, the latter capturing the evanescent nature of the mood swing. The syndrome is reviewed in detail by Stein (1982). Crying spells are the hallmark of the maternity blues and are reported in 50–70% of women. Often there is a very brief cry due to emotion in the first few hours after delivery, and this is accompanied by feelings of happiness or tears of joy, but around 10% of women describe feeling acutely depressed, strange or depersonalised immediately after delivery.

A rather more severe prolonged spell of weeping sometimes occurs between the third and fifth day, and this weepiness is usually associated with an altered mood, although the mood is not necessarily depressed. Anxiety, elation, irritability or a state of emotional lability may accompany these weeping spells. Common reasons given for the weeping include feelings of rejection by the husband or nursing staff, or minor ailments in the baby or themselves. Illness in a new-born baby usually takes precedence over all other causes of maternal anxiety, while among multigravid women, the reason given for the weeping usually revolves around the other children at home.

More severe depressive feelings, sometimes with a violent or bizarre content and reminiscent of the thought pattern observed in depressive illness, occur in around 10% of women and are more common among those with previous depression (Stein, 1980). This more intense depression usually lasts only for a few hours and rarely for the whole day, but may recur in bouts on two or three successive days. Elation is present in over 80% of women on day 1, but this falls to 40% by day 4, although a few women are elated every day. This elation falls far short of hypomania. Emotional lability, particularly on the blues day, is common, as are insomnia, dreaming and even nightmares, and 10% report hypnopompic hallucinations. Rapid eye movement and stage 4 sleep are decreased in pregnancy, but may show a rebound increase on nights 2 and 3 postpartum (Karacan *et al*, 1969).

Irritability with angry feelings often directed at the husband or hospital staff are common, while transient negative feelings towards the baby and an early lack of maternal affection can be elicited in up to 40% of women, but these usually resolve without any adverse consequences (Robson & Kumar, 1980). Although forgetfulness, confusion and poor concentration are common complaints, psychometric testing has failed to detect any objective measure of cognitive impairment, nor are there any significant electroencephalogram (EEG) changes (Melges, 1968). A mild headache, generally bilateral and frontal, occurs in around a third of women, usually between days 3 and 6, and this appears to be more common among those women with a previous or family history of migraine (Stein, 1984).

For most women, the maternity blues is a brief acute episode lasting for no more than a few hours for one or two days only, but a few women may have a rather more continuous pattern of disturbance. Just occasionally a very severe, brief, almost psychotic episode occurs for two to three days as a part of the maternity blues, and this was the original "milk fever". The only established clinical associations with the maternity blues are anxiety and depression during late pregnancy, previous premenstrual tension, and subsequent postnatal depression. Parity, social factors and obstetric complications do not appear to be related.

Hormonal and biochemical hypotheses

The rather fixed time interval of three to four days after delivery, combined with the organic affective picture and the lack of significant psychosocial correlates, suggest the possibility of an underlying biological cause. There are numerous studies that attempt to correlate the severity of the blues with a particular hormone or substance, but so far no single cause has emerged (for review see George & Sandler, 1988). The progesterone deficiency hypothesis, which proposes that the sharp drop in progesterone levels following delivery causes both the maternity blues and postnatal depression, has recently received some support from a large study based on salivary progesterone levels. Harris *et al* (1994) found a significant correlation between salivary progesterone and mood in the maternity blues, as measured on the Stein Scale (Stein, 1980). There was a weak but significant association between mood and higher antenatal salivary progesterone, lower concentrations shortly after delivery, and greater decreases in concentration from antenatal to postnatal values. There was no association between salivary cortisol and mood. Salivary progesterone is an accurate measure of free plasma progesterone, and as this study was based on a large sample (120 women, 9645 saliva samples) the findings are likely to be reliable. Plasma progesterone (which reflects total rather than free progesterone) did not correlate in this study or in the study by O'Hara *et al* (1991).

Oestrogen levels also drop sharply after delivery, but the change fails to correlate with mood disturbance apart from an association with sleep disturbance (Nott *et al*, 1976). Oestrogen may modulate the function of monoamines, and Cookson (1985) has suggested that the fall in oestrogen leads to central dopaminergic changes, causing postpartum psychoses. Wieck *et al* (1991) administered the apomorphine challenge test, a measure of dopaminergic receptor function on the fourth postpartum day, to a group of high-risk women and found evidence of increased dopamine receptor sensitivity among women who became psychotic. There are also isolated case reports of administered oestrogen being abruptly stopped during the puerperium, and the withdrawal triggering a psychosis. When stilboesterol was used to suppress lactation it was thought to diminish the severity of the blues (Hamilton, 1962).

Cortisol may also be an important hormone because its level rises slowly during pregnancy, rises abruptly during labour and then falls. Elevated plasma cortisol levels are among the most consistent endocrine changes found in depression, and the labile mood changes of the maternity blues resemble the dysphoria observed in Cushing's disease. An association between the blues and elevated plasma cortisol has been reported by Okano *et al* (1987). Levy (1987) descibed a syndrome similar in frequency and severity to the maternity blues following major surgery, but in this case there are only changes in cortisol levels and not in the sex hormones. During the early puerperium over 80% of women are dexamethazone non-suppressors (Greenwood & Parker, 1984), yet only one study has reported an association between postpartum mood and the prepartum cortisol levels (Handley *et al*, 1980). A transient biochemical hypothy-roidism has been described between the fifth and tenth month postpartum, but these minor biochemical abnormalities in thyroid function do not appear to be associated with either the maternity blues or postnatal depression. There are, however, a few reports describing beneficial effects of dessicated thyroid extract in relapses of puerperal psychoses (Hatotani *et al*, 1983). If hypothyroidism is detected in cases of postnatal depression, it should be treated.

Physiological changes occurring around the third or fourth postpartum day may also be relevant because this is the time the mood changes occur. Colostrum changes to milk, and body weight continues to rise for the first three postpartum days, but then begins to be lost abruptly around the fourth day; the onset of this weight loss is often synchronous with the blues episode (Stein, 1980). The weight loss is between 0.5 and 1.0 kg daily between days 4–6, but the severity of the mood disturbance shows no correlation with the magnitude of the weight loss. Similar abrupt weight losses have also been described in some patients with bipolar illness at the same time as their mood switch (Crammer, 1959). Amine hypotheses of the maternity blues propose that changes in the biogenic amines found in depression may also occur during the maternity blues. Thus, the levels of free and total plasma tryptophan, the precursors of brain serotonin, correlate with the mood disturbance during the blues (Stein *et al*, 1976; Handley *et al*, 1980; Gard *et al*, 1986), but these changes are unlikely to be causal because administering tryptophan to blues subjects has no beneficial effect (Harris, 1980). Platelet MAO (George & Wilson, 1981) and platelet beta-adrenoreceptors (Best *et al*, 1985) both show some correlation with mood changes in the maternity blues. Beta endorphin levels are elevated during pregnancy, rise further during labour and afterwards fall rapidly (Newnham *et al*, 1984), but levels correlate only with pain and not with mood. After delivery, a myriad of different biochemical and hormonal changes begin to revert back to their prepartum levels. Whatever the relevant changes are, they should be greater during the first two postpartum weeks because this is the period of highest risk, and they should be similar to those causing affective illness, because most postpartum syndromes are affective disorders of one sort or another.

Measurement

Although a few specific instruments have been devised to assess postnatal disorders, most research workers have relied on the standard rating scales used in non-puerperal disorders. A postpartum psychosis can only be reliably assessed with interview methods, and for the purposes of research the Present State Examination and the Schedule for Affective Disorders (SADS; Endicott & Spitzer, 1978) are the most appropriate. Self-rating methods can be used to measure postnatal depression, and the Edinburgh Postnatal Depression Scale (Cox *et al*, 1987) is a reliable and sensitive instrument consisting of 13 items. The scale is simple to use and may be given to mothers in the community by health visitors as a screening instrument.

Studies have mainly been concerned with establishing links between the various biochemical parameters and the mood changes. Stein (1980) described a 13-item scale comprising mainly neurotic symptoms, and Pitt (1973) described a shorter scale of eight items. The scale of Kennerly & Gath (1989) is somewhat longer, is administered daily and consists of a mood adjective checklist.

The most popular method for measuring premenstrual symptoms is the Moos Menstrual Distress Questionnaire (Moos, 1968), which has 47 symptoms grouped into eight separate factors. These are: pain, concentration, behavioural change, autonomic reactions, water retention, negative affects (mainly depression), arousal, and control. It can be administered daily for a whole cycle or once only during the premenstrual phase. The Premenstrual Assessment Form (Halbreich *et al*, 1982) is administered on one occasion only, but has detailed questions on affective symptoms that permit the premenstrual syndrome to be subtyped.

Pregnancy

Pregnancy is generally held to be a time of maternal well-being, but individual reactions vary so widely that generalisations are meaningless. Depression starting during pregnancy is about a third as common as depression starting postnatally (Kumar & Robson, 1984). The first and third trimesters are most commonly affected, while the middle trimester is usually a time of maternal well-being. Depression in pregnancy may be more socially determined than postnatal depression. In one study of hospitalised cases, life events were associated with depression in pregnancy but not postnatal depressions (Brockington *et al*, 1990). Fortunately, depression during pregnancy responds well to low doses of tricyclics, for example, amitriptyline 30–50 mg. Higher doses are best avoided because they tend to cause hypotension and fainting.

New cases of psychotic illness arising during pregnancy are uncommon. Clouston (1896) was only able to collect 15 cases over a 15-year period, and estimated they comprised only 1% of admissions. Psychotic illness during pregnancy is managed as in non-pregnant individuals, but lithium and benzodiazepines are relatively contraindicated. ECT is not contraindicated, but it should only be used if absolutely necessary, the risks being associated with the anaesthesia rather than with the ECT itself. Patients with psychoses during pregnancy should be admitted, and it may occasionally be necessary to hospitalise a severe schizophrenic for the duration of her pregnancy. The effects of psychotropic drugs taken in early pregnancy (teratogenic affects) and their effects in late pregnancy on newborn infants are shown in Table 21.1. More detailed information is given in Briggs *et al* (1990).

Vomiting during pregnancy, particularly the more severe hyperemesis gravidarum, is a condition of unknown aetiology and severe complications such as Wernicke's encephalopathy may rarely occur. Wolkind & Zajdicek (1978) found an association with anxiety, depression and feelings of lack of support from close relatives. How psychological factors influence vomiting is uncertain, but admission to hospital, often without any specific therapy, is usually helpful, possibly because this reduces anxiety.

Psychodynamic aspects

Psychotherapists have taken a keener interest in the psychological effects that pregnancy has in normal women, than in the bizarre mental processes found in the puerperal psychoses. Analysts such as Bibring (1959) considered pregnancy to be a maturation crisis. Pines (1972) pointed out that a first pregnancy is a point of no return in feminine development, even if the pregnancy ends in a miscarriage or abortion. Pregnancy becomes a testing point for the mother–daughter relationship because a woman must become the mother to her own child, yet remain the child of her own mother.

Table 21.1 Effects of psychoactive drugs in pregnancy and on the new-born

Drug	Teratogenicity	Effect on the new-born
Tricyclics	No established link with teratogenicity. Because of extensive experience during pregnancy they are probably the drug of first choice.	Tachycardia, muscle spasms and convulsions in neonates occasionally reported.
MAOIs including moclobemide	No evidence of harm in humans but manufacturers recommend avoidance, unless compelling reasons. Phenelzine teratogenic in animals.	Note traditional MAOIs (e.g. phenelzine) may interact with drugs used in labour such as pethidine.
Selective serotonin reuptake inhibitors (fluoxetine, paroxetine, sertraline)	No evidence of teratogenicity in animals. Not studied in humans therefore effects are unknown and best avoided.	
Neuroleptics	No established teratogenic effects.	Administered in the last trimester may cause extrapyramidal symptoms in the infant, excessive crying, hypertension, hyperreflexia.
Lithium	Cardiovascular abnormalities if administered in first trimester. Previous risks may have been overestimated but should be avoided in pregnancy.	Neonatal goitre, lithium toxicity, hypotonia and cyanosis.
Benzodiazepines	Possible association with cleft palate with first trimester use.	Depressed neonatal respiration, neonatal drowsiness, hypotonia and withdrawal symptoms.

Table 21.1 cont.

Drug	Teratogenicity	Effect on the new-born
Anti-epileptics (NB. Pregnant women with epilepsy are at an increased risk of seizures and some obstetric complications, so anti-epileptics cannot easily be stopped.)		
Phenobarbitone	Congenital malformations.	Neonatal bleeding may be a complication. Ensure prophylactic vitamin K.
Phenytoin	Teratogenic. Congenital malformations.	
Barbiturates	Growth retardation. Facial dysmorphism.	Withdrawal symptoms.
Carbamazepine	Neural tube defects. Also cranio-facial defects. Thought to have lowest risk if used as monotherapy.	Ensure prophlyactic vitamin K.
Ethosuxemide	Reported cases of malformation: risks higher when combined with other drugs.	Ensure prophylactic vitamin K.
Valproate	Teratogenic. Spina bifida. CSM recommends screening for neural tube defects.	
Ensure adequate folate therapy during pregnancy with all anti-epileptics.		
Other drugs Beta blockers	Intra-uterine growth retardation.	Neonatal hypoglycaemia and bradycardia: risk is greater with severe hypertension.
Mepobromate	Cleft lip and other severe abnormalities.	

An alternative view was given by Winnicott (1960) who highlighted the importance of narcissism: "in many ways a pregnant woman is encouraged by her own body to be interested in herself". He postulated that this narcissism persists after delivery. The focus of this narcissistic concern switches from the mother to the baby through the mechanism of projective identification, possibly because the baby has until recently been part of the mother. In another well-known paper, Winnicott (1958) described how the weeks that immediately precede childbirth and the first few weeks afterwards are times of heightened emotional sensitivity.

Liedloff (1975) emphasised loss. There is loss of the pregnant status, loss of income, and in some cases loss of self-esteem derived from a job. Depression occurring after a second or later pregnancy can sometimes be accounted for by unresolved sibling rivalry, with the mother identifying strongly with the new-born infant; the older child reminds the mother of her own siblings and so becomes the target of hostile feelings (Abarbanel, 1983).

Melges (1968) reported on the themes discussed during psychotherapy in 100 women with postnatal depression. As expected, conflict over mothering was most frequent (68%), together with ambivalent identification for the patient's mother (49%) and difficulties in the practical tasks of mothering (30%). Primary hostility to the baby, however, was rare (2.4%), although secondary hostile feelings were observed in 14% of subjects. Object loss was only present in 10% of the women. Dynamic factors probably play only a limited role in the aetiology of postnatal illness, but some acquaintance with the way women with postnatal depression perceive their difficulties may be helpful in therapy.

Cross-cultural aspects

Most cultures acknowledge the need to provide special care for the newly delivered mother. Pilsbury (1978) described the Chinese custom of "doing the month" after delivery, when women should avoid washing, going outside, being blown by the wind, going to another person's home, having sex, reading or crying. Japanese women often return to the mother's house before delivery and stay there for a month afterwards, even if this means leaving the marital home. It is of interest that lower rates of postnatal depression and maternity blues have been reported among Japanese women (Okano *et al*, 1991). Jamaican women are strictly isolated for nine days, and then rather less strictly for a further 30 days, while Indian women are isolated for 40 days. Nigerian mothers and their babies are sometimes placed in a special hut within the family compound and looked after by the baby's grandmother.

Postnatal depression appears to be ubiquitous and equally prevalent in European and African cultures. One study found the prevalence of postnatal depression in rural Uganda to be 10%, while the same interviewer using the same diagnostic criteria found a rate of 13% in Scotland, although the Scottish women had rather more guilt and self-blame (Cox, 1983). Puerperal psychoses are equally common in non-Western countries, but reports from Africa and India appear to include more cases of schizophrenia and organic disorder, possibly because malnutrition and infectious illnesses remain common in these countries. In one report from Senegal, a third of all admissions to the mental hospital were for postpartum psychoses (Collomb *et al*, 1972).

Still birth

A still birth is a devastating event; as many as one in a 100 women will leave hospital without a live baby. In two published series, almost all the women had typical grief reactions (Woolf & Nielson, 1970; Forrest *et al*, 1982). The pattern is usually one of initial shock, commonly followed by numbness, disbelief and denial. Guilt was a prominent feature as women search desparately for an explanation, and some women criticise themselves over-harshly for minor peccadillos during pregnancy, such as drinking alcohol, eating the wrong food, or not strictly following their doctor's advice. Sometimes there is anger directed at the obstetric team, particularly if some intervention had failed. Women may have recurrent nightmares during which they relive their experiences during labour, with the clinical picture showing some resemblance to post-traumatic stress disorder. Only a minority succumb to a prolonged postnatal depression. Even among those who have recovered, anniversary reactions of a depressive type are common.

Despite much early distress, the few available studies do not suggest there are many long-term psychiatric sequelae. Clarke & Williams (1979) found that although depression was more common at three months postpartum, by six months the rate was no higher than women with live babies. By three years, half the primigravid women had become pregnant again, but multigravid women tended to become over-protective towards their other children and a few sought sterilisation (Woolf & Nielson, 1970). Husbands are just as distressed by the loss, but tend to compensate by throwing themselves into their work rather than grieving openly. Adverse long-term effects were noted after the birth of anencephalic or hydrocephalic still-born babies in around half the women 10 to 20 years later. These women continued to suffer from unresolved grief, depression and anxiety (Morris *et al*, 1984). Factors contributing to these prolonged reactions were a failure on the part of doctors to provide a comprehensive explanation for the cause of the still birth, and a lack of emotional support during the first few months after the loss. Lewis & Page (1978) also suggested that a few women are so profoundly affected that the still birth has lifelong and sometimes detrimental effects on the way other children are regarded and the subsequent family life.

Management of still birth

Little attention was given to women who had suffered a still birth until comparatively recently. Most left hospital as soon as possible to avoid painful contact with women who had live births. Those who have to remain in hospital for medical reasons are usually nursed on antenatal wards. Savage (1988) described an active management programme and stressed the role of the consultant obstetrician. This is because almost all women will be keen to know the medical reason for their loss and to see whether anything can be done to prevent a recurrence. Women should therefore be offered an appointment with their consultant obstetrician a few weeks following discharge to discuss the probable cause and possible future management. Further interviews with paediatricians, pathologists and genetic counsellors may also be required depending on the cause. In the immediate day or two after the loss, some women will wish to see their dead child, have a photograph, take a lock of hair or talk to their chaplain to arrange the funeral, but others may not wish to have any contact. Giles (1970) found that about half of the women wished for contact and half did not, or as one of the patients in his series put it, "that every woman would want to [have contact], though it would break her heart".

Counselling with a professional after a still birth may help to diminish the severity of the grief reaction, but most women prefer to seek support from fellow sufferers through organisations such as the Stillbirth and Neonatal Death Society (SANDS) rather than more formal psychotherapy. In a controlled study, Forrest *et al* (1982) showed that counselling significantly decreased the psychiatric morbidity at six months, but by 14 months 80% of the subjects were recovered, and there was no difference between those who received counselling and those who did not.

Miscarriage

Spontaneous abortion or miscarriage is very common and occurs in around one pregnancy in five, but its psychiatric sequelae have been little studied. There is good agreement that psychosis is extremely rare, and figures of 0.2–0.4 per 1000 (Tietze & Lewitt, 1972) and 0.3 per 1000 (Brewer, 1977) are reported. This makes the disorder about a tenth as frequent as puerperal psychosis and is probably not significantly elevated over the base rate for psychosis. However, depressive reactions are common. Thus at one month after the miscarriage about half of the women had depression: four times the expected rate. Depression was more common among those with no previous children (Friedman & Gath, 1989). The picture was of a typical grief reaction with guilt feelings. Some women still believed they were pregnant, or that the diagnosis of miscarriage was a mistake, or that they had twins and only one of these had died. Turner *et al* (1991) described a special miscarriage clinic, and found that at one month 75% of attenders reported a depressive reaction, mainly of unresolved grief, but 21% had a more prolonged reaction, suggesting that women with a miscarriage should be offered counselling routinely.

Termination of pregnancy

The topic has recently been extensively reviewed by Zolese & Blacker (1992). Around one in five pregnancies in England and Wales are terminated with a therapeutic abortion. The mortality for women is now very low (3.5 per 100 000), although the rates for major complications are 0.3–2.1%, and for minor complications 5–10%, these figures being quite high. Psychiatric sequelae are more difficult to quantify and there may be other confounding variables. For example, women seeking a termination are more likely to have relationship difficulties or other psychopathology than those who continue with their pregnancies.

The largest reported study (more than 6500 cases) was the collaborative study between the Royal College of General Practitioners and the Royal College of Obstetricians (Frank *et al*, 1985). Three weeks after the termination, psychiatric morbidity was present in 2.5% of the sample, with only 1.2% requiring psychiatric treatment. Rates for depression were 2.6 times higher among women with a past history of depression. Only two cases were hospitalised, both subjects with schizophrenia in which the link with the operation was questionable. In other studies the rates for neurotic and affective disorders were around 10–20%, which is similar to the population base rates, indicating that the operation probably has little effect in triggering depression.

Older studies highlighted the prevalence of guilt feelings, but as these studies were conducted during an era when society frowned on abortion, and the operation was often unsafe, such findings are not surprising. A later study by Greer *et al* (1976) identified guilt in 37% of women prior to the operation; 15% three months post-operatively; and 7% after two years. Kumar & Robson (1978) observed that guilt arising from a previous termination was associated with postnatal depression in some cases. Also it is not uncommon to hear women presenting with an affective disorder later in life express remorse concerning an earlier termination. Payne *et al* (1976) observed a sociocultural effect among women in Boston. Highest levels of post-abortion guilt were found among Catholic women, intermediate levels among the Protestants, and lowest levels in the Jewish women, a finding reflecting the attitudes of the respective religions to abortion. In the same study a poor relationship with the patient's mother was also associated with post-abortion guilt feelings. Lask (1975) identified a pattern of loss, regret, guilt and self-reproach analogous to a mourning process in some women. Two other subgroups may also have an adverse reaction:

older multiparous women with other children at home who have made a strong identification with the maternal role (Lask, 1975); and women who have the termination on medical grounds (Donnai & Harris, 1981) because their own health is at risk, or because of some foetal abnormality. These women experience a typical bereavement reaction as for a wanted child. However, for the majority of women a termination represents the resolution of a temporary life crisis and is a "willed-for loss" (Zolese & Blacker, 1992) in contrast to the unwanted loss of a miscarriage, and this may partially explain why the prevalence of depression is so much higher following a miscarriage.

Premenstrual syndrome (PMS)

Many women describe an exacerbation of mental symptoms in the week or ten days prior to menstruation, with a relatively asymptomatic phase in the first two weeks after menstruation. The main psychological symptoms of PMS are depression, irritability and lethargy, but a wide variety of other symptoms may also occur, as shown in Table 21.2. Depressive symptoms are usually associated with weeping, but the mood tends to be labile in contrast to the more continuous depressed mood encountered in a depressive illness. In other cases there is a picture of atypical depression with hypersomnia, food cravings and a reactive mood, and rarely there may be a picture resembling a Kleine–Levin syndrome (see page 1200) with premenstrual hypersomnia, hyperphagia and hypersexuality. In some women the depression is associated with agitation and anger, which may reach a peak about two days before the onset of menstruation. There is a considerable overlap with affective disorder as around two-thirds of women presenting to PMS clinics give a lifetime history of affective disorder (Halbreich & Endicott, 1985) or have scores corresponding to psychiatric caseness on the General Health Questionnaire (Clare, 1983).

Irritability in PMS is associated with both irrationality and impatience, while spouses may report increased anger, vindictiveness, and temper tantrums in their wives. There may be profound lethargy, impaired efficiency, clumsiness and a tendency to drop things. Rates for sick-leave, domestic and work accidents are also higher. There is an increased rate of attempted suicide, and admission rates for affective disorders, but not for schizophrenia, are higher (Dalton, 1984).

Rather less common psychological symptoms include brief psychotic episodes, alcohol cravings (with occasional drunken bouts), food cravings (particularly for sweet-tasting foods) and heightened sexual urges (which may occasionally result in promiscuity). The disorder is also accompanied by a variety of somatic symptoms such as breast pain. This is explained by water retention, although objective studies of premenstrual weight gain suggest this effect is small (Bruce & Russell, 1962). Frontal headache is also frequent and headache is more common among those with a previous history or family history of migraine, although PMS headaches are generally relieved by minor analgesics and are not true migraines.

Definition and classification of PMS

Dalton (1984) offered a succinct definition as "the recurrence of symptoms during the premenstruum, with their absence in the post menstruum". Until recently the premenstrual syndrome was considered too trivial a disturbance for classification as a psychiatric disorder. ICD–10 does not include it as a psychiatric disorder, but as one of the menstrual cycle-related disorders in the gynaecological section. DSM–IV does not give PMS the full status of a psychiatric disorder either, but instead includes it in a chapter entitled "Criteria, sets and axes, provided for further study". Instead of giving 'diagnostic criteria' (because it is not fully recognised as a disorder), only "Research criteria for premenstrual dysphoric disorder" are published and these are given in Box 21.2.

Table 21.2 Frequency of individual symptoms in premenstrual syndrome on first consultation (n = 610)

Symptom	Frequency (%)
Depression	71
Irritability	56
Tiredness	35
Headaches	33
Bloatedness	31
Breast tenderness	21
Tension	19
Violence	13
Suicidal feelings	6
Anxiety/panic	5
Fits	3
Psychotic episodes	3
Skin lesions	3
Vertigo	2
Alcoholic craving	2
Asthma	1.5
Urinary symptoms	1
Ear, nose and throat lesions	0.7
Eye lesions	0.7

Adapted from Dalton (1984), with permission.

Epidemiology and aetiology

Around 20–40% of women experience some premenstrual symptoms, but only 5% report that the symptoms have some impact on their work or lifestyle (Severino & Molin, 1989). Rees (1953) estimated that symptoms were severe in 5%, moderate in 16%, but detectable in 80% of women. Although the syndrome can present at any age after puberty, it is usually more severe and presents for treatment among those over 30, and may be most severe in the 5–10 years prior to the menopause.

Because the syndrome does not occur before puberty or following the menopause or an ovariectomy, it has been suggested that the hormones involved in ovulation may be causal. Which ovarian hormone is responsible? The progesterone deficiency hypothesis (Dalton, 1984) suggests that there is an absolute or relative deficiency of progesterone, while Israel (1938), who first described the disorder, believed that an excess of oestrogen was responsible. Other theories involve the oestrogen/ progesterone ratio, prolactin, the biogenic amines, pyridoxine, nutrition, prostaglandins and allergy (see Severino & Molin, 1989). There is also some evidence that genetic factors are important. In a large Finnish study, over 70% of the daughters of mothers with PMS also had PMS (Kantero & Widholm, 1971). A large twin study of PMS estimated the hereditability of the symptoms to be between 0.5 and 0.7 (Van den Akker *et al*, 1987) and this observation has been replicated in a more recent twin study (Condon, 1993). Psychosocial stress, life events and relationship difficulties may all increase symptoms, while conversely, good relationships may have some protective effect, but psychosocial factors are probably not the primary cause.

Management

PMS acts as a convenient umbrella to cover many of life's troubles. Thus, the initial evaluation should always seek to exclude any coexisting psychiatric disorder, particularly depression, relationship problems, and other social problems, and whenever possible the diagnosis should be confirmed by asking the patient to chart her symptoms prospectively.

Severino & Molin (1989) reviewed over 50 treatments, all of which claimed to be successful, but this is hardly surprising as the placebo response rate is somewhere between 40–90%. They recommend that simpler non-medical remedies should always be tried first. These include simple psychotherapy, educating the patient and her partner about the nature of PMS, making appropriate changes in lifestyle, increasing exercise, and the avoidance of caffeine and alcohol during the premenstrual phase. A reduction in salt intake is indicated if fluid retention is a problem. Among women with weight gain a thiazide diuretic may be helpful, but diuretics do not help women who only complain of bloatedness (O'Brien,

---

Box 21.2 DSM–IV research criteria for premenstrual dysphoric disorder

A. In most menstrual cycles during the past year, five (or more) symptoms should be present during the luteal phase, should remit within a few days of onset of the follicular phase, and should be absent in the week post menses, with one of the symptoms being 1, 2, 3 or 4.

1. depressed mood
2. anxiety, tension
3. affective lability
4. irritability, anger or increased interpersonal conflicts
5. decreased interest
6. poor concentration
7. lethargy, easy fatigue ability
8. change in appetite, over-eating, specific food cravings
9. hypersomnia or insomnia
10. a subjective sense of being overwhelmed or out of control
11. other physical symptoms, breast tenderness or swelling, headaches, joint or muscle pain, a sensation of bloating, weight gain.

B. Interferes with work, school or social activities.

C. Not due to an exacerbation of another DSM–IV disorder such as major depressive disorder, panic disorder, personality disorder or dysthymia.

D. The diagnosis should be confirmed by prospective daily rating of two consecutive cycles.

Adapted with permission from DSM–IV. Copyright 1994 American Psychiatric Association.

1993). The National Association for the Premenstrual Syndrome recommends a dietary regime that aims to avoid fluctuations in blood sugar level, if not actual hypoglycaemia. They suggest that meals should have high starch content and little or no sugar, and should be taken frequently, preferably at intervals of less than three hours. Some patients claim benefit from proprietary remedies, such as magnesium, or the fatty acids linoleinic and linolenic acids (oil of evening primrose). Vitamin B6 is not quite the harmless remedy it was once thought to be because if taken in excess it may cause peripheral neuropathy presenting with unstable gait, numbness of the hands and peri-oral numbness. Rigorous trials for all of the above remedies are lacking, and so their effectiveness (if any) is unproven.

Two recent controlled trials have shown beneficial effects for clomipramine in doses of 25–75 mg daily (Sundblad *et al*, 1992) and for fluoxetine 20 mg daily (Menkes *et al*, 1992), suggesting a possible role for serotonin in the origin of PMS. Women with mainly physical symptoms may benefit from a potassium-sparing diuretic such as spironolactone. The complaint of mastodynia sometimes responds well to bromocriptine, although vomiting is a common side-effect. Mefenamic acid, a prostaglandin synthetase inhibitor that is more often used in dysmenorrheae, may sometimes be helpful in PMS, but as the drug can cause blood dyscrasias it should be used sparingly.

Some patients report an improvement in their PMS when they are taking the oral contraceptive pill, but this is not routinely used in the management of PMS. Hormonal therapies have recently become popular and Dalton (1984) advocated the use of progesterone. As the hormone is rapidly degraded in the liver it has to be administered rectally in the form of suppositories. Unfortunately, even though repeated controlled trials have failed to confirm that progesterone has any beneficial effects, the treatment remains popular. Magos *et al* (1986) reported some success with oestradiol implants, although in these studies placebo response rates were also very high. In cases with decreased libido, the addition of testosterone implants have been tried. Hormone implants tend to wear off after a few months and symptoms reappear unless the implant is repeated. A medical ovariectomy using a gonadotrophin releasing hormone (GnRH) analogue will also alleviate PMS, but this method is far too drastic for routine clinical use because of the risk of osteoporosis (Mortola *et al*, 1991). Danazol may also block the ovarian cycle and may be helpful in some cases of PMS, but its use is presently still experimental (O'Brien, 1993).

The menopause

The main hormonal change of the menopause is a sharp fall in oestrogen levels resulting in a compensatory rise in FSH and LH. The symptoms most likely to be caused directly by oestrogen deficiency are hot flushes, night sweats, insomnia, and atrophic vaginitis, which may result in sexual problems and, after some years, osteoporosis (Utian, 1972). General population studies have failed to demonstrate any significant excess of minor psychological symptoms at around the time of the menopause, but there is evidence that fatigue and depression may be more severe in the five premenopausal years than in the year after the menopause (Ballinger, 1975).

Psychological and social factors make an important contribution to psychiatric morbidity at this time. Thus the early psychoanalysts adopted a rather negative view of the menopause, emphasising loss of femininity, loss of reproductive potential, as well as fears of ageing. More recently psychotherapists have taken a more optimistic view: for example, Prados

(1967) believed that the menopause may be a time of stability and satisfaction. In those Asian cultures where increased age is linked to a higher social status (e.g. India), the only menopausal symptoms reported regularly were menstrual changes. In Japan menopausal complaints are uncommon. Psychosocial changes occurring in mid-life may also independently contribute to psychiatric morbidity (Ballinger, 1990), particularly children leaving home (the so-called empty nest syndrome), worries about work, difficulties with adolescent children, ailing husbands, and ageing parents. Menopausal status itself was not found to be a factor contributing to depression in one community study of women in this age group (Cooke, 1985).

Controversy remains as to whether perimenopausal changes contribute to the increased prevalence of affective disorder in women of middle age. Kraepelin (1906) first proposed the concept of involutional melancholia, in which the presumed cause of the depression was ovarian involution, but later retracted the idea, believing that the increasing prevalence might best be explained solely by the effect of increasing age (Kraepelin, 1921). Although most studies fail to demonstrate an increased admission rate at the time of the menopause, Eagles & Whalley (1985) found that the greatest difference between rates for female to male admissions for affective disorder was between the ages of 45–55. This suggests that whatever was responsible for the difference between men and women with regard to admissions for affective disorder, it was greatest at this time. At one time it was thought that hysterectomy itself could cause depression; for example, in the study by Barker (1968) there were more psychiatric referrals following hysterectomy (all causes) than following cholecystectomy. However, a population-based study showed a general improvement in psychiatric morbidity following hysterectomy when pre- and post-operative measures of mood were compared (Gath *et al*, 1982). Obviously for some women depression may start for the first time after hysterectomy, but this is not the usual pattern.

There are definite medical indications for hormone replacement therapy (HRT), particularly following oophorectomy when HRT may help prevent osteoporosis, premature heart disease or stroke, or among women who may be at increased risk of these diseases even without oophorectomy. HRT is also helpful for those with hot flushes, insomnia and atrophic vaginitis. The role of HRT in the treatment of minor psychiatric disturbance is rather more controversial, with some gynaecologists enthusiastically advocating its use (Khaw, 1992) while most psychiatrists remain unconvinced (Ballinger, 1990). There is, however, general agreement that it is of little use in major depression or other serious psychiatric illnesses.

Women presenting with almost any mental symptom at this time will have been well briefed by the popular press that they must be suffering from some hormone deficiency, and therefore should take hormone replacement therapy. The doctor's task is to clarify the patient's main source of distress, whether this is due to social and relationship difficulties, affective disorder, or possibly a hormonal contribution. Montgomery *et al* (1987) showed that oestrogen implants in menopausal women led to a more rapid resolution of depression and anxiety, although by four months there was no difference between active hormonal treatment and placebo. Standard antidepressive therapy should be used for those with major depression, but a small number of women presenting in the perimenopausal years with cyclical depressions coinciding with their premenstruum may benefit from hormonal implants.

Acknowledgements

I would like to thank Dr Louis Appleby and Dr Robin Jacobson for their helpful advice and comments on an earlier draft of this chapter, and Ms Eka Lee for her assistance with Box 21.1 and Table 21.1.

References

Abarbanel, J. (1983) The revival of the sibling experience during the mother's second pregnancy. *Psychoanalysis of the Child*, **38**, 353–379.

Agrawal, P., Bhatia, M. S. & Malik, S. C. (1990) Post partum psychosis: a study of indoor cases in a general hospital psychiatric clinic. *Acta Psychiatrica Scandinavica*, **81**, 571–575.

American Psychiatric Association (1994) *Diagnostic and Statistical Manual of Mental Disorders* (4th edn) (DSM–IV). Washington, DC: APA.

Appleby, L. (1991) Suicide during pregnancy and in the first post partum year. *British Medical Journal*, **302**, 137–140.

Ballinger, C. B. (1975) Psychiatric morbidity and the menopause. Screening of a general population sample. *British Medical Journal*, iii, 344–346.

—— (1990) Psychiatric aspects of the menopause. *British Journal of Psychiatry*, **156**, 773–787.

Barker, M. (1968) Psychiatric illness after hysterectomy. *British Medical Journal*, **2**, 91–95.

Best, N. R., Cowen, P. J., Elliott, J. M., *et al* (1985) Changes in imipramine and α2 adreno-receptor binding sites in the early puerperium. *British Journal of Clinical Pharmacology*, **19**, 555.

Bibring, G. (1959) Some considerations of the psychological processes in pregnancy. *Psychoanalytic Study of the Child*, **14**, 113–121.

Brewer, C. (1977) Incident of post abortion psychosis: a prospective study. *British Medical Journal*, **1**, 467–477.

Briggs, G., Freeman, R. K. & Yaffe, J. (1990) *A Reference Guide to Foetal and Neonatal Risk. Drugs in Pregnancy and Lactation* (3rd edn). Baltimore: Williams & Wilkins.

Brockington, I. F., Winokur, G. & Dean, C. (1982) Puerperal psychosis. In *Motherhood and Mental Illness* (eds I. F. Brockington & R. Kumar), pp. 37–69. London: Academic Press.

——, Martin, C., Brown, G. W., *et al* (1990) Stress and puerperal psychosis. *British Journal of Psychiatry*, **157**, 331–334.

Bruce, J. & Russell, G. F. M. (1962) A study of weight changes and balances of water, sodium and potassium. *Lancet*, **2**, 267–271.

Clare, A. W. (1983) Psychiatric and social aspects of premenstrual complaint. *Psychological Medicine*, **13** (suppl. 4), 1–58.

Clarke, M. & Williams, A. J. (1979) Depression in women after perinatal death. *Lancet*, **i**, 916–917.

Clouston, T. S. (1896) *Clinical Lectures on Mental Diseases* (4th edn). London: Churchill.

Coghill, S. R., Caplan, H. L., Alexandra, H., *et al* (1986) Impact of maternal postnatal depression on cognitive development of young children. *British Medical Journal*, **292**, 1165–1167.

Collomb, H., Guena, R. & Diop, B. (1972) Psychological and social factors in the pathology of childbearing. *Foreign Psychiatry*, **1**, 77–89.

Condon, J. T. (1993) The premenstrual syndrome: a twin study. *British Journal of Psychiatry*, **162**, 481–486.

Cooke, D. J. (1985) Psychosocial vulnerability to life events during the climacteric. *British Journal of Psychiatry*, **147**, 71–75.

Cookson, J. C. (1985) Neuroendocrinology of mania. *Journal of Affective Disorders*, **8**, 233–241.

Cooper, P. J., Campbell, E. A., Kennerley, H., *et al* (1988) Non-psychotic disorder after childbirth: a prospective study of prevalence, incidence, course and nature. *British Journal of Psychiatry*, **152**, 799–806.

Cox, A. D. (1988) Maternal depression and impact on children's development. *Archives of Diseases in Childhood*, **63**, 90–95.

Cox, J. L. (1983) Postnatal depression: a comparison of African and Scottish women. *Social Psychiatry*, **18**, 25–28.

—— (1988) The life event of childbirth; Socio-cultural aspects of post natal depression. In *Motherhood and Mental Illness*, 2 (eds R. Kumar & I. F. Brockington). London: Wright.

——, Connor, Y. & Kendell, R. E. (1982) Prospective study of the psychiatric disorders of childbirth by personal interview. *British Journal of Psychiatry*, **140**, 111–117.

——, Holden, J. M. & Sagovsky, R. (1987) Detection of postnatal depression: Development of the 10-item Edinburgh Postnatal Depression Scale. *British Journal of Psychiatry*, **150**, 782–786.

——, Murray, D. & Chapman, G. (1993) A controlled study of the onset, duration and prevalence of postnatal depression. *British Journal of Psychiatry*, **163**, 27–31.

Crammer, J. L. (1959) Water and sodium in two psychotics. *Lancet*, **i**, 1122–1126.

Dalton, K. (1971) Prospective study into puerperal depression. *British Journal of Psychiatry*, **118**, 689–692.

—— (1984) *The Premenstrual Syndrome and Progesterone Therapy* (2nd edn). Chicago, IL: Year Book Medical Publishers.

—— (1985) Progesterone prophylaxis used successfully in postnatal depression. *The Practitioner*, **229**, 507–508.

Da Silva, L. & Johnstone, E. C. (1981) A follow up study of severe puerperal psychiatric illness. *British Journal of Psychiatry*, **139**, 346–354.

Davidson, J. & Robertson, E. (1985) A follow up study of post partum illness 1946–1978. *Acta Psychiatrica Scandinavica*, **71**, 451–457.

Dean, C. & Kendell, R. E. (1981) The symptomatology of puerperal illnesses. *British Journal of Psychiatry*, **139**, 128–133.

——, Williams, R. J. & Brockington, I. F. (1989) Is puerperal psychosis the same as bipolar manic depression disorder? A family study. *Psychological Medicine*, **19**, 637–647.

Donnai, D. & Harris, R. (1981) Attitudes of patients after genetic termination of pregnancy. *British Medical Journal*, **282**, 621–622.

D'Orban, P. T. (1979) Women who kill their children. *British Journal of Psychiatry*, **134**, 560–571.

Dowlatschahi, D. & Paykel, E. S. (1990) Life events and social stress in puerperal psychosis: absence of effect. *Psychological Medicine*, **20**, 655–662.

Eagles, J. M. & Whalley, L. J. (1985) Ageing and affective disorders. The age at first onset of affective disorders in Scotland 1969–1978. *British Journal of Psychiatry*, **147**, 180–187.

Edwards, D. R. L., Porter, S. A. M. & Stein, G. S. (1994) A pilot study of postnatal depression using two retrospective rating instruments. *Journal of Psychosomatic Research*, **38**, 111–118.

Endicott, J. & Spitzer, R. L. (1978) A diagnostic interview: the Schedule for Affective Disorders and Schizophrenia. *Archives of General Psychiatry*, **35**, 837–844.

Enoch, M. D. & Trethowan, W. H. (1979) The couvade. In *Uncommon Psychiatric Syndromes* (2nd edn), pp. 63–76. Bristol: John Wright.

Esquirol, J. E. D. (1845) *Des Maladies Mentale. A Treatise on Insanity* (transl. E. K. Hunt, 1965). New York: Hafner.

Forrest, G. C., Standish, E. & Baum, J. D. (1982) Support after perinatal death: a study of support and counselling after perinatal bereavement. *British Medical Journal*, **285**, 1475–1479.

Frank, P. I., Kay, C. R., Winsgrave, S. J., *et al* (1985). Induced abortion operations and their early sequelae. *Journal of the Royal College of General Practitioners*, **31**, 473–477.

Friedman, T. & Gath, D. (1989) The psychiatric consequences of spontaneous abortion. *British Journal of Psychiatry*, **155**, 810–813.

Gard, P. R., Handley, S. L., Parsons, A. D., *et al* (1986) A multivariate investigation of post partum mood disturbance. *British Journal of Psychiatry*, **148**, 567–575.

Garvey, M. J., Tuason, V. B., Luming, A. E., *et al* (1983) Occurrence of depression in the post partum state. *Journal of Affective Disorders*, **5**, 97–101.

Gater, R., Dean, C. & Morris, J. (1989) The contribution of childbearing to the sex differences in first admission rates for affective psychoses. *Psychological Medicine*, **19**, 719–724.

Gath, D., Cooper, P. & Day, A. (1982) Hysterectomy and psychiatric disorder: I. Levels of morbidity before and after hysterectomy. *British Journal of Psychiatry*, **140**, 335–350.

George, A. J. & Wilson, K. C. M. (1981) Monoamine oxidase activity and the puerperal blues syndrome. *Journal of Psychosomatic Research*, **25**, 409–413.

—— & Sandler, M. (1988) Endocrine and biochemical studies in puerperal mental disorders. In *Motherhood and Mental Illness* (eds. R. Kumar & I. F. Brockington), pp. 78–104. London: Wright.

Gibson, E. & Klein, F. (1961) *Murder: a Home Office Research Unit Report.* London: HMSO.

Giles, P. F. H. (1970) Reactions of women to perinatal death. *Australian and New Zealand Journal of Obstetrics and Gynaecology,* **10**, 207–210.

Glaser, Y. I. M. (1962) A unit for mothers and babies in a psychiatric hospital. *Journal of Child Psychology and Psychiatry,* **3**, 53–60.

Gooch, R. (1829) Puerperal psychosis. In *Three Hundred Years of Psychiatry* (1963) (eds R. Hunter & I. Macalpine), pp. 768–800. Oxford: Oxford University Press.

Greenwood, J. & Parker, G. (1984) The dexamethasone suppression test in the puerperium. *Australian and New Zealand Journal of Psychiatry,* **18**, 282–284.

Greer, H. S., Lal, C. S., Lewis, S. C., *et al* (1976) Psychological consequences of therapeutic abortion. Kings Termination Study III. *British Journal of Psychiatry,* **128**, 74–79.

Halbreich, U., Endicott, J., Schacht, S., *et al* (1982) The diversity of premenstrual changes as reflected in the premenstrual assesssment form. *Acta Psychiatrica Scandinavica,* **65**, 46–65.

—— & —— (1985) Relationship of premenstrual dysphoric changes to depressive disorders. *Acta Psychiatrica Scandinavica,* **77**, 331.

Hamilton, J. A. (1962) *Postpartum Psychiatric Problems.* St Louis: Mosby.

—— (1982) The identity of post partum psychosis. In *Motherhood and Mental Illness* (eds I. F. Brockington & R. Kumar), pp. 1–17. London: Academic Press.

Handley, S. L., Dunn, T. L., Waldron, G., *et al* (1980) Tryptophan, cortisol and puerperal mood. *British Journal of Psychiatry,* **136**, 498–508.

Hannah, P., Adams, D., Lee, A., *et al* (1992) Links between early post partum mood and post-natal depression. *British Journal of Psychiatry,* **160**, 777–780.

Harris, B. (1980) Prospective trial of L-tryptophan in the maternity blues. *British Journal of Psychiatry,* **137**, 233–235.

——, Lovett, L., Newcombe, R. G., *et al* (1994) Maternity blues and major endocrine changes: Cardiff puerperal mood and hormone study II. *British Medical Journal,* **308**, 949–953.

Harvey, I. & McGrath, G. (1988) Psychiatric morbidity in spouses of women admitted to a mother and baby unit. *British Journal of Psychiatry,* **152**, 506–510.

Hatotani, N., Nomura, J., Yamaguchi, T., *et al* (1983) Clinical endocrine studies of post partum psychoses. In *Neurobiology of Periodic Psychoses* (eds N. Hatotani & J. Nomura), pp. 93–104. Tokyo: Igateu-Shoin.

Hays, P. (1978) Taxonomic map of the schizophrenias, with special reference to puerperal psychosis. *British Medical Journal,* **2**, 755–757.

Israel, R. S. (1938) Premenstrual tension. *Journal of the American Medical Association,* **110**, 1721–1723.

Janssen, B. (1964) Psychic insufficiences associated with childbearing. *Acta Psychiatrica Scandinavica,* **39** (suppl. 172), 41–56.

Kadramas, A., Winokur, G. & Crowe, R. (1980) Postpartum mania. *British Journal of Psychiatry,* **135**, 551–554.

Kantero, R. L. & Widholm, O. (1971) A statistical analysis of the menstrual patterns of 8000 Finnish girls and their mothers: IV. Correlations of menstrual traits between adolescent girls and their mothers. *Acta Obstetric Gynecologica Scandanavica,* **14** (suppl), 7–18.

Karacan, I., Williams, R. L., Hursch, C., *et al* (1969) Some implications for the sleep pattern for post partum emotional disorder. *British Journal of Psychiatry*, **115**, 929–932.

Karnosh, L. J. & Hope, J. M. (1937) Puerperal psychoses and their sequelae. *American Journal of Psychiatry*, **94**, 537–550.

Katona, C. L. E. (1982) Puerperal mental illness; comparison with non-puerperal controls. *British Journal of Psychiatry*, **141**, 447–452.

Kendell, R. E. (1985) Emotional and physical factors in the genesis of puerperal mental disorders. *Journal of Psychosomatic Research*, **29**, 3–11.

—, Rannie, D., Clarke, J. A., *et al* (1981) The social and obstetric correlates of psychiatric admission in the puerperium. *Psychological Medicine*, **11**, 341–350.

—, Chalmers, J. C. & Platz, C. (1987) Epidemiology of puerperal psychosis. *British Journal of Psychiatry*, **150**, 662–673.

Kennerly, H. & Gath, D. (1989) Maternity blues. I. Detection and measurement by questionnaire. *British Journal of Psychiatry*, **155**, 356–362.

Khaw, K. T. (1992) Hormone replacement therapy. *British Medical Bulletin*, **48**, 249–276.

Kleiner, G. J. & Greston, W. M. (1984) Overview of demographic and statistical factors. In *Suicide in Pregnancy* (eds G. J. Kleiner & W. M. Greston), pp. 23–40. Littleton, MA: John Wright.

Klompenhouwer, J. C. & Van Hulst, A. M. (1991) Classification of post partum psychoses. *Acta Psychiatrica Scandinavica*, **84**, 255–281.

Kraepelin, E. (1906) Lecture 1 – Introduction: Melancholia. In *Lectures on Clinical Psychiatry* (revised and edited by T. Johnson). New York: Balliere, Tindall & Cox.

— (1921) *Manic Depression, Insanity and Paranoia* (transl. R. M. Barclay, ed. G. M. Robertson). Edinburgh: E. & S. Livingstone.

Kumar, C. & Robson, K. (1978) Previous induced abortion and antenatal depression in primiparae: Preliminary report of a survey of mental health in pregnancy. *Psychological Medicine*, **8**, 711–715.

Kumar, R. & Robson, K. (1984) A prospective study of emotional disorders in childbearing women. *British Journal of Psychiatry*, **144**, 35–47.

Lask, B. (1975) Short term psychiatric sequelae to therapeutic termination of pregnancy. *British Journal of Psychiatry*, **126**, 173–177.

Levy, V. (1987) The maternity blues in post partum and post operative women. *British Journal of Psychiatry*, **151**, 368–372.

Lewis, E. & Page, A. (1978) Failure to mourn a stillbirth: An overlooked catastrophe. *British Journal of Medical Psychology*, **51**, 237–241.

Liedloff, P. (1975) *The Continuum Concept*. London: Gerald Duckworth.

Magos, A. L., Brincat, M. & Studd, J. W. W. (1986) Treatment of the premenstrual syndrome by subcutaneous oestradiol implants and cyclical norethisterone: placebo controlled study. *British Medical Journal*, **292b**, 1629–1633.

Main, T. F. (1958) Mothers with children in psychiatric hospital. *Lancet*, **ii**, 845–847.

Marcé, L. V. (1858) *Traité de la Folie des Femmes Enceintes, des Nouvelles Accouchées et des Nourrices*. Paris: Bailliere.

Margison, F. (1982) The pathology of the mother–child relationship. In *Motherhood and Mental Illness* (eds I. F. Brockington & R. Kumar), pp. 191–122. London: Academic Press.

—— & Brockington, I. F. (1982) Psychiatric mother and baby units. In *Motherhood and Mental Illness* (eds I. F. Brockington & R. Kumar), pp. 223–238. London: Academic Press.

Martin, M. E. (1958) Puerperal mental illness. A follow-up study of 75 cases. *British Medical Journal*, **2**, 773–777.

Melges, F. T. (1968) Postpartum psychiatric syndromes. *Psychosomatic Medicine*, **30**, 95–108.

Meltzer, E. S. & Kumar, R. S. (1985) Puerperal mental illness, clinical features and classification: a study of 142 mother-and-baby admissions. *British Journal of Psychiatry*, **147**, 647–654.

Menkes, D. B., Taghavi, E., Mason, P., *et al* (1992) Fluoxetine treatment of severe premenstrual syndrome. *British Medical Journal*, **305**, 346–347.

Montgomery, J. C., Brincat, M., Appleby, L., *et al* (1987) Oestrogen and testosterone implants on psychological disorders in the climacteric. *Lancet*, *i*, 297–298.

Moos, R. H. (1968) The development of a Menstrual Distress Questionnaire. *Psychosomatic Medicine*, **30**, 853–857.

Morris, J., Tew, B. & Lawrence, K. M. (1984) Long term reactions following a stillbirth with a congenital abnormality: A preliminary report. *Zeitschrift fur Kinderchirurgie*, **39** (suppl. 2), 117–119.

Mortola, J. F., Girton, L., Fischer, U., *et al* (1991) Successful treatment of severe premenstrual syndrome by combined use of gonadrotropic-releasing hormone against and estrogen/progestin. *Journal of Clinical Endocrinology and Metabolism*, **72**, 252A-D.

Murray, L., Cooper, P. J. & Stein, A. (1991) Post natal depression and infant development. *British Medical Journal*, **302**, 978–979.

Newnham, J. P., Dennett, P. M., Ferron, S. A., *et al* (1984) A study of the relationship between circulating ß-endorphin like immunoreactivity and post partum 'blues'. *Clinical Endocrinology*, **20**, 169–177.

Nott, P. H., Franklin, M., Armitage, C., *et al* (1976) Hormonal changes and mood in the puerperium. *British Journal of Psychiatry*, **128**, 379–383.

Oates, M. (1988) The development of an integrated community orientated service for severe post natal mental illness. In *Motherhood and Mental Illness 2* (eds R. Kumar & I. F. Brockington), 133–158. London: Wright.

O'Brien, P. M. S. (1993) Helping women with premenstrual syndrome. *British Medical Journal*, **307**, 1471–1475.

O'Hara, M. W., Schlechte, J. A., Lewis, D. A., *et al* (1991) Prospective study into post partum blues. *Archives of General Psychiatry*, **48**, 801–806.

Okano, T., Nomura, J., Makita, I., *et al* (1987) Clinico-endocrine studies of the maternity blues. *Annual Report of the Pharmacopsychiatry Research Foundation*, **18**, 294–301.

——, ——, Koshikawa, N., *et al* (1991) Cross-cultural study of the maternity blues and post partum depression. *Japanese Journal of Clinical Psychiatry*, **33**, 1051–1058.

Paffenbarger, R. S. Jr (1964) Epidemiological aspects of postpartum mental illness. *British Journal of Preventative and Social Medicine*, **18**, 189–195.

Paykel, E. S., Emms, E. M., Fletcher, J., *et al* (1980) Life events and social support in puerperal depression. *British Journal of Psychiatry*, **136**, 339–346.

Payne, E. C., Kravitz, A. R., Notamen, M. T., *et al* (1976) Outcome following therapeutic abortion. *Archives of General Psychiatry*, **33**, 725–733.

Pilsbury, B. L. K. (1978) "Doing the month." Confinement and convalescence of Chinese women after childbirth. *Social Science and Medicine*, **12**, 11–22.

Pines, D. (1972) Pregnancy and motherhood: interaction between fantasy and reality. *British Journal of Medical Psychology*, **45**, 333–343.

Pitt, B. (1968) Atypical depression following childbirth. *British Journal of Psychiatry*, **114**, 1325–1335.

— (1973) 'Maternity blues'. *British Journal of Psychiatry*, **122**, 431–433.

Prados, M. (1967) Emotional factors in the climecterium of women. *Psychotherapy and Psychosomatics*, **15**, 231–244.

Protheroe, C. (1969) Puerperal psychoses: a long term study 1927–1961. *British Journal of Psychiatry*, **115**, 9–30.

Pugh, T. F., Jerath, R. K., Schmidt, W. M., *et al* (1963) Rates of mental disease related to childbearing. *New English Journal of Medicine*, **268**, 1224–1228.

Rees, L. (1953) The premenstrual tension syndrome and its treatment. *British Medical Journal*, **1**, 1014–1016.

Rehmann, A., St Clair, D. & Platz, C. (1990) Puerperal insanity in the 19th and 20th centuries. *British Journal of Psychiatry*, **156**, 861–865.

Reik, T. (1931) *Ritual.* London: Hogarth Press.

Robson, K. M. & Kumar, R. (1980) Delayed onset of maternal affection after childbirth. *British Journal of Psychiatry*, **136**, 347–353.

Samuels, M. P., McClaughlin, W., Jacobsen, R. R., *et al* (1992) Fourteen cases of imposed upper airway obstruction. *Archives of Disease in Childhood*, **67**, 162–170.

Savage, G. H. (1875) Observations on the insanity of pregnancy and childbirth. *Guy's Hospital Reports*, **20**, 83–117.

Savage, W. (1988) The active management of perinatal death. In *Mother and Mental Illness 2. Causes and Consequences* (eds R. Kumar & I. F. Brockington), pp. 247–269. London: Wright.

Severino, S. K. & Molin, M. L. (1989) *Premenstrual Syndrome. A Clinician's Guide.* New York: Guilford.

Shah, D. K., Wig, N. N. & Akhtar, S. (1971) Status of post partum illness in psychiatric nosology. *Indian Journal of Psychiatry*, **13**, 14–20.

Silbermann, R. M., Beenen, F. & De Jong, H. (1975) Clinical treatment of postpartum delirium with perphenazine and lithium carbonate. *Psychiatrica Clinica*, **8**, 314–326.

Stein, G. S. (1980) The pattern of mental change and body weight change in the first post partum week. *Journal of Psychosomatic Research*, **24**, 165–171.

— (1982) The maternity blues. In *Motherhood and Mental Illness* (eds I. F. Brockington & R. Kumar), pp. 119–154. London: Academic Press.

— (1984) Headaches in the first post partum week and their relationship to migraine. *Headache*, **21**, 201–205.

—, Milton, F., Bebbington, P., *et al* (1976) Relationship between mood disturbance and free plasma tryptophan in post partum women. *British Medical Journal*, **2**, 451.

—, Gath, D. H., Bucher, J., *et al* (1991) The relationship between post natal depression and mother child interaction. *British Journal of Psychiatry*, **158**, 46–52.

Stewart, D. E., Klompenhouwer, J. L., Kendell, R. E., *et al* (1991) Prophylactic lithium in puerperal psychosis: the experience of three centres. *British Journal of Psychiatry*, **158**, 393–397.

Strecker, E. A. & Ebaugh, F. C. (1926) Psychoses occurring during the puerperium. *Archives of Neurological Psychiatry*, **15**, 239–252.

Sundblad, C., Modigh, K., Anderseh, B., *et al* (1992) Clomipramine effectively reduces premenstrual irritability and dysphoria: a placebo controlled trial. *Acta Psychiatrica Scandinavica*, **85**, 39–47.

Surtees, P. G., Dean, C., Ingham, J. C., *et al* (1983) Psychiatric disorder in women from an Edinburgh community: association with demographic factors. *British Journal of Psychiatry*, **142**, 238–246.

Tetlow, C. (1955) Psychoses of childbearing. *Journal of Mental Science*, **101**, 629–639.

Thuwe, I. (1974) Genetic factors in puerperal psychosis. *British Journal of Psychiatry*, **125**, 378–385.

Tietze, C. & Lewitt, S. (1972) Joint program for the study of abortion: Early complications of legal abortion. *Studies in Family Planning*, **3**, 97.

Trethowan, W. H. & Conlon, M. F. (1965) Couvade syndrome. *British Journal of Psychiatry*, **111**, 57–60.

Turner, M. J., Flannelly, G. M., Wingfield, M., *et al* (1991) The miscarriage clinic: an audit of the first year. *British Journal of Obstetrics and Gynaecology*, **98**, 306–398.

Utian, W. H. (1972) The true clinical features of the menopause and post-oophorectomy, and their response to oestrogen therapy. *South African Medical Journal*, **46**, 732–737.

Van den Akker, O. B., Stein, G. S., Neale, M. C., *et al* (1987) Genetic and environmental variation in the menstrual cycle: histories of two British samples. *Acta Genetica Medica Gemollogica (Rome)*, **36**, 541–548.

Watson, J. P., Elliott, S. A., Rugg, A. J., *et al* (1984) Psychiatric disorder in pregnancy and the first postnatal year. *British Journal of Psychiatry*, **144**, 453–462.

Wieck, A., Kumar, R., Hirst, A. D., *et al* (1991) Increased sensitivity of dopamine receptors and recurrence of affective psychoses after childbirth. *British Medical Journal*, **303**, 613–616.

Winnicott, D. W. (1958) Primary maternal preoccupation. In *Through Paediatrics to Psychoanalysis* (ed. D. W. Winnicott), pp 300–305. London: Hogarth Press.

—— (1960) The theory of the parent–infant relationship. *International Journal of Psychoanalysis*, **61**, 585–595.

Wolkind, S. & Zajdicek, E. (1978) Psycho-social correlates of nausea and vomiting in pregnancy. *Journal of Psychosomatic Research*, **22**, 1–5.

Woolf, J. R. & Nielson, P. E. (1970) The emotional reaction to stillbirth. *American Journal of Obstetrics and Gynaecology*, **108**, 73–77.

World Health Organization (1992) *The ICD–10 Classification of Mental and Behavioural Disorders*. Geneva: WHO.

Yarden, P. E., Max, M. D. & Eisenbach, Z. (1966) The effect of childbirth on the prognosis of married schizophrenic women. *British Journal of Psychiatry*, **112**, 491–499.

Zolese, G. & Blacker, C. V. R. (1992) The psychological complications of abortion. *British Journal of Psychiatry*, **160**, 742–749.

22 Organic psychiatric disorders

Robin Jacobson & Michael Kopelman

History • Syndrome definition • Classification • Syndromes with regional connections • Symptoms with regional connections • Assessment • Delirium • Dementia

---

Organic psychiatry is concerned with disorders of cognition, behaviour and affect arising from disorders of brain function. Lishman (1987) considered that it embraces the psychiatric problems of patients with neurological disorders and the psychological consequences of extra-cerebral diseases, toxic, metabolic and endocrine, that indirectly affect the brain. It also addresses the neuroscientific aspects of patients with certain general psychiatric disorders, where it overlaps with biological psychiatry. Organic psychiatry focuses on the cerebral mechanisms of psychological functioning and cognitive skills and abilities, and the ways in which pathological processes disturb them. The knowledge and application of techniques derived from psychiatry, neurology, neuro-psychology, pharmacology and medicine are essential to clinical practice. Nevertheless, the intricate reality of the patient's abnormal psychic experience and relationships is not disregarded. The developmental, psycho-social and cultural context of the individual is closely integrated into his/her assessment and treatment.

Organic psychiatry should be distinguished from two related fields, neuropsychology and biological psychiatry. Neuropsychology investigates the cognitive organisation of mental processes and functions, and their disturbances in brain-damaged patients. Neuropsychologists examine the assets and deficits of patients with brain disorders by psychological tests designed to characterise and quantify dysfunction and to guide rehabilitation. Biological psychiatry focuses on the structural, physiological and neurochemical abnormalities underlying primary psychiatric disorders such as depression and schizophrenia, in which no brain abnormality is proven (or consistently demonstrated). Organic psychiatry, on the other hand, deals with the (cognitive and behavioural) effects of known brain or neuroendocrine disease.

A comprehensive approach to organic psychiatry requires the integration of biological factors with the personal, family and social context and the consequences of brain damage. The burden on patients, relatives and carers is often severe, requiring a multidisciplinary approach to the patient and his family, as after head injury (Jacobson, 1995) and in dementia (Burns & Levy, 1994). Organic psychiatry depends critically, not only on developments in aetiology, pathogenesis and brain repair mechanisms, but also on the integration of diverse clinical investigative and treatment approaches.

History

The history of organic psychiatry has oscillated, in the main, between *localisationist* and *holistic* phases. The former developed in the early 19th century when the phrenologists Gall & Spurzheim (1809) speculated that the cerebral convolutions reflected the juxtaposition of many discrete cerebral organs, each serving a particular psychological function. Early advances in aphasia by Broca (1861) and Wernicke (1874) led to the flowering of the localisation approach by the "diagram makers" who sought to explain aphasia. In this era, Meynert (1867) described the motor and sensory cortex, and Hughlings Jackson (1875) observed contralateral focal seizures. Lissauer (1890) and Freud (1891) described agnosia, and Liepmann (1900) described apraxia. Opponents of this localisation approach to higher mental functions included Hughlings Jackson, whose schema of a hierarchy of functions with a 'dissolution' and a regression to lower levels of function, incorporating positive and negative symptoms, after brain damage, supplied an essentially unitary view of the patient. Globalist accounts of mental function developed further in the early 20th century critiques by Marie, Head and Goldstein of narrow localisationist theories of language. In 1929, Lashley's theory of mass action proposed that the cortex was undifferentiated and equipotential for cognitive abilities, their degree of impairment depending on the extent but not localisation of brain damage. More recently, localisationist or modular (Shallice, 1988) approaches have predominated.

Classical neuropsychiatric disorders were described and the syndromatic approach clarified at the turn of the century. Huntington's chorea was described in 1872, Wernicke's encephalopathy in 1881, Korsakoff's syndrome in 1887 and Pick's disease in 1892. Alzheimer (1907) described the disease that bears his name. The term delirium was introduced by Celsus in the first century AD, but Hippocrates' work was rich in descriptions of delirium, which remained a stable psychiatric category until the 19th century (Berrios, 1981).

The prevailing view that individual physical diseases gave rise to their own specific insanities was challenged by Chaslin in 1895 and Bonhoeffer in 1909, who redefined confusion and delirium as the stereotyped manifestations of acute brain failure (Berrios, 1981). Bonhoeffer (1909) recognised that, irrespective of type, different forms of insult or injury led to a narrow repertoire of stereotyped responses ('exogenous reaction types'), notably delirium.

In the 19th century, the growth of neurology and neuropathology shaped the view that mental diseases are brain diseases, while psychological systems of explanation came to receive an enormous boost from debate over the nature of hypnosis and hysteria. Charcot's physical explanation of hypnosis and hysteria clashed with, and later yielded to, Bernheim's psychogenic conception, which was expanded by Janet (Micale, 1990). In this context, Freud developed psychodynamic theory. The early 20th century witnessed only modest advances in organic psychiatry, due largely to the emergence of psychoanalysis and social psychiatry, the influence of Lashley and Gestalt psychology, and the move away from localisation to descriptive approaches to psychosis.

Organic psychiatry then lay fallow until after the Second World War. Three major studies in different nations then examined the relationship of cognitive dysfunction to the localisation of missile wounds (Luria, 1947; Semmes *et al*, 1960; Newcombe, 1969). Geschwind (1965) rediscovered the important descriptions of the 19th century 'behavioural' neurologists and relaunched the study of higher cortical functions. Luria (1966) constructively softened the localisation–holistic polarisation and began to elucidate frontal lobe functioning.

Advances in the description of behavioural syndromes have been immensely aided by the new technologies of brain-imaging and the localisation of brain lesions. Arteriography, air encephalography and isotope brain scanning heralded the era of computerised tomographic (CT) brain scanning. The CT brain scan revolutionised neurology by revealing the immediate localisation, nature and natural history of a lesion. The behavioural correlates of lesions and the structural basis of psychological deficits were now open to safe non-invasive study. New advances in cerebral blood flow measurement, positron emission tomography (PET), single photon emission computerised tomography (SPET), and nuclear magnetic imaging and spectroscopy promise to enhance further both theory and clinical practice. The complementary approaches of neuro- and psychopharmacology hold much promise for the clarification and treatment of organic disorders.

The work of the neuropsychiatrist or organic psychiatrist is primarily concerned with the psychiatric manifestations and complications of neurological disorders, whereas that of the neurologist is mainly with the diagnosis and treatment of specific lesions or diseases. Both deal with acute organic reactions, and each with different manifestations and referral patterns of patients with chronic organic reactions. The organic psychiatrist is primarily concerned with the aetiological diagnosis and management of specific organic disorders/syndromes (e.g. delirium, dementia), the management of secondary behaviours (e.g. depression after head injury or stroke, psychosis in epilepsy or dementia), the prevention of secondary complications, support for relatives and carers, and the coordination of care in hospital and in the community. The organic psychiatrist will sometimes assess an organic contribution to functional disorders, and issues of compensation.

Syndrome definition

'*Acute organic reaction*' and '*chronic organic reaction*' are the terms best used for the first major division of organic psychiatric disorders (Lishman, 1987). The terms imply the type of abruptness and onset, and to some extent the main symptoms and the likely duration of disorder, but not the ultimate prognosis. Acute symptoms may be due to delirium (acute confusional state), a focal neurological deficit or psychiatric disorder; whereas chronic symptoms may be due to dementia, a focal neurological deficit, or psychiatric illness.

Delirium

Delirium or acute organic reaction is also known as acute confusional state, toxic psychosis, and acute organic psychosis. This syndrome is characterised by disorientation in time and place, and by global cognitive impairment of acute onset and relatively brief duration, particularly involving an impairment of attention and consciousness. Clouding of consciousness, which results in disturbances of attention and awareness, is the cardinal clinical feature. Other core features include disturbances of cognition (perception, thinking and memory), the sleep–wake cycle and psychomotor behaviour (Lipowski, 1990). Delirium is due to a widespread disturbance of cerebral metabolism. It is a common feature of physical illness or drug intoxication, especially in the elderly. While potentially reversible, delirium may herald death and requires urgent attention. Delirium must be distinguished from dementia, a chronic syndrome: see below and Table 22.1.

DSM–IV (American Psychiatric Association, 1994) and ICD–10 (World Health Organization, 1992) virtually equate the terms delirium and acute organic reaction, whereas in the UK the term delirium has formerly been used for a more disturbed type of acute organic reaction: "a syndrome of impairment of consciousness which is accompanied by intrusive abnormalities derived from the fields of perception and affect" (Lishman, 1987).

Subacute organic reactions

These have a less sudden onset than acute disorders, a longer course, and a mixture of acute and chronic symptoms.

Confusion

Confusion may be defined as the lack of customary clarity and coherence of thought, perception, understanding, or action. The confusion of delirium is due largely to impairment of consciousness, whereas disruption of thought processes underlies that found in chronic organic reactions such as dementia. Confusion may occur in functional psychoses and in focal neurological disorders such as aphasia. The specific meaning of the term in organic psychiatry contrasts with its meaning in other settings.

Clouding of consciousness

This describes the mildest stage of impairment of consciousness that is detectable clinically, on the continuum from full awareness to coma (Lishman, 1987). Traditionally an essential feature of delirium, the term 'clouding of consciousness' has been dropped from current American definitions of delirium, for there is no generally accepted definition of consciousness, and 'clouding' is an even vaguer term. The term is little more than a metaphor referring to the set of cognitive and attentional deficits that constitutes the core of the syndrome of delirium.

Coma

Coma represents the extreme of a graded continuum of impairment of consciousness in which the patient is in a state of unarousable unrespon-siveness (Plum & Posner, 1980). The patient is incapable of sensing or responding adequately to external stimuli or inner needs, shows little or no spontaneous movement apart from respiration, and no evidence whatever of mental activity (Lishman, 1987). The Glasgow Coma Scale (Teasdale & Jennett, 1974), in which four grades of eye opening, five of the 'best verbal response' and five of the 'best motor response' are charted in individual patients, is used to assess grades of impairment of consciousness (see page 1048).

Stupor

Stupor refers to a clinical syndrome of akinesis and mutism, but with evidence of relative preservation of conscious awareness (Lishman, 1987). Loose and inconsistent use has bedevilled the term, which has sometimes incorrectly referred to an impairment of consciousness; sometimes to a syndrome ("akinetic mutism") characteristic of mid and upper brain-stem lesions; and sometimes to a superficially similar state due to functional psychiatric illness. DSM–IV defines stupor as a state of unresponsiveness with immobility and mutism. Its clinical features are discussed on page 1000. It is one form of *organic catatonic disorder. Mutism* is a condition in which a person does not speak or attempt spoken communication despite preservation of an adequate level of consciousness. It may sometimes be the only abnormality in otherwise normal behaviour.

Dementia

Dementia is defined as an acquired global impairment of intellect, memory and personality, but without impairment of consciousness (Lishman, 1987). It is persistent (unlike delirium), occurs in an alert patient without clouding of consciousness (which excludes delirium), has a global disturbance of higher mental function, and causes impairment of function (with loss of occupational, social and personality competence). It is caused by physical disease, without implying a specific physical cause. Although many dementias are progressive and untreatable, about 15% of those diagnosed in patients under the age of 65 referred to specialist centres are reversible with treatment (Marsden, 1985; Lishman, 1987). Dementia may be complicated by delirium. Table 22.1 compares the two disorders.

A variety of diagnostic guidelines are available for the diagnosis of dementia. DSM–IV requires that the patient has impaired ability to learn new information or to recall previously learned information, associated with one or more of the following cognitive disturbances: aphasia, apraxia, agnosia and disturbance in executive functioning (planning, organising, sequencing, abstracting) sufficient to compromise social or occupational functioning, with a course characterised by gradual onset and continuing cognitive decline. Loss of a single capacity or intellectual function such as memory or speech, however devastating, is not sufficient. The DSM–IV definition has several limitations. Firstly, the requirement that all demented patients have memory loss excludes disorders such as Pick's disease, which has preserved memory in the early and middle phases of the illness (Cummings & Benson, 1992). The dementia due to Pick's disease is classified separately within the dementia rubric. Secondly, personality change, a diagnostic feature in DSM–III–R (American Psychiatric Association, 1987) and one of several non-cognitive aspects of dementia (Absher & Cummings, 1994), has been relegated to an associated feature and disorder in DSM–IV "because of its relative lack of specificity for dementia". Yet personality change is the hallmark of dementia of frontal-lobe type (see page 1014). Thirdly, social and occupational impairments are hard to define and quantify; they vary with the demands of circumstances and level of support for any given disability. Fourthly, by also excluding aetiological non-organic factors, the pseudodementias are excluded (see page 1015).

Difficulties in the early detection of dementia are reviewed by Henderson (1994).

Personality and behavioural disorders due to brain disease, damage and dysfunction (ICD–10)

Brain disease, damage or dysfunction often results in persistent personality changes or behavioural disorders, either lifelong if they originate in childhood, or more usually representing a change or accentuation of a

Table 22.1 Differential diagnosis of delirium and dementia

Feature	Delirium	Dementia
Onset	Acute	Usually insidious
Duration	Transient (hours to weeks)	Persistent (months to years)
Course	Fluctuating over hours; worse at night, lucid intervals	Stable over days
Conscious level/ awareness	Depressed	Normal
Alertness	Abnormally low or high	Usually normal
Attention	Impaired, causing distractibility; fluctuates	Relatively normal
Sleep–wake cycle	Disrupted; often drowsy during day, insomnia at night	Usually normal
Orientation	Impaired	Impaired
Language	Incoherent, hesitant, slow or rapid	Anomia common
Memory:		
1° or working	Shortened	Impaired
2° or short-term	Impaired	Impaired
Perception	Frequent illusions and hallucinations	Normal early; agnosia, misidentifications and hallucinations later
Thinking	Disorganised, delusional	Impoverished
Mood	Agitation or fear common	Apathy or disinhibition common
Autonomic changes	Common	Unusual
Psychomotor changes	Common	Uncommon
EEG	Diffuse slow-wave activity	Mild slowing (but varies with aetiology)

previous trait. Changes in the control of emotions and impulses and in motivation and social judgement are most typical, leading to affective instability, euphoria, aggressive outbursts, social indiscretion, inability to plan or persevere with goal-directed activity, marked apathy and indifference, or suspiciousness with paranoid ideation. Cognitive deficits are mainly or exclusively of frontal lobe type. The terms "organic personality disorder" (ICD–10) or "personality change due to a general medical condition" (DSM–IV) are used. This disorder usually occurs with strictly focal brain damage.

The existence of a personality pattern specifically associated with epilepsy is controversial. Patients with complex partial seizures arising from a temporal lobe focus tend towards humourless sobriety, circumstantiality and religiosity (the three most discriminating traits) (Waxman & Geschwind, 1975). These interictal personality changes may occur, however, in other epileptic and psychiatric disorders (Master *et al*, 1984).

Placidity often accompanies frontal or bilateral limbic system lesions, as in the Kluver-Bucy syndrome and Korsakoff's syndrome. Irritability and apathy are the characteristic personality changes found in Huntington's disease, probably the result of disrupted caudate–frontal connections.

Reduced control over aggression may occur in patients with temporal lobe epilepsy; with tumours in the medial temporal, septal and hypothalamic areas; following birth trauma, head injury and intracerebral infections; and in habitually aggressive offenders with electroencephalogram (EEG) abnormalities, including the controversial syndrome of "episodic dyscontrol" (see page 1039).

ICD–10 includes the "post-encephalitic syndrome" and the "post-concussional syndrome" here, whereas DSM–IV relegates the latter to a category of proposed disorders requiring refinement of the criteria set. ICD–10 includes a right hemisphere organic affective disorder in its category for "other organic personality and behavioural disorder".

The amnesic syndrome

This is best defined as "an abnormal mental state in which memory and learning are affected out of all proportion to other cognitive functions in an otherwise alert and responsive patient" (Victor *et al*, 1971). Korsakoff's syndrome refers, by modern convention, to those cases of an amnesic syndrome that result from chronic or subacute on chronic nutritional deficiency, most commonly resulting from alcohol misuse. Note that there is no reference to either "short-term memory" or "confabulation" in these definitions. ICD–10 describes "organic amnesic syndrome", and DSM–IV "amnestic disorder due to a general medical condition" as well as "substance-induced persisting amnestic disorder".

Organic hallucinosis (ICD–10) or psychotic disorder due to a general medical condition (DSM–IV)

This refers to a syndrome of prominent persistent or recurrent hallucinations, usually visual or auditory, occurring in a setting of clear consciousness, attributable to a specific organic factor. Insight is variable; any delusions that occur are secondary to the hallucinations. Common causes are: use of hallucinogens; sensory deprivation and seizures; and alcohol withdrawal and hallucinosis. These are coded separately in ICD–10 and DSM–IV.

Organic catatonic disorder (ICD–10) or catatonic disorder due to a general medical condition (DSM–IV)

This is a disorder of diminished or increased psychomotor activity associated with catatonic symptoms. The extremes of psychomotor disturbance may alternate. Common causes are brain tumours, encephalitis, hypercalcaemia, liver failure and diabetic ketoacidosis.

Organic delusional (schizophrenia-like) disorder (ICD–10)

This encompasses paranoid and schizophreniform disorders due to specific organic factors. Persistent or recurrent delusions and criteria for assuming an organic aetiology are required. Hallucinations, thought disorder and isolated catatonic phenomena may be present. Consciousness and memory must not be affected. Examples include amphetamine psychosis (Connell, 1958) and the chronic schizophrenia-like psychosis of temporal lobe epilepsy. DSM–IV describes prominent hallucinations or delusions in the category "psychotic disorder due to a general medical condition".

Organic mood (affective) disorders (ICD–10)

These disorders reveal persistent depressed mood, or elevated, expansive or irritable mood, or a mixed affective state, that is directly due to a specific organic factor rather than an emotional response to the patient's knowledge of having a concurrent disorder or its symptoms. Common causes include drugs, thyroid disease, Cushing's syndrome, cancer and anterior left hemisphere strokes. DSM–IV classifies a corresponding "mood disorder due to a general medical condition".

Organic anxiety disorder (ICD–10)

Recurrent panic attacks or generalised anxiety or both conditions develop from a specific organic factor in this disorder. Examples include hypoglycaemia, thyroid disorders, phaeochromocytoma, drug intoxication and withdrawal, and seizures. DSM–IV includes obsessions and compulsions as well as prominent anxiety and panic attacks in the category "anxiety disorder due to an general medical condition".

ICD–10 also describes "organic dissociative disorder", "organic emotionally labile (asthenic) disorder", "mild cognitive disorder", and "other" and "unspecified disorders". DSM–IV additionally includes sexual dysfunction and sleep disorder due to a general medical condition in relevant sections.

Classification

Organic psychiatric disorders can be subdivided using three criteria:

(1) whether the impairment of intellectual or psychological function is generalised or focal;
(2) whether the disorder is acute or chronic;
(3) whether the underlying dysfunction is functional (e.g. pseudo-dementia) or neurological (Marsden, 1985).

The principles of classification of organic psychiatric disorders turn crucially on the central distinction between the concepts of syndrome and disease, and the further need to separate organic and functional disorders. A syndromal approach is based purely on a set of observed associations of symptoms and signs, is largely atheoretical, and does not include notions of aetiology, pathology, course and treatment response, which are intrinsic to the concept of disease. The nosology of organic disorders wavers uneasily between a syndromal and an aetiological approach (Lindesay *et al*, 1990). The move towards a syndrome-oriented and operational approach to classification, which eschews theoretical orientation, was expounded in DSM–III–R. Loose, colloquial terms, such as confusion and senility, have been abandoned in recent classifications. ICD–10 has adopted diagnostic guidelines for categorisation and a syndrome-oriented approach like DSM–III–R.

The major heading "Organic mental disorders" has been eliminated from DSM–IV "because it implies that the other disorders in the manual do not have an organic component". In DSM–IV, the three sections "Delirium, dementia, and amnestic and other cognitive disorders", "Mental disorders due to a general medical condition", and "Substance-related disorders" are distinguished. The term 'cognitive' is now preferred to 'organic' for dementias and delirium, and 'organic' is omitted from the other disorders. The term 'cognitive disorder' is preferred (Spitzer *et al*, 1992), but cognitive impairment is not invariably present in this group of conditions, and there are frequently changes in behaviour as well as in cognition (Absher & Cummings, 1994).

By contrast, ICD–10 retains the term organic, without equating the organic/non-organic distinction with disorders having or not having a biological basis.

In both ICD–10 and DSM–IV, the three major organic or cognitive disorders are delirium, dementia and the amnestic syndrome. Both classifications include specific categories for the dementias of Pick's, Creutzfeld-Jakob, Huntington's, Parkinson's and HIV diseases.

Syndromes with regional connections

Frontal lobe syndrome

Frontal lobe lesions may cause profound personality changes, but IQ, memory and other cognitive functions are commonly preserved (Stuss & Benson, 1986). One of the first case reports was of Phineas Gage, a reliable railroad foreman who became profane, irritable and irresponsible after recovery from an accident when an iron bar was blown through his frontal lobes.

The outstanding personality change in the frontal lobe syndrome is disinhibition, with euphoria, over-familiarity, tactlessness, overtalkativeness, and inappropriate sexual conduct. Patients may also display impulsive behaviour, irritability and aggressive outbursts, childish excitement or silliness ('moria') with inappropriate jokes, puns or pranks ('Witzelsucht'). Insight, especially concern for the future and for the consequences of actions, is limited, leading to gross errors of judgement. Mood is elevated with a shallow and fatuous euphoria rather than a true elation. Euphoria is generally episodic, often superimposed on a background of profound apathy, indifference and lack of motivation, and marked slowing of psychomotor activity. Some patients no longer carry out the necessary activities of daily living (dressing, washing, eating, elimination), but these can be performed upon coaxing or may occur at any time or place without regard for the social consequences. Medial frontal lesions may produce akinesia, which may progress to stupor, and incontinence with or without distress. Other patients reveal impairments of abstract reasoning, creativity, problem-solving and mental flexibility, jumping to premature conclusions. Patients may answer correctly questions requiring judgement, yet seem unable to govern their actions by the same verbal rule. They perform normally on externally-driven tasks, but very poorly at self-motivated learning. Impeccable behaviour during examination may conceal impaired judgement and comportment, which only emerges in the less structured settings of everyday life.

Concentration, attention, the ability to maintain a behavioural set without perseveration (Luria, 1966), and to initiate cognitive strategies as tested by generating lists of words, are disrupted. Loss of the ability to shift cognitive set, as revealed in the Wisconsin Card Sorting Test, occurs in many cases of frontal lesion, perhaps particularly in those involving dorsolateral lesions (Milner, 1963). Sequencing of behaviour and temporal-order judgements are impaired. Planning, problem-solving, performance on simultaneous (dual) tasks and self-motivated learning are compromised. Other evidence of a frontal lobe lesion includes adversive focal seizures, ipsilateral optic atrophy or anosmia, grasp reflex, and Broca's aphasia.

Blumer & Benson (1975) described two distinct frontal lobe syndromes: a "pseudodepressed" type, characterised by apathy with lack of initiative and indifference, sometimes attributed to convexity lesions; and a "pseudo-psychopathic" type marked by disinhibition with euphoria, irritability, impulsivity and antisocial behaviour, tending to follow orbitofrontal pathology. Memory can also be involved, resulting in either impoverished recall of past memories or florid confabulation (Kopelman, 1991).

Clinically a mixture of frontal lobe symptoms is more common than a pure set, and occasionally large 'silent' lesions can be accommodated with little clinical disturbance. In an individual patient the localisation, size, type and course of the lesion will determine the clinical picture, which in turn will be coloured by the previous personality and age of onset. The manifestations of bilateral frontal lobe disease are more dramatic than those of unilateral lesions, which can be subtle and elusive (Mesulam, 1986). Common causes of the frontal lobe syndrome include vascular disease, tumours, head injury, multiple sclerosis, dementia and occasionally infections.

Temporal lobe syndromes

A variety of syndromes can occur with temporal lobe lesions, depending on whether the left or right lobe is affected, whether one or both lobes are involved, and whether or not there is associated epilepsy. Lesions restricted to the temporal poles may also be "silent".

Dominant temporal lesions may produce a sensory (Wernicke) aphasia alone, which may be mistaken for dementia. More posterior lesions may impair visual aspects of language, producing alexia and agraphia. Non-dominant temporal lobe lesions may yield few symptoms or signs, or sometimes visuospatial problems.

Bilateral medial temporal lobe lesions, involving the hippocampus, produce a severe and selective amnesic syndrome. Unilateral lesions rarely produce spontaneous complaints, probably because the intact hippo-campus can compensate in part. Modality-specific memory loss, affecting verbal material on the dominant side and non-verbal material (such as places, faces, music and drawings) on the non-dominant side, is usually only revealed by special testing.

Personality disturbance may occur similar to that following frontal lesions, but is usually associated with intellectual and neurological deficits.

Emotional instability, aggression and paranoid states are common, and depersonalisation and sexual disorders may occur. Schizophreniform, schizo-affective and affective psychoses are well recognised complications of temporal lobe lesions, especially epilepsy. There is support for an association of schizophrenia-like psychoses and left-sided epileptic foci. The wide variety of focal seizures and their complications due to temporal lobe lesions are discussed on page 1033. The single most important sign of a deep temporal lobe lesion is a contralateral upper quadrantic hemianopia.

The *Kluver-Bucy syndrome* follows *bilateral* ablations or lesions of the medial and lateral temporal lobes including amygdalae, unci and hippocampi. Originally described in monkeys, its human analogue includes:

(1) excessive oral tendencies including bulimia;
(2) placidity and loss of fear or anger with apathy and pet-like compliance;
(3) visual agnosia, and sometimes prosopagnosia;
(4) hypermetamorphosis or an irresistible impulse to touch objects in sight;
(5) altered sexual activity (Lilly *et al*, 1983).

Common causes are Pick's disease and herpes simplex encephalitis. Individual features such as binge-eating may occur in Alzheimer's disease (Burns *et al*, 1990).

The *amnesic syndrome* (as defined above) refers to a pattern of memory impairment in which performance at digit, word, or block span and other tests (as examples of 'primary' or working memory) is preserved, while new learning ('secondary' memory) is severely impaired (see Box 22.1). The patient experiences severe difficulty in recalling or recognising material acquired in previous learning episodes or experiences ('explicit' memory).

There may also be a variable degree of retrograde amnesia (loss of memories initially acquired before the onset of the amnesic disorder). General knowledge of the world ('semantic' memory) may be affected to variable degrees. Knowledge of how to use language is characteristically preserved, but the name of the present Prime Minister will usually be forgotten. However, skill learning (procedural memory) and the facilitation of responses to the previous 'priming' of material may also be preserved: taken together, these are known as 'implicit' memory.

An amnesic syndrome can result from a variety of underlying pathologies – nutritional deficiency resulting from alcohol, malnutrition or malabsorption syndromes (Korsakoff's syndrome), infection (such as herpes simplex encephalitis or TB meningitis), head injury, anoxia, vascular lesions (thalamic infarction or subarachnoid haemorrhage), or deep midline tumours.

Box 22.1 Aspects of memory processes

Primary or working memory
Holds information for a few seconds only, in which it can be rehearsed, processed, or utilised for tasks such as speech comprehension
Tested in span tests or 'short-term' forgetting tasks
Impaired in focal temporal-parietal lesions and in global cortical atrophy

Secondary memory
Large capacity; information is 'consolidated' from primary to secondary memory; rate of forgetting is relatively slow
Explicit or *episodic* memory refers to recall of incidents or events
Semantic memory refers to factual or conceptual knowledge
Implicit memory refers to learning of which the subject may not have conscious awareness, e.g. classical conditioning, 'priming', memory for perceptuo-motor skills or procedures.
Each of these components can have an *anterograde* (current) and *retrograde* (remote) aspect.
Anterograde amnesia results from damage involving the limbic circuits. Retrograde amnesia may result from damage to the temporal or frontal cortex. Secondary memory is impaired in the 'amnesic syndrome' and in global dementia.

Consistent with the above, a Korsakoff patient will show severe impairment in new learning as well as a variable, but often extensive (two decades or more), retrograde loss (Kopelman, 1995). Other cognitive functions will be relatively intact, although disorders on frontal and visuospatial tests are commonly found (Jacobson *et al*, 1990; Kopelman, 1991). The patient may appear rather apathetic and indifferent to his or her environment, aside from occasional episodes of irritability, and he or she will stick to a fairly rigid daily routine. He or she will learn the way around the hospital or institution, but will remember remarkably little from day to day. On the other hand, Victor *et al* (1971) remarked that 25% of Korsakoff patients show recovery through time, 50% show some degree of improvement, and 25% do not change; clinical observation suggests that improvement can still occur a considerable time after onset of the disorder. A striking feature is that, following the Wernicke episode, these patients often lose any interest in further alcohol intake.

Korsakoff (1889) himself noted that a common feature in such patients is the confusion of the temporal sequence of events, and 'confabulation' commonly consists of real memories jumbled up and recalled inappropriately. More recent studies have distinguished spontaneous or 'fantastic' confabulation from 'provoked' or momentary confabulation, which consists of fleeting intrusion errors or distortions in response to a memory test (Berlyne, 1972; Kopelman, 1987). Spontaneous confabulation appears to result from frontal lobe pathology (Stuss *et al*, 1978; Kapur & Coughlan, 1980), whereas momentary confabulation may be a normal response to a 'weak' or failing memory. Spontaneous confabulation is occasionally seen in the early (acute) stage of the Wernicke–Korsakoff syndrome, but is seldom seen in the later stages. Momentary confabulation can be found in approximately 50% of Korsakoff patients, but neither spontaneous nor momentary confabulation is pathognomic of Korsakoff's syndrome.

Parietal lobe syndromes

Parietal lobe lesions may produce a complex and florid variety of cognitive deficits (Critchley, 1953). Lesions of either parietal lobe may yield visuo-spatial difficulties including constructional apraxia, visuospatial agnosia (see below) and disturbance in the perception of spatial relationships.

Topographical disorientation is revealed by difficulty in learning or recalling the way around, for example, a ward to which the patient has recently been admitted.

Lesions of the dominant parietal lobe produce conduction aphasia or anomia. Anterior lesions may be associated with motor dysphasia, and posterior lesions with sensory dysphasia. Apraxia, finger agnosia and right–left disorientation may also occur.

Non-dominant parietal lobe lesions produce disturbances of the body image and of external space, particularly involving the contralateral side. These include: denial of disability ("anosognosia"); neglect of the left half of space (for example, when drawing, walking or driving); dressing dyspraxia; visuospatial disorganisation, which may lead to difficulties with driving, using machinery, or laying a table; and visuospatial agnosia.

Anterior parietal lesions encroach on primary sensory cortex causing contralateral cortical sensory loss, which is marked by intact perception of pain, temperature, touch or vibration, but inability to interpret these sensations. As a result there is loss of recognition of objects by palpation ("astereognosis"), of figures written on the hand ("agraphaesthesia"), and defective tactile localisation (sensory extinction) or discrimination of two stimuli. Visual inattention may also occur. Posterior lesions cause a contralateral lower quadrantic hemianopia.

Occipital lobe lesions are characterised by contralateral homonymous defects. Less common are complex visual recognition disorders such as alexia without agraphia, colour agnosia, prosopagnosia and complex visual hallucinations.

Corpus callosum lesions cause intellectual deterioration with a pattern reflecting damage to adjacent lobes and callosal disconnection.

Diencephalic and brain-stem lesions

An amnesic syndrome and hypersomnia are the most characteristic symptoms of lesions of the deep midline structures. Amnesia occurs with lesions distributed around the third ventricle, cerebral aqueduct, and posterior hypothalamus. It appears that lesions in the mammillary bodies, mammillo-thalamic tract and anterior thalamus are critical in disrupting memory processes (Mair *et al*, 1979; Von Cramon *et al*, 1985; Mayes *et al*, 1988). Somnolence and hypersomnia, which suggest posterior midbrain or brain-stem lesions, may progress to stupor or coma.

Generalised intellectual decline secondary to hydrocephalus, a rapidly progressive dementia and a frontal-type syndrome are other presentations. Raised intracranial pressure with headache and papilloedema are found in most obstructive lesions, but focal neurological signs may be absent. Endocrine and other neurological signs may indicate hypothalamic and thalamic involvement respectively.

Symptoms with regional connections

Aphasia

Aphasia denotes the loss or impairment of language caused by brain damage (Benson, 1979). Historically, language disorders were the first disorders of higher cortical function to be correlated with focal brain lesions. In 1861, Broca demonstrated frontal lobe damage in a 'speechless' patient. Four years later, Broca reported left hemisphere dominance for language, which is now well-established in 95–99% of right-handers and in 60–70% of left-handers (Milner, 1975; Benson, 1979). The classification of aphasias began in 1874 with Wernicke's clinical and pathological distinction between two types of aphasia, motor and sensory. A proliferation of classification schemes then developed around this dichotomy.

Aphasic syndromes suggest a location or type of pathology but do not invariably result from pathology in a given site; no single symptom within a syndrome has localising value (Benson, 1979). Aphasias can be divided clinically and anatomically into syndromes involving the primary language cortex (the perisylvian area) and those involving other cortical or subcortical centres. Patients with disturbed repetition have perisylvian pathology, whereas repetition is spared by surrounding cortical lesions. Most aphasics also fall into two clinical types based on their conversational speech: *non-fluent* and *fluent* aphasias. Non-fluent aphasia is associated with pathology anterior to the major central sulcus (e.g. motor (Broca's) aphasia), while fluent aphasia indicates pathology posterior to it (e.g. sensory (Wernicke's) aphasia).

There are three perisylvian aphasic syndromes – primary motor (Broca's), primary sensory (Wernicke's) and conduction aphasia.

Primary motor (Broca's expressive) aphasia

Spontaneous speech is non-fluent, with decreased output (<50 words per minute, often found to be <10), increased effort to produce words (with grimacing and gestures), with the choice of wrong words, dysarthria leading to mispronunciation, and a disturbance of rhythm (dysprosody). The phrase length is short, often with single words. Telegraphic speech, which refers to the utterance of meaningful nouns and verbs and omission of prepositions and adjectives, is meaningful despite few words (e.g. "wife come hospital tonight"). Perseveration is common. Comprehension is relatively intact, but repetition seriously impaired. Naming is usually poor but is helped by prompting. Reading and writing are invariably affected. Accompanying features include right hemiplegia (over 80% of cases), an apraxia affecting the non-paralysed left side, and sometimes sensory loss and visual field defects occur. Pathology involves the dominant posterior-inferior frontal lobe (Broca's area).

Primary sensory (Wernicke's receptive) aphasia

This differs dramatically from motor aphasia. The key features of sensory aphasia are impaired comprehension and fluent paraphasic speech with defective repetition. The sensory (Wernicke's) aphasic patient speaks effortlessly and without hesitation, sometimes even excessively (logorrhea). Articulation, phrase length and prosody are normal. Speech content, however, is filled with empty phrases and circumlocutions with few meaningful nouns and verbs. The major types of error are: literal or phonemic *paraphasias* (substitutions within language), in which a similar sounding phoneme is substituted for the correct one (e.g. hen for pen); and verbal or semantic paraphasias, in which an incorrect word is substituted (e.g. mother for wife); or meaningless nonsense words (neologisms). Rapid unintelligible speech is termed jargon aphasia (e.g. "she wants to give me the subjective vocation to maintain the vocation of perfect impregnation simbling"). Naming ability is usually poor and, in contrast to motor aphasia, prompting rarely helps. Auditory comprehension is invariably impaired, often to the point that the patient understands very little. Writing and reading (both aloud and for comprehension) are impaired. Where reading is relatively intact, the term 'pure word deafness' is used. A lack of accompanying neurological signs sometimes leads to misdiagnosis as psychosis or confusion. Pathology lies in the dominant temporal lobe in the posterior–superior portion of the first temporal gyrus.

Conduction aphasia

The hallmark of conduction aphasia is impairment of repetition of speech out of proportion to all other deficits. Following Warrington & Shallice

(1969), many neuropsychologists have interpreted this disorder as reflecting a specific deficit within short-term or working memory.

Borderzone or transcortical aphasic syndromes

The outstanding characteristic of the transcortical or borderzone aphasias is an intact or relatively good ability to repeat spoken language despite serious aphasia. Pathology is located outside the perisylvian region, in the vascular borderzone between the territory of the middle cerebral artery and those of the anterior or posterior cerebral arteries. Further details of these disorders are discussed by Benson (1979) and Lishman (1987).

Anomic aphasia (nominal aphasia)

In anomic aphasia, confrontation naming is affected more than any other language function. Low frequency names or words are particularly affected. Anomia raises the possibility of a focal left hemisphere lesion, although the location may vary, and it is an early symptom in dementia. It occurs occasionally in hysteria, and may be the only residue of recovered aphasia.

Global aphasia

Language loss encompasses expressive, receptive, nominal and conductive components, with lesions including and extending beyond both Wernicke's and Broca's areas.

Alexia

Alexia is an acquired inability to comprehend written language caused by brain damage. Alexia with agraphia (parietal–temporal alexia) implies both letter and numerical blindness plus word blindness, and all aspects of writing are affected. Alexia without agraphia implies impaired reading while writing and spelling are intact. The hallmark of this syndrome is the paradoxical inability of the patient to read the words he has just written. Spelled words are recognised, in sharp contrast to parietal–temporal alexia. Associated findings include right homonymous hemianopia and colour anomia. Pathology involves the left inferior medial occipital region and splenium of the corpus callosum.

The neuropsychological classification of acquired reading disorders includes letter-by-letter dyslexia, surface dyslexia, and deep dyslexia (Patterson, 1981; Howard *et al*, 1992). Letter-by-letter dyslexia is accompanied by pronounced slowness in reading, and probably results from a visual processing deficit. The clinical diagnosis is usually alexia without agraphia. Surface dyslexia is characterised by a particular difficulty in reading irregular words (e.g. 'PINT') but not regular words (e.g. 'MINT'). It probably results from a semantic memory deficit, is usually accompanied by a naming deficit, and often results from left temporal lobe lesions (e.g. in herpes encephalitis). Deep dyslexia results from a deficit of grapheme–phoneme conversion or of the phonological system itself. It is diagnosed by a particular difficulty in reading non-words (e.g. 'RINT') and associated impairments in reading abstract words, in working memory, and in other aspects of language. There is often widespread cortical atrophy or pathology in such patients.

The language impairment in Alzheimer-type dementia

This depends on the stage of disease and disturbances in other psychological functions, such as memory and perception. Anomia is the first obvious abnormality and rapidly worsens. Naming errors are made resulting in semantic substitutions (e.g. chair for table) and circumlocutions (e.g. of a snowman: "It's cold, it's a . . . man . . . cold . . . frozen"). Spontaneous speech and vocabulary are impoverished.

Later symptoms include simplified syntax, reliance on stock phrases, impaired comprehension and writing, verbal perseveration, vague and meaningless content, and paraphasias. Finally, language is incoherent, and occasionally patients are mute (Morris, 1991). Changes correspond to the more posterior types of aphasia, such as transcortical sensory or Wernicke's aphasia. The later picture resembles global aphasia (Miller, 1989).

Apraxia

Apraxia is defined as the inability to carry out voluntary skilled movement, not attributable to weakness, akinesia, incoordination, sensory loss, intellectual deterioration, poor comprehension or uncooperativeness (Heilman & Rothi, 1985).

Two principal types of apraxia were recognised in Liepmann's original description in 1900. *Ideational apraxia* implies that the patient fails to carry out coordinated sequences of actions correctly, such as folding a letter, inserting it into an envelope, and stamping it; however, each separate component of the sequence can be successfully performed. This contrasts with *ideomotor apraxia*, in which the patient fails to perform when asked on actions that can usually be performed spontaneously, such as waving good-bye, or stirring a cup of tea. Ideational apraxias occur in dementia and with lesions of the corpus callosum. Ideomotor apraxias occur with lesions of the dominant left hemisphere. In *orobuccal apraxia*, learned skilled movements of the face, lips, tongue, cheeks, larynx and pharynx are compromised. Lesions of the inferior frontal region and the insula are reponsible.

Dressing difficulties

This problem is often loosely called dyspraxia, and occurs in several different clinical syndromes:

(1) in association with profound unilateral neglect, only the non-neglected side being bathed, toileted, and dressed;
(2) in delirium, dementia and schizophrenia – patients may wear multiple layers of clothing inappropriate to the weather;
(3) a syndrome of true body–garment disorientation or dressing dyspraxia may occur, with difficulty relating the spatial form of garments to that of the body. Examples of this include difficulty orienting an arm to a sleeve, wearing one's shirt on one's leg, putting on clothes backwards, and difficulty doing up ties, zips, buttons and laces.

Right-sided or bilateral parieto-occipital lesions are commoner than left-sided lesions (Cummings, 1985; Lishman, 1987).

Constructional apraxia

Often synonymous with visuospatial agnosia, this is primarily a disorder in the execution (praxis) of actions that involve a spatial dimension. The spatial organisation of actions is altered, without any apraxia for individual movements (Lishman, 1987). Typical difficulties occur in driving, using machinery, laying a table and drawing. Drawing and copying abilities are particularly vulnerable and are therefore the basis of many diagnostic tests. The quality of errors depends on the laterality of the (parietal) lesion, and whether the lesion is focal, or diffuse as in Alzheimer's disease (Moore & Wyke, 1984; McCarthy & Warrington, 1990; Kirk & Kertesz, 1991).

Agnosia

Agnosia is a disorder of recognition of objects that cannot be attributed to sensory defects, mental deterioration, attentional disturbances, aphasic misnaming or to unfamiliarity with the object. An agnosic patient must be shown to have intact primary sensory perception and intact ability to name the object once it has been recognised. The failure of recognition usually afflicts a single sensory modality: vision, hearing or touch. Three distinct processing stages of visual object recognition have been identified. Objects are analysed for their visual sensory properties (either occipital lobe); then for the formation of a percept (apperception) (lateralised to the right parietal lobe); and the third stage (lateralised to the left hemisphere, occipito-temporal region) assigns meaning to a percept (association) (McCarthy & Warrington, 1990). For example, in visual agnosia an object cannot be named by sight but is identified by other means, such as touch or hearing (see Humphreys & Riddoch, 1987).

Prosopagnosia

This describes the inability to recognise familiar faces. Patients usually see faces as faces but cannot identify whose face they are viewing. In extreme form the patient cannot recognise his own face in a mirror. It is important to distinguish prosopagnosia from the Capgras symptom, in which the patient believes that familiar persons have been replaced by physically identical doubles or impostors. A posterior right hemisphere lesion is common to all cases, but most cases have bilateral involvement (Ellis & Young, 1990).

Reduplicative paramnesia

Patients with this symptom incorrectly describe the place that they are in, and further maintain that a familiar place exists simultaneously in several different locations. Bilateral frontal pathology is found in most cases (McCarthy & Warrington, 1990).

Speech dominance and handedness

The relationship of speech dominance to handedness can be determined in different ways:

(1) by the carotid amytal test;
(2) by the proportions of cerebral lesions producing dysphasia;
(3) by studies using unilateral electroconvulsive therapy (ECT).

These various techniques give broadly consistent results – 95% of right-handers are left-hemisphere dominant and 5% are right-hemisphere dominant; 70% of lefthanders are left-hemisphere dominant, 15% are right-hemisphere dominant, and 15% show a bilateral pattern of speech representation (see Kopelman, 1982; McManus, 1985).

There is evidence that lefthanders may show a better prognosis following cerebrovascular accidents involving language processes (Subirana, 1958), but that there may be a higher prevalence of psychosis in mixed and lefthanders (Lishman & McMeekan, 1976). It is important to be aware of the figures for speech dominance in determining the side used for unilateral ECT. McManus (1985) provided a detailed genetic model of the relationship of handedness and language dominance to dysphasia.

A commonly employed assessment procedure to determine the pattern of hand preference in an individual is the Annett Handedness Questionnaire (Annett, 1970).

The *Gerstmann syndrome* results from dominant parietal lobe lesions and includes finger agnosia, right–left disorientation, dyscalculia and dysgraphia. These four components can appear with other deficits and often fail to cluster together, and so do not really constitute a true 'syndrome'. Finger agnosia is shown by the bilateral loss of ability to recognise, name or select individual fingers, either on the patient's own body or another body (Lishman, 1987). In right–left disorientation, the patient cannot carry out instructions which involve an appreciation of right and left. Dyscalculia has many possible causes and occurs with lesions in various sites. If a patient cannot do simple additions and subtractions in the absence of sufficient dementia or dysphasia, suspect a left parietal lesion.

Body image disturbances

The body image or body schema is a subjective model of the body, acquired during development from physiological, psychological, social and cultural influences.

Organic psychiatric illness may produce bilateral or unilateral disturbances of the body image. Bilateral body image disturbances are commoner with left cerebral lesions than right, are usually restricted to finger agnosia or right–left disorientation and rarely autotopagnosia. *Autotopagnosia* is the inability to recognise, name or point on command to various body parts on the patient's own or on other bodies, while other external objects are dealt with normally. Left parieto-occipital lesions are necessary, but bilateral lesions are more common.

Unilateral body image disturbances are commoner with right hemisphere lesions than left, and therefore more often affect the left side of the body. Unilateral unawareness and neglect also most often affect the left side of the body, with a spectrum of disorders ranging from mild inattention to unawareness and active neglect (Critchley, 1953), due to right parietal lobe lesions, usually acute strokes. *Hemisomatagnosia* denotes neglect of one side of the body.

Anosognosia implies lack of awareness of disease. First described for left hemiplegia by Babinski in 1914, it ranges in degree from lack of concern to frank denial of disability. It is much commoner for left than right hemiplegic limbs. The term is also used generically for lack of insight into other disabilities, such as sensory (Wernicke's) asphasia, amnesia in Korsakoff's syndrome, and cortical blindness (Anton's syndrome).

Anomalous and false bodily experiences and morbid emotional attitudes towards parts of the body are discussed by Cutting (1990) and Lishman (1987).

Visuospatial deficits

Cerebral lesions produce a variety of disorders of spatial perception that are difficult to classify, as they affect various mental functions such as perception, memory, attention, motor action, symbolisation and "central spatial representation" (McCarthy & Warrington, 1990).

In *visual disorientation*, the ability to localise objects in space by vision alone is impaired (Lishman, 1987). Bilateral occipito-parietal lesions are responsible.

Visuospatial agnosia implies failure on tasks which demand explicit analysis of the spatial properties of a visual display. Errors include a failure to copy drawings or construct patterns with blocks, misalignment of words on a page, and spatial bias. Unilateral visual neglect may lead the patient to fail to make left turns, or lose his way on familiar routes. Visuospatial agnosia results from lesions in the parietal lobes, and is more common and severe with lesions of the right lobe than the left.

Loss of topographical memory impairs the ability to recall or recognise routes, buildings or places. The difficulties occur with both visual and tactile maps, suggesting a modality-unspecific defect in the appreciation of extrapersonal space. While bilateral parietal lobe lesions are often found, a unilateral right postero-medial lesion may be sufficient to produce the syndrome (Landis *et al*, 1986).

Organic delusions

Four groups of organic delusion have been proposed: simple persecutory, complex persecutory, mood-congruent, and delusions associated with specific neurological lesions or neuropsychological deficits (Cummings, 1985; Cutting, 1987).

Simple delusions are poorly systematised and usually transient, occurring in patients with cognitive deterioration as in delirium and dementia, and tend to respond to treatment. Fleeting paranoid delusions, elicited and modified by current stimuli, occur in delirium (Lipowski, 1990). Delusions of theft, suspicion and infidelity occur in Alzheimer's disease, but paranoid ideation short of delusions is more common (Burns *et al*, 1990). *Complex delusions* are more bizarre, systematised and stable than simple ones. They may occur in delirium with two main themes: belief in imminent misadventure to others, or in bizarre happenings in the immediate vicinity (Cutting, 1987). Compared with schizophrenic delusions, organic delusions are more likely to involve others as victims of the imagined drama. Complex delusions also occur in dementia (e.g. belief that a pet had been burned, belief that she was changing into a man) and include primary delusions, persecutory delusions, morbid jealousy, and the Capgras symptom. Other causes include epileptic psychoses, herpes encephalitis, and subcortical or limbic lesions.

The content of delusions may be associated with the laterality of the lesion. Left hemisphere damage may produce primary delusions and systematised persecutory delusions that are often indistinguishable from those of schizophrenia. Right hemisphere damage is associated with delusional reduplication of place, time and object, and delusional misidentification of people, as in the Capgras symptom (Cutting, 1990).

The onset of delusions in middle or late life should prompt a particular search for an organic cause. Organic hallucinosis and organic mood syndrome are described on page 962, and organic personality change on page 959.

Assessment

History-taking

A careful history taken from close relatives or friends is essential to establish the mode of onset of the disorder, the nature and duration of symptoms and their subsequent course. The patient's own account of his symptoms will frequently be distorted by confusion, memory lapses, inconsistency, denial and lack of insight. Early changes include memory loss, behaviour disturbances, disruption of daily living (dressing, eating, handling money), mood and physical symptoms. Was the onset over hours, suggesting an acute organic reaction, or over months or years, implicating a chronic organic state? Are there symptoms suggesting focal pathology such as those of raised intracranial pressure (headaches, nausea, vomiting and ataxia), stroke-like events, a stepwise deterioration, or seizures? Incontinence and fluctuations in symptoms and behaviour should be asked about. Nocturnal worsening or restlessness indicates clouding of consciousness; episodic abnormal behaviour of sudden onset and ending may suggest epilepsy; and changes in behaviour inconsistent with the setting can imply organicity. Attention to past medical and family history, drugs, alcohol and toxic exposure is important. The handedness of the patient should be determined to assess cerebral dominance for speech.

The formal psychiatric history remains important, to distinguish functional and organic illness, to clarify premorbid patterns of functioning (and stress reactions) and the current social and family structure, and to detect other aetiological factors, such as abnormal illness behaviour.

A thorough physical examination is required; 12% of admissions to psychiatric hospital have physical signs of illness directly contributing to their mental disorders (Lishman, 1987). The elderly are especially vulnerable, with about a third having medical disorders complicating dementia (Lipowski, 1990). Physical examination alone may detect treatable organic disorders.

Neurological examination may be surprisingly negative in organic patients. Subtle signs include clumsiness, motor impersistence, minor Parkinsonian or gait abnormalities, and exaggerated jaw jerk (in pseudobulbar palsy).

The mental state examination

This begins with the patient's appearance and general behaviour. Pallor, loss of weight, and disorders of facial expression, posture, movement and standards of self-care suggest organicity. Look for slow or hesitant responses, perseveration and poor grasp. Is he impulsive, disinhibited, insensitive, or neglectful of dress or hygiene? Does he tire unduly? Nursing observations of ward behaviour may reveal: indifference to events, bewilderment, a puzzled expression, aimless wandering, restlessness, stereotypies, loss of way, memory lapses, occasional transient losses of consciousness, aggressive, suspicious or paranoid behaviour, feeding or dressing difficulties, binge-eating and incontinence.

Speech

The interview may reveal minor incoherence, wandering off the point, or perseverative or paraphasic errors. The patient may deny his difficulties, evade questions, or rationalise his failures. Speech may reveal a poverty of content, restriction of theme, concrete thinking, or impaired reasoning ability.

Mood

Abnormalities include inappropriate placidity and lack of concern, coupled with mild disinhibition or euphoria; or agitated hostile moods; or shifts between the two as in delirium. In early dementia, a quiet perplexity or emotional lability prevails. An empty, shallow quality to emotional expression also suggests organicity. Other signs include blunting of affect and the *catastrophic reaction*, in which failure at a previously accomplished task elicits an intense emotional reaction with crying, negativity, withdrawal or hostility.

Thought content

The effects of cognitive impairment on the direction, detail, coherence and integration of thought noted above vary with the expected level of intelligence. Ideas of reference and delusions of persecution are common, but are often poorly elaborated, vague, shallow, and transient or inconsistently related. Anxious, depressive and hypochondriacal ideas frequently occur along with perceptual distortions, illusions and hallucinations.

Cognitive assessment

(Adapted from Institute of Psychiatry, 1987; see also Hodges, 1994.) The main aim is to establish the level of consciousness and to determine whether one or more intellectual functions are impaired. The patient's premorbid level of intellect must be estimated from his educational and occupational attainment, or from formal tests. Cognitive assessment must be adjusted according to the previous and current intellectual state, and the examiner should have a good understanding of the limitations of the tests he uses and of the normal range of replies. The patient's answers to questions and behaviour should be carefully recorded to allow later evaluation of change. Aphasia and perseveration, in which the patient repeats a previous response to a subsequent stimulus, may each cause the patient's intellectual performance to be underestimated.

In all patients, whether or not organic cerebral disease is suspected, the following tests should be administered.

Orientation. What day of the week is it? What is the time of day? What is the date – day, month, year? Where are you now? What is this place, street, town, county? Who are you? What is your age and date of birth?

Attention and concentration. Is attention easily aroused and sustained? Is he easily distracted? Can he concentrate? Ask him to give in reverse order the days of the week or months of the year. Record and time subtraction of serial 7s from 100, but interpret the response cautiously as attention, memory, and calculating ability are required. Assess the forward and backward digit span (delivered evenly and at one-second intervals).

Memory. The ability to recall information immediately and after a delay should be assessed. Compare the patient's account of his life with that given by others. Assess the patient's knowledge of past public events and recent news events. Assess memory for recent general information: names of present monarch, of his/her children, of the Prime Minister, and the President of the US. Examine his memory for recent personal events such as admission to hospital, and in particular for the temporal sequence of recent events. Test the ability to repeat a name and address immediately and five minutes later.

Record any selective impairment in memory for special incidents, periods, or themes in the patient's life. Retrograde and anterograde amnesia must be distinguished in relation to the onset of an acute disorder. Note any evidence of confabulation or false memories and the patient's attitude to his memory difficulties.

Intelligence. Note the discrepancy between the expected level of intelligence, estimated from the educational and occupational attainment, and performance during the above tests, which may indicate deterioration. An extended cognitive examination and formal IQ assessment are then indicated.

Further examination for suspected organic cerebral disorder

Testing must not tire the patient and may need to be spread out over several sessions. The examiner must be sensitive to the patient's reaction to failure, adapt tests to his general level of intelligence and note that one disability may mask another (e.g. it is difficult to detect dyspraxia in a dysphasic patient).

A simple screening routine is helpful at the start of the examination. Firstly, note the patient's level of cooperation. Then make a preliminary assessment of his level of conscious awareness. Thirdly, assess language function briefly by estimating his conversational speech; asking him to name a series of common objects, like a pen, watch or key; presenting him with written commands to point to objects; asking him to write down the names of objects to which you point. Next assess the patient's memory, in particular his new learning ability (a sensitive indicator of cerebral disorder), and then his spatial and constructional ability by asking him to draw simple figures.

Level of conscious awareness. Record any evidence of drowsiness, diminished awareness of the environment, or fluctuations in level of consciousness. Minor impairment may be suspected from a vague, inert or hesitant manner, or from performance in tests of attention and memory above. Judgement of the passage of time is often inaccurate.

Is the patient alert or dull, awake or drowsy? Assess his capacity for sustained attention by asking him to signal whenever designated letters appear in a spoken list, or to cancel specific letters in a designated script. If somnolent, can he be roused to full or only partial awareness? If his attention cannot be sustained, does he drift back into sleep or does his attention wander? Are his eyes open or shut, fixed or following movement? The level of consciousness should be recorded by defining the nature of the stimulus required to evoke responses, such as eye opening. Evidence for delirium, coma or stupor should be specified in detail.

Language

Six separate aspects of speech function must be assessed. These are motor aspects, comprehension, repetition, word-finding, reading and writing.

Motor aspects. Note the quality of spontaneous speech and that in response to questions. Is there any disturbance of articulation (dysarthria)? Does he use freely flowing phrases or sentences, or hesitant, one or two-word groupings separated by pauses? Does he have difficulty finding words, or use circumlocutions (phrases where a single word would suffice)? Does he use wrong words, neologisms (e.g. I've not norter with a verker), or paraphasias (e.g. lemon = demmun, snail = stale)? Is his grammar incorrect (e.g. the boy hit the ball on the head)? Are words omitted and sentences cut short in the telegram style (e.g. girl give flower teacher)? Is speech incomprehensible (jargon aphasia)? Observe for perseverative errors of speech, such as repetition of phrases just spoken (echolalia), of terminal words or phrases (palilalia) (e.g. I'm not so well today, today, today . .), or of a terminal syllable (logoclonia). Note the content of speech (the meaning conveyed, circumlocutions, and errors).

Look for discrepancies between spontaneous speech and replies to questions, between conversational speech and automatic speech or the naming of serials (e.g. days of the week), and between formal and emotional speech.

Comprehension. This must be assessed separately, whether or not speech production is impaired. Can he point correctly on command to one of several objects in view? Can he respond to yes/no questions, carry out simple commands (e.g. close your eyes), or more complex instructions involving the understanding of prepositions (e.g. point to the window, then to the ceiling; put a key between the paper clip and coin)?

Repetition of speech. Can the patient repeat precisely digits, words, short phrases, or long sentences?

Word finding (anomia). Ask the patient to name both common and uncommon objects, object parts (e.g. a watch, the strap, hands, buckle), body parts, and colours. In visually impaired subjects naming can be tested by sentence completion (e.g. "you write with a . . .").

Writing. Can he write spontaneously and to dictation? What are his errors? Is copying better preserved than writing to dictation? Is spelling out loud better than that on paper? Test more than just the patient's signature and address, which may be relatively intact.

Reading. Can he read out loud and perform simple written commands? Failing this, can he read aloud single letters or words? Does he comprehend what he reads?

Verbal fluency. This should be assessed, even in patients with no other language disturbance, since it is sensitive to frontal lobe lesions. Ask the patient to name as many words as possible in one minute beginning with a particular letter, or as many different animals.

Memory functions. Full examination of memory functions will always be required. Special attention should be focused on recent memory and learning ability, both verbal and visuospatial. The latter is tested by asking the patient to reproduce simple figures after a five-minute interval.

Visuospatial and constructional difficulties. Test the patient's ability to judge the relationships between objects in space, to estimate distances, to indicate the nearer of two objects, and to point out objects in the room with his eyes shut. Can he connect two dots by a straight line, bisect a straight line, draw simple geometric figures, or copy a series of line drawings of increasing complexity?

Ask the patient to draw a house, a clock face with hands, and a rough map of Great Britain, observing for hemispatial neglect or crowding into one part. Test the ability to construct simple designs with sticks or matches.

Visual agnosia. Can the patient describe what he sees, and identify objects and persons? Ask him to name an object in view such as a pen or key, describe its use, or if dysphasic indicate its use. If he fails, can he identify it by touch? Can he name or match colours, grasp the meaning of a whole picture, or recognise familiar faces (by pointing out a named person in a group, or naming photographs of relatives or well-known figures)?

Dyspraxia. Test the patient's ability to carry out purposeful movements to command (e.g. holding out arms, crossing legs, sticking out tongue). Test each hand separately for opening and closing of the hand. Ask him to gesture, salute, wave goodbye, or threaten somebody, and then to imitate a gesture (do this after me); to mime the use of an imaginary object (show me how to use a comb or toothbrush); to demonstrate the use of an actual object (show me how to open and close a door, use a key, use a can opener); and finally to perform complex coordinated sequences of movement (e.g. pour water from a sealed bottle).

Frontal executive function tests (Hodges, 1994)

Initiation: verbal fluency tests (described above) include letter fluency, category fluency (animals, vegetables), and the supermarket fluency test.

Abstraction: proverbs, similarities, and cognitive estimates. Observe for concrete interpretation of proverbs, but note that educational level and cultural background influence the response. Concrete verbal responses are also given by schizophrenic patients.

The *similarities test* involves asking subjects in what way two conceptually linked items are alike, starting with simple pairs such as "apple and banana", "shirt and dress", and progressing to more abstract pairs such as "plant and animal". Patients with frontal deficits or dementia make concrete interpretations.

A formal test is the Cognitive Estimates Test, which requires common-sense judgements to answer various questions, e.g. "What is the height of the Post Office Tower?" A correct reply is within the range 100–800 feet. Each answer is scored for unusual or extreme responses.

Response inhibition and set-shifting

Alternating sequences. The examiner produces a short sequence of alternating square and triangular shapes. The patient is asked to copy the sequence, and then to continue the pattern. Patients with frontal lobe deficits repeat one of the shapes rather than alternate the pair.

Go–No–Go test. The patient is asked to place a hand on the table and to raise one finger in response to a single tap, while holding still in response to two taps from the examiner's unseen finger.

Motor sequencing. Test the patient's sequencing ability in the Luria three-step (fist, edge, palm hand movements) and alternating hand movements test (Lishman, 1987).

Formal tests. The Trail Making Test includes two parts: in part A, the patient must connect randomly arranged numbers in numerical sequence. In part B, the test is to draw a line connecting numbers and letters in an alternating ordinal sequence, e.g. from 1 to A, to 2 to B, to 3 to C, and so on.

Other tests

Number functions. If patients fail on the serial 7s test, give them simpler addition and subtraction problems. Test the ability to handle money properly. Can he read or write numbers of more than two digits?

Topographical disorientation. Does the patient lose his way about the ward, or get into the wrong bed? Can he locate different rooms on the ward or at home, and describe familiar routes?

Right–left disorientation. Can he point to objects or parts of his own or the examiner's body, both on the left and on the right? Can he touch his right ear with his left hand?

Body image disturbances. Ask him to name, move on command or point to individual fingers or other body parts. Is one side of the body neglected in bimanual tasks, washing, grooming or dressing? When touched symmetrically and simultaneously on both sides, does he fail to report the stimulus on one side? Does he ignore, show lack of concern or deny the disability of an injured body part?

Dressing difficulties. Does the patient show undue difficulty in dressing and undressing, or get muddled when inserting limbs into clothing?

Other general indications, insight and judgement. Observe for lability of mood, euphoria or catastrophic reaction. Were emotional responses exaggerated, flat or lacking? Ask the patient what he thinks is wrong, and about his understanding of the problems that have been identified (whether by him or by others). Does he show appropriate concern about his symptoms or mistakes during tests? Is he evasive; does he minimise, deny or excuse his problems? Is his judgement good when discussing financial or domestic matters? To what extent does he recognise his need to rely on help and advice from others?

Patients who lack insight or show lack of concern, or even denial of their disabilities, tend to have organic lesions, whereas excessive concern in the absence of objective memory loss usually indicates an anxiety or depressive state.

Examination of the mute or apparently inaccessible patient

Assess separately (with the help of an informant) the following features: to what extent can the patient dress, feed himself, or manage hygiene? When aroused does he briefly become alert and verbally responsive? Assess his response to graded stimulation. Are the eyes open or shut? If open, are they watchful and do they follow moving objects? If shut, do they resist passive opening? Observe the physical posture at rest. Is it constrained, or bizarre, or suggestive of possible delusions? What happens after passive movement? Observe the facial expression and its emotional reaction. Are there spontaneous or abnormal movements? Test the musculature for tone, rigidity, negativism, waxy flexibility, automatic obedience, echopraxia. After recovery examine for memory of events that occurred during stupor.

If mute, is mutism elective, confined to some situations, or some persons but not others? Is the patient himself disturbed by it? Distinguish mutism from severe motor dysphasia, dysarthria, aphonia, poverty of speech or psychomotor retardation. Is partial vocalisation preserved, are emotional utterances possible, or can simple yes/no answers be given? Can he articulate (whisper or make lip movements of speech), phonate, grunt or cough? Does he speak occasionally, or respond after a long delay?

A detailed neurological examination is required, focusing on the level of conscious awareness, evidence of raised intracranial pressure and of diencephalic or upper brain stem pathology: thus examine for papilloedema, equality and reactivity of the pupils, quality of respiration, long tract signs, and conjugate reflex eye movements on passive head rotation.

Summary

Table 22.2 summarises the assessment of the cognitive state. The important point is to ensure that a basic screening of all the subheadings has been done. More detailed testing is the province of properly qualified neuropsychologists, and the assessment can be regarded as a 'screening' process (Kopelman, 1994).

Table 22.2 Summary assessment of the cognitive state

In frankly psychotic or obviously neurotic states where an organic disorder is not suspected, it is sufficient to assess orientation in time, place and person, concentration and attention, and immediate and delayed recall of a name and address (or knowledge of three recent news events). Where an organic disorder is suspected, each aspect of cognitive function (see under 'sub-headings') should be sampled along the lines suggested. This table is not fully comprehensive, and the more detailed assessment of deficits more commonly seen in neurological than psychiatric practice, such as apraxia and agnosia, is described in the text. When reporting your findings, do try to order them under subheadings. The assessment of the cognitive state should be viewed as a 'screening' procedure, and is certainly no substitute for proper neuropsychological assessment by a psychologist.

Subheading	Example items	Comments
Orientation	Time, place, person ± age, ± date of birth, ± duration of present admission/ delay since last out-patient visit	The sense of personal identity is commonly lost in psychogenic amnesia, but seldom in organic disorders except for profound dementia. Age orientation is commonly impaired in amnesia, dementia, and schizophrenia, underestimates being more common than overestimates.
Attention/ concentration	Days of week forwards/backwards Months of year forwards/backwards Digit span forwards/backwards Subjective assessment of concentration by the patient and the examiner (Serial 7s)	Attention is a complex psychological function encompassing such components as simple and choice reaction time, speed of information processing, sustained attention (vigilance), selective attention, and dual-task processing. The tests suggested to the left measure speed of information processing, and the other components are best measured by formal psychological tests. Commonly used, the Serial 7s test confounds attention, memory, and mental calculation. Digit span forward is also a measure of 'primary' or 'working' memory, which is spared in the amnesic syndrome.

Subheading	Example items	Comments
Memory		
General or public information	Description of three recent news events (e.g. accidents, catastrophes, political or sports events) (3 points) / Queen's full name and title (1 point) / Number of children she has (1 point) / Names of her four children (1 point if all correct) / Current PM (1 point) / Previous PM (1 point) / President of US (1 point) / Previous President (1 point) / Years of Second World War (2 points)	These items are taken from the Gresham Questionnaire and when scored out of 12, give good differentiation between patients who have amnesia or dementia and healthy controls or depressed patients.
(semantic memory)		Subjects should be asked for details of recent news events (and also personal memories, below). Mildly impaired patients may be able to give an outline of events (scoring 1/2 mark each), but not any detail.
Remote and recent personal (or 'auto-biographical') memories (facts and incidents)		This is important to sample, but usually will already have been done in the course of obtaining the psychiatric history. Ask, for example, about recent incidents in hospital. / NB. the terms 'remote' and 'recent' are immensely preferable to 'long-term' and 'short-term' which are used in different ways by different disciplines.
Current (or new) learning	Name and address / – immediate: repeat up to five times until subject recalls completely correctly / – delayed: five minutes	Use a standard procedure on each occasion of testing. for example: / Mr John Brown / 12 Brighton Road (8 items) / Edinburgh, Scotland / Record patient's score (out of 8) at each learning trial and at delayed recall.

Subheadings	Example items	Comments
	Paragraph recall	Read the subject a short paragraph of several lines of fairly concrete information, e.g. a brief story, and test recall immediately and at a half hour delay. Note any intrusion errors ('momentary confabulation').
	Copy designs and recall at five minutes' delay	Other tests, e.g. recall of paired associates or pictures, can also be incorporated.
Language		
Naming	Readily available items of clothing, furniture, desk utensils, including more global names (e.g. jacket/watch) and more specific items (e.g. lapel/winder), which are generally more difficult. Doctor's name and other staff or patients in ward/department.	An impairment of naming and word-finding is an early feature of dementia and the most common dysphasic deficit found in psychiatric practice.
Comprehension	Ask subject to follow a single-stage instruction (e.g. 'use your right hand to touch the tip of your nose'), 2-staged instruction ('...left ear then right ear'), 3-staged instruction ('...left knee, left ear, tip of nose'), and 4-staged instruction ('...right ear, left knee, tip of nose, left ear').	Record how complex an instruction (i.e. how many 'stages') the subject can follow correctly. Will be impaired in early dementia.
Expression	Assess for dysphasia and dysarthria	
Repetition ('conduction')	Repeat 'The cow jumped over the moon'/'The rain in Spain falls mainly on the plain'.	Impaired in dementia, and occasionally in left temporo-parietal lesions.

Subheadings	Example items	Comments
Reading and writing	Get subject to read short paragraph and write a brief sentence.	Specific reading deficits require formal neuropsychological assessment.
Disorders of form and content	Pressure of speech, flight of ideas, 'clang' associations, and poverty of speech.	Should have been noted already but, if not, should be remarked upon here.
Mental calculation	Ask the subject to perform simple additions/subtractions/divisions/ multiplications of varying difficulty e.g. 6+4 27+18 6x3 12x13 19–6 51–13 12/3 108/9	Graduate level of difficulty to subject's ability. If necessary, present the subject with money and get him or her to work out appropriate change for a given price of article. These simple calculations tend to give a better impression of the subject's capacity than 'serial 7s'.
Drawing and copying	Clock face Draw a house Copy a star, cube or abstract design	Draw circle and ask subject to fill in numbers and hands to current time (tell subject what current time is). Can indicate perceptual and perceptuomotor deficits, constructional apraxia, or unilateral neglect. Look for omissions/distortions/displacements/intrusions.
Other agnosic or apraxic deficits	Visual agnosia, motor apraxia or dressing apraxia	These are not part of the routine cognitive assessment, as they are seen relatively seldom in psychiatric practice except as part of a global dementia. *Agnosia* refers to a disorder in the recognition of objects independent of any primary sensory or naming deficit. *Apraxia* refers to an inability to carry out a voluntary skilled movement not attributable to to a primary sensory or motor deficit. Right/left disorientation and astereognosis can also be noted here. See text.

Subheading	Example items	Comments
Frontal function		
Verbal fluency	Ask subject to give as many words in a minute beginning with the letter F, then A, then S. Or, as many words as possible from a given category, for example, animals.	For FAS verbal fluency, normal subjects score 30+ in total. 20–30 suggests mild frontal dysfunction. Scores less than 20 suggest large frontal lesions or moderately severe dementia. (Note – non-frontal lesions can sometimes produce impairment on this and other 'frontal' tests. Hence, they are sometimes called 'executive' tests.)
Abstracting ability	Ask subject to interpret proverbs and /or to estimate measurements such as the height of the Telecom Tower, the size of the British population, or the height of the average Englishwoman.	Patients with frontal lesions sometimes, but by no means always, give 'concrete' interpretations of proverbs and/or grossly aberrant cognitive estimates.
Luria's motor tests	Make a fist, slicing movement, and slapping movement with the hand in sequence to the words 'punch', 'cut', 'slap' and ask the subject to mimic. Then get the subject to carry on in sequence by himself/herself.	These movements are often poorly coordinated in patients with frontal lesions.
Behavioural observations	Apathetic, unkempt, irritable, disinhibited, emotionally labile, loss of social graces.	May have been noted under 'Appearance and behaviour' (above), but should be considered here in relation to test findings.
(Primitive reflexes)		(Part of physical examination, and not very specific for frontal pathology.)

Taken from Kopelman (1994) in the *British Journal of Hospital Medicine*, **52**, 277–281, with permission.

Psychological tests

Only brief mention can be made here. Fuller accounts of modern psychological assessments can be obtained from Walsh (1987), Ellis & Young (1988), Shallice (1988), McCarthy & Warrington (1990), Morris & McKiernan (1994) and Lezak (1995).

It has become customary to estimate premorbid IQ using a reading test – the National Adult Reading Test (Nelson, 1982). Current intelligence is most commonly assessed using the Wechsler Adult Intelligence Scale – Revised (WAIS–R; Wechsler, 1981). Alternatives include the Standard Progressive Matrices (Raven *et al*, 1977), and the Mill Hill Vocabulary Test, which is commonly used alongside them.

The Wechsler Memory Scale – Revised (Wechsler, 1987) is probably the best known, internationally available assessment of memory, although it is lengthy and does not contain any assessment of recognition memory. Hence it can usefully be supplemented by the Warrington Recognition Memory Test (Warrington, 1984). Other tests such as the California Verbal Learning Test (Delis *et al*, 1991) are also available. The Rivermead Behavioural Memory Test purports to measure aspects of 'everyday' memory (Wilson, 1987). There are relatively few published (as opposed to research) tests of retrograde memory, but the Autobiographical Memory Interview (Kopelman *et al*, 1990) may be useful in this regard.

Tests of language include the Boston Naming Test, the Graded Naming Test (McKenna & Warrington, 1983), the Token Test, and the Reporters Test.

There are many tests of frontal function, which tend to correlate poorly with one another once the effects of age and IQ have been partialled out (Kopelman, 1991). Tests of frontal function include measures of verbal fluency (Benton, 1968), the Wisconsin Card Sorting Test and Modified Card Sorting Test (Nelson, 1986), the Cognitive Estimates Test (Shallice & Evans, 1978) and the Tower of London Test (Shallice, 1982).

Computerised methods of assessment of cognitive function have been developed. The Cambridge Neuropsychological Test Automated Battery (CANTAB) assesses visual memory, attention, spatial working memory and planning. Based on animal tests of cognitive functions with proven neural substrates, CANTAB is sensitive to deficits in patients with Alzheimer's and Parkinson's diseases (Robbins & Sahakian, 1994).

Interviews for rating behavioural abnormalities in dementia and other neuropsychiatric disorders have been developed. The Present Behavioural Examination (PBE; Hope & Fairburn, 1992) is a structured interview administered to the patient's main carer to obtain detailed and reliable measures of specific behavioural abnormalities in the following categories: mental health, walking (including wandering), eating, diurnal rhythms, aggression, sexual behaviour, incontinence and individual behavioural abnormalities (e.g. plucking, searching, mumbling, 'obsessionality'). Other behavioural rating scales for use in neuropsychiatric patients are reviewed by Folstein (1991) and Kluger *et al* (1994).

Cognitive scales

A number of scales, such as the Mini Mental State Examination (MMSE; Folstein *et al*, 1975), the Newcastle Dementia Scale (Blessed *et al*, 1968), and CAMDEX (Roth *et al*, 1986), have been developed to screen or assess cognitive function. While these scales are not strictly diagnostic tests, they are extremely useful in grading the severity of cognitive impairment, particularly in dementing disorders (Kluger *et al*, 1994). Scores on these scales have been shown to correlate with one another, and also with the number of post-mortem plaques and/or tangles and particularly with neuronal cell loss in Alzheimer's disease. The uses and limitations of the MMSE are discussed by Anthony *et al* (1982), Roman *et al* (1993) and Hodges (1994). Population-based norms for the MMSE by age and educational level are published by Crum *et al* (1993).

Imaging

Computerised tomography (CT)

CT of the brain is essential in the investigation of cerebral disorder. It detects most cortical lesions, vascular infarctions, demyelination and white matter change (leucodystrophy), and hydrocephalus. Cerebral atrophy (widened ventricles and enlarged sulci) is often reported in dementia, with the abnormalities increasing as the disease progresses (Jacoby & Levy, 1980; Burns *et al*, 1991). Problems exist, however, with the interpretation of CT scan findings of cerebral atrophy in dementia:

(1) atrophy may occur in many elderly normal subjects (Jacoby *et al*, 1980);
(2) it may be absent in early clinical dementia;
(3) it is not specific to one disorder.

No feature of the CT scan is diagnostic of Alzheimer's disease, but an increase in ventricular size over one year is strongly suggestive. Automated volumetric indices of brain atrophy may discriminate between normal ageing and Alzheimer's disease, even in its mild stages (Förstl & Hentschel, 1994). A frontal distribution of atrophy may suggest Pick's disease, and caudate atrophy Huntington's disease as well as neuroacanthocytosis. Atrophy may occur in psychiatric disorders such as alcoholism, schizophrenia or affective disorder (Jacoby & Levy, 1980; Ron, 1983; Lewis, 1990). Detailed views of the temporal lobes may reveal subtle pathology and improve the discriminating ability of the scan in dementia (Burns & Pearlson, 1994). It is critical that CT scan appearances should be interpreted in conjunction with the *total* clinical picture.

Magnetic resonance imaging (MRI)

MRI (or nuclear magnetic resonance, NMR) is a major advance in imaging structural change. MRI yields fine anatomical detail in several planes, differentiates grey and white matter, outlines major blood vessels and detects small lesions particularly in the posterior fossa and pituitary regions, which are areas poorly visualised by CT. MRI sensitively detects lesions, such as white matter changes and infarcts, assists in the differential diagnosis of focal tissue pathology, and detects and allows quantitative estimations of atrophy, both generalised and focal, such as hippocampal atrophy in Alzheimer's disease (Kesslak *et al*, 1991; Besson, 1994) and cortical volume in schizophrenia (Harvey *et al*, 1993).

Single photon emission computerised tomography (SPET)

SPET assesses brain function by measuring the photon emission from radiotracers, which cross the blood–brain barrier and distribute in proportion to regional cerebral blood flow shortly after intravenous injection. This provides an indirect measure of cerebral metabolic function. The radioactivity involved is a limiting factor and an ethical issue. SPET is cheaper and more widely available then positron emission tomography (PET), which in addition allows the evaluation of brain metabolism. Transmitter receptor studies can be done with both SPET and PET. The applications of SPET in psychiatry are reviewed by Ell & Costa (1992) and Geaney (1994); and of PET by Kennedy & Frackowiak (1994).

EEG

The electroencephalogram (EEG) is used widely when organic disorders are suspected, confirming abnormalities of brain structure and function in about 60% of cases. The EEG reading is symmetrical and usually classified into four characteristic waveforms: delta rhythms at less than 4 Hz, theta at 4–7 Hz, alpha at 8–13 Hz, and beta over 13 Hz.

Focal abnormalities are most consistent with localised disorders such as tumours, abscesses, subdural haematomas or cerebral infarctions; diffuse slowing occurs in toxic and metabolic disorders and in advanced degenerative diseases. The EEG is a sensitive indicator of deranged cerebral metabolism. The degree of bilateral diffuse slowing correlates positively with the degree of cognitive impairment in delirium (Engel & Romano, 1959) and so serial EEGs are useful for monitoring its progress.

Triphasic waves occur in liver failure, high amplitude sharp waves in herpes simplex encephalitis, low voltage activity with posterior slowing in uraemia, acceleration of alpha in hyperthyroidism, and low voltage activity in myxoedema. In delirium tremens the EEG may show fast activity rather than slowing. In toxic delirium associated with drugs, the EEG may show drug-specific patterns of fast-wave activity (antidepressants, benzodiazepines) or slowing (phenothiazines). Localised spike and sharp-wave complexes usually suggest an intracranial cause for delirium.

In very early Alzheimer's disease the EEG is usually normal, but as the disease advances there is progressive slowing of the tracing, with less alpha and beta activity and more delta and theta posteriorly. Multi-infarct dementia is characterised by an asymmetric tracing with focal slowing in over two-thirds of patients, with relative preservation of the alpha rythym (Roberts *et al*, 1978). Pronounced flattening of the EEG suggests Huntington's disease, whereas repetitive spike discharges or triphasic sharp-wave complexes may indicate Creutzfeld-Jakob disease. The latter may yield a floridly abnormal EEG in a patient with mild cognitive impairment, and little change on structural imaging (CT or MRI). In investigating dementia, a normal EEG may be found in early degenerative dementia and pseudodementia, and in 20% of cases with tumours or subdural haematoma. The use and limitations of the EEG are discussed by Lishman (1987), Fenton (1993) and Binnie & Prior (1994). Evoked potentials are reviewed by Philpot (1994).

Delirium

Delirium (acute organic reaction, confusional state, toxic confusional state, acute organic psychosis) occurs in about 10% of all hospitalised patients and in 17–50% of hospitalised elderly patients (Lipowski, 1983; Taylor & Lewis, 1993). In the Eastern Baltimore mental health survey, the point prevalence of delirium in adults aged 18–64 in the community was 0.4%, rising to 1.1% in those aged 55 years and over (Folstein *et al*, 1991). The ICD–10 and DSM–IV diagnostic criteria for delirium are set out in Boxes 22.2 and 22.3.

Clinical features

Traditionally, the cardinal feature of delirium is clouding of consciousness. It manifests as impaired alertness, awareness and attention in a patient who is awake. The impairment is mild but can advance to coma if untreated. Clouding is distinguished from natural drowsiness in that the patient cannot be easily aroused. While ICD–10 retains the term 'clouding of consciousness', yoking it to disordered attention (Box 22.2), DSM–IV eschews the term. In DSM–IV, disturbance of consciousness, which is manifest by a reduced clarity of awareness of the environment, is operationalised by core attentional deficits (see Box 22.3). Reduced attentiveness can range from mild distractibility, losing the thread of conversations and failing to grasp complex details, to reduced interaction, a lack of spontaneous speech, and neglect of bodily needs. Arousal may be raised, with psychomotor overactivity, screaming and excessive reactions to noise and bright lights; or it may be reduced. In either case, patients are unable to focus attention or concentrate.

Box 22.2 ICD–10 diagnostic criteria for delirium

For a definite diagnosis, mild or severe symptoms should be present in *each* of the following areas:

1. Impairment of consciousness and attention (on a continuum from clouding to coma); reduced ability to direct, focus, sustain, and shift attention
2. Global disturbance of cognition (perceptual distortions, illusions and hallucinations; impairment of abstract thinking and comprehension, with or without transient delusions, but typically with some degree of incoherence; impairment of recent memory but relatively intact remote memory; disorientation for time, place and person)
3. Psychomotor disturbances (hypo- or hyperactivity and unpredictable shifts from one to the other; increased reaction time; increased or decreased flow of speech; enhanced startle reaction)
4. Disturbance of the sleep–wake cycle (insomnia, total sleep loss or reversal of the sleep–wake cycle; daytime drowsiness; nocturnal worsening of symptoms; disturbing dreams or nightmares, which may continue as hallucinations after awakening)
5. Emotional disturbances, such as depression, anxiety, irritability, euphoria, apathy, or wondering perplexity

---

The onset of delirium is usually rapid over hours, as after concussion or intoxication, or more gradual over a few days. In the latter case, the patient cannot concentrate or think clearly, universally fails to judge the passage of time, feels anxious and restless, and may be irritable, hypersensitive to light and noise, and drowsy at times, with insomnia or vivid dreams and nightmares, or even transient hallucinations. The patient may try to conceal her confusion by evasion or brief answers to questions, or by complaints and anger. As delirium progresses, the patient becomes more obviously confused. *Confusion* is a term combining impaired attention, muddled thinking, poor grasp of one's situation, forgetfulness and some degree of disorientation for time and place. The patient has difficulty naming the correct day of the week or the date. As delirium advances she may think she is at home instead of in the hospital. She may misidentify doctors and nurses for relatives and friends; this tendency to misidentify the unfamiliar for the familiar is characteristic.

As delirium worsens, the patient becomes increasingly distractible, and either drowsy or hyperalert and excited. She may look inert, sleepy and withdrawn, responding slowly to questions with long pauses between

---

**Box 22.3 DSM–IV diagnostic criteria for delirium due to ...
(indicate the general medical condition)**

1. Disturbance of consciousness (reduced clarity of awareness of the environment) with reduced ability to focus, sustain, or shift attention
2. A change in cognition (such as memory deficit, disorientation, language disturbance) or the development of a perceptual disturbance that is not better accounted for by a pre-existing, established or evolving dementia
3. The disturbance develops over a short period of time (usually hours to days) and tends to fluctuate during the course of the day
4. There is evidence from the history, physical examination or laboratory findings that the disturbance is caused by the direct physiological consequences of a general medical condition

Adapted with permission from DSM–IV. Copyright 1994 American Psychiatric Association.

---

words, and pleading to be left alone. Alternatively, she may be restless, fidgety, scanning the room, and striking out in terror at invisible animals. In either case, attention remains impaired. The patient cannot sustain a train of thought and forgets the question or the beginning of her sentence. Thinking is laboured and slow, or rapid and incoherent. Attempts to get out of bed are common in the more restless patients, and injuries may result. Noisy expressions of fear and screams for help may attend hallucinations, as in delirium tremens (see page 1111).

Reduced responsiveness may shift unpredictably to outbursts of excitement. At any time an excited hallucinating patient may calm down and ask coherent pointed questions about his whereabouts, the time, or his family. These lucid intervals are characteristic of delirium, and occur more often during daylight hours. Sleep–wake cycles are frequently disrupted or reversed, and confusion is often more marked at night.

Illusions and hallucinations may appear, especially at night, most commonly visual but often mixed with auditory and other misperceptions. Perceptual illusions include distortions of shape, size and position of the patient's body and surroundings. Depersonalisation and derealisation are common, but are often poorly expressed. Perceptual abnormalities are usually fleeting and changeable, and are readily interpreted as hostile and persecutory. A merging of dream contents, waking hallucinations and the fragments of true perceptions, is common in delirium, and is recalled after recovery as real experience.

Memory loss

Impairment of memory, with reduced digit span, impaired new learning and defective recall of remote events is an important clinical feature.

One of the earliest symptoms of memory loss is minor forgetfulness or "absent-mindedness" with muddled time sequences, or more striking memory lapses. Loss of topographical memory is often seen, with the patient losing his way when wandering from home or driving to work. An early sign is disorientation for time, and later disorientation for place. The memory deficit is global, affecting all types of material and remote as well as recent events, with failure of new learning a key feature. The memory deficit is also patchy, so that partially correct information may be incorporated into confabulatory answers or delusions. After recovery the patient has partial or total amnesia for the period of confusion, but isolated events, especially vivid hallucinations, may be remembered in detail.

Thinking

Thought processes are either slowed or rapid. In all cases thinking is incoherent, fragmented, illogical and undirected, with poverty of content. The capacity to select and order thoughts to solve problems, plan action, understand a situation and communicate adequately is impaired. Intrusive images lend a dream-like quality, blurring dream and waking imagery, fact and fantasy.

Ideas of reference and paranoid delusions may develop, which tend to be poorly worked out, fleeting, changeable, and readily elicited and modified by the environment.

Speech

Speech is increased or decreased in output and often hesitant or slurred. Sentences are simple, poorly organised, often repetitious with circumlocutions, slips of the tongue and paraphasias. Nominal dysphasia is common and writing is nearly always defective.

Emotion

Lability of emotional expression is common in delirium. Anxiety, depression, irritability, anger, perplexity and suspicion are often observed in varying combinations, intensity and duration. Autonomic arousal often occurs, with tachycardia, sweating, dilated pupils, increased blood pressure and tremor as in delirium tremens.

Psychomotor changes

Psychomotor activity is virtually always disturbed, with two contrasting patterns, but patients may shift between the two. In most patients, spontaneous motor activity is depressed, but some are hyperactive and restless.

Perseverative or repetitive stereotyped motor behaviour may occur, such as aimless plucking at bedclothes or mimicry of familiar activities.

Involuntary movements such as tremor and myoclonus are usually seen in drug withdrawal or metabolic disorders. Rarely, patients are catatonic. Variability in the levels of arousal and awareness, psychomotor activity, and the presence of hallucinations and delusions is characteristic of delirium, both between patients and in the same patient over time. Lipowski (1990) distinguished three patterns of psychomotor activity – hyperactive, hypoactive, and mixed subtypes. Psychomotor overactivity and heightened alertness distinguish the *hyperactive* variant. The most important example is delirium tremens. In the *hypoactive* subtype, psychomotor activity and alertness are reduced, as in Wernicke's encephalopathy and hepatic encephalopathy. In the most common, the *mixed* subtype, shifts occur between states of lethargy and marked excitement, which make it difficult to gauge the correct dose of sedative drug for the patient, with the risk of over- or under-sedation.

Differential diagnosis

Delirium needs to be differentiated from chronic organic disorders, including dementia (see Table 22.1) and the focal organic disorders, and from functional psychiatric disorders, in particular depression, paranoid psychosis and mania. The major distinguishing features of delirium are: mode of onset (rapid); duration (brief; if longer than three months, it is unlikely to be delirium); characteristic symptoms; and EEG findings (usually abnormal; Lipowski, 1990). The first essential distinction to be made is whether delirium results from a neurological cause or complicates a systemic illness.

Causes

The most common causes of delirium (Table 22.3) vary with the age group of the patient, but from teenage years onwards frequently include drug and alcohol intoxication and withdrawal syndromes, and (in the elderly) infections and multiple medications. *Neurological* causes can usually be recognised by the additional presence of focal neurological signs, but diffuse neurological diseases such as encephalitis may yield no focal signs. Space-occupying lesions of the nervous system usually cause headache and focal signs, but brain abscess and midline tumours may present with gradually evolving confusion. Acute onset may indicate brain-stem compression or acute hydrocephalus. *Systemic* causes are usually characterised by the absence of focal neurological signs apart from delirium. Drugs are the commonest cause of confusion, particularly in the elderly. Wernicke's encephalopathy should be considered in patients with a history of alcoholism, malnutrition, and persistent vomiting as in hyperemesis gravidarum. Focal infections may cause confusion in the elderly.

Table 22.3   Causes of delirium (after Lishman, 1987)

Class	Specific causes
Degenerative	Presenile or senile dementias complicated by infection, anoxia, etc.
Space-occupying lesions	Cerebral tumour, subdural haematoma, cerebral abscess
Trauma	Concussion, intracranial haematoma
Infection	Meningitis and encephalitis (viral, bacterial, fungal, protozoal), subacute meningovascular syphilis, septicaemia, malaria, subacute bacterial endocarditis, focal infection (e.g. pneumonia), exanthemata, HIV
Vascular	Acute cerebral thrombosis or embolism, transient cerebral ischaemic attack, subarachnoid haemorrhage, hypertensive encephalopathy, vasculitis (e.g. systemic lupus erythematosus, giant cell arteritis), air and fat embolism
Epileptic	Psychomotor seizures, petit mal status, post-ictal states
Metabolic	Uraemia, liver disorder, electrolyte disturbances, alkalosis, acidosis, hypercapnia, remote effects of carcinoma, porphyria
Endocrine	Diabetic hypoglycaemia or pre-coma; over- or under-activity of thyroid, parathyroid, adrenal; hypopituitarism
Toxic	Drug and alcohol intoxication (incl. therapeutic drugs: salicylate, anticholinergic, lithium and psychotropic drugs), drug withdrawal, chemical toxins, heavy metals, organic toxins
Anoxia	Pulmonary, cardiac, anaemia, carbon monoxide poisoning, post-anaesthetic
Vitamin deficiency	Thiamine (Wernicke's encephalopathy), nicotinic acid (pellagra), B12 and folic acid deficiency
Other	Hypothermia, heat stroke

Investigation

This is an urgent procedure. It involves urea, electrolytes, blood sugar, a full biochemical profile, a blood count, ESR, chest x-ray, electrocardiogram, drug and toxicological screen, blood and urine cultures, a complete infectious diseases screen if indicated, referral to physicians for cerebrospinal fluid examination, and consideration of EEG and imaging studies. Endocrine, vitamin and other tests may be indicated.

Management

The management of delirium has two major aspects, symptomatic and aetiological. The patient with delirium is often agitated and before the appropriate examination can be completed, his cooperation is required. Patients can be calmed by a sympathetic response from medical staff and relatives. Nursing care should be given in a quiet, well-lit room with a dimmed light at night, with facilities for frequent observation. If these steps do not calm the patient, sedation may be required for restlessness, agitation, overactivity and/or fear. An oral or intramuscular major tranquilliser such as haloperidol is suitable in most cases, but contraindicated in alcohol withdrawal states where it may provoke fits. Chlormethiazole or diazepam are then the drugs of choice. Tranquillisers can sometimes exacerbate an abnormal mental state or disguise neurological signs of deterioration (see page 1113).

Treatment of the underlying cause is crucial, and presupposes accurate diagnosis, which may take time. Management begins with identification and correction of hypoxia, hypoglycaemia, hypothermia, or dehydration. Parenteral thiamine should be given to patients in whom there is any suspicion of Wernicke's encephalopathy. Adequate nutrition, fluid intake and electrolyte balance must be provided. Subsequent treatment depends on the underlying cause.

Prognosis

The outcome of delirium includes full recovery, usually within a week or so, but sometimes after several weeks or months; or secondly, progression to stupor and coma, or cardiovascular collapse and death in up to 25% of patients. Thirdly, some patients pass through a subacute organic syndrome before recovering. This is a transitional cognitive, affective, behavioural or mixed disorder in a state of full alertness, such as an amnesic syndrome after delirium due to Wernicke's encephalopathy or head injury. Fourthly, delirium may progress to an irreversible organic brain syndrome (e.g. Wernicke's encephalopathy to Korsakoff's syndrome). Lastly, delirium may occasionally trigger a functional psychosis. Even after recovery, the disturbance associated with delirium may result in job loss and be socially destructive. The five-year cumulative mortality may be as high as 50%, and mortality depends more on the underlying medical disorder than on the presence of delirium (van Hemert *et al*, 1994).

Stupor

Stupor refers to a clinical syndrome of akinesis and mutism (see above) but with evidence of relative preservation of conscious awareness (Lishman, 1987). There is profound lack of responsiveness. The eyes may be open and apparently watchful, with the patient directing his gaze towards the examiner and the eyes following moving visual stimuli. When the eyes are shut they may resist passive opening. Strong painful stimuli may produce blinking or evasive action. Although spontaneous movement is typically absent, tremors, twitching or motor stereotypies can occur. The resting posture may be awkward or meaningful in the context of psychotic experience. Reflexes are often normal. Complete mutism is the rule, but patients may grunt, cough, mutter or rarely sing. In light stupor, feeding is possible, sphincters are intact, and commands may elicit simple responses.

The principal causes are schizophrenia (31%), depression (25%), organic (20%: dementia, delirium, tumour or cyst, neurosyphilis, post-encephalitic, post-epileptic), neurosis or hysteria (10%), or uncertain (14%) (Joyston-Bechal, 1966). The exclusion of neurological causes is essential, particularly raised intracranial pressure and mid-brain or upper brain-stem lesions. Changes from initial to final diagnosis are common, particularly from a psychiatric to a neurological diagnosis; certain clinical features aid this differential diagnosis (Altshuler *et al*, 1986).

In stupors due to functional psychiatric disorders, feeding ability and the sphincters may be partially preserved, the facial expression may react to events, and respiration and the pupils are normal. Schizophrenic stupor is essentially catatonic, but catatonic signs are diagnostically non-specific.

In depressive stupor there is severe psychomotor retardation, sadness and hopelessness in posture or expression, and silent tears may be shed, but consciousness is retained. Manic stupor is very rare, with an affect of elation. Hysterical stupor occurs under stress, usually with signs of conversion. It often fluctuates and there is complete passive dependence on others (see also page 19).

In organic stupors, the patient is immobile yet seemingly alert, with full eye movements, and can occasionally be aroused to move ('coma vigil'); alternatively, the patient appears apathetic and somnolent and has oculomotor abnormalities. The former pattern is seen with lesions at the base of the brain anteriorly, the latter with brain-stem lesions. Stupor may also occur in metabolic and endocrine disorders, and in intoxications (alcohol, barbiturates, psychotropic drugs).

In one psychiatric hospital series, almost half the cases resolved in one week, a fifth lasted more than a month, but all patients with prolonged stupor had severe brain damage (Joyston-Bechal, 1966). On recovery, the recollection of the mute period is absent in organic subjects, poor in affective patients, and often intact in schizophrenics.

Dementia

Dementia is the major cause of long-term disability in old age. The point-prevalence of dementia in those over the age of 65 years ranges from 3–8% (on average 5% in the UK), and is 15% in those over 80, with a relative excess of dementia of Alzheimer type (DAT) among women, and of vascular dementia among men (Jorm *et al*, 1987; Livingston, 1994). The prevalence rate of dementia doubles with every five years of age after 65. Rates for the "treated incidence" of dementia vary between 1.9–2.6 per 1000 for men and 2.1–4.1 for women over 60 years of age, but are about 10–16 per 1000 for both sexes in field surveys (Cooper, 1991). The incidence of dementia in a Liverpool community study confirmed by a three-year follow-up was 9.2/1000 cases per year, broken down into Alzheimer-type (6.3), vascular (1.9) and alcohol-related (1.0). Rates approximately trebled with every ten years of age, and the prognosis for organic 'subcases' was poor (Copeland *et al*, 1992).

The distinction between dementia occurring before the age of 65 (presenile dementia) and that occurring after (senile dementia) was based on the assumption that the causes were different. Although the expression and course of diseases may vary with age, the major findings in demented patients of all ages are broadly similar, and the age-specific incidence rates are unimodally distributed (Cooper, 1991), so that the distinction is arbitrary.

Two principal patterns of intellectual impairment have been described in dementia (Cummings & Benson, 1992). The first reflecting *cortical* dysfunction occurs in the majority; the second, *subcortical* dementia, is less common, but there is a considerable overlap in clinical presentation.

The cortical pattern of intellectual decline includes loss of language, learning, perception, calculation and praxis skills, and manifests as aphasia, amnesia, agnosia, acalculia and apraxia. The subcortical pattern results from disordered motivation, mood, attention, and arousal, revealed by psychomotor slowing, memory loss, affective disorders, and impaired problem-solving (Cummings, 1986). Cortical dementias produce neuropathological changes involving primarily, but not exclusively, association cortex and the medial temporal lobes, as in Alzheimer's disease and selected strokes. The subcortical pattern results from lesions in the basal ganglia, thalamus and brain stem, as in Huntington's and Parkinson's diseases. Mixed subcortical–cortical patterns occur in multiple sclerosis, stroke, severe head injury, Creutzfeld-Jakob disease and neoplastic causes.

Differential diagnosis

Dementia must be distinguished from delirium (see Table 22.1), from focal neurological (see chapter 23) or organic syndromes (see chapter 24), and from psychiatric disorders.

Functional psychiatric disorder masquerading as dementia, or pseudo-dementia, occurs in about 9% of cases of 'dementia', most often due to depression and rarely schizophrenia, hypomania, paraphrenia, hypochondriasis, hysteria and the Ganser state (Lishman, 1987). Subjective complaints of memory loss are more related to depressed mood than to objective memory performance, particularly in the elderly (Bolla *et al*, 1991; O'Brien & Beats, 1994). The differentiation between anxious preoccupation with memory and other mental functions, depression and dementia can be difficult in psychiatric settings. Two follow-up studies have revealed that a third to a half of patients discharged from psychiatric units were wrongly diagnosed initially as demented. They proved on follow-up to have had neurotic or personality disorders (Nott & Fleminger, 1975), or affective disorders alone or associated with static or transient organic reactions, or Parkinson's disease (Ron *et al*, 1979).

In the elderly, dementia must be distinguished from age-associated memory impairment (AAMI) or minor degrees of forgetfulness that accompany ageing (benign senescent forgetfulness), in which the recall of names and places is variably impaired while the recall of experiences

Table 22.4 Prevalence of different causes of dementia in adults referred for evaluation of progressive intellectual deterioration

Cause	Prevalence (%)
Alzheimer's disease (presumed)	39
Multi-infarct dementia	13
Alcoholic dementia	8
Metabolic disorders	4
Hydrocephalus	4
Cerebral neoplasms	3
Huntington's disease	2
Infections	1
Toxic conditions	1
Post-traumatic	1
Post-anoxic	0.2
Parkinson's disease	0.1
Subdural haematoma	0.1
Miscellaneous	11
Dementia associated with a psychiatric disorder (pseudodementia)	9
Not demented	2

Data based on 708 patients from eight world-wide series (Marsden, 1985).
Note that Lewy body dementia has subsequently been shown to account for up to 20% of patients with dementia at autopsy. AIDS-dementia complex is not included in this series.

remains intact, and the activities of daily life are not impaired (Kral, 1962). Criteria for AAMI have been proposed, which include age over 50 years, subjective complaints of forgetfulness, performance on well-standardised memory tests at least one standard deviation below the normal values of young adults, gradual dysfunction in the activities of daily living, and absence of dementia or significant medical or psychiatric problems (Crook *et al*, 1986). The concept is reviewed by O'Brien & Beats (1994).

The early symptoms and signs of progressive dementia are often indistinguishable from AAMI, and the two may lie on a cognitive continuum (Rediess & Caine, 1993). AAMI is thought not to progress to definite dementia, but this may depend on Apolipoprotein E4 status (Feskens *et al*, 1994).

Causes

The possible causes of dementia are listed in Table 22.4, along with the frequency with which the various causes were found among a total of 708 patients from a worldwide series, in which most patients were below the age of 65 (Marsden, 1985).

The so-called primary dementias include Alzheimer's disease, Pick's disease, Huntington's disease (chorea) and Creutzfeld-Jakob disease. The most frequent cause of dementia, Alzheimer's disease, is diagnosed by exclusion.

Potentially treatable causes of dementia are found in approximately 15% of patients below the age of 65, but in under 5% of those over 65 presenting with intellectual impairment. About half of the treatable patients have pseudodementia; the others have treatable tumours, haematoma, hydrocephalus, metabolic or infective disorders. Among the 'incurable' disorders, vascular dementia associated with hypertension, alcoholic dementia and AIDS-related dementia may be amenable to therapy.

There are few studies of causes of dementia in Third World countries. The prevalence of dementia in Shanghai in people over the age of 55 is 4.6% (Zhang *et al*, 1990), and in the Chinese islet of Kinmen 3.5%, rising with age, and falling with years of education (Liu *et al*, 1994). In Nigeria, however, 'senile' dementia is virtually unknown, perhaps because the elderly are usually a survival elite (Henderson, 1986). Toxic, nutritional and infective causes of organic reactions are more common, and found in younger subjects.

Alzheimer's disease

Alzheimer's disease is strictly speaking a pathological diagnosis, which is not usually made during life. The DSM–IV diagnostic criteria for dementia of the Alzheimer's type are set out in Box 22.4. ICD–10 primarily requires a decline in both memory and thinking sufficient to impair activities of daily living, which is of insidious onset, slow deterioration and has a minimum duration of symptoms and impairments of six months. The

---

Box 22.4 DSM–IV diagnostic criteria for dementia of the Alzheimer's type

A. The development of multiple cognitive deficits manifested by both:
   (1) memory impairment (impaired ability to learn new information or to recall previously learned information)
   (2) one (or more) of the following cognitive disturbances:
      (a) aphasia
      (b) apraxia
      (c) agnosia
      (d) disturbance in executive functioning

B. The cognitive deficits in criteria A1 and A2 each cause significant impairment in social or occupational functioning and represent a significant decline from a previous level of functioning

C. The course is characterised by gradual onset and continuing cognitive decline

D. The cognitive deficits in criteria A1 and A2 are not due to any of the following:
   (1) other central nervous system conditions that cause progressive deficits in memory and cognition (e.g. cerebrovascular disease, Parkinson's disease, Huntington's disease, subdural hematoma)
   (2) systemic conditions that are known to cause dementia
   (3) substance-induced conditions

E. The deficits do not occur exclusively during the course of delirium

F. The disturbance is not better accounted for by another Axis I disorder

Adapted with permission from DSM–IV. Copyright 1994 American Psychiatric Association.

---

accuracy of the clinical diagnosis is high if a careful history and examination as well as strict diagnostic criteria are used, such as the 'gold standard' of McKhann *et al* (1984).

Three phases in Alzheimer's disease have usually been described (Sjogren, 1952; Lishman, 1987), although a variable pattern is common. In the earliest stages the patient complains of forgetfulness and difficulty in naming and word-finding. This may be accompanied by disorders of visuospatial skills, particularly evident if the patient uses these skills for his or her profession (e.g. technical drawing). Such features may commonly be accompanied by some degree of depression in reaction to the cognitive impairment or some considerable degree of performance anxiety, or both.

In the second stage, these impairments become more severe and are accompanied by other 'focal' features such as apraxia, agnosia, comprehension difficulties, and a failure in mental calculation. There may be personality changes or the development of psychotic, particularly paranoid, symptoms, or both.

In the terminal stages, the disorder is characterised by the patient becoming mute, stuporose, wasted and incontinent, leading eventually to death. The loss of the sense of personal identity occurs in the later stages of the disorder.

In terms of the memory concepts outlined in Box 22.1, neuropsychological studies have demonstrated deficits in both working memory and secondary memory. The working memory deficit is particularly characterised by what Baddeley (1990) termed a "dysexecutive syndrome", involving difficulty monitoring incoming information when there are two or more tasks in hand. The secondary memory deficit involves the characteristic impairment of explicit or episodic memory, and there are both retrograde and anterograde components to this memory loss. There is controversy concerning the extent to which implicit memory is spared in Alzheimer dementia, but there is agreement that semantic memory is more extensively affected than in the amnesic syndrome. Alzheimer patients, however, contrast with patients who have so-called semantic dementia, involving a relatively selective deficit of semantic memory (Hodges *et al*, 1992).

The cardinal neuropathological features of Alzheimer's disease are the presence of neuritic plaques and neurofibrillary tangles at post-mortem or cortical biopsy. Both can occur in normal ageing, but the tangles are most commonly confined to the hippocampi in normal ageing, and become much more widespread and prevalent in dementia. The quantity of plaques and tangles has been shown to relate to ante-mortem measures of the degree of cognitive impairment. In addition, there is granulo-vacuolar degeneration in the hippocampi, aluminium and amyloid deposition, hyaline degeneration, and loss of neurons and synaptic connections, as well as depletion of the acetylcholine, noradrenaline, and serotonin neurotransmitter systems. There is evidence that the reduction in neuronal counts and synaptic connections and/or the degree of cholinergic depletion may be better correlated with measures of ante-mortem cognitive function than are the counts of plaques and tangles. Lewy bodies, which are characteristic of Parkinson's disease, have been described in the cortex of about 20% of cases of Alzheimer's disease.

The aetiology of the disorder remains a topic of intense research interest. Most recently, considerable attention has been addressed to the possible genetic contribution for two reasons. Firstly, there is commonly a family history, especially in younger cases. If a member of the family is affected, the chances of getting the disorder are greater the younger the age of onset in the affected member, and the greater the number of first-degree relatives who have been affected (Heston *et al*, 1981). Secondly, an anomaly of the beta-amyloid gene has been identified on chromosome 21 in cases in whom there was a strong family history. Isoleucine was substituted for valine at codon 717 of the gene for amyloid precursor protein (APP) (Goate *et al*, 1991). Other substitutions in the same codon, together with other mutations in the same region, have also been identified (Harrison, 1991; Mullan, 1992), in all accounting for about 5% of the families.

Two other genes, called the presenilin (PS) genes, have been discovered. Presenilin-1 on chromosome 14 harbours an estimated 70% of the disease-causing mutations, making it the major gene for familial presenile AD. The PS-1 gene (originally S-182) is predicted to be an integral membrane protein with at least seven transmembrane domains. At least 22 missense mutations (e.g. Met 146 Leu) have been found in over 40 chromosome 14 linked families of various ethnic origins (Sherrington *et al*, 1995; Van Broeckhoven, 1995).

A third gene for presenile AD maps to chromosome 1 in the Volga-German AD families, in which AD is the result of a founder effect (Levy-Lehad *et al*, 1995). This gene, called presenilin-2 (PS-2), has been identified and is a minor cause of presenile AD. At least one other genetic locus is suspected for presenile AD.

Linkage studies implicate markers on chromosome 19, coding for poly-morphisms of apolipoprotein E (Rubinsztein, 1995). The possession of the e4 allele of apolipoprotein E (ApoE4) is a major risk factor in the development of late-onset Alzheimer's disease, both sporadic and familial (Strittmatter & Roses, 1995; Rubinsztein, 1995). Population studies suggest a dose–response relationship between the number of e4 alleles and the prevalence of late-onset Alzheimer's disease. Research into putative non-genetic aetiological factors continues nonetheless, including the possible role of toxins such as aluminium, an anomaly of the tau protein, or a 'slow' viral infection.

Hyperphosphorylation of the tau protein, a microtubule stabiliser, results in axonal breakdown and deposition of paired helical filaments (PHF) (Harrington & Wischik, 1994; Trojanowski *et al*, 1994). Severity of cognitive impairment correlates with the deposition of PHF-tau and inversely with the amount of normal, soluble tau in the medial temporal lobes. ApoE3 and E4 may be involved in beta-amyloid deposition and the protection of tau from hyperphosphorylation (Anderton, 1994).

Recently, an animal model of Alzheimer's disease has been developed. Transgenic mice over-expressing human mutant APP progressively develop the pathological hallmarks of Alzheimer's disease, including amyloid deposits, neuritic plaques, synaptic loss, astrocytosis and gliosis with regional specificity resembling that of the human disease. The absence of tangles in these mice suggests a primary role for APP/β-amyloid in the genesis of Alzheimer's disease and could provide a preclinical model for testing therapeutic drugs (Games *et al*, 1995).

Box 22.5 Proposed operational criteria for senile dementia of Lewy-body type (McKeith *et al*, 1992)

1. Fluctuating cognitive impairment affecting both memory and higher cortical functions (such as language, visuospatial ability, praxis or reasoning skills). Fluctuation is marked, with occurrence of both episodic confusion and lucid intervals, as in delirium

2. At least one of the following:
   (i) visual and/or auditory hallucinations, usually accompanied by secondary paranoid delusions
   (ii) mild spontaneous extrapyramidal features or neuroleptic sensitivity syndrome
   (iii) repeated unexplained falls and/or transient clouding or loss of consciousness

3. Despite the fluctuating pattern the clinical features persist over a long period of time (weeks or months). The illness progresses, often rapidly, to an end stage of severe dementia

4. Exclusion of any underlying physical illness adequate to account for the fluctuating cognitive state

5. Exclusion of past history of confirmed stroke and/or evidence of cerebral ischaemic damage by brain-imaging

---

The rate of progress of the disorder is very variable. Once a patient has been admitted, the life expectancy is usually less than two years (Roth, 1955; Blessed & Wilson, 1982), but the time taken to reach this point may vary from approximately two years to over ten. Cases in whom there is a significant degree of language impairment at an early stage usually show faster deterioration than those who do not, and some studies indicate that cases with a younger age of onset deteriorate more quickly.

The depletions of the various neurotransmitters have given rise to particular interest because of the implications that they have for replacement therapy. Cholinergic depletion has been found to be the most consistent and severe loss in Alzheimer's disease, and it is known that cholinergic-blocking drugs impair memory in healthy subjects (Rosser *et al*, 1984; Kopelman & Corn, 1988). Various attempts have been made to replace acetylcholine by administering cholinergic precursors, choline, or anticholinesterases to Alzheimer patients. Although some success has been claimed, the results indicate no more than fairly minimal degrees of improvement for a variable length of time in a proportion of patients (Eagger *et al*, 1991, 1994), before relentless deterioration.

Senile dementia of Lewy-body type

Lewy bodies (LBs) are hyaline, eosinophilic intraneuronal inclusion bodies which are characteristically found in the substantia nigra of patients with Parkinson's disease. They are also found in the cerebral cortex of patients with dementia. It is unclear whether the combination of dementia and cortical LBs represents a distinct clinicopathological entity, a variant of Parkinson's disease, or a variant of Alzheimer's disease. This uncertainty is reflected in the variety of terms used to describe cases, which are characterised by LBs and variously by dementia, Parkinsonism, hallucinations, confusional states, neuroleptic sensitivity and unexplained falls, and a fluctuating course (McKeith *et al*, 1992; Förstl *et al*, 1993). Operational criteria for the diagnosis of LB dementia have been proposed (Box 22.5); diagnostic confusion could occur with vascular dementia or delirium secondary to other causes.

Hospital autopsy series suggest that LB dementia may account for up to 20% of dementia presentations in the elderly. About 12% of Alzheimer patients may reveal LBs at autopsy. They are more likely than Alzheimer patients to exhibit Parkinsonian features, frontal cerebral atrophy, and loss of neurons in the basal nucleus of Meynert and the substantia nigra (Förstl *et al*, 1993). The apolipoprotein E4 genotype may be associated with LB dementia.

Vascular dementia

At the turn of the century, arteriosclerosis was regarded as the major cause of senile dementia. The concept of arteriosclerotic dementia fell into disuse, however, when cerebral blood flow studies showed that cerebrovascular disease resulted in focal areas of cortical infarction, rather than a diffuse strangulating reduction in cerebral blood flow. Tomlinson *et al* (1970) demonstrated that at least 50–100 ml of brain tissue had to be infarcted before vascular dementia occurred. As a result, vascular disease came to be regarded as a rare cause of dementia.

The advent of CT and MRI scanning has, however, revealed an increasing frequency of ischaemic abnormalities in the deep white matter of patients with dementia, demonstrating that much smaller volumes of ischaemic damage may cause dementia, and reviving interest in subcortical arteriosclerosis as an important cause of vascular dementia.

The principal ICD–10 categories of vascular dementia will be described.

Vascular dementia of acute onset usually follows a succession of strokes or a single large infarction.

Multi-infarct dementia (MID) is characterised by abrupt episodes of hemiparesis, sensory changes, dysphasia and focal syndromes from strokes, with a fluctuating course and a *stepwise* deterioration in intellectual functioning. Nocturnal confusion, relative preservation of personality, emotional lability, somatic complaints and depression are more common in MID, but not diagnostic. Focal neurological signs and symptoms are present, including pseudobulbar palsy (with dysarthria, dysphagia and emotional incontinence), ataxia and small-stepped gait, usually associated with hypertension. An acute onset with stepwise deteriorating course and a 'patchy' distribution of deficits distinguishes MID from other dementias. The Hachinski *et al* (1975) ischaemia index has been widely used to distinguish MID and Alzheimer's disease, which may overlap in 20% of patients. The most discriminating clinical variables (stepwise deterioration, evidence of cerebrovascular disease and focal neurology) are enshrined in DSM–IV diagnostic criteria and the revised ischaemia score of Ettlin *et al* (1989) for vascular dementia.

Many cases of MID result from multiple widespread cerebral emboli from the heart or extra-cranial arteries.

Subcortical vascular dementia has a complex pathogenesis, which depends on the combination and siting of lacunar infarcts with more diffuse subcortical arteriosclerotic ischaemia of deep white matter. The cerebral cortex is usually preserved and this contrasts with the clinical picture, which may closely resemble Alzheimer's disease. The *lacunar state* follows the rupture of hypertensive micro-aneurysms or is secondary to other widespread vascular disease.

Binswanger's disease is a slowly progressive dementia associated with subacute progression of focal neurological deficits in chronically hypertensive patients. The clinical signs include a small-stepped wide-based gait, pseudobulbar palsy, pyramidal and Parkinsonian signs, incontinence, and fluctuating mental changes (poor concentration and memory, abulia, bradyphrenia and emotional lability). Deep white matter demyelination and loss results from diffuse ischaemic damage, with hydrocephalus "ex vacuo". Lacunar infarcts are frequently present. Diffuse or patchy white matter translucencies (*leukoaraiosis*) in periventricular regions on the CT or MRI scan reflect demyelination of presumed ischaemic origin.

Subcortical white matter ischaemia may be a more important cause of vascular dementia than multiple cortical infarcts. In patients thought to have MID clinically, leukoaraiosis is found in at least three-quarters, and in at least a fifth of cases leukoaraiosis is found on CT without evidence of cortical infarction (Brown, 1993).

Huntington's disease

An autosomal dominant disorder of choreiform movements and subcortical dementia, Huntington's disease (HD) has a prevalence of about 4–9 cases per 100 000 in the UK (Quarrell *et al*, 1988). The onset is insidious, with a mean age between 35 and 44 years; however, 4% begin under 20 years of age (juvenile form) and 7–11% appear after the age of 60. The interval between onset and diagnosis is about eight years; the average duration is 13–16 years, with wide variation. Some patients survive for up to 30 years (Martin & Gusella, 1986; Harper, 1991; Watt & Seller, 1993).

Two-thirds of living HD patients present with chorea and a third with mental changes (Walker *et al*, 1981). Chorea consists of muscle jerks randomly distributed in space and time, brief in duration and unpredictable in appearance. Chorea is part of a wider motor disturbance in HD, which frequently includes dystonia, rigidity, bradykinesia, and decreased voluntary movement. It is these other movement disorders that compromise function most. Eye movements are also abnormal. Dysarthria and dysphagia worsen as the disease progresses. Less common, except in juvenile HD, are cerebellar dysfunction, upper motor neurone signs, epilepsy and myoclonus. Chorea usually involves all body parts, unlike tardive dyskinesia. Its severity may vary from restlessness with mild, intermittent exaggeration of gesture and expression, fidgetiness of the hands and unstable, dance-like gait, to a continuous flow of disabling, violent movements (Lakke, 1981). Chorea increases progressively early on, later tending to plateau, in contrast to the continued progression of the other motor features. Late-onset cases commonly present with chorea and few other features of HD.

Folstein (1989) and Watt & Seller (1993) used standardised diagnostic criteria to establish a prevalence of psychiatric disorder in HD of 66–73%. There were five main psychiatric syndromes: behaviour and personality disorder (irritability, violence, suspicion, apathy) which often appears first (40% of patients), major affective disorder (41%: 32% depressive, 9% bipolar), minor depression, dementia, and conduct disorder in the offspring of affected families. All but the last are genetically linked. Paranoid and schizophreniform psychoses occurred in up to 12% of patients, and suicide in 8%. Familial association of affective disorder was found in some HD families. Minor depression and behaviour disorder were associated with the onset of physical signs of HD, while major affective disorder and schizophrenia were not (Watt & Seller, 1993).

Initial misdiagnosis of HD is common; psychiatric misdiagnosis is commoner than neurological, especially for schizophrenia or paranoid psychosis where the chorea may be ascribed to fidgetiness, "mannerisms" or drug side-effects. Conversely, up to 15% of patients notified as HD prove to have other neurological diagnoses, including Parkinsonism, tardive dyskinesia and Alzheimer's disease (Folstein, 1989).

The subcortical dementia has an insidious onset, with apathy and inefficiency in everyday life. Intellectual abnormalities include impaired concentration, conceptual tracking, organisation of thought and visuo-spatial skills, including map-reading (Cummings, 1986). Memory loss is usually mild to moderate, with impaired new learning and only a mild degree of retrograde amnesia. Judgement is often severely impaired, but insight is commonly retained until late. Aphasia may occur (Gordon & Illes, 1987), but apraxia and agnosia are notably absent, in striking contrast to Alzheimer's and other cortical diseases.

Social effects

The slow progression of motor symptoms, prominent dementia and psychiatric complications produce an immense burden on the family. The effects of HD include lower social class, poor educational attainment, difficulty in holding down employment for more than five years after onset, and loss of independence (Tyler, 1991). The distress suffered by the patient arises from the disease state itself, from the implications for children, and from previously observing the experiences of HD sufferers.

Families are often disorganised with personality disorders, alcoholism, depression, violence, marital breakdown, suicide, criminality and sexual disturbance. Carers are stressed in proportion to the rate of adversive behaviour of HD patients, who often refuse external help. The extended family may shun the branch with an affected member, keeping the disease 'secret'.

The experience of being at an initial 50% risk of HD breeds anxiety, insecurity, symptom-searching, denial and survivor guilt, with a history of depression in 35% (Watt & Seller, 1993); but most people at risk come to terms with their status and achieve a reasonable quality of life (Folstein, 1989).

Aetiology

HD shows genetic linkage to the G8 marker, localising the gene to the short arm of chromosome 4 (Gusella *et al*, 1983). Recently the gene has been identified (IT15). It contains an excessive (usually above 40) and unstable number of trinucleotide or triplet (CAG) repeats at one end (Huntington's Disease Colloborative Research Group, 1993). Its predicted product, which does not resemble any known protein, is termed 'Huntingtin'. The length of the trinucleotide repeat and the age of onset are inversely correlated, regardless of the sex of the transmitting parent (Snell *et al*, 1993). Affected children of affected fathers have an age of onset 8–10 years earlier than their fathers, while those of affected mothers have an age of onset similar to their mothers. Patients with disease of paternal origin have more triplet repeats in the gene than those whose disease has been maternally transmitted (Snell *et al*, 1993). These observations provide a molecular substrate for genetic 'anticipation' (Ross *et al*, 1993). The clinical consequences of isolating the gene for HD are discussed by Harper (1993*a*).

Pathology

The key lesions are progressive atrophy of the caudate nuclei (evident on CT brain scan) and putamen with spiny cell loss and astrocytic proliferation. Ventricular dilation and cerebral atrophy occur, both maximally affecting the frontal areas. Reduced levels of gamma aminobutyric acid (GABA) in the striatal projection pathways in the basal ganglia and substantia nigra (but not frontal cortex) are found in HD patients (DiFiglio, 1990). Because GABA is known to inhibit dopamine release, excessive dopamine may be released from an intact nigrostriatal system on to a reduced population of striatal neurons, resulting in motor disinhibition, which provokes chorea (Quarrell, 1991). Levels of met-enkephalin, substance P, cholecystokinin and choline acetyltransferase are also reduced. In early HD, loss of inhibitory GABA and met-enkephalin striatal fibres to the lateral globus pallidus may increase inhibition of the subthalamic nucleus, which in turn results in disinhibition of thalamo-cortical fibres, causing chorea (Albin *et al*, 1989). Excitotoxic amino acid neurotoxicity has been more recently implicated (DiFiglio, 1990).

Management

The aims of management are to preserve the patient's mobility and independence; to treat concurrent medical illness; and to provide long-term support for the families and primary carers.

Drugs play a small part in the overall management of the patient. Chorea may be controlled initially with neuroleptic drugs, such as haloperidol in doses of no more than 10 mg/day (Barr *et al*, 1988) or tetrabenazine, but these may make the patient functionally worse. Benzodiazepines may help. The use of other drugs is reviewed by Morris & Tyler (1991).

HD patients have special care needs, for they are not demented like Alzheimer's disease patients. They may have preserved insight and memory until the end, hidden behind grotesque chorea. Day care and specialised residential accommodation may be needed. Hospital care lasts on average 4–7 years to death (Simpson & Johnston, 1989; Tyler, 1991).

Genetic counselling is the only method available for curtailing the disease. It aims to reduce the numbers born carrying the HD gene, and does influence couples at risk for HD, who tend to have fewer children after counselling (Harper & Tyler, 1991). The population prevention of HD requires accurate case ascertainment and genetic registers, as well as genetic counselling (European Community Huntington's Disease Collaborative Study Group, 1993). Many attempts have been made to identify carriers; molecular genetics holds most promise (Harper, 1993*b*). Despite the possibility of stigmatisation in employment, insurance and personal relationships, 56–84% of the relatives at 50% risk intend to request predictive testing, but about 40% drop-out during pre-test counselling. About half of those with a positive test result become depressed (Meissen *et al*, 1988; Harper *et al*, 1991).

Creutzfeld-Jakob disease: prion diseases

Creutzfeld-Jakob disease (CJD), along with scrapie in sheep, bovine spongiform encephalopathy ("mad cow disease"), and Kuru and Gerstmann-Straussler syndrome in man, belongs to a group of slow virus dementias or spongiform encephalopathies. All of these are degenerative diseases of the central nervous system (CNS), with long incubation periods. Once manifested, the disease usually progresses swiftly, without remission and uninfluenced by treatment, to death within months. All the diseases are transmissible, including familial cases. The transmissible agent or virus-like particle has characteristics unique to this group of diseases (usually small, very resistant to disinfection and lacking in immune or tissue culture response). It may not contain nucleic acid. This has prompted the name *prion* (proteinaceous infectious particle) (Prusiner, 1982).

The pathology of CJD includes neuronal degeneration with astrocytic glial proliferation and status spongiosus (spongy appearance of the grey matter). The cortex is almost always involved, with additional variable involvement of the basal ganglia, thalamus, cerebellum, brain stem and spinal cord. This has given rise to subvarieties of CJD and diverse clinical features. The onset is usually between 40 and 60 years of age, affecting men and women equally. CJD presents with early neurotic or psychotic changes or neurological signs, or both, and progresses rapidly to a dementia, with spasticity, ataxia, extrapyramidal signs, muscle atrophy and seizures. Myoclonic jerks frequently occur.

The cerebrospinal fluid is usually normal. The CT brain scan usually reveals a minor degree of atrophy, but can be normal. The EEG shows characteristic triphasic sharp wave complexes, which are periodic in the late stages.

CJD occurs sporadically, but 5–15% of cases have an autosomal dominant inheritance. A key process in the development of CJD is conversion of prion protein PrPc, a harmless host-encoded glycoprotein normally found in neuronal membranes, to a protease-resistant form (scrapie prion protein, PrPsc). Conversion occurs either by direct interaction of PrPc with PrPsc or, in the case of sporadic or hereditary spongiform encephalopathies, by a rare event that sparks off the self-replicating, catalytic conversion of PrPc to PrPsc. In prion disease, the infectivity titre cannot increase and the disease cannot progress without the recruitment of host-coded prion protein. Prion theory is reviewed by Prusiner (1992) and Collinge & Palmer (1994).

Dementia of frontal lobe type and Pick's disease

Dementias characterised by specific impairments in frontal and temporal lobe functions, frontotemporal dementia or dementia of frontal lobe type (DFT), have now been recognised (Neary *et al*, 1994). In the Lund study of 158 cases of dementia investigated clinically and neuropathologically, 10% received the pathological diagnoses of DFT, 2.5% of Pick's disease, while a further 3.8% of cases had Alzheimer's and other diseases with predominant frontal lobe involvement (Brun, 1987; Gustafson, 1987). Neary *et al* (1988) found that 19% of dementia patients met clinical criteria for DFT.

In the Lund series, DFT and Pick's disease had similar average ages of onset (53–56 years) and slowly progressive courses with average survivals of 8 years and 11 years respectively, each with a wide range. The estimated heritability for each illness was 50%.

The onset of each disorder is insidious, with personality change (loss of judgement, personal and social awareness, lability, inappropriate jocularity), disinhibition, social misconduct, lack of insight followed by apathy, stereotypy and echopraxia. Less common features are rigidity in daily routine, persistent pain and features of the Kluver-Bucy syndrome. Speech invariably reveals poor verbal fluency, limited output, echolalia and eventual mutism. Memory loss is variable and less severe than in Alzheimer's disease (Baldwin & Förstl, 1993).

Frontotemporal or frontal atrophy on CT, in the presence of the characteristic clinical features, supports a diagnosis that can only be confirmed at autopsy. The EEG is normal. SPET scans show selective reduction of emission from the frontal lobes (Neary *et al*, 1988).

The characteristic neuropathology of Pick's disease includes balloon cells (neurons) with argentophilic intraneuronal inclusions (Pick bodies) and eosinophilic inclusions (Hirano bodies), but not in all cases. DFT shows neither change, but only non-specific degeneration of the grey matter. Both disorders reveal neuronal and myelin loss, and astrocytic gliosis in the cortex and white matter. Plaques and tangles are conspicuously absent. At autopsy or cortical biopsy, some DFT cases will reveal spongiform encephalopathy, and others Lewy-body dementia and Alzheimer's disease.

DFT may be linked to Diogenes syndrome, a disorder presenting with senile self-neglect, often in the absence of obvious psychiatric illness or intellectual decline, and formerly viewed as the end-stage of a personality disorder (Orrell & Sahakian, 1991; see also page 769).

Tumours and mass lesions

Brain tumours may present with dementia, particularly slowly-growing deep midline tumours or tumours of the corpus callosum or frontal lobes.

Frontal meningiomas are important to detect as they are benign and potentially curable. Chronic subdural haematoma is another treatable cause of dementia, in which the head injury may have been remote, mild or forgotten. Hydrocephalus is usually due to tumours, particularly in the posterior fossa, obstructing the cerebral aqueduct and thereby cerebrospinal fluid (CSF) flow. Features of raised intracranial pressure (such as headaches and papilloedema) and non-cognitive focal signs may be absent. Colloid cysts of the third ventricle, pineal masses and parapituitary tumours may present with dementia only. Most causes of dementia due to mass lesions or raised intracranial pressure are easily diagnosed from the MRI or CT scan.

In *communicating hydrocephalus*, the block is not within the ventricular system but in the subarachnoid space, usually around the basal cisterns. Patients present with subacute progressive dementia, which is treatable. A history of headache, ataxia and gait disturbance is usual, but signs of raised intracranial pressure may be absent. The combination of dementia, urinary incontinence and gait disorder in the absence of routine evidence of raised intracranial pressure suggests the syndrome of *normal pressure hydrocephalus*, which may respond to ventricular drainage. The condition may develop many years after meningitis, severe head injury with bleeding, or subarachnoid haemorrhage.

Pseudodementia

This term describes a syndrome of disordered intellectual function, which mimics dementia, that can occur in patients with primary psychiatric illness. The interactions of depression and dementia were reviewed by Mahendra (1985), who argued that the concept of pseudodementia is no longer logically sustainable. In recovered depressive patients without initial dementia, a third suffer persistent cognitive impairment and 12–79% subsequently develop degenerative dementia over 2–18 years, suggesting that the term 'pseudodementia' is unclear and misleading (Bulbena & Berrios, 1986; Emery & Oxman, 1992; Rabins & Pearlson, 1994). 'Dementia syndrome of depression' and 'depression-induced cognitive impairment' are alternative terms.

Pseudodementia accounts for about 9% of patients under the age of 65 referred to neurologists for suspected dementia (Marsden, 1985). The commonest cause is depression, particularly in the elderly (Kiloh, 1961), but depressed mood may not be evident. The clinical picture may resemble Alzheimer's disease.

The distinction may be difficult, but the correct diagnosis of depression is often suggested by a history of acute onset with the absence of memory loss or intellectual decline before the onset of depressive symptoms; and by the presence of depressed mood during admission, a history of previous affective disorder and abnormal premorbid personality (Ron *et al*, 1979).

Depressed patients often complain about their cognitive difficulties much more than seems justified by their performance on intellectual tests. In contrast, the truly demented patient rarely complains appropriately, and his affect is labile and shallow. The depressed patient is often inconsistent during the history-taking, and often answers "Don't know" to questions rather than being wrong, or even fails to attempt an answer (Wells, 1979).

Variability in performance during testing, particularly improvement with encouragement, is characteristic, especially on tasks of similar difficulty. Memory loss for recent and remote events may be equally severe, and gaps for specific periods or events are common. In contrast, the organic patient provides near-miss or confabulatory answers to questions or furnishes facile excuses for his failure; produces a consistently poor performance on tests; and usually shows relative sparing of early memories. Physical investigations are generally unhelpful in the distinction of depression and dementia, but neuropsychological tests may be helpful. Caine (1981) found that attention, detail analysis, spontaneous elaboration and speed of mental processing were specifically impaired in depressive pseudodementia. Cognitive impairment was reported in 70% of elderly depressives, particularly in memory and latency of response, to a degree comparable to Alzheimer's disease, but with a different pattern of errors (Abas *et al*, 1990). Confirmation of diagnosis follows improvement in intellectual functioning with antidepressant therapy.

Diagnosis is more difficult when depressive illness complicates dementia. At least one depressive symptom is found in almost two-thirds of Alzheimer patients, of whom a quarter are rated as clinically depressed (Burns *et al*, 1990). Even when depression is treated, cognitive impairment may remain (Abas *et al*, 1990).

The other main varieties of pseudodementia, including the Ganser syndrome, hysterical pseudodementia and simulated dementia, are discussed on page 691.

Investigations

The age, history, and clinical findings dictate the selection of tests for dementia. Investigations essential in all patients are aimed at excluding reversible causes of dementia. These include: a full blood count and film; ESR; blood sugar; thyroid, liver and renal function tests; calcium; serology; vitamin B12 and folate; chest and skull x-rays; CT or MRI brain scans; ECG and EEG; and neuropsychological testing.

In selected patients, further investigations will be required: CSF examination for cells, protein and oligoclonal bands, HIV antibodies, infectious diseases screen, autoantibodies and immunoglobins, serum copper and caeruloplasmin, jejunal biopsy (Whipple's disease), drug and toxin screen, cerebral angiography and blood flow studies. Brain biopsy and metabolic screening are rarely required. Ideally, every patient with dementia should have a CT or MRI scan to exclude treatable intracranial pathology (focal lesions and hydrocephalus), but scanning is less likely to influence management in the elderly patient with a history of degenerative dementia.

References

Abas, M. A., Sahakian, B. J. & Levy, R. (1990) Neuropsychological deficits and CT scan changes in elderly depressives. *Psychological Medicine*, **20**, 507–520.

Absher, J. R. & Cummings, J. L. (1994) Cognitive and noncognitive aspects of dementia syndromes: an overview. In *Dementia* (eds A. Burns & R. Levy), pp. 59–76. London: Chapman & Hall.

Albin, R. L., Young, A. B. & Penny, J. B. (1989) The functional anatomy of basal ganglia disorders. *Trends in Neurosciences*, **12**, 366–375.

Altshuler, L. L., Cummings, J. L. & Mills, M. J. (1986) Mutism: review, differential diagnosis, and report of 22 cases. *American Journal of Psychiatry*, **143**, 1409–1414.

Alzheimer, A. (1907) Uber eine eigenartige, Erkrankung der Hirnrinde. *Allg. Z. Psychiat. Psych-Gerichtl*, ixiv, 146–148. Translated by Jarvik, L. & Greenson, H. (1987) About a peculiar disease of the cerebral cortex. *Alzheimer Disease and Associated Disorders*, 7–8.

American Psychiatric Association (1987) *Diagnostic and Statistical Manual of Mental Disorders* (3rd edn, revised) (DSM–III–R). Washington, DC: APA.

—— (1994) *Diagnostic and Statistical Manual of Mental Disorders* (4th edn) (DSM–IV). Washington, DC: APA.

Anderton, R. (1994) Apolipoprotein E and Alzheimer's disease. *Alzheimer's Review*, **5**, 97–101.

Annett, M. (1970) A classification of hand-preference by association analysis. *British Journal of Psychology*, **61**, 303–321.

Anthony, A. C., LeResche, L., Niaz, U., *et al* (1982) Limits of the 'Mini-Mental State' as a screening test for dementia and delirium among hospital patients. *Psychological Medicine*, **12**, 397–408.

Baddeley, A. D. (1990) *Human Memory: Theory and Practice*. Hillsdale, NJ: Lawrence Erlbaum.

Baldwin, B. & Förstl, H. (1993) Pick's disease – 101 years on. Still there, but in need of reform. *British Journal of Psychiatry*, **163**, 100–104.

Barr, A. N., Fischer, J. H., Koller, W. C., *et al* (1988) Serum haloperidol concentration and choreiform movement in Huntington's disease. *Neurology*, **38**, 84–88.

Benson, D. F. (1979) *Aphasia, Alexia and Agraphia*. Edinburgh: Churchill Livingstone.

Benton, A. L. (1968) Differential behavioural effects in frontal lobe disease. *Neuropsychologia*, **6**, 53–60.

Berlyne, N. (1972) Confabulation. *British Journal of Psychiatry*, **120**, 31–39.

Berrios, G. E. (1981) Delirium and confusion in the 19th century; a conceptual history. *British Journal of Psychiatry*, **139**, 439–449.

Besson, J. A. O. (1994) Magnetic resonance imaging and spectroscopy in dementia. In *Dementia* (eds A. Burns & R. Levy), pp. 427–436. London: Chapman & Hall.

Binnie, C. D. & Prior, P. F. (1994) Electroencephalography. *Journal of Neurology, Neurosurgery and Psychiatry*, **57**, 1308–1391.

Blessed, G., Tomlinson, B. E. & Roth, M. (1968) The association between quantitative measures of dementia and of senile change in the cerebral grey matter of elderly subjects. *British Journal of Psychiatry*, **114**, 797–811.

—— & Wilson, I. D. (1982) The contemporary natural history of mental disorder in old age. *British Journal of Psychiatry*, **141**, 59–67.

Blumer, D. & Benson, D. (1975) Personality changes with frontal and temporal lobe lesions. In *Psychiatric Aspects of Neurologic Disease* (eds D. F. Benson & D. Blumer), pp. 151–170. New York: Grune & Stratton.

Bolla, K. I., Lindgren, K. N., Bonaccorsy, C., *et al* (1991) Memory complaints in older adults – fact or fiction. *Archives of Neurology*, **48**, 61–65.

Bonhoeffer, K. (1909) Exogenous psychoses. In *Themes and Variations in European Psychiatry* (eds S. R. Hirsch & M. Shepherd), pp. 47–52. Bristol: John Wright.

Broca, P (1861) Remarques sur le siege de la faculte du langage articule suivie d'une observation d'aphemie. *Bulletin de la Societe de Anatomy*, **6**, 330.

Brown, M. M. (1993) Vascular dementia. *Alzheimer's Review*, **3**, 57–62.

Brun, A. (1987) Frontal lobe degeneration of non-Alzheimer type. I: Neuropathology. *Archives of Gerontology and Geriatrics*, **6**, 193–208.

Bulbena, A. & Berrios, G. (1986) Pseudodementia: facts and figures. *British Journal of Psychiatry*, **148**, 87–94.

Burns, A., Jacoby, R. & Levy, R. (1990) Psychiatric phenomenology in Alzheimer's disease. *British Journal of Psychiatry*, **157**, 72–94.

——, ——, Philpot, M., *et al* (1991) Computerised tomography in Alzheimer's disease. *British Journal of Psychiatry*, **159**, 609–614.

—— & Levy, R. (1994) *Dementia*. London: Chapman & Hall.

—— & Pearlson, G. (1994) Computed tomography. In *Dementia* (eds A. Burns & R. Levy), pp. 407–426. London: Chapman & Hall.

Caine, E. D. (1981) Pseudo-dementia; current concepts and future directions. *Archives of General Psychiatry*, **38**, 1359–1364.

Collinge, J. & Palmer, M. S. (1994) Prion diseases. In *Dementia* (eds A. Burns & R. Levy), pp. 835–853. London: Chapman & Hall.

Connell, P. H. (1958) *Amphetamine Psychosis*. Maudsley Monograph No. 5. London: Chapman & Hall.

Cooper, B. (1991) The epidemiology of dementia. In *Psychiatry in the Elderly* (eds R. Jacoby & C. Oppenheimer), pp. 574–585. Oxford: Oxford University Press.

Copeland, J. R. M., Davidson, L., Dewey, M. E., *et al* (1992) Alzheimer's disease, other dementias, depression and pseudo-dementia. Incidence and three year outcome in Liverpool. *British Journal of Psychiatry*, **161**, 230–239.

Critchley, M. (1953) *The Parietal Lobes*. London: Edward Arnold.

Crook, T. H., Ferris, S. H., Whitehouse, P., *et al* (1986) Age-associated memory impairment: proposed diagnostic criteria and measures of clinical change. *Developmental Neuropsychology*, **2**, 261–276.

Crum, R. M., Anthony, J. C., Bassett, S. S., *et al* (1993) Population-based norms for the Mini-Mental State Examination by age and educational level. *Journal of the American Medical Association*, **269**, 2386–2391.

Cummings, J. L. (1985) *Clinical Neuropsychiatry*. Orlando: Grune & Stratton.

—— (1986) Sub-cortical dementia: neuropsychology, neuropsychiatry and pathophysiology. *British Journal of Psychiatry*, **149**, 682–697.

— & Benson, D. F. (1992) *Dementia: A Clinical Approach* (2nd edn). London: Butterworth-Heinemann.

Cutting, J. (1987) The phenomenology of acute organic psychosis: comparison with acute schizophrenia. *British Journal of Psychiatry*, **151**, 324–332.

— (1990) *The Right Cerebral Hemisphere and Psychiatric Disorder*. Oxford: Oxford University Press.

Delis, C. C., Massman, P. J., Butters, N., *et al* (1991) Profiles of demented and amnesic patients on the California Verbal Learning Test: implications for the assessment of memory disorders. *Psychological Assessment*, **3**, 19–26.

DiFiglio, M. (1990) Excitotoxic injury of the neostriatum; a model for Huntington's disease. *Trends in Neuroscience*, **13**, 286–289.

Eagger, S. A., Levy, R. & Sahakian, B. J. (1991) Tacrine in Alzheimer's disease. *Lancet*, **337**, 989–992.

—, Richards, M. & Levy, R. (1994) Long-term effects of tacrine in Alzheimer's disease: an open study. *International Journal of Geriatric Psychiatry*, **9**, 643–647.

Ell, P. J. & Costa, D. C. (1992) The role of nuclear medicine in neurology and psychiatry. *Current Opinion in Neurology and Neurosurgery*, **5**, 863–869.

Ellis, A. W. & Young, A. W. (1988) *Human Cognitive Neuropsychology*. Hove: Lawrence Erlbaum.

Ellis, H. D. & Young, A. W. (1990) Accounting for delusional misidentifications. *British Journal of Psychiatry*, **157**, 239–248.

Emery, V. O. & Oxman, T. E. (1992) Update on the dementia spectrum of depression. *American Journal of Psychiatry*, **149**, 305–317.

Engel, G. & Romano, J. (1959) Delirium, a syndrome of cerebral insufficiency. *Journal of Chronic Disease*, **9**, 260–277.

Ettlin, T. M., Staehelin, H. B., Kischka, U., *et al* (1989) Computed tomography, electroencephalography, and clinical features in the differential diagnosis of senile dementia: a prospective clinicopathologic study. *Archives of Neurology*, **46**, 1217–1220.

European Community Huntington's Disease Collaborative Study Group (1993) Ethical and social issues in presymptomatic testing for Huntington's disease. *Journal of Medical Genetics*, **30**, 1028–1034.

Fenton, G. W. (1993) Electroencephalography. In *The Principles and Practice of Geriatric Psychiatry* (eds J. Copeland, D. Blazer & M. Abou-Saleh), pp. 459–466. Chichester: John Wiley.

Feskens, E., Havekes, L., Kalmijn, S., *et al* (1994) Apoloprotein E4 allele and cognitive decline in elderly men. *British Medical Journal*, **309**, 1202–1205.

Folstein, M. F. (1991) Rating scales for use in the elderly. *Current Opinion in Psychiatry*, **4**, 591–595.

—, Folstein, S. E. & McHugh, P. R. (1975). 'Mini-mental state'. A practical method for grading the cognitive state of patients for the clinician. *Journal of Psychiatric Research*, **12**, 189–198.

—, Basset, S. S., Romanoski, A. J., *et al* (1991) The epidemiology of delirium in the community: the Eastern Baltimore Mental Health Survey. *International Psychogeriatics*, **3**, 169–176.

Folstein, S. (1989) *Huntington's Disease: A Disorder of Families*. Baltimore: John Hopkins Press.

Förstl, H., Burns, A., Luthert, P., *et al* (1993) The Lewy-body variant of Alzheimer's disease: clinical and pathological findings. *British Journal of Psychiatry*, **162**, 385–392.

— & Hentschel, F. (1994) Contribution to the differential diagnosis of dementias: neuroimaging. In *Reviews in Clinical Gerontology* (ed. R. C. Baldwin), pp. 56–80. London: Edward Arnold.

Freud, S. (1891) *Zur Aufassung der Aphasien*. Wien: Deuticke.

Gall, F. & Spurzheim, G. (1809) Research on the nervous system in general and on that of the brain in particular. [Reprinted in K. Pribram (1969) *Brain and Behaviour (vol 1)*. *Mood States and Mind*. Harmondsworth: Penguin.]

Games, D., Adams, D., Alessandri, R., *et al* (1995) Alzheimer-type neuropathology in transgenic mice over-expressing V717F b-amyloid precursor protein. *Nature*, **373**, 523–527.

Geaney, D. P. (1994) Single photon emission tomography. In *Dementia* (eds A. Burns & R. Levy), pp. 437–456. London: Chapman & Hall.

Geschwind, N. (1965) Disconnection syndromes in animals and man. *Brain*, **88**, 585–644.

Goate, A., Chartier-Harlin, M. C., Mullan, M., *et al* (1991) Segregation of a missense mutation in the amyloid precursor protein gene with familial Alzheimer's disease. *Nature*, **349**, 704–706.

Gordon, W. P. & Illes, J. (1987) Neurolinguistic characteristics of language production in Huntington's disease: a preliminary report. *Brain and Language*, **31**, 1–10.

Gusella, J. F., Wexler, N. S., Conneally, P. M., *et al* (1983) A polymorphic DNA marker genetically linked to Huntington's disease. *Nature*, **306**, 234–239.

Gustafson, L. (1987) Frontal lobe degeneration of non-Alzheimer type: II. Clinical picture and different diagnosis. *Archives of Gerontology and Geriatrics*, **6**, 209–223.

Hachinski, V. C., Iliff, L. D., Zilhka, E., *et al* (1975) Cerebral blood flow in dementia. *Archives of Neurology*, **32**, 632–637.

Harper, P. S. (1991) The natural history of Huntington's disease. In *Huntington's Disease* (ed. P. S. Harper), pp. 127–139. London: W. B. Saunders.

— (1993a) Clinical consequences of isolating the gene for Huntington's disease. *British Medical Journal*, **307**, 397–398.

— (1993b) A specific mutation for Huntington's disease. *Journal of Medical Genetics*, **30**, 975–977.

— & Tyler, A. (1991) Genetic counselling in Huntington's disease. In *Huntington's Disease* (ed. P. S. Harper), pp. 337–371. London: W. B. Saunders.

—, Morris, M. & Tyler, A. (1991) Predictive tests in Huntington's disease. In *Huntington's Disease* (ed. P. S. Harper), pp. 373–413. London: W. B. Saunders.

Harrington, C. R. & Wischik, C. (1994) Molecular pathobiology of Alzheimer's disease. In *Dementia* (eds A. Burns & R. Levy), pp. 209–238. London: Chapman & Hall Medical.

Harrison, P. J. (1991) Alzheimer's disease and the b-amyloid gene. *British Medical Journal*, **302**, 1478–1479.

Harvey, I., Ron, M. A., du Boulay, G., *et al* (1993) Reduction of cortical volume in schizophrenia on magnetic resonance imaging. *Psychological Medicine*, **23**, 591–604.

Heilman, K. M. & Rothi, L. J. (1985) Apraxia. In *Clinical Neuropsychology* (eds K. M. Heilman & E. Valenstein), pp. 131–150. Oxford: Oxford University Press.

Henderson, A. S. (1986) The epidemiology of Alzheimer's disease. *British Medical Bulletin*, **42**, 3–10.

— (1994) Early detection. In *Principles and Practice of Geriatric Psychiatry* (eds J. R. M. Copeland, M. T. Abou-Saleh & D. G. Blazer), pp. 267–271. Chichester: John Wiley.

Heston, L. L., Mastri, A. R., Anderson, E., *et al* (1981) Dementia of the Alzheimer type: clinical genetics, natural history, and associated conditions. *Archives of General Psychiatry*, **38**, 1085–1090.

Hodges, J. R. (1994) *Cognitive Assessment for Clinicians*. Oxford: Oxford University Press.

—, Patterson, K., Oxbury, S., *et al* (1992) Semantic dementia. Progressive fluent aphasia with temporal lobe atrophy. *Brain*, **115**, 1783–1806.

Hope, T. & Fairburn, C. (1992) The present behavioural examination (PBE): the development of an interview to measure current behavioural abnormalities. *Psychological Medicine*, **22**, 223–230.

Howard, D., Patterson, K., Wise, R., *et al* (1992) The cortical localisation of the lexicons. Positron emission tomography evidence. *Brain*, **113**, 1768–1782.

Hughlings Jackson, J. (1875) On the scientific and empirical investigation of epilepsies. In *Selected Writings of John Hughlings Jackson*, pp. 162–273. London: Hodder & Stoughton.

Humphreys, G. & Riddoch, M. J. (1987) *To See But Not to See: A Case Study of Visual Agnosia*. Hove: Lawrence Erlbaum.

Huntington's Disease Collaborative Research Group (1993) A novel gene containing a trinucleotide repeat that is expanded and unstable on Huntington's disease chromosomes. *Cell*, **72**, 971–983.

Institute of Psychiatry (1987) *Psychiatric Examination. Notes on Eliciting and Recording Clinical Information in Psychiatric Patients* (2nd edn). Oxford: Oxford University Press.

Jacobson, R. R. (1995) The post-concussional syndrome: Physiogenesis, psychogenesis and malingering: An integrative model. *Journal of Psychosomatic Medicine*, **39**, 675–693.

—, Acker, C. F. & Lishman, W. A. (1990) Patterns of neuropsychological deficit in alcoholic Korsakoff's syndrome. *Psychological Medicine*, **20**, 321–334.

Jacoby, R. J. & Levy, R. (1980) Computed tomography in the elderly: 2. Senile dementia: diagnosis and functional impairment. *British Journal of Psychiatry*, **136**, 256–269.

—, — & Dawson, J. M. (1980) Computed tomography in the elderly: 1. The normal population. *British Journal of Psychiatry*, **136**, 249–255.

Jorm, A. F., Korten, A. E. & Henderson, A. S. (1987) The prevalence of dementia: a quantitative integration of the literature. *Acta Psychiatrica Scandinavica*, **76**, 465–479.

Joyston-Bechal, M. P. (1966) The clinical features and outcome of stupor. *British Journal of Psychiatry*, **112**, 967–981.

Kapur, N. & Coughlan, A. K. (1980) Confabulation and frontal lobe dysfunction. *Journal of Neurology, Neurosurgery and Psychiatry*, **43**, 461–463.

Kennedy, A. M. & Frackowiak, R. S. J. (1994) Positron emission tomography. In *Dementia* (eds A. Burns & R. Levy), pp. 457–474. London: Chapman & Hall.

Kesslak, J. P., Nalcioglu, O. & Cotman, C. W. (1991) Quantification of magnetic resonance scans for hippocampal and parahippocampal atrophy in Alzheimer's disease. *Neurology*, **41**, 51–54.

Kiloh, L. G. (1961) Pseudo-dementia. *Acta Psychiatrica Scandinavica*, **37**, 336–351.

Kirk, A. & Kertesz, A. (1991) On drawing impairment in Alzheimer's disease. *Archives of Neurology*, **48**, 73–77.

Kluger, A., Reisberg, B. & Ferris, S. H. (1994) Rating scales. In *Dementia* (eds A. Burns & R. Levy), pp. 355–378. London: Chapman & Hall.

Kopelman, M. D. (1982) Speech dominance, handedness and electro-convulsions. *Psychological Medicine*, **12**, 667–670.

—— (1987) Two types of confabulation. *Journal of Neurology, Neurosurgery and Psychiatry*, **50**, 1482–1487.

—— (1991) Frontal dysfunction and memory deficits in the alcoholic Korsakoff syndrome and Alzheimer-type dementia. *Brain*, **114**, 117–137.

—— (1994) Structured psychiatric interview: assessment of the cognitive state. *British Journal of Hospital Medicine*, **52**, 277–281.

—— (1995) The Korsakoff syndrome. *British Journal of Psychiatry*, **166**, 154–173.

—— & Corn, T. H. (1988) Cholinergic "blockade" as a model for cholinergic depletion: a comparison of the memory deficits with those of Alzheimer-type dementia and the alcoholic Korsakoff syndrome. *Brain*, **111**, 1079–1110.

——, Wilson, B. A. & Baddeley, A. D. (1990) *The Autobiographical Memory Interview*. Bury St Edmunds: Thames Valley Test Company.

Korsakoff, S. S. (1889) Psychic disorder in conjunction with peripheral neuritis (transl. by M. Victor & P. I. Yakovlev, 1955). *Neurology*, **5**, 394–406.

Kral, V. A. (1962) Senescent forgetfulness: benign and malignant. *Canadian Medical Association Journal*, **86**, 257–260.

Lakke, P. W. F. (1981) Classification of extrapyramidal disorders. Proposal for an international classification and glossary of terms. *Journal of Neurological Sciences*, **51**, 313–327.

Lashley, K. (1929) *Brain Mechanisms and Intelligence*. Chicago: University of Chicago Press.

Landis, T., Cummings, J. L., Benson, F., *et al* (1986) Loss of topographical familiarity: an environmental agnosia. *Archives of Neurology*, **43**, 132–136.

Levy-Lehad, E., Wijsman, E. M., Nemens, E., *et al* (1995) A familial Alzheimer's disease locus on chromosome 1. *Science*, **269**, 970–973.

Lewis, S. W. (1990) Computerised tomography. *British Journal of Psychiatry*, **157** (suppl. 9), 16–24.

Lezak, M. D. (1995) *Neuropsychological Assessment* (3rd edn). Oxford: Oxford University Press.

Liepmann, H. (1900) Das Krankheitsbild der Apraxie (motorische Asymbolie). *Monatsschrift fur Psychiatrie und Neurologie*, **8**, 15–44.

Lilly, R., Cummings, J. L., Benson, F., *et al* (1983) The human Kluver-Bucy syndrome. *Neurology*, **33**, 1141–1145.

Lindesay, J., MacDonald, A. & Starke, I. (1990) *Delirium in the Elderly*. Oxford: Oxford University Press.

Lipowski, Z. J. (1983) Transient cognitive disorders (delirium, acute confusional states) in the elderly. *American Journal of Psychiatry*, **140**, 1426–1436.

—— (1990) *Delirium: Acute Brain Failure in Man*. Springfield, IL: Charles C. Thomas.

Lishman, W. A. (1987) *Organic Psychiatry: The Psychological Consequences of Cerebral Disorder* (2nd edn). Oxford: Blackwell Scientific.

—— & McMeekan, E. R. L. (1976) Hand preference patterns in psychiatric patients. *British Journal of Psychiatry*, **129**, 158–166.

Lissauer, H. (1890) Ein fall von Seelenblindheit nebst einem Beitrag zur Theorie derselben. *Archiv fur Psychologie*, 21, 222–270.

Liu, H. C., Chou, P., Lin, K. N., *et al* (1994) Assessing cognitive abilities and dementia in a predominantly illiterate population of older individuals in Kinmen. *Psychological Medicine*, 24, 763–770.

Livingston, G. (1994) The scale of the problem. In *Dementia* (eds A. Burns & R. Levy), pp. 21–35. London: Chapman & Hall.

Luria, A. R. (1947) *Traumatic Aphasia* (transl. 1970). The Hague: Mounton Press.

—— (1966) *Higher Cortical Functions in Man*. London: Tavistock.

McCarthy, R. A. & Warrington, E. K. (1990) *Cognitive Neuropsychology: A Clinical Introduction*. London: Academic Press.

McKeith, I. G., Perry, R. P., Fairbank, A. F., *et al* (1992) Operational criteria for senile dementia of Lewy body type (SDLT). *Psychological Medicine*, 22, 911–922.

McKenna, P. & Warrington, E. K. (1983) *The Graded Naming Test*. Windsor: Nelson.

McKhann, G., Drachman, D., Folstein, M., *et al* (1984) Clinical diagnosis of Alzheimer's disease: report on the NINCDS-ADRDA work group under the auspices of the Dept. of Health and Human Services Task Force on Alzheimer's Disease. *Neurology*, 34, 939–944.

McManus, I. C. (1985) Handedness, language dominance and aphasia: a genetic model. *Psychological Medicine*, Monograph Supplement 8.

Mahendra, B. (1985) Depression and dementia: the multi-faceted relationship. *Psychological Medicine*, 15, 227–236.

Mair, W. P. G., Warrington, E. K. & Weiskrantz, L. (1979) Neuropathological and psychological examination of two patients with Korsakoff's psychosis. *Brain*, 102, 749–783.

Marsden, C. D. (1985) Assessment of dementia. In *Handbook of Clinical Neurology (Vol. 2): Neurobehavioural Disorders* (ed. J. A. M. Frederiks), pp. 221–232. Oxford: Elsevier Science.

Martin, J. B. & Gusella, J. F. (1986) Huntington's disease: pathogenesis and management. *New England Journal of Medicine*, 313, 1267–1276.

Master, D. R., Toone, B. K. & Scott, D. F. (1984) Interictal behaviour in temporal lobe epilepsy. In *Advances in Epileptology: XVth Epilepsy International Symposium* (eds R. Porter, A. Ward, R. Mattson, *et al*), pp. 557–565. New York: Raven Press.

Mayes, A. R., Meudell, P. R., Mann, D., *et al* (1988) Location of lesions in Korsakoff's syndrome: neuropsychological and neuropathological data on two patients. *Cortex*, 24, 367–388.

Meissen, G. J., Myers, R. H., Mastromauro, C. A., *et al* (1988) Predictive testing for Huntington's disease with use of a linked DNA marker. *New England Journal of Medicine*, 318, 535–542.

Mesulam, M.-M. (1986) Editorial. Frontal cortex and behaviour. *Annals of Neurology*, 19, 320–325.

Meynert, T. H. (1867) Der Bau der Grosshirnrinde und seine ortlichen Verschiedeheiten. *VJ. Schr. Psychiatrie*, i, 77–93.

Micale, M. S. (1990) Hysteria and historiography; the future perspective. *History of Psychiatry*, 1, 33–124.

Miller, E. (1989) Language impairment in Alzheimer-type dementia. *Clinical Psychology Review*, 9, 181–195.

Milner, B. (1963) Effects of different brain lesions on card sorting. *Archives of Neurology*, **9**, 90–100.

—— (1975) Psychological aspects of focal epilepsy and its neurosurgical management. In *Advances in Neurology*, vol. 8 (eds D. Purpura, J. Penry & R. Walter), pp. 299–321. New York: Raven Press.

Moore, V. & Wyke, M. A. (1984) Drawing disability in patients with senile dementia. *Psychological Medicine*, **14**, 97–105.

Morris, M. & Tyler, A. (1991) Management and therapy. In *Huntington's Disease* (ed. P. S. Harper), pp. 205–249. London: W. B. Saunders.

Morris, R. G. (1991) Cognition and ageing. In *Psychiatry in the Elderly* (eds R. Jacoby & C. Oppenheimer), pp. 58–88. Oxford: Oxford University Press.

—— & McKiernan, F. (1994) Neuropsychological investigations of dementia. In *Dementia* (eds A. Burns & R. Levy), pp. 327–354. London: Chapman & Hall.

Mullan, M. (1992) Familial Alzheimer's disease: second gene locus located. *British Medical Journal*, **305**, 1108–1109.

Neary, D., Snowden, J. S., Northen, B., *et al* (1988) Dementia of frontal lobe type. *Journal of Neurology, Neurosurgery and Psychiatry*, **51**, 353–361.

——, —— & Mann, D. M. A. (1994) Dementia of frontal lobe type. In *Dementia* (eds A. Burns & R. Levy), pp. 815–822. London: Chapman & Hall.

Nelson, H. E. (1982) *The National Adult Reading Test*. Windsor: NFER-Nelson.

—— (1986) A modified card sorting test sensitive to frontal lobe deficits. *Cortex*, **12**, 313–324.

Newcombe, F. (1969) *Missile Wounds of the Brain: A Study of Psychological Deficits*. Oxford: Oxford University Press.

Nott, P. N. & Fleminger, J. J. (1975) Presenile dementia: the difficulties of early diagnosis. *Acta Psychiatrica Scandinavica*, **51**, 210–217.

O'Brien, J. T. & Beats, B. (1994) Benign senescent forgetfulness and age-associated memory impairment. In *Dementia* (eds A. Burns & R. Levy), pp. 295–308. London: Chapman & Hall.

Orrell, M. W. & Sahakian, B. J. (1991) Dementia of frontal lobe type. *Psychological Medicine*, **21**, 553–556.

Patterson, K. (1981) Neuropsychological approaches to the study of reading. *British Journal of Psychology*, **72**, 151–174.

Philpot, M. (1994) The neurophysiology of dementia. In *Dementia* (eds A. Burns & R. Levy), pp. 371–386. London: Chapman & Hall.

Plum, F. & Posner, J. B. (1980) *Diagnosis of Stupor and Coma* (2nd edn). Philadelphia: Davis.

Prusiner, S. B. (1982) Novel proteinaceous particles cause scrapie. *Science*, **216**, 136–144.

—— (1992) Molecular biology of prion disease. *Science*, **252**, 1515–1522.

Quarrell, O. (1991) The neurobiology of Huntington's disease. In *Huntington's Disease* (ed. P. S. Harper), pp. 141–178. London: W. B. Saunders.

——, Tyler, A., Jones, M. P., *et al* (1988) Population studies of Huntington's disease in Wales. *Clinical Genetics*, **33**, 189–195.

Rabins, P. D. & Pearlson, G. D. (1994) Depression induced cognitive impairment. In *Dementia* (eds A. Burns & R. Levy), pp. 667–679. London: Chapman & Hall.

Raven, J. C., Court, J. H. & Raven, J. (1977) *Manual for the Standard Progressive Matrices*. London: H. K. Lewis.

Rediess, S. & Caine, E. D. (1993) Aging-associated cognitive changes. How do they relate to the diagnosis of dementia? *Current Opinion in Psychiatry*, **6**, 531–536.

Robbins, T. W. & Sahakian, B. J. (1994) Computer methods of assessment of cognitive function. In *Principles and Practice of Geriatric Psychiatry* (eds J. R. M. Copeland, M. T. Abou-Saleh & D. G. Blazer), pp. 205–209. Chichester: John Wiley.

Roberts, M. A., McGeorge, A. P. & Caird, F. I. (1978) Electroencephalography and computerized tomography in vascular and non-vascular dementia in old age. *Journal of Neurology, Neurosurgery and Psychiatry*, **43**, 903–906.

Román, G. C., Tatemichi, T. K., Erkinjutti, T., *et al* (1993) Vascular dementia: diagnostic criteria for research studies. *Neurology*, **43**, 250–260.

Ron, M. A. (1983) The alcoholic brain. CT scan and psychological findings. *Psychological Medicine*, Monograph Supplement 3.

—, Toone, B. K., Garralda, M. E., *et al* (1979) Diagnostic accuracy in presenile dementia. *British Journal of Psychiatry*, **134**, 161–168.

Ross, C. A., McInnis, M. G., Margolis, R. L., *et al* (1993) Genes with triplet repeats: candidate mediators of neuropsychiatric disorders. *Trends in Neuroscience*, **16**, 254–260.

Rosser, M. N., Iverson, L. L., Reynolds, G. P., *et al* (1984) Neurochemical characteristics of early and late onset types of Alzheimer's disease. *British Medical Journal*, **288**, 961–964.

Roth, M. (1955) The natural history of mental disorder in old age. *Journal of Mental Sciences*, **101**, 281–301.

—, Tym, E., Mountjoy, C., *et al* (1986) CAMDEX: A standardised instrument for the diagnosis of mental disorder in the elderly with special reference to the early detection of dementia. *British Journal of Psychiatry*, **149**, 698–709.

Rubinsztein, D. C. (1995) Apoliprotein E: a review of its roles in lipoprotein metabolism, neuronal growth and repair and as a risk factor in Alzheimer's disease. *Psychological Medicine*, **25**, 223–229.

Semmes, J., Weinstein, S., Ghent, L., *et al* (1960) Somatosensory changes after penetrating brain wounds in man. Cambridge, MA: Harvard University Press.

Shallice, T. (1982) Specific impairment of planning. *Philosophical Transactions of the Royal Society of London*, **B298**, 199–209.

— (1988) *From Neuropsychology to Mental Structure*. Cambridge: Cambridge University Press.

— & Evans, M. E. (1978) The involvement of the frontal lobes in cognitive estimates. *Cortex*, **14**, 294–303.

Sherrington, R., Rogaev, E. L., Liang, Y., *et al* (1995) Cloning of a gene bearing missense mutations in early-onset familial Alzheimer's disease. *Nature*, **375**, 754–760.

Simpson, S. A. & Johnston, A. W. (1989) The prevalence and patterns of care of Huntington's chorea in Grampian. *British Journal of Psychiatry*, **155**, 799–804.

Sjogren, T. (1952) A genetic study of Morbus Alzheimer and Morbus Pick. *Acta Psychiatrica et Neurologica Scandinavica*, suppl. 82, 9–66.

Snell, R. G., MacMillan, J. C. F., Cheadle, J. P., *et al* (1993) Relationship between trinucleotide repeat expansion and phenotypic variation in Huntington's disease. *Nature Genetics*, **4**, 1–6.

Spitzer, R. L., First, M. B., Williams, J. B. W., *et al* (1992) Now is the time to retire the term "Organic mental disorders". *American Journal of Psychiatry*, **149**, 240–244.

Strittmatter, M. J. & Roses, A. D. (1995) Apoliprotein E and Alzheimer's disease. *Proceedings of the National Academy of Sciences*, **92**, 4725–4727.

Stuss, D. T., Alexander, M. P., Liberman, A., *et al* (1978) An extraordinary form of confabulation. *Neurology*, **28**, 1166–1172.

— & Benson, D. F. (1986) *The Frontal Lobes*. New York: Raven Press.

Subirana, A. (1958) The prognosis of aphasia in relation to cerebral dominance and handedness. *Brain*, **81**, 415–425.

Taylor, D. & Lewis, S. (1993) Delirium. *Journal of Neurology, Neurosurgery and Psychiatry*, **56**, 742–751.

Teasdale, G. & Jennett, B. (1974) Assessment of coma and impaired consciousness: a practical scale. *Lancet*, **2**, 81–84.

Tomlinson, B. E., Blessed, G. & Roth, M. (1970) Observations on the brains of demented old people. *Journal of Neurological Science*, **11**, 205–242.

Trojanowski, J. Q., Schmidt, M. L., Shin, R.-W., *et al* (1994) PHF tau (A68): from pathological marker to potential mediator of neuronal dysfunction and degeneration in Alzheimer's disease. *Clinical Neuroscience*, **1**, 184–191.

Tyler, A. (1991) Social and psychological aspects of Huntington's disease. In *Huntington's Disease* (ed. P. S. Harper), pp. 179–203. London: W. B. Saunders.

Van Broeckhoven, C. (1995) Presenilins and Alzheimer disease. *Nature Genetics*, **11**, 230–232.

van Hemert, A. M., van der Mast, R. C., Hengeveld, M. W., *et al* (1994) Excess mortality in general hospital patients with delirium: a 5-year follow-up of 519 patients seen in psychiatric consultation. *Journal of Psychosomatic Research*, **38**, 339–346.

Victor, J., Adams, R. D. & Collins, G. H. (1971) *The Wernicke-Korsakoff Syndrome*. Philadelphia: F. A. Davis.

von Cramon, D. Y., Hebel, N. & Schuri, U. (1985) A contribution to the anatomical basis of thalamic amnesia. *Brain*, **108**, 993–1008.

Walker, D. A., Harper, P. S., Wells, C. E. C., *et al* (1981) Huntington's chorea in South Wales: a genetic and epidemiological study. *Clinical Genetics*, **19**, 213–221.

Walsh, K. (1987) *Neuropsychology: A Clinical Approach* (2nd edn). Edinburgh: Churchill Livingstone.

Warrington, E. K. (1984) *The Recognition Memory Test*. Windsor: NFER-Nelson.

— & Shallice, T. (1969) The selective impairment of auditory verbal short-term memory. *Brain*, **92**, 885–896.

Watt, D. C. & Seller, A. (1993) A clinico-genetic study of psychiatric disorder in Huntington's chorea. *Psychological Medicine*, Monograph Supplement 23.

Waxman, S. G. & Geschwind, N. (1975) The interictal behaviour syndrome of temporal lobe epilepsy. *Archives of General Psychiatry*, **32**, 1580–1586.

Wechsler, D. (1981) *Wechsler Adult Intelligence Scale – Revised*. New York: Psychological Corporation.

— (1987) *Wechsley Memory Scale – Revised*. New York: Psychological Corporation.

Wells, C. E. (1979) Pseudo-dementia. *American Journal of Psychiatry*, **136**, 895–900.

Wernicke, K. (1874) *Der aphasische Symptomkomplex*. Breslau.

Wilson, B. A. (1987) *Rehabilitation of Memory*. New York: Guilford Press.

World Health Organization (1992) *The ICD–10 Classification of Mental and Behavioural Disorders*. Geneva: WHO.

Zhang, M., Katzman, R., Salmon, D., *et al* (1990) The prevalence of dementia and Alzheimer's disease in Shanghai, China: Impact of age, gender and education. *Annual of Neurology*, **27**, 428–437.

23 Psychiatric aspects of neurological disorders

Jonathan Bird & Mary Robertson

Epilepsy ● *Management of epilepsy* ● *Head injury* ● *Cerebrovascular disease* ● *Multiple sclerosis* ● *Miscellaneous neurological disorders* ● *Carcinoma* ● *Infectious diseases* ● *Movement disorders*

"Men ought to know that from the brain, and from the brain only, arise our pleasures, joys, laughter and jests, as well as our sorrows, pains, griefs and tears. It is the same thing which makes us mad or delirious, inspires us with dread and fear, brings sleeplessness, inopportune mistakes, aimless anxieties, absent mindedness and acts that are contrary to habit. These things that we suffer all come from the brain, when it is not healthy." Hippocrates (circa 400 B.C.)

A distinction between psychiatric and neurological disorders of the brain cannot realistically be made (Rogers, 1985; David, 1993). Organic and biological causes of classically psychiatric disorders are increasingly being uncovered, while the importance of intra- and interpersonal factors in the causation and maintenance of neurological disorders is increasingly recognised. Neuropsychiatry is a discipline based on the understanding of the relationship between brain and behaviour. It tends to use organic investigations such as neuropathology, neuroanatomy, neurophysiology, imaging, etc., but this by no means excludes an understanding of the importance of psychological and social aspects of causation and effect (Davison, 1990; Ron, 1994).

Epilepsy

Epilepsy is the quintessential neuropsychiatric disorder, one in which it is impossible to separate psychological from physical issues. It has proved to be one of the great teaching grounds in the understanding of brain function (Gowers, 1893; Penfield, 1967).

In 1876 Hughlings Jackson wrote: "An epileptic discharge is defined as an occasional, sudden, excessive, rapid and local discharge of some part of the cerebral hemisphere". Although the question of "what is epilepsy?" is complex, the basic definition has only three elements:

(1) Paroxysmal abnormalities of the electrical activity of the brain (seen on EEG).

(2) Associated abnormality of brain function, at the same time as the electrical discharge.

(3) A tendency to recurrence.

The first and second elements together form a seizure, the third makes it epilepsy. This section will first describe the clinical features of seizures, and second the associated psychiatric phenomena.

Epidemiology

About 2% of the population will have one or more seizures at some time in their life, but 0.5% will have active epilepsy requiring or receiving long-term treatment. It is the second commonest neurological problem after migraine. Males have a slightly higher prevalence. The age of onset is: 0–10 years in 30%, 11–20 years in 25%, 21–30 years in 20% and over 30 in 25%. It can be seen that the late teens and early 20s are the peak age of onset in adult life (Shorvon, 1990; Chaplin *et al*, 1992). The differential diagnosis of epilepsy is shown in Box 23.1.

Aetiology

The main causes of epilepsy are as follows:

Unknown – 75% (includes "mental handicap", mesial temporal sclerosis, heterotopia)
Cerebrovascular – 9%
Post-traumatic – 7%
Neoplasm – 5% (35% for those over the age of 35 at onset)

Epilepsy may be an inherited disorder, especially if generalised. There are also a number of familial forms such as benign rolandic epilepsy. If one

---

Box 23.1 Differential diagnosis of epilepsy

Cardiovascular:
Syncope, orthostatic hypotension, dysrhythmias (especially Romano-Ward syndrome or prolonged QT interval) aortic stenosis, transient ischaemic attacks
Hypoglycaemia
Migraine
Narcolepsy and cataplexy
Night terrors and sleep walking
Pseudo epileptic attacks (non epileptic attack disorder)
Hysterical amnesia and fugue
Toxic and metabolic disorders (including drugs and alcohol).

Box 23.2 Causes of epilepsy presenting at different ages

Neonatal (first month)
  Birth injury – anoxia or haemmorhage; congenital abnorm-
  alities; metabolic disorders – hypoglycaemia, hypocalcaemia,
  etc.
Infancy (1–6 months)
  As above; infantile spasms
Early childhood (6 months to 3 years)
  Febrile fits; birth injury; infection; trauma; poisons and
  metabolic defects; cerebral degeneration
Childhood and adolescence
  Idiopathic or primary epilepsy; birth injury; trauma; infection;
  cerebral degeneration
Early adult life
  Trauma; tumour; idiopathic or primary epilepsy; birth injury;
  infection; cerebral degeneration
Late adult life
  Vascular disease; trauma; tumour; cerebral degeneration

---

parent has epilepsy the risk for the child is about 3%. If both a parent and
a grandparent have epilepsy the risk is about 10%. The causes of epilepsy
are many and depend to some extent on the age of onset (see Box 23.2).
Some of the rarer causes of epilepsy are shown in Table 23.1.

Prognosis

About 70% of those having a first seizure will have a further seizure, but
50% of those will have less than ten seizures in their lives. Prognosis for
further seizures is much worse if the EEG is abnormal. Thirty per cent of
patients who are seizure free for five years will have further seizures when
taken off anti-epileptic drugs.

Classification

It has proved difficult to classify the epilepsies, although the Commission
of the International League Against Epilepsy (1989) (ILAE) has reached a
consensus, producing an International Classification of Epilepsies, Epileptic
Syndromes, and Related Seizure disorders (ICES). Involving classification
into four major groups, i.e. localisation-related (focal, local and partial),
generalised, undetermined, and special syndromes, this is a rather
unsatisfactory and controversial attempt to carve nature at the joints.
However, the ILAE has achieved more success, and more clinical usefulness,
in classifying seizures rather than epilepsy. Seizures may be either partial

Table 23.1 Rarer causes of seizures

Neurological diseases	Systemic diseases
Lipid storage diseases	Pulmonary insufficiency
Leucodystrophies	Anoxia
Demyelinating diseases	Hypocalcaemia
Spinocerebellar degeneration	Hypoglycaemia
Tuberous sclerosis	Pyridoxine deficiency
Sturge-Weber syndrome	Amino acid abnormalities
Cysticercosis	Water intoxication
Arteriovenous malformation	Renal failure
Subdural haematoma	Liver failure
Syphilis	Reye's syndrome
	Addison's disease
	Acute intermittent porphyria
	Drug withdrawal
	Drug intoxication
	Lead and other poisoning

(focal) or generalised. Partial seizures may become secondarily generalised. Partial seizures are either simple (without impaired consciousness) or complex (with impaired consciousness). These divisions are relevant in terms of aetiology, management and prognosis and are regarded as very important distinctions (see Table 23.2).

Generalised seizures have no aura or warning; sudden loss of consciousness (even if very brief) is invariable. An aura (warning) is evidence of partial seizures, demonstrating the importance of careful history taking and obtaining witness statements.

Stages of a seizure

Prodromata may occur for some hours or days before a fit and are not necessarily evidence of partial seizures. These consist of non-specific and rather vague mood changes or a sense of unease. Their cause is unclear, they may possibly be due to deep seated focal seizure activity or, conversely, due to some other change in brain state which subsequently sets the scene for a seizure to occur.

The aura (like a breath, a breeze before a storm) consists of acute perceptual, mood or behavioural changes and may occur alone, without further development or generalisation. The aura is, in itself, a focal seizure. It is likely to indicate the region of brain involved. Further spread of the abnormal epileptic activity results in a form of Jacksonian march – with characteristic progression of symptoms and signs and eventually a loss of consciousness as the discharge becomes generalised and involves the deeper

Table 23.2 International classification of epileptic seizures

---

I. Partial seizures (seizures beginning locally)
  A. Simple partial seizures (consciousness not impaired)
    1. With motor symptoms
    2. With somatosensory or special sensory symptoms
    3. With autonomic symptoms
    4. With psychic symptoms
  B. Complex partial seizures (with impairment of consciousness)
    1. Beginning as simple partial seizures and progressing to impairment of consciousness.
      a. With no other features
      b. With features as in A.1–4
      c. With automatisms
    2. With impairment of consciousness at onset.
      a. With no other features
      b. With features as in A.1–4
      c. With automatisms
  C. Partial seizures secondarily generalised.
II. Generalised seizures (bilaterally symmetrical and without local onset)
  A. 1. Absence seizures
      2. Atypical absence seizures
  B. Myoclonic seizures
  C. Clonic seizures
  D. Tonic seizures
  E. Tonic–clonic seizures
  F. Atonic seizures
III. Unclassified epileptic seizures (inadequate or incomplete data).

(Adapted from *Epilepsia*, 1981; 22, 489–501, with permission.)

subcortical structures. The study of auras and focal seizures in relation to neuropathology and surgery has added to the understanding of functional neuroanatomy (Penfield, 1967).

In adults the usual form of generalisation is to a tonic/clonic seizure – initial rigidity with respiratory arrest, followed by generalised jerking movements. In children "absences" with flickering eyelids and mild twitching on occasion (petit mal) is the typical form of generalised seizure but rarely continues after the age of 20 and very rarely starts after this age. The term "Petit Mal" should only, properly, be used for such seizures accompanied by 3 Hz spike and wave EEG changes. "Atypical" absence attacks may be similar but show slower spike or polyspike and wave discharges.

Post-ictal abnormalities may give a clue to the focus. Paralysis of a limb (Todd's Paresis) indicates focal motor epilepsy; dysphasias and other focal impairments can occur but may be more misleading as to the origin of the seizure. Confusion, headache and muscle pains are common non-specific post-ictal changes. Occasionally more prolonged amnesic episodes, confusional, delirious and fugue states may occur.

Ictal phenomena

The nature of the aura is often the most important factor indicating the site of the focus (Palmini & Gloor, 1992). About 80% of adult seizures are of focal origin and start as partial complex seizures (although the aura may be very brief). Some are clinically generalised from the beginning even though the EEG shows a brief focal origin.

About 75% of focal seizures originate in the temporal lobes and of these, 80% are in the deep mesial temporal structures particularly the amygdala and hippocampus (Currie *et al*, 1971). Fifteen to twenty per cent of focal seizures originate in the frontal lobes, about 5% in the parietal lobes and about 3% in the occipital lobes. The "typical" auras of these regions are described in Table 23.3. It can be seen that close observation of the seizure, its nature and duration may allow a considerable degree of localisation of the focus, although rapid spread is likely to make it different to be precise. The absolute start of the seizure is undoubtedly the most important indicator. Behavioural or experiential changes may precede EEG changes and are

Table 23.3 Typical epileptic aura by origin

Temporal lobe	75% of partial seizures	
	Mesial	(Amygdala, hippocampus) – 80% of temporal seizures
		Rising epigastric aura, déja vu, fear, derealisation
		Motionless stare, oro-alimentary automatisms
	Lateral	Auditory and visual illusions
		Dreamy state, dysphasia if dominant lobe
	Posterior	Dizziness, vomiting, complex visual hallucinations
Frontal lobe	20% especially 'Supplementary Motor Area'	
	Motor automatisms – "fencing" posture, adversive eye and head movement, speech arrest or bizarre vocalisation (e.g. singing)	
	Bilaterally coordinated limb movements (e. g. clapping)	
	Contralateral clonic Jacksonian march if motor strip	
	Brief, dramatic, nocturnal seizures are typical, with immediate recovery	
	Misdiagnosed often as "hysterical"	
Parietal lobe	Sensory auras, tingling, numbness, sense of movement	
	Visual distortions and formed hallucinations	
Occipital lobe	Fleeting visual phenomena – scotomata, flashes, simple hallucinations	

likely to indicate a deeper origin, for example the amygdala or cingulate gyrus.

Temporal lobe seizures are not only the most common, but also the most likely to be mistaken for a 'psychiatric' disorder, due to the appearance of atypical emotion (especially fear) as well as the possible presence of auditory or visual misperceptions and hallucinations. Derealisation and depersonalisation may cause diagnostic confusion and can be difficult to distinguish from panic disorder. It appears that the mesial temporal lobes are involved in integrating sensory input, memory and emotion and in creating a sense of self. Paroxysmal disturbance of this region is therefore likely to result in disorders of particular interest to the psychiatrist (Gloor, 1990).

Frontal lobe seizures are less common than temporal lobe seizures, although probably more widespread than previously realised. Most frontal seizures involve motor activity, the patient may have no experienced aura because of the immediate loss of consciousness. They are often very brief and frequent. However, seizures arising particularly in the cingulate region may give rise to affective changes as well as complex automatisms similar to those seen in temporal lobe epilepsy. Frontal seizures with an unclear precise origin may cause bimanual/bipedal automatisms such as clapping or stamping, associated with complex verbalisations such as singing and at times with other semi-purposive automatisms (e.g. sexual manipulation) and may therefore earn the epithet "functional" or "hysterical". The 'Supplementary Motor Area' of the mesial/frontal lobe may be the origin of such seizures.

Parietal and occipital seizures are still less common, often due to a progressive lesion and are less likely to be seen by the psychiatrist. However, the abnormal perceptions (somatic, sensory and visual) may be misdiagnosed as "functional". Of course, they are functional disturbances but as this term is usually taken to signify "non-organic", perhaps the correct term should be "organic cause not yet discovered".

Visual hallucinations may be seen in both posterior temporal and occipital seizures. Temporal seizures cause complex visual hallucinations (e.g. Lilliputian) while occipital seizures cause simple visual hallucinations such as flashes or spectra, and scotomata in the opposite half field.

Psychoses associated with epilepsy

The psychoses associated with epilepsy are best divided into those related to the seizure and those seen inter-ictally in people with epilepsy. The former are usually brief, the latter chronic. Seizure-related psychoses may be either ictal or post-ictal.

Ictal psychoses

Ictal psychoses include automatisms and non-convulsive status and are the result of ongoing paroxysmal brain discharges. Automatisms are part of the seizure, associated with clouded or absent consciousness and usually show simple, repetitive movements or wandering with confusion and irritation. In 80% they last less than five minutes and very rarely they last more than an hour.

Non-convulsive status may be due to simple partial status (usually with motor manifestations), Petit mal status or complex partial status. Petit mal status (also called absence status) can start at any age and is associated with altered consciousness, myoclonic flickering of the eyelids and generalised three per second spike and wave discharges on the EEG.

Complex partial status results in mental confusion and psychosis with a fluctuating level of consciousness which may be associated with complex automatisms, episodic hallucinations and marked mood changes which may be mis-diagnosed as a "functional" psychosis. Early and energetic treatment with intravenous diazepam is important as persistent intellectual deficit has been reported after prolonged complex partial status (Fagon & Lee, 1990). The EEG is diagnostic and is an early and essential investigation in confusional psychoses.

Post-ictal psychoses

Post-ictal psychoses are poorly studied and loosely defined in spite of their relative frequency. Post-ictal confusion with accompanying EEG slow wave changes is common, and may, on occasions, last up to a few hours. Post-ictal psychoses are traditionally divided into two forms, fugues and twilight states. The fugue is a prolonged episode of wandering, altered behaviour, amnesia and impaired consciousness and it may last for hours or even days. The EEG is often free of ictal or post-ictal changes. It appears likely that the fugue is a dissociative phenomenon provoked by the seizure. Twilight states are particularly characterised by abnormal subjective experiences (perceptual and affective), and are also associated with cognitive impairment and perseveration. Paranoid hallucinatory disturbances may also be present. Electroconvulsive therapy may be dramatically effective treatment if this state does not resolve itself. Such twilight states may be due to sub-ictal, focal paroxysmal activity detectable with depth electrodes and this observation has been used to support the notion of an epileptic origin for the Episodic Dyscontrol syndrome.

Chronic inter-ictal psychosis

There is no doubt that psychoses which are phenomenologically indistinguishable from schizophrenia have an increased prevalence in people with temporal lobe epilepsy (Logsdail & Toone, 1988; Savard *et al*, 1991; Mace, 1993). The risk is about 3%. Commonly the presentation is of a chronic paranoid hallucinatory psychosis with first rank symptoms. Certain features in the history, however, distinguish them from schizophrenia (Toone *et al*, 1982); there is no increased family history of schizophrenia, usually a good pre-morbid personality with less personality deterioration and a warmer affect. There is also an increased incidence of neurological abnormality on examination. Typically, the psychosis emerges 10–15 years after the onset of epilepsy and there may be a reduction in the severity of the epilepsy as the psychosis develops. Risk factors include alien tissue lesions (hamartomas), an aura of fear, being left handed, having a mesial temporal focus and onset of epilepsy in adolescence (Taylor, 1975). It is now established that a left temporal focus is particularly associated with psychosis, as was initially demonstrated by Flor-Henry (1969), with 62% having a left temporal focus, 15% a right temporal focus and 23% bilateral foci. The suggestion by Flor-Henry that right temporal foci are associated with affective psychosis has not been confirmed, and bipolar illness is no more frequently associated with epilepsy than would be expected in the general population.

Aetiological theories concerning the schizophrenia of epilepsy fall into three groups. The kindling hypothesis suggests that there is frequent or constant sub-ictal paroxysmal activity in the mesial temporal structures which leads to the progressive establishment of abnormal limbic connections, eventually resulting in the symptoms of schizophrenia. It is, for instance, possible that the frequent association of ictal fear or rage with ordinary sensory input would result eventually in established paranoid delusions about the significance of everyday occurrences. The second hypothesis suggests that impairment of brain functioning, for example, due to an alien tissue lesion, first causes epilepsy and then the psychosis. Third, there may be a psychodynamic relationship, the effect on the individual of frequent abnormal experiences in the form of auras eventually resulting in the individual believing them and accepting a psychotic view of reality.

Management of the psychoses of epilepsy is the same as for other psychoses, although sulpiride may be a more appropriate anti-psychotic drug since it appears to be less epileptogenic than other neuroleptics. Reduction in anti-epileptic medication may be possible and appropriate if the epilepsy has been under good control.

Occasionally, transient psychoses with hallucinations, delusions, irritability and restlessness may occur when the epilepsy is brought under control, for example by a new anti-epileptic or surgery (Trimble, 1992). At this time the EEG may become normal, which is known as 'forced normalisation'. Treatment with ECT or reduction of anti-convulsant medication may be necessary. This form of 'alternating psychosis' is rare (although possibly more common in those with learning disability) but of interest.

Epilepsy and mood

Ictal emotion

Fear is the commonest ictal emotion (Daly, 1958), and even when it is not recalled by the patient, witnesses may report that he or she appeared terrified. However, sudden severe depression of mood has often been reported in relation to temporal seizures (or even partial complex status). Rarely, elation of mood is experienced, as described by Dostoevsky with his own seizures. Ictal emotions tend to lack clear, understandable precipitants, start and stop suddenly and have a hard, primitive, unvarying 'organic' quality to them which 'functional' mood disorders lack.

Depressed or altered mood may be seen both in prodromal and post-ictal stages. Of course, after a seizure, patients may be understandably distressed about the implications of the attack.

Inter-ictal mood disorder

Depression and anxiety are the commonest inter-ictal psychiatric disorders occurring in 15–45% of patients, which may not necessarily be greater than in any disabled population. However, affective psychosis and manic–depressive disorder seem to show a normal incidence. The risk of suicide is 3 to 5 times greater in people with epilepsy than in the general population.

It is not clear whether inter-ictal mood disorders are particularly associated with any form or focus of epilepsy, and conflicting results have been obtained in different surveys. Associated features include high anxiety and high hostility scores, an 'endogenous' picture in 40%, a relationship with a long history of epilepsy and currently taking phenobarbitone (Robertson *et al*, 1987, 1994).

The relationship between depression and epilepsy is likely to be multi-factorial and due to a mixture of the factors shown in Box 23.3.

The management of depression with epilepsy will include exploration of all the above issues and making appropriate alteration in anti-epileptic medication as well as counselling and psychotherapy. If antidepressants are required they must be used with awareness that all current antidepressants (except perhaps MAOIs) are potentially epileptogenic, and

---

Box 23.3 Factors contributing to the development of depression in epilepsy

Reaction to the 'label' and implications of the diagnosis.
Reaction to social, work and family problems.
Prodromal affect.
Part of the aura.
Ictal or post-ictal.
Related to seizure activity reduction.
Associated with other psychiatric disorders of epilepsy (e.g. psychosis).
Drug effects, either depression due to anti-convulsants or seizures due to antidepressants.

there is little clear information about the use of the new antidepressants such as the SSRIs. Interestingly, ECT may be an effective treatment, even in those still having natural seizures, although the patient's anticonvulsants may well increase the seizure threshold.

Pesonality and epilepsy

The individual with epilepsy was traditionally thought of as "spiritless, stupid, unsociable, slow to learn and bewildered", as the Roman physician Aretaeus wrote: however, he also recognised that this might be "either from the nature of the disease or from wounds during the attack". The debate about whether any enduring personality characteristics are due to the brain disorder or are secondary to the social, medical and other effects of epilepsy has continued since then. During the Dark Ages epilepsy was widely thought to be due to possession by demons, even though Hippocrates had declared it to be the result of brain malfunction in 400 B.C.; the witchhunters guide (Malleus Malleficorum) instructed its readers in ways to distinguish between natural and spiritual manifestations, in a fashion rather similar to current-day lists of the distinguishing features of true and pseudo epileptic seizures.

The enlightened neurological physician, Gowers, wrote in 1893 that any personality deterioration in epilepsy was a direct result of the frequency of seizures. However, at that time, the Degeneracy Theory of Morel held sway; this regarded epilepsy as the reflection of a hereditary stigma, part of the inevitable decline across the generations of certain families afflicted with moral insanity, mental illness, idiocy and dementia. Epilepsy was seen as a manifestation of that decline and as such showed an association with particular personality attributes. The "Epileptic Personality" was regarded as pedantic, circumstantial, religiose, critical, irritable and "viscous" (sticky) in thought. The "epileptic" was also said to show characteristic facies, unflatteringly described by Kraepelin in 1904.

Such views of the epileptic personality grew out of asylum practice (where psychiatrists looked after epileptics), rather than the emerging view from the London neurologists (Russell-Reynolds, Gowers, Hughlings Jackson) based on private practice, that epilepsy was not necessarily associated with any personality change.

A more enlightened view developed and it was argued that such personality changes as might occur in people with epilepsy were due to stigmatisation, institutionalisation and medication, especially bromides and barbiturates, or were the result of the brain damage or inherited mental handicap which also causes the epilepsy.

However, in the 1940s and 1950s, epileptologists began to identify patients with temporal lobe seizures more reliably (from EEG) and to postulate that personality disorder could arise due to persistent temporal lobe seizure discharges (Geschwind, 1965). In the 1970s Bear & Fedio (1977) published an influential paper detailing the results of a questionnaire study of patients with epilepsy and their relatives. The questionnaire was based on a literature search of all reports of psychiatric changes in patients with complex partial seizures. The results indicated that patients with temporal lobe epilepsy tended to show humourless sobriety, dependence, circumstantiality, obsessionality, preoccupation with religious and pseudo-philosophical concerns and irritability. A right temporal focus was said to be associated with emotionality and with hypergraphia (writing a great deal) (Okanura *et al*, 1993), whilst a left temporal focus was said to be associated with a ruminative intellectual tendency. When patients' questionnaires were compared with those of their relatives, right temporal lobe patients tended to improve on the description of their activities ("polishers") while left temporal lobe patients tended to over-report bad traits ("tarnishers").

Certain particular elements of the "temporal lobe personality syndrome" – circumstantiality/viscosity, deep and ponderous emotionality, a hyper-ethical attitude and hyposexuality were seen as opposite to traits associated with the Kluver–Bucy syndrome of bilateral disconnection of the medial temporal lobes (Lilly *et al*, 1983). The temporal lobe syndrome has thus been termed "temporal hyperconnection" and might result from chronic excessive neuronal activity in the temporo-limbic structures, perhaps having a kindling effect (Geschwind, 1979). However, there are criticisms of this work and other studies have thrown doubt on the proposed special relationship with temporal lobe epilepsy. It seems likely that only a sub-group of patients with temporal lobe epilepsy show this syndrome. Viscosity has recently been shown to be associated with left temporal foci and seen as an inter-ictal language disturbance (Rao *et al*, 1992).

Other seizure types do not seem especially related to any particular personality type, but the effects of developing epilepsy at an important stage of personality development, family attitudes, difficulty finding work and the effects of medication would all have a bearing on the individual's reaction to the diagnosis and personality. A combination of dependency, poor social skills, interrupted education, over-sedation, parental over-protectiveness, low self-esteem and popular prejudice is likely to lead to social isolation, frustration and despondency.

Aggression and epilepsy

There continues to be considerable debate about whether aggressive behaviour is seen more commonly in people with epilepsy than in a normal control population. Confounding factors include the presence of brain damage, lower social class and stigmatisation. Pathological aggression occurs in 4–50% of patients with epilepsy, a range which demonstrates questionable validity. The rate of criminal offences is three times higher than in the general population and the rate of epilepsy in the prison population is 0.72% (compared with 0.5% in the general population), although prison population variables (particularly IQ and social class) may explain the difference. The crimes committed by people with epilepsy are usually non-violent. If there is any significant relationship between epilepsy and violence, it may be of three types – ictal, possibly ictal and probably not ictal.

Ictal violence

Violence may be done to others in a seizure. This has usually been provoked by poor handling of a confused ictal or post-ictal patient, possibly because someone simply got in the way of convulsing arms or because of fearful hitting out by the patient if roughly restrained. Very rarely (in 13 out of 4500 seizures (Currie *et al*, 1971); one out of 434 patients (Rodin, 1973)) violent behaviour occurs as part of an automatism or post ictal state. Ictal violence as a result of an automatism is usually poorly directed, purposeless, fragmentary, simple and repetitive as well as very brief. It may consist of a continuation of a behaviour instigated before the seizure onset. Criteria for determining that a criminal act was done during a seizure are detailed in Box 23.4; this may be important for medico-legal purposes.

Possibly ictal – the Episodic Dyscontrol syndrome

There has been persistent debate about whether or not deep (particularly amygdala) paroxysmal discharges which do not show on the scalp EEG could cause episodes of violent dyscontrol and whether impulsive outbursts of violent or potentially violent behaviour could be a form of partial epilepsy (Mark & Ervin, 1970; Bach-Y-Rita *et al*, 1971; Maletzky, 1973). There have been several case reports of such disturbances seen on depth electrode recordings, although populations studied have not always been normal and have sometimes been prisoners. Also the electro-physiological activity of the normal amygdala is very poorly understood. The disorder has, however, gained diagnostic respectability, appearing in the DSM–IV as 'Intermittent Explosive Disorder'.

Box 23.4 Criteria for determination that a criminal act was ictal (Fenwick, 1990)

Confirmed clinical history of epilepsy, preferably with abnormal EEG and a history of automatisms.
Lack of apparent motivation, planning or pre-meditation.
Little attempt to conceal the crime or to escape.
Brief duration (usually less than a few minutes).
Inappropriate behaviour is evident.
Evidence of impaired or altered consciousness from witnesses.
Amnesia for the behaviour.

The generally accepted features of such disorders include:

(1) Sudden, paroxysmal onset ("Uncontrollable storms of aggression"; Maletzky, 1973).

(2) Behaviour is grossly out of proportion to any stress, precipitant or provocation (usually showing serious assault or destruction of property and usually related to a close family member).

(3) Subsequent genuine remorse.

(4) Hazy recollection only (or amnesia) for the episode.

(5) It is out of character, and between episodes there is no generalised aggressiveness.

This syndrome is significantly associated with a history of developmental delays and specific learning difficulties, previous head injury, epilepsy and there may be non-specific EEG changes (e.g. temporal sharp wave abnormalities or posterior sharp waves). There is also sometimes a family history of violence and epilepsy. Those with episodic dyscontrol disorder may also show a chaotic personal, social and work history. The condition also is discussed on page 782.

Management involves the use of anti-epileptic drugs (particularly carbamazepine although no satisfactory trial exists) and psychological approaches to the control and the avoidance of aggression. Benzodiazepines may make the problem worse. Lithium, neuroleptics and propranolol have been advocated by some.

Probably not ictal

Epilepsy may be associated with criminal (violent or non-violent) behaviour for several reasons which are not directly related to the seizure. These will include:

(1) Organic brain disorder (e.g. frontal or temporal lobes), which may lead both to epilepsy and to offence behaviour.

(2) Epilepsy leads to social rejection, stigmatisation and hence to frustration and offence behaviour.

(3) Adverse social factors (low social class, non-accidental injury, violent families) result both in offending and in an increased incidence of epilepsy.

(4) A tendency to antisocial behaviour (e.g. alcohol abuse, reckless driving) leads both to offences and to brain injury causing epilepsy.

Non-epileptic attack disorders (pseudo seizures, hysterical seizures)

The distinction between epileptic seizures and non-epileptic ('hysterical') seizures has taxed doctors since Roman times. Twenty per cent of patients with apparently intractable epilepsy have non-epileptic attacks, although they may have a combination of true and pseudo epilepsy. Patients with true epilepsy are, indeed, among the most likely to have pseudo seizures. Non-epileptic attack disorders describes a heterogeneous group, with a wide spectrum of morbidity. Different forms of non-epileptic seizure may present to different specialists. Pseudo-epileptic status will usually present to general physicians in an acute fashion, while neurologists are likely to see patients with pseudo seizures of a 'generalised' form. Psychiatrists tend to see those with brief 'partial complex'-like attacks and special centres more often assess or manage those with an intractable combination of epilepsy and non-epilepsy. The views of these professionals differ and lead to difficulty in achieving a consensus overview (Betts, 1990). When distinguishing between epileptic and non-epileptic seizures, neurologists tend to list clinical findings (negative in non-epileptic seizures) and psychiatrists tend to list historical and psychodynamic features (positive in non-epileptic seizures). The distinction is summarised in Table 23.4. At times, however, it may seem impossible to decide whether an individual's attacks are epileptic or not and Landouzy's term "hystero epilepsy" seems closest to the truth (Leis *et al*, 1992).

Post ictal

True confusion is rare, the patient may laugh or smile (it may not be an unpleasant feeling) or may recall events during the seizure in detailed fashion.

Investigations

(1) EEG (e.g. ambulatory monitoring). This is normal during and after an attack, although movement artefact may make interpretation difficult. Also, very localised true epileptic attacks may show no surface abnormality. The continuation of the alpha rhythm during an attack in which consciousness is apparently lost almost always indicates a non-epileptic attack. However, brief frontal seizures may be very difficult to pick up on an EEG. Video-telemetry may be invaluable here, in which clinical acumen can be applied to observation of the detailed nature of the attack even if the EEG is obscured.

(2) Serum prolactin. After generalised seizures, the level is usually over 1000 iu/ml, in partial attacks it may be 500 iu/ml, but in non-epileptic attacks it is usually normal, although it can be somewhat raised (Dana-Haeri *et al*, 1983). Prolactin levels taken within 20 minutes of the start of the seizure may be helpful in generalised attacks but less helpful in partial ones. Frontal lobe seizures may be particularly difficult to distinguish on this basis. The use of prolactin levels has not been as helpful as was initially hoped.

Management

The earlier a diagnosis of non-epileptic seizures is made the better, as reinforcement of illness behaviour with drugs or medical attention can be

Table 23.4 Features more often found in non-epileptic seizures

History	Previous psychiatric disorder
	Family history of psychiatric disorder
	Deliberate self-harm
	Sexual maladjustment
	Hysterical personality is present in only a few (perhaps less than 25%)
Current state	Presence of affective disorder
	Intense current psychosocial stressors
The attack	Emotional precipitant, with evidence of primary or secondary gain. Gradual onset, with a prolonged warning
	Wide range of often bizarre events and behaviour (e.g. talking, screaming, struggling)
	Pelvic thrusting is particularly characteristic, as well as unresponsiveness in the absence of significant motor activity
	Varied, not stereotyped attack pattern
	Lack of true tonic and then clonic movements
	Suggestibility (regarding starting, stopping and changing nature)
	Tongue biting, incontinence and injury are rare but certainly can occur
	Nocturnal episodes may occur and the EEG will demonstrate this as an arousal phenomena not occurring during sleep itself
	Left-sided (non-dominant) somatosensory symptoms and signs may be more frequent

avoided. Once it is established (preferably with an EEG) that the attacks are non-epileptic, gradual withdrawal of anti-epileptic, probably as an in-patient is advised. The attitude of ward staff should be one of "benign neglect" so far as the attacks are concerned, and the family and other patients in the ward must also learn that this is the correct approach. Considerable psychotherapeutic discussion with patient and family will be necessary if the diagnosis of "epilepsy" has been long established. The patient must be reassured that reducing anti-epileptics is not only safe but positively beneficial as it returns control to the individual and reduces sedation. A family-based, cognitive and behavioural approach to the change in diagnosis is usually best. This can be combined with psychotherapeutic exploration of the patient's past, when (apparently increasingly) a history of sexual abuse may be uncovered. However, the presence of non-epileptic seizures must not be taken as proof of childhood sexual abuse and uncovering a history of such abuse is no guarantee of cure. A drug-assisted interview using diazepam or sodium amylobarbitone may help to access the patient's problems. If an "attack" is videoed, this can be shown to the patient and discussed, using it as part of a therapeutic programme. Occasionally "attacks" may be provoked by suggestion.

Cognitive function in epilepsy

Cognitive functioning in people with epilepsy may be impaired by drug intoxication (Thompson & Trimble, 1982), non-convulsive status and possibly by sub-clinical paroxysmal discharges such as hippocampal spike activity. It is clear that brief petit mal absence attacks may go unnoticed by the patient or those nearby and yet can significantly impair registration of memory at the time. The same may apply to brief focal discharges. Post-ictal amnesia and partial amnesias may be misdiagnosed as a dementing process, especially if frequent seizures leave the individual in an almost continuous post-ictal state.

Inter-ictal cognitive impairment and decline are much debated issues (Brown & Reynolds, 1981). It is very clear that epilepsy need not be related to any intellectual impairment. There have been many famous people who have suffered from epilepsy and these include the generals Julius Caesar, Alexander the Great and Napoleon, the writers Dostoevsky, Tennyson, Lewis Carroll, Edward Lear, Kierkegaard, the mathematicians Newton and Pascal, artists such as Van Gogh and a number of religious leaders. Taken as a whole, patients with epilepsy have a normal mean IQ, provided that cases of epilepsy associated as a secondary phenomenon with brain damage (congenital or otherwise) are excluded. Inter-ictal cognitive impairment may be the result of sedative anti-epileptic drugs, interrupted and poor education, parental attitudes and personal reactions to the illness.

However, specific memory and learning deficits can be associated with specific epilepsies, for example, verbal memory impairment with left temporal lobe epilepsy, and impaired attention with generalised epilepsy. The main determinant of cognitive impairment is the aetiology of the epilepsy. Early onset, length of illness and frequency of seizures are weakly related to cognitive impairment.

"Epileptic dementia" (progressive decline in cognitive function) primarily related to the epilepsy may occur in a very small proportion of cases. It is debatable whether it occurs at all or is due to medication, underlying organic factors or additional pathology. It does seem, however, that there are rare cases of patients with epilepsy, usually of early onset, long duration and high severity who show an inexorable but slow intellectual decline, usually associated with severe personality deterioration. This is more common in patients with a known brain lesion and may be associated with reduced reserves due to brain damage, resulting in early dementia.

Psychological induction and inhibition of seizures

A very high proportion (92%) of people with epilepsy identify psychological states as precipitants or facilitators of their seizures, especially tension, depression, tiredness and being over-excited (Antebi & Bird, 1993). More specifically, there are many single case reports of particular affective and cognitive stimuli which can directly provoke reflex seizures in susceptible individuals, for example mental arithmetic, playing cards or chess, reading specific lines, even looking at a safety pin in one famous case. It seems likely that there is an interaction between the presentation of the specific stimulus and the current state of the individual.

A few patients with epilepsy (perhaps 2%, although this figure depends on the sample) are able to induce their own seizures by some conscious act of will – such as waving a hand in front of the eyes or flickering the eyelids to simulate photic flashing.

Alternatively, many patients (20%) actively avoid situations which put them at risk and 25% of patients with an aura feel that they can abort their seizures by some act of will, such as the sudden diversion of attention or by concentration on some cognitive task.

Management of epilepsy

Inevitably, the main line of management in epilepsy is with anti-epileptic drugs (AEDs) (Reynolds, 1981; Chadwick, 1994). These are dealt with in detail in *College Seminars in Learning Disability* (Russell, 1997) and *College Seminars in Clinical Psychopharmacology* (King, 1995) and will not be covered here. The following section covers general principles of management and psychological methods.

When, why and how to treat

First, it must be established that the patient has epilepsy. If only one seizure has occurred, many clinicians would not prescribe an AED. However, if the EEG is abnormal there is an 80% chance of recurrence and there are many indications that the more seizures a person has, the more difficult they will be to control. The correct method of instigating AED therapy is to discuss the risks and benefits with the patient, taking into account their life and work situation. Patients must then be allowed to decide for themselves. All treatment is a trade-off between therapeutic and adverse effects.

A patient should always be started on only one AED, and this should be changed, in an overlapping fashion, for one other drug if the first is shown to be ineffective at a therapeutic level or because of unacceptable side-effects. The initiation of AED therapy must be discussed at length with the patient and family and a system of regular dosing must be worked out. Careful initial follow-up is needed. The choice of specific AED may be important, as some seizure types can be exacerbated by certain AEDs, for example, generalised absence attacks by phenytoin, myoclonic epilepsy by vigabatrin. The first choice for most adult seizure types is either sodium valproate or carbamazepine. Phenytoin and phenobarbitone are no longer first choice AEDs. Initial adverse effects can be minimised by slow introduction and the avoidance of toxic levels. Drug level monitoring is most useful for phenytoin, but of rather less use for other AEDs except perhaps for carbamazepine.

In addition to drug treatment, a supportive and informative psychotherapeutic approach is vital, both for the patient and the family. The implications of epilepsy such as not driving, work restrictions, changed attitudes of teachers and employers, relationships with the family, as well as legal matters, and low self-image are legion and are likely to require several exploratory sessions. Altering a patient's lifestyle may be advisable, for example reducing alcohol intake, regular sleeping and eating times, and care with the use of the oral contraceptive pill and other medication.

Psychological treatment methods

Psychological treatment methods in epilepsy have been largely ignored, which is understandable in the face of the excellent success of AED therapy. However, 10–20% of patients will not be adequately controlled with AEDs and, apart from the consideration of surgical approaches, such as selective amygdalo-hippocampectomy, psychological approaches are the only other treatment. As well as the avoidance of known psychological precipitants of seizures, a number of more specific psychological and behavioural approaches may be effective in some patients (Goldstein, 1990).

Reward management in which overt or covert (fantasised) rewards are used positively to reward reduced seizure frequency.

Self-control strategies – many patients use or can be encouraged to develop the sort of seizure inhibition strategies already described. Specific relaxation training, combined with desensitisation and various interventions during the aura period may also be effective.

Conditioning procedures – in which the antecedents of seizures are closely studied and a behavioural approach then used.

Biofeedback – biofeedback of a variety of EEG rhythms (e.g. a sensorimotor rhythm, alpha rhythm, paroxysmal activities) can be attempted.

Psychotherapy – both individual and group psychotherapeutic approaches may well lead to improved life adjustment and reduced seizure frequency.

Head injury

Head injury has been called the "silent epidemic", resulting as it does in 10% of all visits to Accident and Emergency Departments and in severe permanent disability in 0.1% of the population. The incidence of head injuries is 1500 per 100 000 population each year, 130 of these cases being of sufficient severity to result in lasting cognitive deficit and 17 resulting in severe physical and cognitive deficit. Males are affected twice as often as females and it is the cause of 15–20% of deaths between the ages of 5 and 25 in the United Kingdom.

Head injury rehabilitation is primarily a neuropsychiatric problem, even though many patients, even with severe disabilities, do not present themselves to medical and psychiatric services, hence the relative silence of the epidemic.

Pathophysiology

The characteristic disabilities of traumatic brain injury (TBI) can largely be predicted from an understanding of the mechanics of head injury as they affect the functional anatomy of the brain (Strich, 1969; Hume-Adams *et al*, 1991; Miller, 1993).

Primary injury

Primary damage to the brain occurs as a result of either rotational or horizontal acceleration or deceleration.

Rotational acceleration/deceleration occurs when there is an abrupt transfer of energy to the head as it accelerates suddenly and then is stopped by contact with a hard object. The brain is tethered at the brain stem and so oscillates around the central axis, resulting, first, in diffuse shearing of long central fibres and micro haemorrhages in the corpus callosum and rostral brain stem. Injury is microscopic but widespread and is termed diffuse axonal injury, which eventually leads to Wallerian degeneration of axons in the subcortical white matter and atrophic enlargement of the ventricles in severe head injuries. Second, the rotational acceleration/deceleration causes centrifugal pressure waves to spread out so that the poles of the brain undergo repeated buffeting against the skull and tentorium, especially where there are sharp edges or corners. The frontal poles, orbital frontal regions, temporal poles and medial temporal structures are therefore particularly damaged. The brain stem and mid brain may also be contused by the rim of the foramen magnum and the tentorial edge.

Horizontal acceleration/deceleration injury will also cause contusion at the site of the injury (coup) and on the opposite side (contre-coup).

Secondary injury

Secondary injury to the brain can be the result of various factors. Haemorrhage (subdural, extradural and at times intra-cerebral) may occur and, along with reactive brain swelling and acute fluid collections, can result in raised intra-cranial pressure with a coning of the brain stem. Later development of obstructive or communicating hydrocephalus may occur.

Other peripheral injuries can have a secondary effect on brain function, particularly hypotensive shock due to peripheral bleeding, anoxia due to respiratory or cardiovascular injury and fat emboli due to fracture of long bones.

Thus a common accumulation of injuries to the frontal and temporal poles, orbital frontal region, corpus callosum and brain stem tegmentum lead to the characteristic sequelae of TBI which will be described below.

Coma, post-traumatic amnesia and other indicators of outcome

Outcome after head injury has been extensively studied, but often without using standardised criteria or comparable severity of injury. Two main criteria of injury–severity have emerged: the Glasgow Coma Scale (GCS) and the length of post traumatic amnesia (PTA).

The GCS is an accumulative 15 point scale (15 = fully alert) based on responsiveness in the three areas of eye opening, gross motor activity and verbalisation (see Table 23.5). If accurately recorded, it gives some indication of outcome. A score of 15 at 24 hours after injury is associated in only 6% with a bad outcome (death, vegetative state or severe disability), while a score of 3 at 24 hours indicates an 80% chance of bad outcome (Jennett *et al*, 1981)

Post-traumatic amnesia (PTA, Anterograde Amnesia) is probably a measure of diffuse axonal injury and is one of the best later indicators of severity of injury and likely outcome, except where severe localised damage has occurred (Wilson *et al*, 1994). PTA is the time from injury to restoration of normal, continuous memory. This does not include islets of memory, but will include the length of the period of coma and confusion as a minimum. A PTA of between one and 24 hours is regarded as moderate and over 24 hours as severe. The length of PTA correlates very roughly with eventual outcome, a PTA of more than 24 hours being likely to be associated with some permanent disability, usually of cognition or personality. However, long-term follow-up shows that there is a rather weak correlation between detailed measures of cognitive outcome and these rather coarse measures of severity. Lishman (1987) suggests that a PTA of less than an hour predicts return to work within a month, a PTA of less than a week within four months and a PTA of more than a week predicts invalidism for a year as well as a 50–70% prevalence of severe psychiatric and intellectual disability at five year follow-up.

Other methods used in an attempt to assess severity include slowing of the EEG rhythms, slowed conduction velocity of somatic and brain stem auditory evoked responses and MRI scan results. However, severe and disabling focal damage and slow crushing damage can occur without a coma or a PTA. Retrograde (pre-traumatic) amnesia is of little relevance and tends to shrink with time. If memory for the injury is not impaired at all, post-traumatic stress disorder may be more likely to occur. Dense and very prolonged retrograde amnesia is likely to be psychogenic.

Table 23.5 The Glasgow Coma Scale

		Score
Eye opening	Spontaneous	4
	To speech	3
	To pain	2
	None	1
Motor response	Obedience to commands	6
	Localisation of pain	5
	Withdrawal	4
	Flexion to pain	3
	Extension to pain	2
	None	1
Verbal response	Orientated	5
	Confused conversation	4
	Inappropriate words	3
	Incomprehensible sounds	2
	None	1

Recovery stages

Recovery from TBI occurs in a characteristic sequence of stages. The patient passes from coma into unresponsive vigilance with a return of gross wakefulness. Mute responsiveness follows, with the patient responding to simple instructions. The next stage is a confusional state with severe attentional disturbance, confabulation, denial, perseveration, agitation, disordered sleep and considerable emotional lability at times. Acute hysterical or paranoid features may be present. Subsequent improvement will progress to independence in self-care and increasingly independent intellectual and social functioning.

Neuropsychiatric sequelae

In patients who do not recover fully, and during the lengthy recovery phase in those who do, characteristic disturbances are seen due to dysfunction in the areas of brain usually affected by TBI, as described above.

Frontal polar damage leads to poor judgement and insight, apathy and impaired problem solving. There is often no understanding of the impact of the disability on others. Orbito-frontal damage results in impaired social judgement with impulsivity, excitability, lack of tact and childishness. Temporal lobe damage will result in memory loss and speech difficulties, it may also lead to irritability and aggressive dyscontrol. Diffuse axonal injury characteristically leads to slowed thinking, impaired arousal and drive, poor concentration and attention as well as poor cognitive endurance due to disruption of the many subcortical connections, leading to a picture similar to the subcortical dementias. Attentional problems are the commonest single complaint in head injury rehabilitation.

Many patients will also have idiosyncratic disabilities due to the particular areas of brain which have been directly injured (usually by coup or contre-coup injury or by penetrating injury). Some patients will have a disproportionately severely affected limbic system, with the neocortical limbic structures being more damaged than elsewhere, which may result in major disruption of affect and behaviour but without formal neurological impairment or significant cognitive deficit. Damage to the left hemisphere tends to lead to more severe deficits, especially of language and calculation ability.

Psychological reactions, such as depression, anxiety states and irritability, often occur as understandable responses to the changes wrought by the injury to life style, employment and family. Pre-morbid personality, family support, understanding employers and appropriate psychiatric and psychological management are vital in diminishing these reactions. It is clear that the population who suffer head injuries are not a normal population, there is a high incidence of pre-existing developmental learning difficulty and personality disorder since head injuries are more likely to happen to those who drive recklessly, drink too much or get involved in fights.

Definite psychotic disorder may emerge after TBI. Schizophreniform disorders occur more often than by chance (about 2.5%) and purely paranoid psychoses in a further 2%. Psychotic depression occurs in only 1% and very few manic-depressive disorders are seen apparently as a result of TBI. Most series also report a raised suicide rate, as a late complication following head injury.

A fascinating variety of true 'Hysterical' disorders which have an organic basis may appear for the first time in diffuse brain injury, particularly due to anoxia (Eames, 1992). Specific neuropsychiatric and neurological sequelae also include anosmia (the olfactory nerves are particularly vulnerable), other cranial nerve deficit (especially ophthalmoplegias, deafness, visual field defects) and complex movement disorders due to a combination of brain stem, cerebellar and cortical dysfunctions (e.g. the coarse shoulder muscle tremor of red nucleus damage, balance problems, rigidity, slowness and weakness). Communication difficulties may be profound and involve complex dysarthrias, 'pseudobulbar' disorders and impaired intonation, which can combine with impaired facial mobility and a variety of subtle perceptual difficulties to result in severely damaged social skills.

Post-traumatic epilepsy (PTE) falls into two groups (Caveness *et al*, 1979). Early seizures are those which occur in the first week and are seen in 2–5% of cases of TBI. These early seizures are usually focal and reflect acute brain injury. About a quarter of cases will go on to develop the second category, late PTE, which develops after one week. Only 3% of those without early PTE develop later fits. Depressed fracture (15% risk) and intra-cranial haematoma (35% risk) are the other factors which significantly predict late PTE. Fifty per cent have their first fit in the first year after injury (peak at six months) and 80% in the first four years. Development of late PTE is significantly associated with a worse psychological and social prognosis.

Age at injury will significantly affect prognosis. Older people have a relatively poor outcome for mortality and intellectual impairment (Goldstein *et al*, 1994). Children may be more resilient but vulnerable to developmental delays as a result of specific injury, leading to complex and ongoing interaction between the effects of injury and the developing brain. Behavioural disturbances, particularly over-activity and explosive outbursts may be seen as well as specific learning difficulties (Kinsella *et al*, 1991). There is an increasing recognition of the potentially damaging long-term effects of TBI in childhood, but this remains an under-recognised problem and an under-researched area. The sequelae of injury therefore depend on multiple factors (Box 23.5).

Post-concussional syndrome

After an apparently minor TBI, with brief or even no loss of consciousness, a troublesome but characteristic group of symptoms may occur, usually immediately or within the first two weeks. This is termed post-concussional syndrome (Lishman, 1988). There appear to be two groups of symptoms.

The first group appear within the first seven to 14 days, becoming less prominent later. The symptoms include headache (found in 39%), dizziness (27%), fatigue (23%), hypersensitivity to noise (17%) and difficulty concentrating (15%). It is thought there may be a physical cause for these symptoms – particularly otological (labyrinthine) and cerebral possibly due to cerebral circulation changes and microhaemorrhages. Investigations such as brain stem auditory evoked responses and MRI scans may show changes.

The second group of symptoms appear after the first 14 days and may continue for several weeks. These include anxiety (23%), insomnia (21%), irritability (12%), subjective memory impairment (10%) and depression (6%). These symptoms may be more psychologically determined, being more related to premorbid personality, current stresses, social factors and compensation issues.

Fifty-seven per cent of people after such head injuries have symptoms (especially headache and dizziness) for up to two months, but only 1% are symptomatic after one year. An individual's expectations of sequelae may have powerful effects (Mittenburg *et al*, 1992). The management of those with minor head injuries and post-concussional syndrome is symptomatic and patients should be offered early advice and reassurance about what to expect and when it is best to return to work, which should not be so early as to result in failure nor so late as to risk invalidism.

Chronic traumatic encephalopathy (punch drunk syndrome)

Repeated rotational TBI, particularly as seen in less successful boxers, can result in chronic traumatic encephalopathy (or punch drunk syndrome or dementia pugilistica) (Johnson, 1969; Casson *et al*, 1984). This syndrome is less likely to occur with vertical TBI as may happen in footballers who 'head' the ball frequently. Chronic traumatic encephalopathy consists of characteristic neurological and psychiatric features with typical neuropathological findings. There is severe neurofibrillary tangle formation with less prominent plaque formation than in Alzheimer's dementia, although recent immunocytochemical studies have shown extensive beta protein (plaque) deposits in severe cases. Cortical and cerebellar atrophy and cavum septum pellucidum are seen on scanning, even before any clinical symptoms appear.

The neurological symptoms result from cerebellar, pyramidal and extrapyramidal damage. Dysarthria, poverty of movement and facial immobility are seen early, followed by ataxia, tremor and spasticity. The main psychiatric features include dementia, apathy, irritability and disinhibition. Paranoid features, in particular and morbid jealousy may develop (Johnson, 1969). Progression of neurological and psychiatric features occasionally happens even when the boxing has stopped. Very rarely improvement occurs.

Social and family sequelae

As all those involved in the rehabilitation of the head injured will know, the injury is done to the whole family. TBI results in a huge burden of care, largely borne by the immediate relatives. Stress within the family is usually due to the behavioural, personality and cognitive changes and not due to physical handicap (Weddell *et al*, 1980; Tellier *et al*, 1990). After severe TBI only 50% can be left in charge of the home for any time. There are major role changes for spouses, and the financial strain may be unbearable. Social isolation often results for the whole family.

Box 23.5 Aetiological factors in TBI sequelae

Brain injury: amount and location
Development of post-traumatic epilepsy
Age
Premorbid personality (includes constitution, psychiatric
   history, IQ, physical disorder and alcohol ingestion)
Psychological reaction to the injury
Family, social and work factors
Compensation issues
Appropriateness of rehabilitation measures

It has consistently been shown that the disinhibition of anger and disruptive or childish behaviour are the most damaging changes and the child of a parent with TBI is especially at risk of developing emotional and behavioural problems (Urbach & Culbert, 1991). Studies which have compared the effects of TBI on the family with the effects of other injuries (e.g. spinal injury) consistently show that TBI is more damaging. The burden of care on the family is exacerbated by the lack of facilities for proper rehabilitation and of professionals trained in this field.

Rehabilitation

The process of rehabilitation after head injury must start early and continue late. It is best carried out by a comprehensive head injury team, a single medical and paramedical grouping who are involved in the initial triage of all TBI patients and can carry on with the acute management, early and continuing assessment and long-term rehabilitation. Such a team can reduce the need for admissions, concentrate on appropriate cases, provide training, offer consistent advice to the patient and family and engage in proper research, as well as providing appropriate and comprehensive rehabilitation programmes (Box 23.6). The team should include a neurosurgeon, neuropsychiatrist, nurses, neuropsychologist, social workers, physio-therapists, occupational therapists, speech therapists, cognitive therapists, and teachers. Head injuries result in a wide variety of different disabilities, each requiring its own specific therapeutic measures. Movement and tone problems require physiotherapy and occupational therapy, and this may sometimes be combined with anti-spasticity drugs such as baclofen and dantrolene. Baclofen is the most widely used but should be introduced cautiously as it may exacerbate epilepsy and can result in an organic psychosis. Dantrolene may be less effective but has fewer neuropsychiatric adverse effects. Recently the injection of Botulinum toxin into affected muscle groups has shown some success. Speech and communication difficulties may be helped by the speech therapists, and this may involve retraining in language and writing skills, the use of communication aids, speech therapy for dysarthrias, dysprosody, intonation and volume problems.

Deficits in the activities of daily living require careful *in vivo* assessment and diplomatic management by trained occupational therapists and nurses accustomed to working with head injury patients, since the combination of emotional fragility and unrealistic self-judgement with variable motivation can be difficult to handle. Social skills may be deficient and social skills groups are sometimes useful as well as individual behavioural programmes.

Cognitive deficits should be carefully assessed, both by a neuropsychologist for detailed psychometry and by an occupational therapist for skills of daily living in the home environment. The results in the two settings may be very different. This information is needed to plan therapy from a baseline and for measuring outcome. Cognitive rehabilitation includes re-education, compensation (for permanent deficits) and substitution of new methods of functioning. Memory aids and strategies, as well as computer retraining techniques may be used. In some cases carefully graded training in problem solving is helpful.

Severe behaviour disorders have been successfully treated using consistent token economy behavioural modification techniques (Wood & Eames, 1981). Some behaviour disorders are partly the result of learning a poor coping mechanism in the early period after the injury and may also result from a lack of proper rehabilitation. Specialised head injury rehabilitation units are needed for successful management provided in a consistent and controlled fashion.

Drug therapy is best avoided when possible. This is because excessive or unusual adverse effects can occur in those with TBI. A number of drugs have been used in a rather experimental way. There are claims that vasopressin may improve attention, bromocriptine improve speed of thinking, and stimulants such as the amphetamines or diethylpropion briefly improve alertness. Episodic dyscontrol may be reduced by carbamazepine. Sedative antidepressants, tranquillisers and anti-convulsants (particularly phenytoin) should only be used if necessary. However post-traumatic psychosis and depression must be properly treated with medication in the usual fashion. Prophylactic anti-convulsants, preferably carbamazepine or valproate, should probably be given if one or more of the poor prognostic indicators are present (early seizures, depressed fracture, intra-cranial haemorrhage).

The team will need to involve the family and offer family support at every stage and careful discharge planning will be required. Work assessment with the help of a Disablement resettlement officer and Employment rehabilitation centre may be very helpful. "Headway", the National Head Injuries Association, a self-help organisation for those with TBI and their families, can offer support and respite day care in some centres.

Prognosis

After severe TBI, improvement is usually relatively rapid over the first six months, leading sometimes to unrealistic expectations for the longer term

---

Box 23.6 A comprehensive service for head injury patients

Acute triage and initial intensive in-patient hospital care
A follow up expert clinic (and team) for all TBI admissions
Intensive and comprehensive rehabilitation after initial recovery
  for some
Long-term sheltered or in-patient accommodation for a few
Family support

in an ill prepared family. There is further slower physical and cognitive recovery over the next 18 months. After two years, further recovery is expected but usually is due to compensation, readjustment and acceptance over the following three years. After five years, little substantial improvement can be expected, although gains produced by a rehabilitation programme may actually multiply (Wilson, 1992). A few TBI patients will never be self-supporting even though they should be given as much independence as possible.

Cerebrovascular disease

Stroke, or cerebrovascular accident, results primarily from atherosclerosis and/or hypertension. It occurs in two forms, infarction or haemorrhage. Brief recurrent episodes are termed transient ischaemic attacks. The nature of the sequelae of a stroke will depend on the main cerebral artery occluded or the area of haemorrhage. After a stroke about 30% show permanent cerebral symptoms, particularly with severe cognitive impairment, 6% develop seizures and 50% die within three years. The account given below will focus on psychiatric and cognitive symptoms.

Non-dominant middle cerebral artery occlusion may cause confusional states with few focal signs except sensory loss, inattention and anosognosia and this may lead to diagnostic difficulties. Occlusion of the anterior cerebral artery may result in global dementia and frontal lobe personality changes. Posterior cerebral artery occlusion causes cortical blindness with denial of disability and at times with alexia without agraphia, while transient confusion is common. Occlusion of the rostral basilar artery can result in bizarre hallucinations, disorientation and somnolence.

Progressive, global dementia with step-wise deterioration is the classical picture of multi-infarct dementia, possibly with multiple lacunar infarcts. Gradually progressive organic personality change may also follow, with the individual showing increasing difficulty in coping with new experiences. Anxious or irritable responses to anything unusual are common and may amount to catastrophic responses, particularly in cerebrovascular dementia. Hypochrondiacal and depressive features may predominate. Eventually, emotional flattening, stereotyped reactions and irritability may be very marked.

Depression is common after stroke, occurring in around one-third of cases and usually lasts for at least six months. Clinical depression must be distinguished from the reasonable resignation in an elderly person, understandable distress at the disability, underlying or exacerbated personality traits, and cognitive impairment with mental slowing. Causation is likely to be multi-factorial, and a premorbid history of anxiety or depression, previously self-sufficient personality and a lack of family support may all contribute. However, stroke causes more depression than other similarly disabling conditions and it has been suggested that left frontal infarcts are particularly associated with the development of depression although not all studies show this (Folstein *et al*, 1977; Robinson & Price, 1982). The relationship may result from subcortical atrophy in the frontal regions (Palmini, 1992). Psychotic disorders occasionally follow a stroke, with paranoid hallucinatory psychoses being associated with right hemisphere damage.

Psychological reactions of various kinds are very likely to occur and may bring stroke patients to the notice of psychiatric services. In particular, inappropriate dependency, regression and loss of confidence and, at times, manipulative behaviour for secondary gain, may be seen. Alternatively, stubborn refusal to recognise the disabilities and allow appropriate rehabilitation may result in exasperated calls for help from carers.

Stroke rehabilitation

Rehabilitation is aimed at promoting recovery and optimising the use of residual function. A number of the principles of stroke rehabilitation overlap with those of head injury rehabilitation, but there are also many fundamental differences. A multi-disciplinary team of committed workers is required, with rehabilitation starting early and proceeding as a lengthy, staged process. The differences are related to the fact that there is more physical disability, more speech disorder and less personality changes in stroke patients. The lesion is also different (focal cortical rather than diffuse axonal), and the patients are usually much older and the disorder likely to get worse rather than better over the long term. Stroke rehabilitation (where it occurs) is generally seen as a neurological rather than a psychiatric speciality. However, psychiatric principles of patient and family support and intervention, along with the appropriate use of psychotropic medication still apply.

Subarachnoid haemorrhage

Subarachnoid haemorrhage affects a younger population than other strokes and the sequelae are more likely to bring the patient to the psychiatrist's attention. The usual cause is a ruptured berry aneurysm, although no cause is found in 15% and angiomas are the cause in 5–10%. Occasionally subarachnoid haemorrhage may apparently be the result of acute or, more usually, prolonged emotional stress, especially in patients with normal angiograms.

Sequelae

Persistent memory and dysphasic disability is found in 40%, with severe problems in 10%. Middle cerebral aneurysms cause the most severe cognitive sequelae. Worsening cognitive sequelae after subarachnoid haemorrhage may be due to normal pressure hydrocephalus which can be relieved by inserting a ventriculo-peritoneal shunt. A severe amnesic syndrome resembling Korsakoff's psychosis may emerge in the days or weeks after haemorrhage but is usually short-lived.

Severe personality impairment occurs in 20% and mild changes in a further 20%. Anterior communicating artery haemorrhage may result particularly in "frontal lobe personality disorder" with disinhibition. However, middle cerebral artery rupture is associated with both cognitive deficit and personality change in the form of loss of drive, withdrawal, irritability, anxiety and "organic moodiness" (shallow, rapidly reactive depression). About 5% are reported to have an improvement in personality becoming less irritable, anxious, gloomy or obsessional.

Depression and anxiety are found in about 25%, particularly in posterior communicating aneurysms which interfere with the blood supply to the hypothalamus. Disabling anxiety and agoraphobia may present as a response to subarachnoid haemorrhage. At times symptoms rather like the post-concussional syndrome (fatigue, headache and dizziness) occur and may be psychologically determined. Psychotic disorders occasionally occur.

Subdural haematoma

Subdural haematoma usually presents either acutely, with stupor or coma together with some evidence of localising signs, or it may present chronically. The cause is usually a head injury although this may be trivial and spontaneous haematomas occur. Chronic onset is usually with headache, poor concentration and memory loss but this may be fluctuating. Progression is to variable levels of consciousness down to coma, with few neurological signs although the pupils are often unequal. Papilloedema is usually absent. Subdural haematoma may present as a progressive generalised dementia and the true cause can be easily missed unless a CT scan is performed. In early cases, surgical evacuation of the haematoma is very successful but cognitive impairment is common if surgery is delayed.

Migraine

Migraine is thought to affect up to 20% of the adult population although only 7% seek medical attention. Precise diagnosis and distinction from tension headaches may be difficult, but unilateral onset, and throbbing headache with nausea, vomiting and photophobia are characteristic; this is termed common migraine. If visual or other neurological auras are present, the headache is a classical migraine. More severe effects may occur, such as brain stem dysfunction with vertigo, ataxia and occipital headache in 'basilar' migraine, hemiplegia in 'hemiplegic' migraine and paralysis of external ocular movement in 'ophthalmoplegic' migraine.

A particularly severe form is cluster headache or migraineous neuralgia. This consists of marked peri-orbital pain with lacrimation, nasal blockage and sometimes a Horner's syndrome. Cluster headaches are so called since attacks occur in bouts lasting several days or weeks, often at the same time each day or night.

Precipitation of attacks may result from various dietary factors such as cheese, red wine, coffee or chocolate. Psychological stress has also been implicated but the headache often occurs after the stress is resolved, for example, weekend and holiday migraines are typical. Menstruation, the pre-menstruum, and the contraceptive pill may provoke attacks.

Earlier suggestions that obsessive or repressed personalities are more prone to migraine, have not been substantiated and although there is a suggestion that people with migraine may be more emotionally reactive they are otherwise a normal cross-section of the population (Wolff, 1963).

Mood changes before and during an attack are very common, particularly anxiety, irritability and fatigue. Depression, slowed mentation and poor concentration often occur. Elevation of mood, either before or after the attacks, has also been reported. Altered level of consciousness, mental confusion and even lapses into unconsciousness (migraineous syncopy) may happen. Dramatic psychiatric symptoms are sometimes seen, including dreamy states, complex hallucinations, amnesia, body image disturbances, autoscopy, forced mood, automatisms and compulsive behaviour. Sacks (1992) illustrates the clinical fascination of migraine to the neuropsychiatrist.

Management

Prophylactic treatment is needed for migraineous headaches occurring as frequently as two or three per month. High dose propranolol (up to 320mg per day) is probably best in those who do not suffer from asthma or heart complaints. Pizotifen may be effective but can cause drowsiness, especially if introduced too rapidly. Methysergide is a potent prophylactic agent but can only be given for up to six months at a time because of the danger of retroperitoneal fibrosis.

Acute episodes may be treated with a variety of ergot derivatives and analgesics, if they are given as soon as an attack starts. Over-use of ergot results, paradoxically, in chronic headache, and can lead to a dependency syndrome. Sumatriptan is an effective acute treatment for migraine, including cluster headaches, but has cardio-vascular contraindications. Biofeedback, acupuncture and other 'alternative' therapies may have a part to play and biofeedback of distal finger temperature has been shown to be effective in controlled trials. Stress management, psychotherapy and behavioural approaches may also be appropriate.

Transient global amnesia

This acute amnesia for recent events but with preservation of alertness and memory for personal identity is thought to be due to reversible ischaemia of the infero-medial temporal lobes (Bolwig, 1968). It is seen in late middle or old age and is associated with a high incidence of cerebro-vascular risk factors. It may be precipitated by various sudden physical, vascular or emotional stresses. Sometimes it is associated with epilepsy, migraine or hippocampal tumours.

The clinical hallmarks (Guidotti *et al*, 1989) are a sudden onset of memory loss for recent events, an inability to register new impressions and retrograde amnesia. Innate abilities (e.g. musical) and personal identity are not lost, but semantic memory and frontal lobe functioning may be affected (Hodges, 1994).

Recovery occurs in less than 24 hours and persistent amnesia for the episode is usually the only deficit. Some may go on to develop transient ischaemic attacks or, rarely, completed stroke (Guidotti *et al*, 1989).

Miscellaneous neurological disorders

Multiple sclerosis

The neuropsychiatric manifestations of multiple sclerosis can be divided into the psychiatric (particularly affective) and the cognitive. The major psychiatric complication in multiple sclerosis is depression (Surridge, 1969). Two-thirds of patients will suffer transient mood changes, significant anxiety and irritability in a year and 30% will suffer from clinical major depression. The lifetime prevalence of major depression is as high as 50%. An increased incidence of bipolar disorder is also seen. The presence of depression does not directly relate to the degree of demyelination seen on the MRI scan but rather to perceived stress. Family history and past history of depression are not related to the development of depression in multiple sclerosis. A model of interaction between organic vulnerability and enhanced effects of environmental stresses is suggested.

Euphoria occurs in only 10% and is correlated with MRI changes. Pathological display of emotion, free of appropriate mood changes, is related to pontine, brain stem and peri-ventricular lesions. Transient manic, schizophreniform or confusional psychoses may relate to the disease process. It is of interest that schizophreniform psychoses are related to MRI changes in the temporal horn or occasionally may be due to high dose steroid therapy. Multiple sclerosis rarely presents with psychiatric symptoms, but if it does neurological signs are usually present as well, for example, in an acute encephalitic onset with confusion (Skegg, 1993).

About half the multiple sclerosis patients attending hospital have cognitive impairment, particularly of memory, attention and abstracting ability. This may be present before any neurological signs appear. Cognitive deterioration is closely related to the course of the disease, with little evidence of deterioration when the disease is stable, and a worse cognitive prognosis in the chronic progressive form of the disease (Bergin, 1957). The severity of the cognitive impairment correlates with the overall extent of pathology seen on MRI scans but direct correlation between particular cognitive deficits and localisation of the pathology is not yet established (Ron & Logsdail, 1989). Ron & Feinstein (1992) point out that psychiatric and cognitive abnormalities are often overlooked, but add considerably to the patient's distress. Psychiatric disorders should be energetically managed in the usual fashion, and antidepressants are likely to be effective for depression. Cognitive rehabilitation, supportive psychotherapy and family support will also be needed.

Systemic lupus erythematosis (SLE)

Over 50% of patients with SLE show neuropsychiatric manifestations, usually later in the disease, but sometimes occurring before the appearance of other symptoms (Baker, 1973). A wide variety of psychiatric presentations may occur, often in brief episodes lasting a few weeks. Multiple neuropsychiatric symptoms may be present sequentially or together. Thirty per cent show organic reactions, usually brief acute confusional states, but occasionally progressive dementia is seen. Functional psychoses (depressive, schizophrenic or manic) occur in 16%, and seizures in up to 50%.

These psychiatric symptoms are almost always directly due to the pathological brain changes (small blood vessel inflammatory changes) although the relationship is not exact. Steroid therapy is rarely the cause of the symptoms and may be effective therapy for them.

Polyarteritis nodosa

Polyarteritis nodosa results from focal arteritis of small and medium blood vessels. Cerebral symptoms occur in 50% at the later stages of the disease. Confusional and delirious states are the most common presentation (Ford & Siekert, 1965).

Motor neurone disease (amyotrophic lateral sclerosis)

This is a slowly progressive disorder with prominent peripheral manifestations (lower motor neurone muscular atrophy and spasticity due to cortical spinal damage). Neuropsychiatric manifestations include pseudo bulbar palsy, with loss of emotional control, spastic dysarthria and dysphagia; and frontal lobe dementia (Neary *et al*, 1990), which may, rarely, be of marked degree with loss of paramedial cortical cells, gliosis and spongiform changes. In many patients milder changes are seen in the cortex and subcortical nuclei.

Depression is understandably found in a proportion of patients but not as frequently as might be expected, since denial of unpleasant emotions is said to be particularly prominent in the personalities of people developing motor neurone disease (Hogg *et al*, 1994), although denial may be a useful stratagem in the face of such a debilitating condition.

Friedreich's ataxia

Friedreich's ataxia is a recessively inherited, spino-cerebellar ataxia, with kyphoscolosis, and pes cavus. There is dysarthria, nystagmus, cerebellar dysfunction, hypotonicity, muscle wasting and weakness. The course of the disorder is slowly progressive. There is no initial cognitive impairment but a mild cognitive decline may occur as a result of the extension of the degenerative process into the cortex and a few familial cases may have mental retardation. Personality changes have been reported, particularly immaturity and asociality. Paranoid schizophreniform disorders, with episodes of nocturnal hallucinosis and confusion may be particularly associated with Friedrech's ataxia, although the evidence is not clear (Davies, 1949).

Myasthenia gravis

Myasthenia gravis is an auto-immune disorder of motor end plates, resulting in abnormal muscle weakness after activity (Sneddon, 1980). The disorder may be significantly aggravated or even precipitated by emotional stress. The symptoms are likely to be socially embarrassing and difficult for others to understand or believe. This leads to more complex psychological reactions in the individual concerned as well as diagnostic confusion. A diagnosis of hysteria or personality disorder is often mistakenly made initially and even after using anticholinesterase drugs, tensilon or neostigmine, the diagnosis may remain in doubt if a placebo response is suggested.

Duchenne muscular dystrophy

Duchenne muscular dystrophy is an X-linked recessive disorder in which there is a pseudohypertrophy of lower leg and then pelvic girdle muscles. Considerable debate has taken place about whether the associated learning difficulties are an organic or environmental part of the disorder. There is no special relationship with other psychiatric disorders.

Dystrophia myotonica

Dystrophia myotonica is an autosomal dominant myopathy characterised by delayed relaxation of skeletal muscles after voluntary contraction (myotonica) – especially of the hands, forearms and facial muscles (Caughey & Myrianthopoulos, 1963). This is accompanied by slowly progressive wasting and weakness and dysarthria. Associated features include cataract, hypogonadism, frontal balding in the male, cardiomyopathy, endocrine anomalies, respiratory arrest after barbiturate anaesthesia and a typical EMG abnormality. Cerebral involvement is shown by a high rate of EEG abnormality with theta and delta waves and sometimes focal sharp wave discharges. Mental symptoms are seen in up to 80%, with mental impairment being moderate or severe in around one-third of the cases. Social and intellectual decline is seen in families affected by the disease, even in those who do not show the myotonica. "Anticipation" refers to worsening of the disorder over successive generations. Personalities are said to be characteristic, with poor initiative (laziness), somnolence, fatigue and apathy, possibly due to diencephalic and perhaps frontal involvement in the disease process.

Normal pressure hydrocephalus

This is also known as communicating hydrocephalus and results from blockage of CSF flow in the subarachnoid space, usually in the basal cisterns (Vanneste, 1994). Unlike obstructive, non-communicating hydrocephalus it is not associated with high intra-ventricular pressure. It may be difficult to distinguish from hydrocephalus ex-vacuo, which is secondary to atrophy as seen in Alzheimer's disease. Normal pressure hydrocephalus may be the result of subarachnoid haemorrhage, head injury or meningitis, but 40% are of unknown cause particularly in patients aged 60 or more.

The characteristic triad of clinical features is the gradual development of mental impairment, unsteady gait and urinary incontinence (Pujol *et al*, 1989). Memory loss, slowing of mental activity, reduced spontaneity and impoverished psychic life are the main mental features, leading eventually to a picture of severe dementia. Falling is common but seizures are rare. Initial presentation with depressive or paranoid symptoms can occur and these may be partially responsive to psychotropic medication (Pujol *et al*, 1989). Headache and papilloedema are not features. Focal neurology signs are absent. The EEG usually shows slow wave activity, and the CT scan ventricular enlargement, peri-ventricular lucency and generally minimal sulcal widening. Intracranial pressure monitoring is the most reliable method of establishing the diagnosis, showing normal or low pressure but with characteristic pressure wave patterns. Improvement after the insertion of a ventriculo-caval shunt may be dramatic, especially if there has been a complete block to subarachnoid CSF flow. Normal pressure hydrocephalus is a differential diagnosis of dementia and resistant or atypical depression, and highlights the importance of ordering a CT or MRI scan in these circumstances.

Behçet's disease

This rare syndrome, caused by a virus, primarily consists of attacks of oral ulceration, genital ulceration and uveitis/iridocyclitis. CNS involvement is occasionally seen and occurs as a late and ominous complication. Headache, fever, brain stem signs and a variety of cortical dysfunctions occur in a relapsing and remitting fashion. Confusion and dementia may develop.

Sarcoidosis

Sarcoidosis, with chronic, disseminated granulomatous lesions, affects the CNS in about 5% of cases (Stern *et al*, 1985). The areas most commonly affected are the cranial nerves and the meninges. The brain substance may be involved, especially the hypothalamus and third ventricular region, resulting in somnolence, obesity, memory problems and personality change. Fatigue and atypical depression also occur. Occasionally profound dementia or hallucinosis are reported. The diagnosis is made with chest x-ray, biopsy of skin lesions and the Kveim Test. Elevated serum angiotension converting enzymes and calcium are also seen, as are abnormal lung function tests. The condition is treated with prednisone, and if it is severe high doses are used, and these may cause psychiatric changes which complicate the picture.

Basal ganglia calcification

About 50% of such cases have a deficiency of parathyroid hormone, and a few are related to chronic renal failure, vascular, anoxic or infective cerebral lesions. However, many cases are idiopathic and a few may be familial. Basal ganglia calcification seen on CT scan is often an incidental and non-significant finding. In more severe cases the changes may be associated with dementia and extrapyramidal motor disorders presenting in people in their fifties or occasionally with a schizophreniform psychosis presenting in those in their thirties. The dementia is subcortical with slowing of mentation, forgetfulness and a lack of focal cortical deficit (Cummings *et al*, 1983). Although dementia and schizophreniform disorders are the commonest psychiatric presentations, and found in 50% of published cases, depression and occasional mania are also seen (Trautner *et al*, 1988).

Fahr's disease (familial basal ganglia calcification) is inherited in an autosomal dominant fashion and begins in early adult life with progressive dementia, convulsions and rigidity (Flint & Goldstein, 1992). Recent doubt has been cast both on the familial nature of the disorder and its relationship particularly with psychotic disorder but also with dementia. In an extensive review, Flint & Goldstein (1992) conclude that it is related to learning disability and pseudo-hypoparathyroidism and is not a distinct disease entity.

Hallervorden-Spatz syndrome

A rare familial disorder with extrapyramidal symptoms (rigidity, dystonia, choreoathetoid movements), dysarthria, myoclonus, tremor, postural difficulties, personality change, outbursts of aggression and a gradually developing dementia. Iron-containing pigment is found in the globus pallidus and substantia nigra. Presentation is usually in childhood, although adult cases are reported. The course is progressive to death in 6–11 years.

Carcinoma

The neuropsychiatric manifestations of carcinoma fall into four categories. In addition are the psychological effects on sufferers and their families and the involvement of stress in precipitating cancer (see *College Seminars in Liaison Psychiatry*).

General effects of brain tumours

General effects of brain tumours are largely due to raised intracranial pressure, including headache, drowsiness, confusion and apathy leading to coma if untreated.

Local effects of brain tumours

Local effects will depend on the nature of the tumour (speed of growth, degree of malignancy) and its location. Rapid growth and malignancy (for example, with gliomas) are associated with more severe mental disturbance but slow growing benign tumours (usually meningiomas) may present with psychiatric symptoms and personality change alone and are more easily misdiagnosed. Multiple tumours (usually secondaries) are associated with a particularly high level of mental symptoms, especially confusion and cognitive impairment.

Frontal and temporal lobe tumours are much more likely to present with mental symptoms than parietal, occipital or infra-tentorial tumours (Hunter *et al*, 1968). Seizures may be a presenting feature, especially in temporal and occipital tumours. In general, there are few reliable relationships between tumour site and psychiatric presentation, but the following may be significant:

Frontal lobe tumours

Often these show very few neurological signs initially but can present with irritability, atypical depression and apathy, memory impairment, cognitive slowing and inertia, or with disinhibition, childishness and euphoria. Urinary incontinence can also occur.

Temporal lobe tumours

These may present with seizures, dysphasia, memory loss, affective disorder or, occasionally, schizophreniform disorders. Complex visual, auditory, olfactory and gustatory hallucinations characteristically result from temporal lobe tumours.

Parietal lobe tumours

These are less likely to cause psychiatric symptoms, but can result in disturbance of body image (which may suggest hysteria), depression and rarely personality change.

Occipital tumours

Occipital tumours are not usually associated with an increased presentation of psychiatric symptoms.

Corpus callosum tumours

These are especially associated with the development of rapid, severe cognitive deterioration. Delusional psychosis, catatonia and stupor may occur.

Hypothalamic and third ventricle tumours

These may present with a marked amnesic confabulatory (Korsakoff) syndrome. Removal of craniopharyngiomas from this region may result in a combination of frontal apathy, subcortical slowing, obesity and somnolence which is particularly resistant to rehabilitation. Cysts of the third ventricle may cause progressive dementia due to obstruction of CSF circulation. The combination of worsening intellectual deficit with hypersomnolence (and sometimes with apparent narcolepsy and even cataplexy) strongly suggests a diencephalic tumour.

Pituitary tumours

Pituitary tumours are said to cause mental slowing and apathy, at times with emotional lability and paranoid ideation. They may also result in multiple endocrine changes and problems due to expansion into the diencephalon and temporal regons.

Non-metastatic complications of carcinoma

Between 5% and 10% of extracranial tumours cause some form of distant neurological or myopathic disorder, with about half being neurological manifestations. This is most frequent with lung cancer. Sensory or sensory-motor peripheral neuropathy, myopathy with bulbar palsy and sub-acute cerebellar degeneration are well established non-metastatic effects. Of particular interest to the psychiatrist are the encephalopathic forms. Degenerative and inflammatory changes are seen and may be the result of an altered immunological state and resultant viral invasion. Limbic encephalopathy causes a Korsakoff-like disorder, but with depression, anxiety and occasionally with hallucinations.

Depression

Depression and suicidal ideation are well established as occasional presenting features of carcinoma, even before a diagnosis has been made. Premonitions of illness may occur up to six months before any physical symptoms in up to 50% of cases. The new development of depression in middle or late life is significantly associated with a subsequent diagnosis of carcinoma.

Diagnosis

The widespread availability of CT and MRI scans has eased the fear of psychiatrists about misdiagnosis of brain tumour as a functional disorder. The main misdiagnoses are dementia, neurotic depression and hysteria. In most studies of the psychiatric use of CT scanning, the number of tumours discovered is very small. However, the issue is of great importance. Meningiomas are particularly problematic as early diagnosis and surgery can be curative but they may only be discovered late, when removal is difficult or permanent injury has resulted. A number of tumours found on CT scanning may be incidental to the psychiatric disorder present. It is still necessary to have a high, but proper, index of suspicion in clinical practice since, clearly, only a small proportion of psychiatric patients can be scanned. However, in cases when there are particular indications (Box 23.7) scanning must be carried out.

Infectious diseases

Infectious diseases are rarely a cause of diagnostic confusion in neuropsychiatry, except for initial presentations of encephalitis and neurosyphilis. It was feared that HIV infection would result in an avalanche of neuropsychiatric manifestations. However, psychiatric and cognitive disorders are almost always confined to late stages of this disorder, at which time other needs are usually more pressing. In developing countries chronic parasitic infections remain prominent causes of neuropsychiatric symptoms. In this account emphasis is placed on the neuropsychiatric aspects; details of the pathogens' life cycles, diagnostic tests and treatments are given in textbooks of medicine.

Encephalitis (particularly herpes simplex)

Encephalitis is usually viral, occasionally pyogenic (meningo-encephalitis) and often the precise aetiology is not clear. The commonest single identifiable cause in the UK is herpes simplex, which may also be the most severe form. Presentation is usually with severe progressive headache, vomiting, papilloedema, reduced level of consciousness and coma. However patients may present with seizures, delirium or psychotic symptoms. Focal neurological signs and psychiatric symptoms, especially those indicative of temporal lobe dysfunction (e.g. dysphasia, auditory hallucinations, bizarre behaviour) are most suggestive of herpes simplex. Initial symptomatology may include catatonia, thought disorder, over-excitement and delusions. It is vital to recognise this disorder since early treatment may be life saving. The mortality is very high. Diagnosis is made with antibody titres, but early use of the EEG demonstrating periodic lateralised epileptiform discharges may give vital clues and this is one of the most important indications for the EEG. Treatment is with acyclovir, an anti-viral agent which should be given even in cases of doubt. Dexamethasone may be helpful when intra-cerebral pressure is raised.

Encephalitides (particularly herpes simplex) carry a high risk of prolonged neuropsychiatric morbidity and also have a high mortality (Kapur *et al*, 1994). At least half the survivors show a prolonged episode of disturbed behaviour with restless distractability and poor social adjustment (Oxbury & MacCallum, 1973). This may slowly improve but many are left with dense amnesias, mood disorders, personality change, Kluver Bucy type symptoms and social disinhibition. Post-encephalitic neuropsychiatric disorders are a small but significant group of the chronic brain-damaged population.

Other identifiable encephalitides include Coxsackie B, Lyme disease (Neuroborreliosis) (Halperin *et al*, 1991) as well as epidemic encephalitis (various types – transmitted by ticks or mosquitoes), equine encephalomyelitis (Eastern or Western USA – mosquito borne), echo, and

---

Box 23.7 Clinical indications for further investigations (CT or MRI scanning) in psychiatric disorders

Atypical presentation, e.g. of depression with marked apathy, schizophrenia with prominent perceptual abnormalities
Lack of response to appropriate treatment
Progressive neurological symptoms (which must, firstly, be examined for)
Episodic dysfunctions (suggesting partial seizures)
Headache
Disturbance of conscious level
Unexplained personality change

cytomegalovirus and the various sub-acute and chronic encephalitic viruses (measles, mumps, rubella). The latter group may cause Sub-Acute Sclerosing Panencephalitis (SSPE) with onset in childhood or adolescence of progressive dementia and mood changes associated with seizures and myoclonic jerks, and with a fatal course usually within 18 months. The EEG indicative of SSPE has complex repetitive generalised high voltage slow wave discharges which are synchronous in all leads and occur at fixed intervals of 5–10 seconds along with involuntary jerks.

Encephalitis lethargica is largely of historic interest, but the dramatic sequelae of the 1918 epidemic is described graphically in the book *Awakenings* (Sacks, 1973). However, occasional sporadic cases are still reported, with marked features of parkinsonism, personality change, tics, stereotypies, echolalia, emotional lability, compulsive behaviour, fugues, oculogyric crises and hallucinatory states (Espir & Spalding, 1956). The putative virus was never isolated although the timing of the onset of some of the cases coincided with influenza epidemics.

Influenza

Influenza very rarely affects the CNS giving rise to an encephalitis. Only Influenza A has been implicated and although encephalitis is rare, benign confusional states, and ocular palsies are described. There are several case reports in the literature. For example, a recent report described two children with encephalitis due to influenza A, and CT scans in both cases showed symmetrical localised hypodense lesions within the thalami and pons (Protheroe & Mellor, 1991). There is no obvious explanation for post-influenzal asthenia, or for the onset of depression and even occasionally mania which may follow in the wake of an influenza epidemic. Recently there has been considerable interest in the role of influenzal infection *in utero* and subsequent development of schizophrenia; this is discussed on page 327.

Syphilis

In developed countries, syphilis is now relatively rare (Catterall, 1977). However, in the absence of routine testing with the VDRL potentially treatable cases may be missed unless there is a high index of suspicion in unusual psychiatric presentations. Syphilis modified by the chance concurrent use of antibiotics for other disorders may be particularly difficult to diagnose.

Syphilis is classically divided into four stages – the localised primary lesion (the chancre), secondary lepto-meningitis, tertiary meningovascular syphilis and the final late stages of tabes dorsalis and general paresis of the insane (GPI). In addition congenital syphilis may affect the newborn infant although the condition may not be diagnosed until childhood or later. The pathology of all stages relates to inflammatory responses with lepto-meningitis, obliterative endartertis and gummas (which are granulomata).

Secondary syphilis may present with headache, lethargy, malaise and slowly progressive forgetfulness and irritability. Occasionally an acute confusional state or seizures develop. Associated cranial nerve phenomena may occur, particularly ophthalmoplegias and the legendary Argyll-Robertson pupil (small, irregular pupils reacting to accommodation but not to light). Tertiary meningovascular syphilis may present with almost any focal neurological disorder from mild headache to stupor, with cranial, particularly third nerve palsies, aphasia, seizures, progressive dementia, hemiplegia and other manifestations of this "protean" disorder.

Tabes dorsalis (degeneration of the different fibres of the dorsal roots) takes the form of a slow development of "lightning pains" which are stabbing severe pains in the legs associated with loss of proprioception causing sensory ataxia. Ocular and pupilliary signs are also often present.

General paresis (or paralysis) of the insane (GPI) is the second late stage disorder of syphilis, occurring 8–15 years after the primary infection in about 20% of untreated cases. Spirochaetes are seen in cortical and sub-cortical tissue in at least 50% of cases. Cerebral atrophy occurs in the anterior two-thirds of the hemispheres. The CSF VDRL test is positive in 100% of cases even in the absence of a serum positive VDRL, although the more sensitive and specific Fluorescent Treponemal Antibody Absorption Test (FTA-ABS) is likely to be positive in the serum.

GPI usually presents with progressive moodiness, reduced emotional control, shallow affect (apathy or mild euphoria), irritability and other frontal lobe personality changes. Forgetfulness, poor concentration and impaired insight also occur. This "simple dementing" form, comprises 50–60% of the cases in the UK (Dewhurst, 1969).

In developing countries a "grandiose" form occurring in 60–70% of cases is most common, presenting with euphoria, irritability, grandiose manner and delusions and hypomanic or manic features. This is seen in only 10% of European cases. A "depressive" form with low mood, melancholic delusions, suicidal thoughts and retardation presents in around 30% of cases. Paranoid schizophreniform and neuraesthenic presentations may also occur. Seizures develop in up to 50% and may be focal. Transient cerebrovascular episodes (e.g. hemiplegia) are seen rarely.

Premorbid personality may play a role in determining the form of presentation, and it has been suggested that the explanation for the raised incidence of grandiose forms in developing countries (as perhaps was the case in Europe in the last century) is that the disease has a raised incidence among those in higher socio-economic groups, while in Europe today, the disease is found more among those in lower socio-economic groups.

Treatment is with high dose penicillin which will usually arrest progress and may lead to some improvement in the mental state. Other psychotropic and supportive measures will also be necessary in most cases.

Human immunodeficiency virus (HIV)

A comprehensive account of HIV is beyond the scope of this chapter, which will focus on areas of most concern to a psychiatrist, particularly the neuropathology, neuropsychiatric and psychosocial aspects.

Neuropathology

The brain is infected very early in the disease and cerebral pathology is found in 90% of patients dying of AIDS. This pathology may be related to opportunistic infections, neoplasms or primary HIV CNS infection. There is often multiple pathology (Table 23.6).

The CNS in early HIV disease

The current evidence is unclear but, in general, there are no early neuropsychological deficits in otherwise asymptomatic HIV infections (Levy *et al*, 1985). A sub-group may have subtle deficits but this may be due to confounding factors (e.g. drug abuse, premorbid IQ, poor education, head injury). There is continuing controversy on this subject but a recent eight year cohort follow-up study in Edinburgh (Egan *et al*, 1992) showed that only slight cognitive decline may take place in HIV-positive patients without other symptoms of AIDS. This slight decline is independent of mood, and has little clinical significance in terms of morbidity or mortality and is not a prognostic indicator. Significant cognitive decline is almost entirely confined to late stages of the disorder. This study, and others, (McAllister *et al*, 1992) have helped to allay the earlier fears (Fenton, 1987) of a rising tide of prolonged HIV dementias in the absence of the AIDS syndrome.

HIV associated dementia

Also known as AIDS dementia complex, HIV encephalopathy and Sub-acute encephalitis, this occurs late in the course of the disease in about 30% of patients and is an "AIDS defining illness". There is usually an insidious onset of difficulty with complex sequential mental activity and slowing of mental processing, along with apathy, mood and personality changes, which may initially be mistaken for depressive illness (Marotta *et al*, 1989). This picture suggests a sub-cortical dementia. Cortical focal deficits and memory loss may be seen but are less common at first. As the disorder progresses to profound dementia, ataxia, dysarthria, social withdrawal and eventually coma and death occur. Zidovudine may slow the progression of the process in early cases. The MRI scan may show white matter abnormalities and focal lesions. The EEG has diffuse slowing and neurophysiological evoked responses may demonstrate impaired sub-cortical function.

Psychosocial aspects of HIV

The psychosocial stresses in patients with HIV may be overwhelming. Reaction to the diagnosis may result in considerable shock. Rejection by family, friends and work may lead to social isolation which further lowers self-esteem. Rejection by at least one confidante was reported in around one-quarter of the subjects studied by King (1989). Loss of loved ones through HIV will also add to the distress. Assessing precisely which factors contribute to the psychiatric morbidity among HIV sufferers has proved difficult because many subjects with HIV also have severe pre-morbid psychopathology, such as intravenous drug use. The haemophilia-HIV population lacks the pre-morbid psychopathology associated with the general HIV population and studies of this group have given some indication of the relevant psychosocial risk factors in HIV subjects which predispose to breakdown. These are (a) a previous history of psychiatric disorder, (b) experiencing recent life events, especially loss, (c) low support from family or friends, (d) lack of a sense of mastery over their life (Dew *et al*, 1990).

The psychosocial sequelae of HIV vary widely in different countries, for example, in Africa rejection is common, but it is much less frequent in Europe and America. This account will be confined to reports from the UK. King (1989) applied the Clinical Interview Schedule to an out-patient sample in London and was able to make an ICD–9 diagnosis (mainly adjustment reactions, neurotic depression, and neurotic anxiety) in around one-third of the cases. A psychiatric diagnosis was correlated with past psychiatric history, worries about health, feeling very unwell, and being unable to work or socialise. There was also a trend for a psychiatric condition to be present for those who have known about their HIV for 12 months or less. Psychiatric disorder was no more common than in other medical settings and King (1989) commented that most patients had adapted surprisingly well to their condition.

Studies which include both in-patients and out-patients with HIV paint a rather more gloomy picture. Seth *et al* (1991) found that 58% had affective disorder, mainly depression but occasional cases of mania, and there were also a few cases with neurotic reactions and personality change. Affective disorders were associated with more serious disease and the presence of pneumocystitis carinii infections. Treatment with zidovudine has also been associated with the precipitation of mania.

The risks for suicide are undoubtedly increased and a 16–36-fold increase has been noted in America (Marzuk, 1991). Suicides are most common among men, and in one series half the subjects had seen the psychiatrist in the previous four days, and around one-half of the subjects were profoundly depressed. Alarmingly, 20% of the suicides occurred on the medical ward (Marzuk *et al*, 1988). The latency between receiving the diagnosis and committing suicide was less than nine months in all cases, and at post-mortem none of the cases was observed to be thin, suggesting

Table 23.6 Neuropathology of HIV

Opportunistic infections	
Viral	Cytomegalovirus (causing encephalitis), ventriculitis, retinitis and inflammation of the choroid plexus in about 20% Herpes simplex, herpes zoster and progressive Multifocal Leuco-encephalopathy due to papavovirus
Fungal	Cryptococcus – with meningoencephalitis, in 5% Candida – with multiple abscesses or meningitis
Parasites	Toxoplasmosis – causing multiple focal necrotic lesions and abscesses in 20%
Neoplasms	Lymphomas: 5%, usually highly malignant, non-Hodgkins B-Cell lymphomas. Epstein-Barr virus may be implicated in the pathogenesis. Kaposi's Sarcoma: may occur, usually as a secondary from elsewhere.
Primary HIV CNS infection	Aseptic meningitis may be an early feature presenting with headache, fever,neck stiffness and cranial nerve palsies. Vasculitis may also develop. Myelopathy, peripheral neuropathy and myopathy may also develop as a result of primary HIV infection. HIV encephalitis with multinucleated giant cells containing viral sequences, distributed multi-focally, in 25%. HIV leucoencephalopathy – diffuse white matter damage with inflammation and demyelination, in 13%.

that suicide occurred early rather than later in the disease. This suggests that suicide was not a terminal event, and that knowledge of the diagnosis has a major impact on suicidal behaviour.

Asymptomatic HIV seropositivity, which is much more common than symptomatic AIDS is associated with a raised rate for attempted suicide, for example, Marzuk (1991) reported a 37-fold increase, but the rates for completed suicide are not known. The time of testing for HIV and the next two to three months are thought to be periods of particular risk, hence the need for counselling at this time.

Psychiatric disorders, seizures and delirious reactions of various types may occur in the later stages, possibly because of secondary pathologies such as fungal infections, toxoplasmosis or CNS lymphoma but may also occur because of HIV alone. Finally the early stages of HIV associated dementia may result in a picture resembling depression.

There has also emerged the group of "worried well", who fear that they have AIDS and are likely to come to psychiatric attention, especially if associated with affective or obsessive–compulsive disorder, which must be treated in their own right (Miller *et al*, 1985).

Psychiatrists are also involved in the management of the psychological effects of AIDS on the family and staff members. An understanding of the importance of counselling and support for those who are rejected and those who have rejected is vital in the management of HIV disease. More specific psychiatric therapy in addition to the anti-viral agents may include neuroleptics and antidepressants although they seem less effective and more likely to cause adverse effects in this group. Psychostimulants have been used to assist cognitive function. Specific cognitive therapies may help the ill as well as the "worried well".

Tuberculosis

Tuberculosis has a long association with psychiatry and was the major cause of mortality in asylums until the advent of chemotherapy for TB. Odegård (1936) showed the mortality for TB among patients with schizophrenia was increased by a factor of 7–9 for men and more than tenfold for women. Resistance to TB was thought to be reduced by poor living conditions prior to admission, poor asylum food and the asthenic constitution.

Epidemiological studies of TB today show that while rates are generally low in most Western countries, there are small pockets, such as in New York, where rates may be rising. TB tends to be a disease confined to the urban poor, the elderly, and those with AIDS; in the UK, immigrants from Asia may be specially vulnerable. Some of the de-institutionalised patients with schizophrenia have joined the ranks of the urban poor and this group may also be at particular risk, as may those still in asylums or in nursing homes, and the disease should always be suspected among those in the high risk groups. Tuberculosis is undoubtedly a major problem in developing countries, and Daniel (1991) estimates that half of the population of the world is infected with *M. tuberculosis*, with 30 million active cases, 10 million new cases and 3 million deaths with TB accounting for 6% of deaths worldwide each year.

Most of these deaths are due to pulmonary TB, and neuropsychiatric presentations are rare. Tuberculosis may infect the meninges resulting in tuberculous meningitis. The CSF characteristically has a high protein, low sugar content and a lymphocytosis. In adults the onset is insidious with a prodromal phase of vague ill health for two to three weeks and then gradual development of anorexia, headache and mental changes such as apathy and irritability. As the disease progresses typical meningeal signs appear, and also some focal signs including oculomotor palsies, ptosis, tremor, hemiplegia and other neurological defects. Papilloedema and choroidal tubercules can be seen in the retina.

TB meningitis may also affect children during a primary infection (i.e. without obvious pulmonary involvement) and present with a febrile fit, or meningitis. Prior to chemotherapy this form of the disease was always fatal but with modern treatment the outcome is often favourable. Williams & Smith (1959) followed 19 adults for four years, and found few lasting cognitive changes although all the patients had amnesia for the first few weeks or months of their illness. Lorber (1961) followed 100 children who survived the illness. Two-thirds recovered completely despite having neurological abnormalities during the acute phase but around a quarter had residual neurological defects including paresis, deafness and blindness which gradually improved although six (6%) with an early onset became profoundly mentally retarded. Occasionally adults develop tuberculomas in their brains and years later develop fits.

Typhoid

This acute infectious disease is caused by Salmonella typhi and rarely paratyphi. Diarrhoea and gastro-intestinal presentation is most frequent, but acute pyrexial confusional states occur in severe cases. In addition, post typhoid psychosis which is often schizophreniform has been reported and is common in Africa as is post typhoid amnesia. Focal cortical symptoms due to meningitis may also occur.

Typhus

This disease is caused by the parasite *Rickettsia prowazekii* carried by the body louse. Epidemics once ravaged Russia and Eastern Europe and were responsible for many of the deaths in the concentration camps in World War II. With improved sanitation the condition has been largely conquered though not completely eradicated. There is direct CNS infection with microscopic nodules in vessel walls and thrombosis. Prior to the introduction of chloramphenicol or tetracycline 60% of those infected died. The disease presents with fever, headache, insomnia, delirium, meningism, focal cortical symptoms, cranial nerve signs and acute delirium alternating with stupor. Cerebellar and peripheral neurological symptoms may occur and survivors often show persistent cortical damage. Other rickettsia cause Q fever, trench fever and rocky mountain spotted fever.

Malaria

Malaria is a protozoan disease transmitted by the bite of the Anopheles mosquito. It is the most important of the human parasitic diseases, affecting approximately 200 million people worldwide and causing approximately one million deaths per annum. Four species of the genus *Plasmodium* (*P. vivax, P. ovale, P. malaria* and *P. falciparum*) are responsible, and most cases of cerebral malaria and fatalities are due to infection by *P. falciparum* (Malignant tertian malaria, black water fever.) The disease has been eradicated from Europe and North America, but remains common in tropical Africa, South America, and parts of South East Asia. Carothers (1953) estimated that 3% of all first admissions to mental hospitals in Kenya were suffering from cerebral malaria. Where malaria is endemic, the disorder should always be considered in the differential diagnoses of psychiatric disorders, and it should also be considered in travellers returning from endemic areas.

Clinical features

The initial symptoms are non-specific, and include lack of wellbeing, headache, fatigue and muscle aching, suggestive of a minor viral illness. In some patients there may also be chest pain, abdominal pain, arthralgia, myalgia and diarrhoea. The classical malarial paroxysms with spikes of fever and rigors at regular intervals are rare. Severe malaria can cause renal failure due to acute tubular necrosis, pulmonary oedema, lactic acidosis, anaemia, jaundice and hypoglycaemia. This account will focus on cerebral malaria and the neuropsychiatric presentations.

Cerebral malaria occurs in around 2% of affected individuals. Sporulata of the parasite cause thrombosis in the cerebral capillaries with haemorrhage and oedema; this results in a diffuse symmetrical encephalopathy and so focal signs are unusual. There may be some passive resistance to head flexion but other signs of meningeal irritation are absent. The eyes may be divergent and a point reflex is common. Muscle tone may be increased or decreased, and tendon reflexes are variable with the plantar being flexor or extensor. Abdominal and cremasteric reflexes are absent. Generalised convulsions occur in 50% of adults with cerebral malaria, and in a higher proportion of children while retinal haemorrhages are present in 15% of patients.

According to Daroff et al (1967) cerebral malaria can present with five different neuropsychiatric syndromes. In order of frequency these are (i) disturbances of consciousness, stupor and coma (most common), acute delirium: (ii) acute psychosis or personality change; (iii) movement disorders with tremors; (iv) a stroke-like syndrome with focal neurological cases; and (v) subacute or chronic cases present with depression or apathy without fever. Increased slow waves may be detected on the EEG in some cases. Acute psychosis and atypical depression in clear consciousness were first reported by Boshes (1947). More recently Prakash & Stein (1990) described the case of a 30-year-old English woman with atypical depression and hypersomnolence which failed to respond to an MAOI. The diagnosis was only suspected at the fourth interview when she described a family holiday in Thailand, in which she mentioned as an aside that she had visited a malaria-infested island, later adding that she had not taken her anti-malaria prophylaxis on returning to the UK. Treatment is with quinine and other anti-malarials.

Trypanosomiasis

Sleeping sickness or African Trypanosomiasis is caused by the *Trypanosome* parasite and is transmitted by the tsetse fly of the genus *Glossina*. An initial febrile illness is followed months or years later by progressive neurological impairment and death. In East Africa the disease is caused by *T.brucei rhodiense* and in West Africa by *T. brucei gambiense*. Insects acquire infection when they ingest blood from mammalian hosts, and after cycles of multiplication in the midgut of the vector, the parasites migrate to the salivary glands, and transmission to humans (or other mammals) takes place during inoculation at the next insect bite. A self-limiting chancre appears at the site of the bite, and there is widespread lymphadenopathy and splenomegaly. Perivascular infiltration of parasites and lymphocytes results in an endarteritis which is responsible for later cerebral damage. Around 20 000 new cases are reported yearly in Africa, and in contrast to malaria the disease tends only to affect the native population in endemic areas, and rarely occurs in tourists.

Stage I disease is characterised by the chancre, malaise, headache, and arthralgias, oedema and hepato-splenomegaly, lymphadenopathy, pruritus, and bouts of high fever lasting several days, separated by afebrile periods. Lymph nodes are said to be moveable, rubbery and non-tender and cervical nodes are visible.

Central nervous system involvement (Stage II disease) is characterised by an insidious development of a variety of neurological symptoms in the form of tremors, incoordination, convulsions, paralysis and confusion, headaches, apathy and daytime somnolence with restlessness at night. A listless gaze accompanies loss of spontaneity and speech becomes halting and indistinct. Extrapyramidal signs include choreiform movements, tremors and fasciculation and a Parkinsonian picture. In the final phase progressive neurological involvement results in coma and death. Treatment is with suramin, pentamidine, and organic arsenicals. The South American variety of trypanosomiasis (Chagas disease) is caused by *T. cruzi* transmitted by the *reduviid* bug. The acute phase generally lasts one month and there is an insidious progression to the secondary stage with cardiomyopathy, myositus, facial swelling and thyroid involvement. CNS involvement is less common but meningo-encephalitis and seizures may occur. Diagnosis is made by detecting antigens to *T. cruzi*, and treatment is with nifurtimox or benznidazole.

Fungal CNS infections

The main agents are cryptococcus, actinomyces and coccidiomycoses and these may cause sub-acute or chronic meningeal symptoms with an insidious onset. A primary psychiatric presentation for these infections is rare. With the advent of AIDS, these infections have become rather more common.

Most respond to antifungal therapies, such as amphotericin B and micanazole.

Toxoplasmosis

The obligate intracellular protozoan *Toxoplasmosis gondii* is responsible for congenital toxoplasmosis (a cause of mental handicap) as well as adult toxoplasmosis. The disease is transmitted in domestic animals (mainly cats), but can be detected in 10% of lamb and 25% of pork prepared for human consumption (Murray, 1991). If meat is not cooked to 60°C or frozen below –20°C cysts remain fully viable, and ingestion of poorly cooked meat remains the most common form of transmission, and infection is often latent or subclinical.

The clinical manifestations of acute toxoplasmosis in adults usually include pyrexia, rashes, headaches and joint pains. They are not very distinctive and are similar to a variety of conditions affecting the lymph glands such as lymphoma, TB, sarcoidosis, Epstein-Barr, Hodgkins and AIDS. The diagnosis is usually made when a patient suspected of having Hodgkins disease is biopsied. Ocular involvement with bilateral retinal involvement occurs in up to 35% of adults affected. Immuno-compromised subjects such as those with AIDS are at special risk.

Infection during pregnancy is a particular hazard because the organism may be transmitted through the placenta. Congenital toxoplasmosis is most severe if the infection occurs early in the first trimester while most infants infected in the third trimester are asymptomatic at birth. Neonatal screening programmes using Guthrie card tests which incorporate an IgM specific for Toxoplasma may help detect cases at birth. A recent study of 600 000 screenings in the USA detected 50 cases giving an incidence rate of a little less than 1/10 000 (Guerina *et al*, 1994). A study of cases presenting to ophthalmological clinics in south London found a much higher rate of ocular toxoplasmosis among subjects born in West Africa (57/100 000) as compared with subjects born in Britain (0.4/100 000) (Gilbert *et al*, 1995). It is estimated that there are 500–600 new cases of congenital toxoplasmosis each year in the UK.

Congenital toxoplasmosis is evident in the first few days of life and presents with seizures, microcephaly, spasticity, opisthotonos, chorio-retinitis, microphthalmus, optic atrophy and other eye lesions and there may be internal hydrocephalus. The liver and spleen may be enlarged with a raised bilirubin and pneumonitis. Calcified nodules may be present on CT scan. Symptoms of the infantile form are similar but do not show cerebral calcification. Mental retardation, which may be severe, is a later manifestation.

A definitive diagnosis is made by isolating toxoplasma in the CSF, but this is often difficult particularly in older children when the diagnosis is suspected on clinical grounds as the cause of mental retardation. In these cases a variety of serological tests including the Sabine-Feldman dye test (for IgG antibody), fluorescent antibody (for a specific anti-toxoplasma IgM antibody) and complement fixative tests are useful. Treatment is with pyrimethamine plus sulphadiazine and all affected infants should be treated to prevent subclinical infection and later recrudescences of infection. In cases of infection diagnosed during pregnancy, women should be offered treatment as well as the possibility of an abortion.

Cysticercosis

Cysticercosis is the result of the encystment of the larvae of *Taenia solium* (pork tapeworm) in the tissues. CNS involvement occurs in 50–70% of the cases. Unselected autopsy studies in Mexico have shown that 2–4% of the population have cerebral cysticercosis, and the disease is now becoming more common in south western parts of the USA because of migration by Mexicans. The disease also occurs in Africa, South East Asia, Eastern Europe and South America. Worldwide it may be the most common cause of neurological disease (Jubelt & Miller, 1989).

Calcified cysts are found in the muscle, skin and various organs and CNS involvement is due to cysts in the brain. These result in seizures, raised intracranial pressure, and meningitis if the cysts are in the meninges. A variety of focal neurological symptoms may also occur depending on the site of the cysts.

Psychiatric sequelae follow as a consequence of the general deterioration in more severe cases, or are due to the associated epilepsy. Dementia, affective disorders and schizophreniform states have been reported (Tavares, 1993). The diagnosis should be considered in anyone with a neurological disorder who has lived in an endemic area. The cysts may be demonstrated by CT and MRI scan. The CSF may show meningitic changes but diagnosis is by specific ELISA antibody tests, and in doubtful cases a biopsy may be necessary. Niclosamide is used to treat the intestinal infections; praziquantel appears to be the first drug to be helpful against cerebral cysts but needs to be administered together with corticosteroids to prevent inflammation; phenytoin may help control fits.

Other worm larvae, *Toxocara* infection (dog and cat round worms), Trichinosis (from pork), Schistosomiasis (bilharzia) and Echinococcosis (hydatid cyst) may rarely affect the CNS.

Whipple's disease

This is a rare multisystem disease with immunological deficits. It presents more commonly among men over 50 with weight loss, lassitude, malabsorption, arthralgia and lymphadenopathy. A slowly progressive dementia with myoclonus, opthalmoplegia and trigeminal neuralgia occurs in some of the reported cases (Halperin *et al*, 1982). The cause is unknown but membrane-bound basilliform bodies are found. Diagnosis is by PAS positive macrophages found on jejunal biopsy. Prolonged antibiotic therapy may sometimes lead to remission.

Movement disorders

Gilles de la Tourette syndrome

Gilles de la Tourette syndrome (GTS) is characterised by both multiple motor and one or more vocal (phonic) tics or noises which occur many times a day in bouts. The number, frequency and complexity of the tics change over time, but are present for more than a year and usually begin before the age of 18 years (see ICD–10 and DSM–IV).

History

The first clear medical description of GTS was made by Itard in France in 1825 when he documented the case of the Marquise de Dampierre. Subsequently she was documented again by Georges Edouard Brutus Gilles de la Tourette (1885), a French neurologist and neuropsychiatrist. He also documented eight other cases of GTS, emphasising the triad of multiple tics, coprolalia and echolalia, which later gained him eponymous fame.

Prevalence, epidemiology and demography

GTS, once thought to be a rarity, is found in all cultures, ethnic and religious groups, presenting with similar clinical characteristics. The exact prevalence of GTS is unknown and depends, at least in part, on the definition, the method of ascertainment and the type of epidemiological investigation undertaken. The generally accepted figure is 0.5/1000 (approximately 110 000 patients in the USA and 25 000 in the UK). The majority of studies agree that it occurs 1.5–3 times more commonly in males than in females and is found in all social classes. There have been several comprehensive reviews of the literature (Kurlan, 1989; Robertson, 1989, 1994) and textbooks which give wide coverage to all aspects of GTS (Cohen *et al*, 1988; Shapiro *et al*, 1978; 1988; Comings, 1990; Chase *et al*, 1992; Kurlan, 1993) .

Clinical characteristics

GTS is essentially a tic disorder, in which both motor and vocal tics occur. A tic is a sudden, rapid, recurrent, nonrhythmic, stereotyped motor movement or vocalisation which is experienced as irresistible, but can be suppressed for varying lengths of time (APA, 1994).

The age of onset of symptoms ranges from two to 15 years, with a mean of seven years. The most frequent initial symptoms involve the eyes, for example, excessive eye-blinking. Although often referred to as a tic disorder, patients with GTS usually demonstrate a variety of complicated movements including forced touching, licking, spitting, jumping, smelling, squatting and a variety of complexities of gait. The onset of vocalisations is usually later than that of the motor tics, with a mean age of onset of 11 years. A variety of utterances are common including sniffing, coughing, throat-clearing, barking, grunting, snorting, low- and high-pitched noises and inarticulate sounds. Coprolalia (the inappropriate uttering of obscenities) occurs in about 30% of clinic patient populations but is uncommon in children or mildly affected cases (2–4%), and it usually has a mean age of onset of 13–14.5 years, disappearing later in up to a third of patients. Overall, coprolalia occurs in less than 10% (APA, 1994). Copropraxia (involuntary and inappropriate obscene gestures) is reported in 1–21% of clinic samples with the palm-backed V sign being common in Europe. Echolalia and echopraxia (copying behaviours) occur in 10–44% of clinic patients. Palilalia (the repetition by the patient of the last word or phrase in a sentence or last syllable of a word uttered by the patient) occurs in 6–15% of patients. These symptoms are common as the syndrome develops into its fullest form, while other more subjective symptoms, such as sensory tics, mental coprolalia and coprographia are only discovered when enquired about directly.

Tics and vocalisations are usually aggravated by anxiety and stress, while sleep, alcohol, relaxation, or concentrating on an enjoyable task usually lead to a temporary disappearance of symptoms. Stimulants such as caffeine, methylphenidate and amphetamines have been implicated in tic exacerbation which may be a dose-related problem (Robertson & Eapen, 1992; APA, 1994). Characteristically, the course of GTS over the person's lifetime is punctuated by the appearance of new tics and the disappearance of older ones. Many GTS symptoms improve and may disappear after adolescence.

Differential diagnosis

Tics are not uncommon in childhood, and the various tic disorders are distinguished on the basis of duration and variety of tics. Transient tic disorder lasts for at least four weeks but less than 12 months, while chronic motor or vocal tic disorder last more than 12 months, but are distinguished from GTS by the requirement that for GTS there should be multiple motor tics and at least one vocal tic (APA, 1994). A syndrome similar to GTS, "acquired Tourettism", has also been reported in association with both short- and long-term neuroleptic use, head injury or carbon monoxide poisoning (Robertson, 1989).

Associated psychopathology

Ever since Gilles de la Tourette himself described the high rates of anxiety and phobia, there has been much interest in the varied psychopathology associated with GTS. It should be noted, however, that published studies show considerable variation in their description of precisely what is associated, and the strengths of these associations, as well as possible underlying mechanisms.

The psychopathology most commonly recognised as characteristic of GTS is obsessionality. Most series of GTS cases report an increased rate of obsessive–compulsive disorder (OCD) and obsessive–compulsive behaviours (OCB). Epidemiologically based studies and family studies have shown raised rates of OCB in first degree relatives. However, the phenomenology observed in GTS subjects shows some difference from the obsessions and compulsions found among those without the disorder. Thus, obsessions among GTS subjects are significantly more often sexual, violent and symmetrical, while touching, counting and self-damaging compulsions are more frequent (Eapen & Robertson, 1994).

Hyperactivity, distractibility and impulsivity are also relatively common in GTS (APA, 1994). There appears to be an association with attention deficit disorder (ADD) (with and without hyperactivity) and rates of 20–90% of ADD are reported in comparison with rates of around 10% in the general population of a similar age. The precise nature of this association is complex and unclear, although there have been recent suggestions that the two disorders may in some cases be genetically related (Robertson & Eapen, 1992).

Around one-third of clinic subjects with GTS manifest self-injurious behaviour (SIB). Rarely the SIB can result in serious injury such as retinal detachment due to head banging, dermatological problems from repetitive skin picking, or orthopaedic problems from knee banging (APA, 1994). In one study the clinical correlates of SIB were found to be increased severity of GTS (as measured by the cumulative number of motor tics), a previous psychiatric history, as well as traits of hostility and obsessionality (Robertson *et al*, 1989). Interestingly some of the mild cases of GTS found in epidemiological studies and relatives of GTS probands may also manifest SIB (Robertson, 1994).

Controlled studies have shown increased rates of depression. Depression is more severe among those with a longer history of GTS, suggesting that it may possibly be reactive to having a chronic, disabling and stigmatising disorder (Robertson *et al*, 1993).

Referral or ascertainment bias may also partly explain the high rates of exhibitionism, discipline problems and other antisocial behaviours found in GTS clinic patients (Robertson, 1989). Comings (1990) consider a variety of other disorders to be associated including dyslexia, learning difficulties, conduct disorders, phobias and panic attacks, mania and manic depressive disorder, schizoid behaviours, alcohol and drug abuse as well as pathological gambling, but the strength or specificity of these associations is unclear.

The IQ in GTS appears to be average but there is often a verbal performance discrepancy of around 15 points (performance being the lower). There are also specific deficits in reading, writing and arithmetic. A recent study has suggested the "intention editor" is dysfunctional in GTS (Baron-Cohen *et al*, 1994), while another investigation has shown specific deficits in attention (Channon *et al*, 1992). The "intention editor", a key mechanism that underlies the will and which begins to function in early childhood, is triggered whenever there are several intentions competing in parallel with each other and is hypothesised to be a subcomponent of the Supervisory Attentional System (Shallice, 1988) which serves inhibition and is subserved by frontal circuits (Robertson, 1994).

Aetiology and pathophysiology

A vulnerability to GTS and related disorders is genetically determined. Good evidence for this comes from the twin study of Price *et al* (1985) involving 43 pairs of same-sex twins in which at least one co-twin had GTS. They reported concordance rates of 53% for monozygotic twins and 8% for dizygotic twins but concluded, however, that non-genetic factors were also important in the expression of GTS (Price *et al*, 1985). It is now recognised that GTS is probably transmitted in an autosomal dominant pattern (Pauls *et al*, 1990; Curtis *et al*, 1992). This vulnerability that the child inherits is for developing a tic disorder, but the precise type or severity of the tic disorder may vary in different generations. However, not all individuals who inherit this vulnerability will express symptoms of a tic disorder. Penetrance in female gene carriers is approximately 70%, but in male carriers is about 99%. The phenotypes of the putative gene may be full blown GTS, chronic motor or vocal tic disorder (APA, 1994), some kinds of OCB (Eapen *et al*, 1993) and perhaps ADD, although this is somewhat controversial. In approximately 10% of those with GTS there is no familial pattern (APA, 1994). It has also been suggested that some prenatal events or exposures such as maternal stress, anti-emetic medication or other unknown agents may lead to changes in the sensitivity of some dopaminergic receptors, and this could partially determine the eventual severity of expression of the diathesis to the GTS (Leckman *et al*, 1990). The majority of chromosomes in GTS are normal although several chromosomal anomalies have been reported (Robertson & Trimble, 1993). Although reports have tentatively assigned the gene to various chromsomes (3, 11, 18), dopamine and D3 receptors, there has been much debate and over 80% of the genome has been excluded.

Early post-mortem (PM) studies have indicated no specific abnormalities. Subsequent PM investigations, however, have suggested decreased 5-hydroxytryptamine and glutamate (especially in the subthalamus) in many areas of the basal ganglia, a reduction in the second messenger cyclic AMP, an increased number of dopamine uptake carrier sites in the striatum (see Robertson, 1994), and a decrease in dynhorphin-like immuno-reactivity in the globus pallidus (Haber & Wolfer, 1992). More recently the involvement of the endogenous opioid system in GTS has attracted further interest (Chappell, 1994). Suggestions for the site of abnormalities have included the limbic forebrain structures, particularly the anterior cingulate cortex, and their inter-relationships with the specific nuclei, periaqueductal grey matter and midbrain tegmentum and the amygdaloid complex. It seems highly likely that several monoamines in different parts of the brain will be implicated (Robertson, 1994).

Other investigations

The EEG is essentially normal in GTS; in particular, there is no evidence of any paroxysmal activity synchronous with the tics. The principal abnormality in the EMG is the absence of the Bereitschafts-potential before the tics. The Bereitschafts-potential probably represents the summed activity of changing firing patterns in preparation for normal movement. This suggests that simple tics are not generated through the normal cortical motor pathways used for skilled movement. Minor abnormalities in the visual and sensory evoked potentials have been found in the range of 90–280 MH which may reflect specific attention deficits observed in some patients. CT scans have not shown any consistent gross abnormalities (Robertson, 1989, 1994). Not unexpectedly, the MRI studies reveal substantially more abnormalities than the CT scan investigations. Abnormalities include primarily those in the basal ganglia and lateral ventricles. These include abnormalities of caudate nucleus size (mostly decrease) and loss of normal caudate asymmetry, abnormalities in the asymmetry of other basal ganglia structures (e.g. putamen and lenticular nucleus), abnormalities in the size of the lateral ventricles and loss of ventricular asymmetry and abnormalities of the corpus callosum (Demeter, 1992; Singer *et al*, 1993; Peterson *et al*, 1993, 1994; Hyde *et al*, 1995). Several abnormalities have also been noted in studies using functional neuro-imaging positron emission tomography (PET) which has demonstrated metabolic and perfusion abnormalities in the basal ganglia, fronto-temporal areas with special reference to the putamen. Single photon emission computerised tomography (SPECT) has shown hypoperfusion in the basal ganglia, thalamus and frontal and temporal cortical areas, as well as in the left putamen-globus pallidus in GTS patients. Although limited due to the small numbers involved, these findings seem to suggest decreased relative metabolic activity and regional cerebral blood flow in the basal ganglia.

Management

Psychosocial measures and pharmacological intervention for the individual, as well as various manoeuvres for helping the family of the patient are all important in managing the condition. For many patients with a mild disorder, explanation and reassurance are often sufficient. In a similar way, the parents of mildly affected children can often be reassured by the diagnosis, explanation about the nature of disorder, information about the self-help groups and booklets for teachers. For the severely afflicted patient, who may have the associated features of ADD, SIB and aggressive behaviours, the management is far from simple.

Although individual psychotherapy may be a useful adjunctive, the tics are not responsive to psychotherapy. While originally it was thought that behaviour therapy was useful in the treatment of tics, it is now not felt to be a useful strategy except in the treatment of the obsessive–compulsive aspects of the disorder, when it can be used alone or in combination with medication.

Chemotherapy is, at present, the mainstay of treatment for the motor and vocal symptoms as well as some of the associated behaviours, and the medications most commonly used for the tics are dopamine antagonists such as haloperidol, pimozide and sulpiride. Extrapyramidal side-effects, sedation and dysphoric states are common with haloperidol, but less so with pimozide. Butyrophenones may also impair concentration and scholastic achievement and cause tardive dyskinesia. Sulpiride has less extrapyramidal problems including tardive dyskinesia and dystonia as well as less cognitive and sedative side-effects compared with haloperidol and pimozide, but gynaecomastia, galactorrhoea, menstrual irregularities and possible depression have been reported. With the neuroleptics these side-effects can be avoided by starting with small doses (e.g. haloperidol 0.25–0.5mg daily) and increasing by 0.5mg every week until a point is reached with maximal benefit and minimal side-effects.

Clonidine is also used with some success and may well be the agent of choice if a child has GTS and ADD. Clonidine has fewer and milder side-effects than the neuroleptics in general but drowsiness, insomnia, dry mouth, headaches and postural hypotension do occur. Clonidine can also be used as a transdermal patch.

Specific serotonin reuptake inhibitors (fluoxetine, fluvoxamine, sertraline, paroxetine) and clomipramine can be used to treat the OCB aspects of the syndrome; augmentation of anti-obsessional effects of, for example, fluvoxamine by neuroleptics (e.g. pimozide) has been reported in patients with obsessive–compulsive disorder and GTS (George *et al*, 1993).

Other medications have been given with success such as the sequential use of opioid agonists and antagonists (Chappell, 1994), fluphenazine, penfluridol, clomipramine, clonazepam, calcium antagonists (nifedipine, verapamil), tetrabenazine, progabide, physostigmine and lithium carbonate (Robertson, 1989). In very severe cases, especially when complicated by OCB and SIB, psychosurgery has been successful.

Wilson's disease

Hepatolenticular degeneration (Wilson's disease) is an uncommon recessively inherited disorder of copper metabolism with a worldwide prevalence of around 1 per 30 000 (Bachmann *et al*, 1979*a,b*). There is an accumulation of copper in the liver, brain, kidney, cornea and bone. It was first described by Wilson (1912) who recognised both hepatic and neurological involvement as well as the familial nature of the disorder. He described the characteristic symptoms which include generalised tremor, dysarthria, dysphagia, muscular rigidity, emaciation, spasmodic contractions, cirrhosis of the liver and emotionalism, and it can present with almost any psychiatric disorder.

The gene for Wilson's disease has been located to the long arm of chromosome 13 (Frydman *et al*, 1985) and recently the gene was cloned (Petruhkin *et al*, 1993). High rates of consanguinous marriage may increase the prevalence, particularly in Japan (Chu & Hung, 1993). Linkage studies among Chinese families in Formosa have shown strong linkage with the gene for esterase D and the retinoblastoma gene. The gene for caeruloplasmin has been located on to chromosome 3, indicating that failure to form the copper protein is not the primary cause.

The exact metabolic defect is uncertain but is possibly due to an inability of hepatic lysozymes to excrete copper that has been cleaved from caeruloplasmin into bile and an inability to store copper due to a deficiency of caeruloplasmin. Copper is deposited in the liver causing a focal necrosis ultimately leading to a coarse nodular post-necrotic cirrhosis. In the kidneys copper is deposited in the tubular epithelial cells resulting in aminoaciduria. Post-mortem studies of the brain show a striking brick-red pigmentation in the basal ganglia as well as spongy degeneration of the putamen leading to the formation of small cavities. Copper is deposited in the pericapillary areas and within the astrocytes. Microscopic studies reveal a loss of neurones axonal degeneration and large numbers of giant multinucleated forms known as Alzheimer cells. Copper is deposited within the astrocytes bound to cerebrocuprein as well as other cerebral proteins, but is absent from neurones and ground substance (Menkes, 1989). In the eye, deposits in the cornea particularly in Descemets membrane are responsible for the characteristic yellow to green to brown Kayser-Fleisher ring . It is almost always associated with neurological or psychiatric disorder.

Presentation, symptoms and signs

Most cases present in the first two decades although it may develop later. Martin (1968) suggested there may be two types: an early onset (7–15 years) which is a more fulminant juvenile type, and a later onset (19–35 years) less fulminant "adult" type. The disease presents with hepatic involvement in half the cases – acute hepatitis, fulminant hepatitis, chronic active hepatitis and cirrhosis. The release of copper may also cause haemolytic anaemia.

The neurological disorder is primarily a disorder of motor function, and there are no sensory symptoms. Tremors and rigidity are common early signs. The tremor may be of the intention type (cerebellar) or it may be due to basal ganglia damage and resemble the alternating tremor of Parkinson's disease. Most commonly it is a bizarre tremor and has been described as "wing beating" (Menkes, 1989). It is generally absent at rest but may be so violent that patients are thrown off balance. Changing the position of the outstretched arms may alter the severity of the tremor. Rigidity and spasms of the muscles are often present. In some cases a typical Parkinsonian rigidity may involve all the muscles. Torticollis, tortipelvis and other dystonic movements may also occur. Spasticity of the laryngeal and pharyngeal muscles may lead to dysarthria and dysphagia. Drooping of the lower jaw accompanied by a gaping smile and drooling are common. Tendon reflexes are increased but extensive plantar responses are rare. Convulsions and coma are also described.

Psychiatric aspects

The nature of the psychiatric disorder in Wilson's disease has been examined in several retrospective series (Dening, 1985; Dening & Berrios, 1989; Akil *et al*, 1991; Huang & Chu, 1992).

Around one-fifth of the cases in one series (Dening & Berrios, 1989) initially presented to the psychiatric clinic. The reported frequency for psychiatric symptomatology varies between the different series from 26% (Dening, 1985) to 65% (Akil *et al*, 1991). The two most frequently observed clinical pictures are (i) affective symptomatology, with emotional lability, incongruity and a picture of neurotic depression, present in 27% of cases (Akil *et al*, 1991; Oder *et al*, 1991); and (ii) a picture of behavioural/personality change, with aggression, irritability, and childish behaviour sometimes accompanied by schizoid, hysterical and psychopathic personality tracts, observed in 45% of the cases in the series of Akil *et al* (1991).

Anxiety, attempted suicide, organic delusional states, catatonia and psychosis have also been reported. In most series, schizophrenia-like psychoses are rare or absent. An exception is in the Chinese population studied by Huang & Chu (1992) who found that 11.3% of their cases presented with psychosis.

Although dementia is a recognised outcome, severe cognitive impairment is rare. Cognitive impairment can be detected particularly among those who are neurologically impaired and those who have abnormalities of the basal ganglia on CT scan (Medalia, 1988). Memory functioning, and impairments in visual function and learning capacity are all affected, but a more recent study has found that motor, psychiatric and memory symptoms are all relatively independent impairments (Medalia *et al*, 1992).

Diagnosis

The diagnosis of Wilson's disease is easy, provided it is suspected (Scheinberg, 1991). The condition should be suspected in any patient under 30 who develops an unexplained CNS disorder, particularly unexplained personality change, cognitive impairment, psychosis, catatonia; and suspicion should be increased if there is any liver disease, or in a patient who has a blood relative with Wilson's disease. The diagnosis is confirmed by the presence of Kayser Fleischer rings and low caeruloplasmin levels. Serum copper is usually low or normal, but serum caeruloplasmin is almost always low. In doubtful cases a liver biopsy may be required and this shows elevated hepatic copper levels. Urinary copper excretion is generally elevated and there may be other evidence of renal disease such as aminoaciduria, as well as evidence of bone disease. Five per cent of cases may have normal serum caeruloplasmin levels. Very rarely, hepatic disorders such as primary biliary cirrhosis will simulate the presence of Wilson's disease. In such situations there are further tests which can discriminate Wilson's disease (Scheinberg, 1991).

It should be remembered that while both corneas should always be inspected for Kayser Fleischer rings, only slit lamp examination is definitive, and their presence is usually, but not always, associated with neurological damage (Willeitt & Kiechl, 1991). CT and MRI studies in Wilson's disease show that ventricular dilation, cortical atrophy and basal ganglia hypodensities are commonly present (William & Walshe, 1981; Starosta-Rubinstein *et al*, 1987). If the diagnosis is confirmed, it is essential to screen the patient's siblings, because asymptomatic cases can be treated prophylactically.

Treatment

Treatment involves the copper chelating agents. The first drug to be used was dimercaprol or British anti-Lewisite (BAL) introduced by Peters *et al* (1945). A more powerful copper chelating agent penicillamine, a breakdown product of penicillin, was discovered by Walsh (1956). A diet restricting foods high in copper (liver, cocoa, chocolate, mushrooms, shellfish, nuts and dried fruits and vegetables) is preferred and penicillamine 1–3 grams daily should be administered, as this prevents virtually every manifestation of the disease. It should be continued for life, as the mortality of those who stop treatment is high. Sensitivity to penicillamine is managed using established protocols, and some success has been claimed for trien (triethylene-tetramine) a new copper chelating agent. Vitamin B6 is required to counteract the anti-pyridoxine action of penicillamine. Hepatic disorder responds less well than neurological or psychiatric disturbance and the response to treatment is variable. Early diagnosis is essential if the disease process is to be reversed.

Sydenham's chorea

Sydenham's chorea, also known as 'St Vitus dance', is characterised by sudden, involuntary, irregular, jerky movements of the extremities, frequently associated with emotional instability and muscle weakness. The onset may be gradual, with complaints that the child is nervous. The patient may become clumsy and stumble, fall or drop objects. There are often complaints from the teachers at school of poor attention and deteriorating handwriting. Facial grimacing and a variety of speech disorders occur. As the chorea becomes more severe, the irregular jerking movements can (rarely) be sufficiently violent to result in injury. Muscle weakness may also be profound. Most of the choreiform movements subside during sleep and are exaggerated by emotions. Characteristically, if the patient is asked to extend the arms, hands and fingers, flexion of the wrists and hyperextension of the metacarpophalangeal joints are observed. The pronator sign may be elicited: following raising of the arms above the head there is gradual pronation of the hands (apposition of the dorsal aspects of the hands). Other signs consist of an inability to hold the tongue still when it is protruded and spasmodic contractions of the hands when the patient intentionally grips objects or the examiner's hands (Amman & Ward, 1982).

Sydenham's chorea is found in 10–30% of children with rheumatic fever (Veasy *et al*, 1987), most commonly in prepubertal girls; it is rare in black and adult populations, although it can reappear in adulthood as chorea gravidarum (Nausieda *et al*, 1980). Obsessive–compulsive symptoms (OCS) have been noted in the context of Sydenham's chorea for some time (Chapman *et al*, 1958). Moreover, a recent controlled study showed that patients scored significantly higher on the Leyton Obsessional Inventory than a rheumatic fever comparison group. Five of the 23 patients with Sydenham's chorea and none of the 14 rheumatic fever subjects obtained obsessional interference scores of 14 or more (Swedo *et al*, 1989). The authors suggested that the high prevalence of obsessive–compulsive features in the disorder supports other evidence linking obsessive–compulsive disorder to the basal ganglia. The same group (Swedo *et al*, 1993) confirmed their earlier findings in a later study, reporting specific OCS in 82% of patients with Sydenham's chorea, as well as increased emotional lability, motoric hyperactivity, irritability and distractibility. Swedo *et al* (1993) also reported antineuronal antibodies in 10 out of 11 children with Sydenham's chorea. Goldman *et al* (1993) described a PET finding of striatal hypermetabolism in a child with the disorder which normalised on clinical recovery, which also further implicates the basal ganglia.

Spasmodic torticollis

Spasmodic torticollis (ST) is the most common focal dystonia (Fahn *et al*, 1987) and is caused by involuntary contractions of the neck muscles resulting in abnormal postures and/or involuntary movements of the head, resulting in a "wry neck" (neck and head rotated and twisted laterally). Patients with the disorder find it very distressing but are generally agreed to suffer no increase of formal psychiatric illness (Sheehy & Marsden, 1982) although obsessive–compulsive symptoms may be more frequent (Jahanshahi, 1991; Bihari *et al*, 1992). Much of the early literature is dominated by attempts to distinguish between organic and hysterical forms of spasmodic torticollis (Meares, 1973). Today hysteria is considered an important differential diagnosis of spasmodic torticollis. Several groups have found that OCS and depression are more common in patients with spasmodic torticollis. Symptomatic improvement with botulinum toxin injection is associated with a significant reduction in depression suggesting that the depression is a consequence of the postural abnormality of the head (Jahanshahi & Marsden, 1988, 1992).

Writer's cramp

Writer's cramp, also one of the focal dystonias (Fahn *et al*, 1987), is characterised by postural cramps of the hand when, for example, the patient attempts to write. Patients with writer's cramp generally suffer no increase of formal psychiatric illness (Sheehy & Marsden, 1982; Grafman *et al*, 1991) but may have difficulty in expressing anger and hostility (Crisp & Moldofsky, 1965). Robertson & Trimble (1988) also demonstrated that patients with writer's cramp had higher hostility than controls on the Hostility and Direction of Hostility Questionnaire.

Dystonia musculorum deformans

Dystonia musculorum deformans can be considered as equivalent to idiopathic generalised dystonia (Fahn *et al*, 1987). The majority have a childhood onset and no associated psychopathology. At one time it was fairly common for patients with dystonia to be misdiagnosed as having a psychiatric disorder (Lesser & Fahn, 1978). Although psychogenic dystonia occurs, it is relatively uncommon and should be diagnosed only if there is clearcut evidence of a conversion reaction or malingering (Fahn *et al*, 1987). Psychogenic dystonia can, however, be severe enough to lead to fixed permanent contractures and warrant surgical procedures (Fahn *et al*, 1987).

Parkinson's disease

Parkinson's disease (PD) is one of the most common neurological disorders of later life with an estimated prevalence of around 1%. The classical neurological manifestations are (i) pill-rolling tremor at a frequency of 4–8 per second, present at rest but disappearing during sleep; the tremor may affect the hands (pronation/supination), jaw, tongue, head or lower limbs; (ii) rigidity affecting the muscles of the limbs, trunk and neck and said to have a "lead-pipe" quality; if tremor is superimposed upon the rigidity then the phenomenon of cog-wheel rigidity may be observed; (iii) hypokinesia which results in poverty of movement (akinesis/bradykinesis) resulting in a slowness in initiating movement; hypokinesia probably explains the mask-like facies and infrequent blinking. Numerous other symptoms may also occur and these include ocular-motor abnormalities, postural changes, flexed posture, festinant gait, excessive salivation, seborrhoea, constipation, subjective sensory disturbance and marked fatigue (Lishman, 1987).

Psychiatric sequelae are common in PD and fall into four main groups: (i) Cognitive decline (global dementia, focal cognitive deficits, drug induced confusional states, depression-related cognitive difficulties); (ii) affective disorders (depressive symptoms, depressive illness meeting diagnostic criteria); (iii) psychotic (depressive psychosis, drug-induced psychosis) (Ring, 1993); and (iv) changes in personality or personality traits (Todes & Lees, 1985).

Depression

An association between PD and depression is well established but it is unclear to what extent the depression is reactive to a serious disabling illness, or whether it is an integral part of the disease process itself. The topic has been reviewed by Brown & Marsden (1984), Ring & Trimble (1991) and more recently by Cummings (1992) and Ring (1993); the descriptions of depression will be collated from these, unless otherwise individually referenced.

Reviewing 26 previous studies, Cummings (1992) reported a mean rate of depression in 40% (range 4–70%). Some of these studies utilised the Beck Depression Inventory to measure depression but this method has been criticised because the scale contains somatic items such as "motor slowing" which may also be part of the motor disorder itself. A more recent study by Dooneief *et al* (1992) found an inception rate for depression of 1.86% per year in PD subjects.

Around half of those with depression satisfy criteria for major depression while slightly less than half qualify for dysthymia or minor depression. It is of interest that minor depression and dysthymia are more closely related to the motor state of PD and also more likely to remit. An older study by Robins (1976) which compared a group of age and sex-matched patients who also had severe disabling diseases (hemiplegia, paraplegia, arthritis) found higher rates of depression among the PD patients than among controls, suggesting that the depression might be a more integral part of the disease process rather than simply being reactive to the disability.

The depression in PD patients shows some minor phenomenological differences from primary major depression. Thus in PD there are high levels of dysphoria, anxiety and pessimism concerning the future, as well as irritability, sadness and suicidal ideation. However, there is rather less in the way of guilt, self-reproach, delusions or hallucinations. Despite a high rate of suicidal ideation, completed suicide appears to be rare.

Risk factors for depression include female gender, a past personal history of depression (but not a family history of depression), bradykinesis, gait instability (rather than tremor dominant syndromes), a greater degree of left brain involvement and an earlier age of onset of the PD (but not current age). The course of the depression has received little attention, but patients with PD can be broadly divided into two groups, one with and one without mood changes, and the groups are relatively stable over time.

The aetiology of this depression is unknown, but it is tempting to speculate on the role of brain monoamines, as both disorders are thought to result from a functional deficiency of central monoamines particularly dopamine and serotonin (5-hydroxytryptamine [5-HT]). The depression seen in PD may be a predictor of future dementia (Stern *et al*, 1993).

Standard antidepressive treatment such as tricyclic antidepressants and ECT appear to be effective in treating the depression (for review see Cummings, 1992). If selegiline (which is a potent MAOI) is being used to treat the Parkinson's disease, SSRIs are contraindicated and tricyclics should be used with caution as well. ECT may alleviate not only the depression but sometimes also the motor symptoms of the PD itself (Lebensohn & Jenkins, 1975; Abrams, 1989).

Thus it would appear that depression in PD is common, but that the true incidence and prevalence are not known. The relationship between the two disorders is complex and with phenomenological differences, and with many factors suggested as being aetiologically significant. The treatment is by conventional methods.

Psychoses

The most common psychotic illnesses in PD are those associated with the anti-PD drugs, and are seen in 30–60% in the late stages of the disorder. Depressive psychosis is also common, with only two schizophrenic psychoses and no manic illnesses being found in a retrospective study of 89 patients (Mindham, 1970). The organic psychoses associated with PD show great variability between individuals, but in general are characterised by affective changes, auditory, visual and olfactory hallucinations, persecutory and paranoid delusions: they are often associated with a past psychiatric history and usually occur within the context of chronic treatment with levodopa or benzhexol. Other psychiatric complications of levodopa include delirium, depression, agitation, hypersexuality, impulsivity, lethargy, anxiety, insomnia and vivid dreams (for review see Robertson, 1990). Clozapine, an antipsychotic without extrapyramidal adverse effects, may prove useful in the treatment of psychosis in the setting of PD although at present the drug is only licensed for use in cases of schizophrenia.

Personality

Reviewing the personality of patients with PD, Todes & Lees (1985) concluded that introspective, over-controlled, anhedonic personality traits together with suppressed agressivity are frequently found, but suggested that it was unclear whether the behavioural patterns were aetiological factors or prodromal symptoms of the disease. In a later study, female PD patients appeared to have a "premorbid personality" characterised by increased hypochondria, depression, hysteria and social introversion on the Minnesota Multiphasic Personality Inventory (Jimenez-Jimenez *et al*, 1992). These personality changes may reflect early symptoms of the PD itself, since motor symptoms only occur once the striatal dopamine content is reduced by at least 80%, and in many cases there is a slow fall in dopamine activity occurring over 20–30 years (Marsden, 1990).

Cognitive disturbances

Cognitive disturbances in PD may be subdivided into generalised global dementia, focal and specific cognitive deficits, drug-induced confusional states and depression-related cognitive difficulties (Ring, 1993).

Dementia. Dementia in PD is rather less common than was once thought, probably having a life-time risk for those over the age of 65 of 10–20%, in comparison with 5–10% of the general population of similar age. Gibb & Luthert (1994) estimate a threefold increased risk over the general population. As in the general population, age is the most important single determinant for the prevalence of dementia among PD subjects. Thus dementia is very rare among those with PD under 40 years, but the prevalence rises to 65% for those over 85 (Mayeux *et al*, 1990). A recent study by Stern *et al* (1993) showed that the risks for dementia were greater for those aged over 70 years, with more severe PD, facial masking as a presenting sign or having developed confusional psychoses while taking levodopa. Typically the patient who has been stable and well maintained for many years on levodopa or a related drug presents with a confusional state, paranoid delusions, visual hallucinations and memory loss. Admission to hospital and stopping the drug lead to some improvement but the underlying dementing picture soon becomes apparent.

In some cases there are more cortical features (temporo-parietal dysfunction) with severe forgetfulness, aphasia, ataxia and agnosia, suggestive of a dementia of the Alzheimer-type (DAT). In other cases the features of subcortical dementia and a fronto-limbic picture are predominant with a pure PD picture of apathy, slowness of thought, depressive symptomatology and rather less memory loss. Ring (1993), however, points out there is little evidence to support the validity of such subgrouping. The neuropathological processes which underlie the cognitive decline are uncertain but are likely to include Alzheimer-like changes, Lewy body disease, cholinergic and dopaminergic deficits as well as the effect of age on the PD process itself.

Focal cognitive deficits. Isolated, focal cognitive deficits are common in PD and may occur in patients without global dementia or depression

(Ring, 1993), and the frontal lobe has been most commonly implicated (Gotham *et al*, 1988; Sagar *et al*, 1988*a*, *b*; Sahakian *et al*, 1988). However, Ring (1993) suggests that the frontal lobe deficits probably also relate to striatal dysfunction. At the stage of mild disability even before treatment commences there may be an impairment on the Wisconsin card sorting test which is known to be sensitive to frontal lobe dysfunction (Lees & Smith, 1983). Cooper *et al* (1991) have shown that even as early as 16 months after the onset of PD there may be significant cognitive deficits including difficulties in immediate recall of verbal memory, cognitive sequencing, working memory, language expression and semantic fluency.

Medication and depression mediated cognitive changes. All the common antiparkinsonian medications may precipitate reversible confusional states. These are most often encountered with anti-muscarinic compounds and selegiline, with elderly PD patients being at greater risk (Ring, 1993). Patients with PD and depression show a greater intellectual decline, with particular problems in frontal lobe tasks.

References

Abrams R (1989) ECT for Parkinson's disease. *American Journal of Psychiatry*, **146**, 1391–1393.

Achte, K. A., Hillbom, E. & Aalberg, V. (1969) Psychoses following war brain injuries. *Acta Psychiatrica Sandinavica*, **45**, 1–18.

Akil, M., Schwatz, J. A., Dutchak, D., *et al* (1991) The psychiatric presentations of Wilson's disease. *Journal of Neuropsychiatry and Clinical Neurosciences*, **3**, 377–382.

Amman, A. J. & Ward, D. W. (1982) Collagen vascular diseases (rheumatic diseases). In *Paediatrics* (Seventeenth Edition) (ed. A M. Rudolf), pp. 431–448. Norwalk Connecticut: Appleton Century Crofts.

Antebi, D. & Bird, J. M. (1993) The facilitation and evocation of seizures. *British Journal of Psychiatry*, **162**, 759–764.

Bachmann, H., Lossner, J. & Biesold, D. (1979*a*) Wilson's disease in the German Democratic Republic. I. Genetics and epidemiology. *Z-Gesamte-Inn-Med*, **115**, 744–748.

—, —, Gruss, B., *et al* (1979*b*) The epidemiology of Wilson's disease in the German Democratic Republic and current problems from the viewpoint of population genetics. *Psychiatr-Neurol-Med-Psychol-Leipz*, **31**, 393–400.

Bach-Y-Rita, G., Lion, J. R., Climent, C. E., *et al* (1971) Episodic dyscontrol: a study of 130 violent patients. *American Journal of Psychiatry*, **127**, 1473–1478.

Baker, M. (1973) Psychopathology in systemic lupus erythematosus. 1. Psychiatric observations. *Seminars in Arthritis and Rheumatism*, **3**, 95–110.

Baron Cohen, S., Cross, P., Crowson, M., *et al* (1994) Can children with Gilles de la Tourette syndrome edit their intentions. *Psychological Medicine*, **24**, 29–40.

Bear, D. M. & Fidio, P. (1977) Quantitative analysis of inter-ictal behaviour in temporal lobe epilepsy. *Archives of Neurology*, **34**, 454–467.

Bergin, J. D. (1957) Rapidly progressing dementia in disseminated sclerosis. *Journal of Neurology, Neurosurgery and Psychiatry*, **20**, 285–292.

Betts, T. (1990) Pseudoseizures: seizures that are not epilepsy. *Lancet*, **336**, 163–168.

Bihari, K., Hill, J. L. & Murphy, D. L. (1992) Obsessive-compulsive characteristics in patients with idiopathic spasmodic torticollis. *Psychiatry Research*, **42**, 267–272.

Bolwig, T. G. (1968) Transient global amnesia. *Acta Neurologica Scandinavica*, **44**, 101–106.

Boshes, B. (1947) Neuropsychiatric manifestations during the course of malaria: experiences in the Mediterranean theater in World War II. *Archives of Neurology and Psychiatry*, **58**, 14–27.

Brown, R. G. & Marsden, C. D. (1984) How common is dementia in Parkinson's disease? *Lancet*, *ii*, 1262–1265.

—— & —— (1987) Neuropsychology and cognitive function in Parkinson's disease: an overview. In *Movement Disorders* (2) (eds C. D. Marsden & Fahn), pp. 99–193. Butterworths.

Brown, S. W. & Reynolds, E. H. (1981) Cognitive impairment in epileptic patients. In *Epilepsy and Psychiatry* (eds E. H. Reynolds & M. R. Trimble). Edinburgh: Churchill Livingstone.

Carothers, J. C. (1953) The African mind in health and disease: a study in ethnic psychiatry. World Health Organization Monograph Series (No. 17). Geneva: WHO.

Casson, I. R., Siegel, O., Sham, R., et al (1984) Brain damage in modern boxers. *Journal of the American Medical Association*, **251**, 2663–2667.

Catterall, R. D. (1977) Neurosyphilis. *British Journal of Hospital Medicine*, **17**, 585–604.

Caughey, J. E. & Myrianthopoulos, N. C. (1963) *Dystrophia Myotonica and Related Disorders*. Springfield, Illinois: Thomas.

Caveness, W. F., Meirowsky, A. M., Rish, B. L., et al (1979) The nature of post-traumatic epilepsy. *Journal of Neurosurgery*, **50**, 545–553.

Chadwick, D. (1994) Epilepsy. *Journal of Neurology, Neurosurgery and Psychiatry*, **57**, 264–277.

Channon, S., Flynn, D. & Robertson, M. M. (1992) Attentional deficits in Gilles de la Tourette Syndrome. *Neuropsychiatry, Neuropsychology, and Behavioral Neurology*, **5**, 170–177.

Chaplin, J. E., Lasso, R. Y., Shorvon, S. D, et al (1992) National general practice study of epilepsy. The social and psychological effects of a recent diagnosis of epilepsy. *British Medical Journal*, **304**, 1416–1417.

Chapman, A. H., Pilkey, L. & Gibbons, M. J. (1958) A psychosomatic study of eight children with Sydenham's chorea. *Pediatrics*, **21**, 582–595.

Chappell, P. B. (1994) Sequential use of opioid antagonists and agonists in Tourette's syndrome (comment). *Lancet*, **343**, 556.

Chase, T. N., Friedhoff, A. J. & Cohen, D. J. (eds (1992) Tourette syndrome: genetics, neurobiology, and treatment. *Advances in Neurology, Volume 58.* New York: Raven Press.

Chu, N. S. & Hung, T. P. (1993) Geographic variations in Wilson's disease. *Journal of Neurological Sciences*, **117**, 1–7.

Cohen, D. J., Bruun, R. D. & Leckman, J. F. (eds) (1988) *Tourette's Syndrome and Tic Disorders. Clinical Understanding and Treatment*. New York: Wiley.

Comings, D. E. (1990) *Tourette Syndrome and Human Behavior*. Duarte, California: Hope Press.

Commission of the International League Against Epilepsy (1989) Proposal for revised classification of epilepsies and epileptic syndromes. *Epilepsia*, **30**, 389–399.

Cooper, J. A., Sagar, H. J., Jordan, N., *et al* (1991) Cognitive impairment in early, untreated Parkinson's disease and its relationship to motor disability. *Brain*, 114, 2095–2122.

Crisp, A. H. & Moldofsky, H. (1965) A psychosomatic study of writer's cramp. *British Journal of Psychiatry*, **111**, 841–858.

Cummings, J. L. (1992) Depression and Parkinson's disease: a review. *American Journal of Psychiatry*, **149**, 443–454.

——, Gosenfeld, L. F., Houlihan, J. P., *et al* (1983) Neuropsychiatric disturbances associated with idiopathic calcification of the basal ganglia. *Biological Psychiatry*, **18**, 591–601.

Currie, S., Heathfield, K. W. G., Henson, R. A., *et al* (1971) Clinical course and prognosis of temporal lobe epilepsy – a survey of 666 patients. *Brain*, **92**, 173–190.

Curtis, D., Robertson, M. M. & Gurling, H. M. D. (1992) Autosomal dominant gene transmission in a large kindred with Gilles de la Tourette Syndrome. *British Journal of Psychiatry*, **160**, 845–849.

Daly, D. (1958) Ictal affect. *American Journal of Psychiatry*, **115**, 97–108.

Dana-Haeri, J., Trimble, M. R. & Oxley, J. (1983) Prolactin and gonadotrophin changes following generalised and partial seizures. *Journal of Neurology, Neurosurgery and Psychiatry*, **46**, 331–335.

Daniel, T. M. (1991) Mycobacterial disease. In *Harrison's Principles of Internal Medicine*. Twelfth edition (eds J. D. Wilson, E. Braunwald, Isselbacher, K. J. *et al*), pp. 637–645. New York: McGraw Hill.

Daroft, R. B., Deller, J. J., Kasil, A. J., et al (1967) Cerebral malaria. *Journal of the American Medical Association*, **202**, 681–682.

David, A. S. (1993) Cognitive neuropsychiatry? *Psychological Medicine*, **23**, 1–6.

Davies, D. L. (1949) Psychiatric changes associated with Friedrich's ataxia. *Journal of Neurology, Neurosurgery and Psychiatry*, **12**, 246–250.

Davison, K. (1990) Miscellaneous topics in neuropsychiatry. *Current Opinion in Psychiatry*, **3**, 117–121.

Demeter, S. (1992) Structural imaging in Tourette syndrome. *Advances in Neurology*, **58**, 201–206.

Dening TR (1985) Psychiatric aspects of Wilson's disease. *British Journal of Psychiatry*, **147**, 677–682.

Dening, T. R. & Berrios, G. E. (1989) Wilson's disease. Psychiatric symptoms in 195 cases. *Archives of General Psychiatry*, **46**, 1126–1134.

Dew, M., Ragni, M. & Nimorwicz, P. (1990) Infection with human immuno-deficiency virus and vulnerability to psychiatric distress: a study of men with haemophilia. *Archives of General Psychiatry*, **44**, 737–744.

Dewhurst, K. (1969) The neurosyphilitic psychoses today: a survey of 91 cases. *British Journal of Psychiatry*, **115**, 31–38.

Dooneief, G., Mirabello, E., Bell, K., *et al* (1992) An estimate of the incidence of depression in idiopathic Parkinson's disease. *Archives of Neurology*, **49**, 305–307.

Eames, P. (1992) Hysteria following head injury. *Journal of Neurology, Neurosurgery and Psychiatry*, **55**, 1046–1053.

Eapen, V., Pauls, D. L. & Robertson, M. M. (1993) Evidence for autosomal dominant transmission in Gilles de la Tourette Syndrome - United Kingdom cohort. *British Journal of Psychiatry*, **162**, 593–596.

—— & Robertson, M. M. (1994) Tourette's syndrome and obsessive–compulsive behaviours. In *Psychiatry in Europe* (eds T. Sensky, C. Katona & S. Montgomery), pp. 48–57. London: Gaskell.

Egan, V., Brettle, R. P. & Goodwin, G. M. (1992) The Edinburgh cohort of HIV-positive drug users – pattern of cognitive impairment in relation to progression of disease. *British Journal of Psychiatry*, 161, 522–531.

Espir, M. L. E. & Spalding, J. M. K. (1956) Three recent cases of encephalitis lethargica. *British Medical Journal*, 1, 1141–1144.

Fagon, K. J. & Lee, S. I. (1990) Prolonged confusion following convulsions due to generalised non-convulsive status epilepticus. *Neurology*, 40, 1689–1694.

Fahn, S., Marsden, C. D. & Calne, D. B. (1987) Classification and investigation of dystonia. In *Movement Disorders (2)* (eds C. D. Marsden & S. Fahn), pp. 332–358. London: Butterworths.

Fenton, T. W. (1987) AIDS-related psychiatric disorder. *British Journal of Psychiatry*, 151, 579–588.

Fenwick, P. (1990) Automatism, medicine and the law. *Psychological Medicine*, Suppl. 17, 12.

Flint, J. & Goldstein, L. H. (1992) Familial calcification of the basal ganglia: a case report and review of the literature. *Psychological Medicine*, 22, 581–595.

Flor-Henry, P. (1969) Psychosis and temporal lobe epilepsy: a controlled investigation. *Epilepsia*, 10, 363–395.

Folstein, M. F., Maiberger, R. & McHugh, P. R. (1977) Mood disorder as a specific complication of stroke. *Journal of Neurology, Neurosurgery and Psychiatry*, 40, 1018–1020.

Ford, R. G. & Siekert, R. G. (1965) Central nervous system manifestations of peri-arteritis nodosa. *Neurology*, 15, 114–122.

Frydman, M., Bonne-Tamir, B., Farrer, L. A., *et al* (1985) Assignment of the gene for Wilson disease to chromosome 13: linkage to the esterase D locus. *Proceedings of the National Academy of Science (USA)*, 82, 1819–1821.

George, M. S., Trimble, M. R. & Robertson, M. M. (1993) Fluvoxamine and sulpiride in comorbid obsessive-compulsive disorder and Gilles de la Tourette Syndrome. *Human Psychopharmacology*, 8, 327–334.

Geschwind, N. (1965) Disconnection syndromes in animals and man. *Brain*, 88, 237–294 & 585–644.

—— (1979) Behavioural changes in temporal lobe epilepsy. *Psychological Medicine*, 9, 217–219.

Gibb, W. R. G. & Luthert, P. J. (1994) Dementia in Parkinson's disease and Lewy Body disease. In *Dementia* (eds A. Burns & R. Levy), pp. 719–737. London: Chapman and Hall.

Gibb, W. R. G., Luthert, P. J., Janota, I., *et al* (1989) Cortical Lewy body dementia: clinical features and classification. *Journal of Neurology, Neurosurgery and Psychiatry*, 52, 185–192.

Gilbert, R. E., Sandford, M. R., Jackson, H., *et al* (1994) Incidence of acute symptomatic toxoplasma retinochoroiditis in south London according to country of birth. *British Medical Journal*, 310, 1037–1040.

Gilles De La Tourette G (1885) Etude sur une affection nerveuse caracterisee par de l'incoordination motrice accompagnee d'echolalie et de copralalie. *Archives of Neurology*, 9, 19–42, 158–200.

Gloor, P. (1990) Experiential phenomena of temporal epilepsy. *Brain*, 113, 1673–1694.

Goldman, S., Amrom, D., Szliwowski, H. B., *et al* (1993) Reversible striatal hypermetabolism in a case of Sydenham's chorea. *Movement Disorders*, **8**, 355–358.

Goldstein, L. H. (1990) Behavioural and cognitive behavioural treatments for epilepsy. *British Journal of Clinical Psychology*, **29**, 257–269.

Goldstein, F. C., Levin, H. S. & Presley, R. M. (1994) Neuro-behavioural consequences of closed head injury in older adults. *Journal of Neurology, Neurosurgery and Psychiatry*, **57**, 961–966.

Gotham, A. M., Brown, R. G. & Marsden, C. D. (1988) 'Frontal' cognitive function in patients with Parkinson's disease 'on' and 'off' levodopa. *Brain*, **11**, 1299–1321.

Gowers, W. R. (1893) *A Manual of Diseases of the Nervous System*. Vol. 2, Second edition. London: Churchill.

Guerina, N. G., Ho Wen, H., Meissner, H. C., *et al* (1994) Neonatal serologic screening and early treatment for congenital toxoplasmosis infection. *New England Journal of Medicine*, **330**, 1858–1863.

Guidotti, M., Anzalone, N. & Morabito, A. (1989) A case-control study of transient global amnesia. *Journal of Neurology, Neurosurgery and Psychiatry*, **52**, 320–323.

Grafman, J., Cohen, L. G. & Hallet, M. (1991) Is focal hand dystonia associated with psychopathology? *Movement Disorders*, **6**, 29–35.

Haber, S. N. & Wolfer, D. (1992) Basal ganglia peptidergic staining in Tourette syndrome. In *Advances in Neurology*, **58**, 145–150. New York: Raven Press.

Halperin, J. J., Landis, D. M. D. & Kleinman, G.M. (1982) Whipple disease of the nervous system. *Neurology*, **32**, 612–617.

——, Volkmann, D. J. & Wu, P. (1991) Central nervous system abnormalities in Lyme Disease. Neuroborreliosis. *Neurology*, **41**, 571–582.

Hodges, J. R. (1994) Semantic memory and frontal executive function during transient global amnesia. *Journal of Neurology, Neurosurgery and Psychiatry*, **57**, 605–608.

Hogg, K. E., Goldstein, L. H. & Leigh, P.N. (1994) The psychological impact of motor neurone disease. *Psychological Medicine*, **24**, 625–632.

House, A., Dennis, M., Warlow, C., *et al* (1990) Mood disorders after stroke and their relation to lesion location. *Brain*, **113**, 1113–1129.

Huang, C. C. & Chu, N. S. (1992) Wilson's disease: clinical analysis of 71 cases and comparison with previous Chinese series. *Journal of the Formosa Medical Association*, **91**, 502–507.

Hume Adams, J., Graham, D. I., Gennarelli, T. A., *et al* (1991) Diffuse axonal injury in non-missile head injury. *Journal of Neurology, Neurosurgery and Psychiatry*, **54**, 481–483.

Hunter, R., Blackwood, W. & Bull, J. (1968) Three cases of frontal meningiomas presenting psychiatrically. *British Medical Journal*, **3**, 9–16.

Hyde, T. M., Stacey, M. E., Coppola, R., *et al* (1995) Cerebral morphometric abnormalities in Tourette's syndrome. *Neurology*, **45**, 1176–1182.

Itard, J. M. G. (1825) Memoire sur quelques fonctions involontaires des appareils de la locomotion de la prehension et de la voix. *Archives of General Medicine*, **8**, 385–407.

Jahanshahi, M. (1991) Psychosocial factors and depression in torticollis. *Journal of Psychosomatic Research*, **35**, 493–507.

—— & Marsden, C. D. (1988) Depression in torticollis: a controlled study. *Psychological Medicine*, **18**, 925–933.

—— & —— (1992) Psychological functioning before and after treatment of torticollis with botulinum toxin. *Journal of Neurology, Neurosurgery and Psychiatry*, **55**, 229–231.

Jennett, B., Snoek, J., Bond, M. R., *et al* (1981) Disability after severe head injury: observations on the use of the Glasgow Coma Scale. *Journal of Neurology, Neurosurgery and Psychiatry*, **44**, 285–293.

Jimenez-Jimenez, F. J., Santos, J., Zancada, F., *et al* (1992) "Premorbid" personality of patients with Parkinson's disease. *Acta Neurologica Napoli*, **14**, 208–214.

Johnson, J. (1969) Organic psychosyndromes due to boxing. *British Journal of Psychiatry*, **115**, 45–53.

Jubelt, B. & Miller, J. R. (1989) Parasitic infections. In *Merrit's Textbook of Neurology*. Eighth edition (ed. L. P. Rowland), pp. 164–175. Philadelphia: Lea & Febiger.

Kapur, N., Barker, S. & Burroughs, E. H. (1994) Herpes simplex encephalitis: Long-time magnetic resonance imaging and neuro-psychological profile. *Journal of Neurology, Neurosurgery and Psychiatry*, **57**, 1134–1342.

Kerr, T. A., Kay, D. W. & Lassman, L. P. (1971) Characteristics of patients, type of accident and mortality in a consecutive series of head injuries admitted to a neurosurgical unit. *British Journal of Preventative and Social Medicine*, **25**, 179–185.

King, D. J. (1995) *College Seminars in Clinical Psychopharmacology*. London: Gaskell.

King, M. B. (1989) Psychosocial status of 192 outpatients with HIV infection and AIDS. *British Journal of Psychiatry*, **154**, 237–242.

Kinsella, G., Packer, S. & Oliver, J. (1991) Maternal reporting of behaviour following very severe blunt head injury. *Journal of Neurology, Neurosurgery and Psychiatry*, **54**, 422–426.

Kirchhoff, L. V. (1991) Trypanosomiasis. In *Harrison's Principles of Internal Medicine*. Twelfth edition (eds J. D. Wilson, E. Braunwald, Isselbacher, K. J. *et al*), pp. 791–794. New York: McGraw Hill.

Kraepelin, E. (1904) *Lectures on Clinical Psychiatry*. New York: W. Wood.

Kurlan, R. (1989) Tourette's syndrome: current concepts. *Neurology*, **39**, 1625–1630.

—— (ed.) (1993) *Handbook of Tourette's Syndrome and Related Tic and Behavioural Disorders*. New York: Marcel Dekker.

Lancet. Editorial (1989) Pseudostatus Epilepticus, *Lancet*, *ii*, 485.

Landolt, A. (1958) Serial EEG investigations during psychotic episode in epileptic patients and during schizophrenic attacks. In *Lectures on Epilepsy* (ed. A. M. Lorenz de Hass), pp. 21–113. Amsterdam.

Lebensohn, Z. M. & Jenkins, R. B. (1975) Improvement of Parkinsonism in depressed patients treated with ECT. *American Journal of Psychiatry*, **132**, 283–285.

Leckman, J. F., Dolnansky, E. S. & Hardin, M. T. (1990) Perinatal factors in the expression of Tourette's syndrome: an exploratory study. *Journal of the American Academy of Child and Adolescent Psychiatry*, **29**, 220–226.

Lees, A. J. (1986) Georges Gilles de la Tourette: the man and his times. *Revue Neurologique* (Paris), **142**, 808–816.

Leis, A. A., Ross, M. A. & Summers, A. K. (1992) Psychogenic seizures: Ictal characteristics and diagnostic pitfalls. *Neurology*, **42**, 95–99.

Lesser, R. P. & Fahn, S. (1978) Dystonia: a disorder often misdiagnosed as a conversion reaction. *American Journal of Psychiatry*, **153**, 349–352.

Levy, R. M., Bredesen, D. E. & Rosenblum, M. L. (1985) Neurological manifestations of the acquired immunodeficiency syndrome (AIDS): experience at UCSF and review of the literature. *Journal of Neurosurgery*, **62**, 475–495.

Lilly, R., Cummings, J. L., Benson, F., *et al* (1983) The human Kluver-Bucy syndrome. *Neurology*, **33**, 1141–1145.

Lishman, W. A. (1987) *Organic Psychiatry. The Psychological Consequences of Cerebral Disorder*. 2nd edn. Oxford: Blackwell Scientific.

—— (1988) Physiogenesis and psychogenesis in the "Post-concussional syndrome". *British Journal of Psychiatry*, **153**, 460–469.

—— (1992) What is neuropsychiatry? *Journal of Neurology, Neurosurgery and Psychiatry*, **55**, 983–985.

Logsdail, S. J. & Toone, B. K. (1988) Post-ictal psychoses – a clinical and phenomenological description. *British Journal of Psychiatry*, **152**, 246–252.

McAllister, R. H., Hearns, M. V., Harrison, M. J. G., *et al* (1992) Neurological and neuropsychological performance in HIV, seropositive men without symptoms. *Journal of Neurology, Neurosurgery and Psychiatry*, **55**, 143–148.

Mace, C. (1993) Epilepsy and schizophrenia. *British Journal of Psychiatry*, **163**, 439–445.

Maletzky, B. M. (1973) The episodic dyscontrol syndrome. *Diseases of the Nervous System*, **34**, 178–185.

Mark, V. H. & Ervin, F. R. (1970) *Violence and the Brain*. New York: Harper and Row.

Marotta, R. & Perry, S. (1989) Early neuropsychological dysfunction caused by HIV. *Journal of Neuropsychiatry*, **1**, 225–235.

Marsden, C. D. (1990) Parkinson's disease. *Lancet*, **335**, 948–952.

Marzuk, P., Tierney, H., Tardift, K., *et al* (1988) Increased risk of suicide in persons with AIDS. *Journal of the American Medical Association*, **259**, 1333–1337.

—— (1991) Suicidal behaviour and HIV illnesses. *International Review of Psychiatry*, **3**, 365–371.

Mayeux, R., Chen, J., Mirabello, E., *et al* (1990) An estimate of the incidence of dementia in idiopathic Parkinson's disease. *Neurology*, **40**, 1513–1517.

Meares, R. (1973) Spasmodic torticollis. *British Journal of Hospital Medicine*, **9**, 235–241.

Medalia, A., Isaacs-Glaberman, K. & Scheinberg, H. (1988) Neuropsychological impairment in Wilson's disease. *Archives of Neurology*, **45**, 1502–1504.

——, Galynker, I., Scheinberg, I. H. (1992) The interaction of motor, memory, and emotional dysfunction in Wilson's disease. *Biological Psychiatry*, **31**, 823–826.

Menkes, J. H. (1989) Disorders of metal metabolism. In *Merritt's Textbook of Neurology*, 8th edn (ed. L. P. Rowland), pp. 538–544. Philadelphia: Lea & Febiger.

Miller, J. D. (1993) Head injury. *Journal of Neurology, Neurosurgery and Psychiatry*, **56**, 440–447.

Miller, D., Green, J., Farmer, R., *et al* (1985) A 'pseudo-AIDS' syndrome following from fear of AIDS. *British Journal of Psychiatry*, **146**, 550–551.

Mindham, R. H. S. (1970) Psychiatric symptoms in Parkinsonism. *Journal of Neurology, Neurosurgery and Psychiatry*, **30**, 188–191.

Mittenburg, W., Digiula, D. V. & Perrin, S. (1992) Symptoms following mild head injury: Expectation as aetiology. *Journal of Neurology, Neurosurgery and Psychiatry*, **55**, 200–204.

Murray, H. W. (1991) Toxoplasmosis. In *Harrison's Principles of Internal Medicine*. Twelfth edition (eds J. D. Wilson, E. Braunwald, Isselbacher, K. J. *et al*), pp. 795–799. New York: McGraw Hill.

Nausieda, P. A., Grossman, B. J., Koller, W. C., *et al* (1980) Sydenham's Chorea: an update. *Neurology* (NY), **30**, 331–334.

Neary, D., Snowden, J. S., Mann, D. M. A., *et al* (1990) Frontal lobe dementia and motor neuron disease. *Journal of Neurology, Neurosurgery and Psychiatry*, **53**, 23–32.

Ødegård, Ø. (1936) Mortality in Norwegian hospitals from 1916 to 1933. *Acta Psychiatrica et Neurologica*, **11**, 323–356.

Oder, W., Grimm, G., Kollegger, H., *et al* (1991) Neurological and neuropsychiatric spectrum of Wilson's disease: a prospective study of 45 cases. *Journal of Neurology*, **238**, 281–287.

Okamura, T., Fukai, M., Yamadori, A., *et al* (1993) A clinical study of hypergraphia in epilepsy. *Journal of Neurology, Neurosurgery and Psychiatry*, **56**, 556–559.

Oxbury, J. M. & MacCallum, F. O. (1973) Herpes simplex virus encephalitis: clinical features and residual damage. *Postgraduate Medical Journal*, **49**, 387–389.

Palmini, A. & Gloor, P. (1992) The localizing value of auras in partial seizures: A prospective and retrospective study. *Neurology*, **42**, 801–808.

Pauls, D. L., Pakstis, A. J. & Kurlan, R. (1990) Segregation and linkage analyses of Gilles de la Tourette's syndrome and related disorders. *Journal of the American Academy of Child and Adolescent Psychiatry*, **29**, 195–203.

Penfield, W. (1967) Epilepsy: the great teacher: the progress of one pupil. *Acta Neurologica Scandinavica*, **43**, 1–10.

Peters, R. A., Stocken, L. A. & Thompson, R. H. S. (1945) British antilewisite (BAL) *Nature* (London), **15**, 656.

Peterson, B., Riddle, M. A., Cohen, D. J., et al (1993) Reduced basal ganglia volumes in Tourette's syndrome using three-dimensional reconstruction techniques from magnetic resonance images. *Neurology*, **43**, 941–949.

——, Leckman, J. F., Duncan, J. S., et al (1994) Corpus callosum morphology from magnetic resonance images in Tourette's syndrome. *Psychiatry Research: Neuroimaging*, **55**, 85–99.

Petruhkin, K., Fischer, S. G., Pirastu, M., Tanzi, R. E., *et al* (1993) Mapping, clonong and genetic characterisation of the region containing Wilson's disease gene. *Nature Genetics*, **5**, 338–343.

Prakash, M. V. A. & Stein, G. S. (1990) Malaria presenting as atypical depression. *British Journal of Psychiatry*, **156**, 594–595.

Price, R. A., Kidd, K. K., Cohen, D. J., *et al* (1985) A twin study of Tourette syndrome. *Archives of General Psychiatry*, **42**, 815–820.

Protheroe, S. M. & Mellor, P. (1991) Imaging in influenza A encephalitis. *Archives of Diseases in Childhood*, **66**, 702–705.

Pujol, J., Leal, S., Fluvia, X., *et al* (1989) Psychiatric aspects of normal pressure hydrocephalus. A report of five cases. *British Journal of Psychiatry*, **154**, 77–80.

Rao, S. M., Devinsky, O., Grofman, J., *et al* (1992) Viscosity and social cohesion in temporal lobe epilepsy. *Journal of Neurology, Neurosurgery and Psychiatry*, **55**, 149–152.

Ray, C. G. (1991*a*) Rubella ("German Measles") and other viral exanthems. In *Harrison's Principles of Internal Medicine*. Twelfth edition (eds J. D. Wilson, E. Braunwald, Isselbacher, K. J. *et al*), pp. 707–709. New York: McGraw Hill.

Ray, C. G. (1991*b*) Mumps. In *Harrison's Principles of Internal Medicine*. Twelfth edition (eds J. D. Wilson, E. Braunwald, Isselbacher, K. J. *et al*), pp. 717–720. New York: McGraw Hill.

Reynolds, E. H. (1981) The management of seizures associated with psychological disorders. In *Epilepsy and Psychiatry* (eds E. H. Reynolds & M. R. Trimble) Edinburgh: Churchill Livingstone.

Ring, H. (1993) Psychological and social problems of Parkinson's disease. *British Journal of Hospital Medicine*, **49**, 111–116.

Ring, H. A. & Trimble, M. R. (1991) Affective Disturbance in Parkinson's Disease. *International Journal of Geriatric Psychiatry*, **6**, 385–393.

Robertson, M. M. (1989) The Gilles de la Tourette Syndrome: The current status. *British Journal of Psychiatry*, **154**, 147–169.

— (1990) The psychiatric aspects of movement disorders. *Current Opinion in Psychiatry*, **3**, 83–89.

— (1994) Gilles de la Tourette Syndrome: an update. *Journal of Child Psychology and Psychiatry*, **35**, 597–611.

—, Trimble, M. R. & Townsend, H. R. A. (1987) Phenomenology of depression in epilepsy. *Epilepsia*, **28**, 364–372.

— & — (1988) Some personality variables in functional neurological disorders. *Behavioural Neurology*, **1**, 23–28.

— & Eapen, V. (1992) Pharmacologic controversy of CNS stimulants in Gilles de la Tourette's Syndrome. *Clinical Neuropharmacology*, **15**, 408–425.

—, Channon, S., Baker, J. E., *et al* (1993) The psychopathology of Gilles de la Tourette syndrome: a controlled study. *British Journal of Psychiatry*, **162**, 114–117.

— & Trimble, M. R. (1993) Normal chromosomal findings in Gilles de la Tourette syndrome. *Psychiatric Genetics*, **3**, 95–99.

—, Channon, S. & Baker, J. (1994) Depressive symptomatology in a general hospital sample of outpatients with temporal lobe epilepsy: a controlled study. *Epilepsia*, **35**, 771–777.

Robins, A. H. (1976) Depression in patients with Parkinsonism. *British Journal of Psychiatry*, **128**, 141–145.

Robinson, R. G. & Price, T. R. (1982) Post-stroke depressive disorders: a follow-up study of 103 patients. *Stroke*, **13**, 635–641.

Rodin, E. (1973) Psychomotor epilepsy and aggressive behaviour. *Archives of General Psychiatry*, **28**, 210–213.

Rogers, D. (1985) The motor disorders of severe psychiatric illness: A conflict of paradigms. *British Journal of Psychiatry*, **147**, 221–232.

Ron, M. A. (1994) Somatisation in neurological practice. *Journal of Neurology, Neurosurgery and Psychiatry*, **57**, 1161–1164.

— & Logsdail, S. J. (1989) Psychiatric morbidity in multiple sclerosis: a clinical and MRI study. *Psychological Medicine*, **19**, 887–895.

— & Feinstein, A. (1992) Multiple sclerosis and the mind. *Journal of Neurology, Neurosurgery and Psychiatry*, **55**, 1–3.

Russell, O. (1997) *College Seminars in Learning Disability*. London: Gaskell.

Sacks, O. (1973) *Awakenings*. London: Duckworth.

— (1992) *Migraine*. London: Picador.

Sagar, H. J., Sullivan, E. V., Gabriele, J. D. E., *et al* (1988*a*) Temporal ordering and short-term memory deficits in Parkinson's disease. *Brain*, **111**, 525–539.

—, Cohen, N. J., Sullivan, E. V., *et al* (1988*b*) Remote memory function in Alzheimer's disease and Parkinson's disease. *Brain*, **111**, 185–206.

Sahakian, B. J., Morris, R. G., Evenden, J. L., *et al* (1988) A comparative study of visuospatial memory and learning in Alzheimer-type dementia and Parkinson's disease. *Brain*, **111**, 695–718.

Savard, G., Andermann, F., Olivier, A., *et al* (1991) Postictal psychosis after complex partial seizures: a multiple case study. *Epilepsia*, **32**, 225–231.

Scheinberg, I. H. (1991) Wilson's disease. In Harrison's Principles of Internal Medicine, 12th edn (eds J. D. Wilson, E. Braun Wald, K. J. Isselbacher, *et al*), pp. 1843–1844. New York: McGraw Hill.

Seth, R., Granville-Grossman, K., Goldmeier, D., *et al* (1991) Psychiatric illnesses in patients with HIV infection and AIDS, referred to the liaison psychiatrist. *British Journal of Psychiatry*, **159**, 347–350.

Shallice, T. (1988) *From Neuropsychology to Neural Structure*. Cambridge: Cambridge University Press.

Shapiro, A. K., Shapiro, E. S., Bruun, R. D., *et al* (1978) *Gilles de la Tourette Syndrome*. New York: Raven Press.

——, ——, Young J. G., *et al* (1988) *Gilles de la Tourette Syndrome (second edition)*. New York: Raven Press.

Sheehy, M. P. & Marsden, C. D. (1982) Writers' cramp – a focal dystonia. *Brain*, **105**, 461–480.

Shorvon, S. D. (1990) Epidemiology, natural history and genetics of epilepsy. *British Medical Journal*, **336**, 93–96

Singer, H. S., Reiss, A. L., Brown, J.,E., *et al* (1993) Volumetric MRI changes in basal ganglia of children with Tourette's syndrome. *Neurology*, **43**, 950-956

Skegg, K. (1993) Multiple sclerosis presenting as a pure psychiatric disorder. *Psychological Medicine*, **23**, 909–914.

Sneddon, J. (1980) Myasthenia gravis: a study of social, medical and emotional problems in 26 patients. *Lancet*, **1**, 526–528.

Starosta-Rubinstein, S., Young, A. B., Kluin, K., *et al* (1987) Clinical assessment of 31 patients with Wilson's disease. Correlations with structural changes on magnetic resonance imaging. *Archives of Neurology*, **44**, 365–370.

Stern, B. J., Krumholz, A. & Johns, C. (1985) Sarcoidosis and its neurological manifestations. *Archives of Neurology*, **42**, 909–917.

Stern, Y., Richards, M., Sano, M., *et al* (1993) Comparison of cognitive changes in patients with Alzheimer's and Parkinson's disease. *Archives of Neurology*, **50**, 1040–1045.

Strich, S. J. (1969) The pathology of brain damage due to blunt head injuries. In *The Late Effects of Head Injury* (eds A. E. Walker, W. F. Caveness & M. Critchley). Springfield, Illinois: Thomas.

Surridge, D. (1969) An investigation into some psychiatric aspects of multiple sclerosis. *British Journal of Psychiatry*, **115**, 749–764.

Swedo, S. E., Rapaport, J. L., Cheslow, D. L., *et al* (1989) High prevalence of obsessive-compulsive symptoms in patients with Sydenham's chorea. *American Journal of Psychiatry*, **146**, 246–249.

——, Leonard, H. L., Schapiro, M. B., *et al* (1993) Sydenham's chorea: physical and psychological symptoms of St Vitus dance. *Pediatrics*, **91**, 706–713.

Tavares, A. M. (1993) Psychiatric disorders in neuro-cysticercosis. *British Journal of Psychiatry*, **163**, 839.

Taylor, D. T. (1975) Factors influencing the occurrence of schizophrenia-like psychosis in patients with temporal lobe epilepsy. *Psychological Medicine*, **5**, 249–254.

Tellier, A., Walker, A. E., Adams, K. M., *et al* (1990) Long term effects of severe penetrating head injury on psychosocial adjustment. *Journal of Consulting and Clinical Psychology*, **58**, 531–537.

Thompson, P. J. & Trimble, M. R. (1982) Anticonvulsant drugs and cognitive functions. *Epilepsia*, **23**, 531–544.

Trimble, M. R. (1992) Behavioural changes following temporal lobectomy, with specific reference to psychosis. *Journal of Neurology, Neurosurgery and Psychiatry,* **55,** 89–91.

Todes, C. J. & Lees, A. J. (1985) The pre-morbid personality of patients with Parkinson's disease. *Journal of Neurology, Neurosurgery and Psychiatry,* **48,** 97–100.

Toone, B. K., Garralda, M. E. & Ron, M. A. (1982) The psychoses of epilepsy and the functional psychoses: a clinical and phenomenological comparison. *British Journal of Psychiatry,* **141,** 256–261.

Trautner, R. J., Cummings, J. L., Read, S. L., *et al* (1988) Idiopathic basal ganglia calcification and organic mood disorders. *American Journal of Psychiatry,* **145,** 350–353.

Urbach, G. & Culbert, J. P. (1991) Head injured parents and their children. *Psychosomatics,* **32,** 24–33.

Vanneste, J. A. L. (1994) Three decades of normal pressure hydrocephalus – are we wiser now? *Journal of Neurology, Neurosurgery and Psychiatry,* **57,** 1021–1025.

Veasy, L. G., Wiedmeier, S. E., Orsmond, G. S., *et al* (1987) Resurgence of acute rheumatic fever in the intermountain area of the United States. *New England Journal of Medicine,* **316,** 421–427.

Weddell, R., Oddy, M. & Jenkins, D. (1980) Social adjustment after rehabilitation: a two year follow-up of patients with severe head injury. *Psychological Medicine,* **10,** 257–263.

White, N. J. & Plorde, J. (1991) Malaria. In *Harrison's Principles of Internal Medicine.* Twelfth edition (eds J. D. Wilson, E. Braunwald, K. J. Isselbacher, *et al*), pp. 782–788. New York: McGraw Hill.

Willeit, J. & Kiechl, S. J. (1991) Wilson's disease with neurological impairment but no Kayser-Fleischer rings. *Lancet,* **337,** 1426.

Wilson, B. (1992) Recovery and compensation strategies in head injured, memory impaired people, several years after insult. *Journal of Neurology, Neurosurgery and Psychiatry,* **55,** 177–180.

Wilson, J. D., Braunwald, E., Isselbacher, K. J., *et al* (eds) (1991) *Harrison's Principles of Internal Medicine.* Twelfth edition. New York: McGraw Hill.

Wilson, J. T. L., Teasdale, G. M. & Hadley, D.M. (1994) Post traumatic amnesia – still a valuable clinical yard stick. *Journal of Neurology, Neurosurgery and Psychiatry,* **57,** 198–201.

Wilson, S. A. K. (1912) Progressive lenticular degeneration: a familial nervous disease associated with cirrhosis of the liver. *Brain,* **34,** 296–509.

Wolff, H. G. (1963) The relation of life situations, personality features, and reactions to the migraine syndrome. In *Headache and Other Head Pain,* 2nd edition. New York: Oxford University Press.

Wood, R. & Eames, P. (1981) Application of behaviour modification in the treatment of traumatically brain-injured adults. In *Applications of Conditioning Theory* (ed. G. Davey). London: Methuen.

World Health Organization (1992) *The Tenth Revision of the International Classification of Diseases and Related Health Problems* (ICD–10). Geneva: WHO.

24 Toxic, metabolic and endocrine disorders

Roger Howells

Alcohol • *Medicinal drugs* • *Drugs of misuse* • *Plants and plant-derived substances* • *Environmental elements and other chemical substances* • *Metabolic and endocrine disorders*

Most toxic, metabolic and endocrine disorders are rare conditions. Collectively, however, they are numerous, and form an important but often unrecognised source of psychiatric morbidity. Presentations range from personality disorder to profound dementia. Behavioural change, mood disturbance, fatigue, and apathy are common. Cognitive change is frequently absent, but when present it can be subtle and easily missed.

It could be argued that the greatest impediment to correct diagnosis is the emphasis that psychiatrists give to diagnosing functional psychiatric syndromes, without sufficient consideration being given to organic syndromes. However, there are other difficulties: tell-tale biochemical, endocrine or toxicological derangements may fluctuate and be missed on isolated screening tests. Physical signs may unfold late or insidiously, or be hidden by the side-effects of medication.

How can routine practice be improved? In this context it is important to "think organic", i.e. it is unwise to assume a 'functional' or 'psychological' aetiology without adequately excluding an organic cause. The practice of attempting to test, or refute, functional diagnoses should be firmly encouraged.

How far should organic investigations be taken? The availability of tests should neither dictate, nor limit the diagnostic inquiry. While it makes no sense to screen every patient for metachromatic leucodystrophy, the clinician should have a mental list of the possible causative conditions and be prepared to apply tests whenever the patient's presentation is suggestive.

What benefits accrue from detecting more organic diagnoses? Firstly, there is the chance of either a cure or the partial reversal of some conditions, removing the necessity for indefinite psychiatric care. Rarer organic disorders are brought into sharper relief and become better managed. If disorders are inherited, other family members usually derive benefit from screening and genetic counselling. Lastly, identification of various linked multi-system conditions is of great importance for their adequate management.

The range of cerebral intoxicants is very diverse but has been drawn together in the form of a simple classification (Box 24.1). As alcohol is

1103

Box 24.1   Intoxicants of the brain with the potential to cause significant psychiatric symptomatology

Alcohol
Medicinal drugs
Drugs of misuse
Plants and plant-derived substances
Environmental elements and other chemical substances

---

associated with the most extensive physical and psychiatric effects it is given prominence in the classification scheme and following account. The term "psychotoxicology" embraces this aspect of neuropsychiatry.

Alcohol

Ethyl alcohol (ethanol) is but one of many psychoactive substances in an alcoholic beverage – these other substances are called *congeners* and include higher alcohols such as amyl alcohol and butyl alcohol, and acetaldehyde. A beverage such as vodka might contain approximately 3 mg/100 ml of congeners, whereas a cognac or bourbon can contain in the region of 250 mg/100 ml (Murphree, 1971). The precise contribution of congeners to the toxicity of alcoholic beverages is at present unclear and, therefore, is of little assistance when gauging the relative effects of different beverages on the brain and behaviour.

The neurological and psychiatric sequelae of alcohol misuse commonly coexist (Box 24.2).

Drunkenness and coma

The classification of alcohol intoxication is similar in DSM–IV (American Psychiatric Association, 1994) and ICD–10 (World Health Organization, 1992). In DSM–IV, the diagnosis "alcohol intoxication" requires that there has been maladaptive behavioural or psychological change following recent alcohol use, along with signs of intoxication (e.g. slurring of speech, incoordination, or impairment of attention or memory) in the absence of other physical or mental disorder. In ICD–10 "acute intoxication" carries a qualification such as uncomplicated or pathological intoxication.

It is well-recognised that alcohol affects individuals differently. The degree of acquired physical tolerance is especially important, but influential factors include age, gender, weight, prior experience with alcohol, learned expectations concerning the effects of alcohol, personality and culture (Nathan & Hay, 1984).

Box 24.2 The neurological and psychiatric sequelae of alcohol misuse (adapted from Adams & Victor, 1989, with permission of The McGraw-Hill Companies)

Group I. Disorders related to alcohol intoxication:
(i)   drunkenness
(ii) coma
(iii) memory blackouts
(iv) pathological intoxication (manie à potu)
(v)   traumatic head injury

Group II. Alcohol dependence syndrome

Group III. Alcohol withdrawal syndromes:
(i)   simple alcohol withdrawal (with or without fits)
(ii) alcoholic hallucinosis – acute/subacute
(iii) alcohol withdrawal delirium (delirium tremens)

Group IV. Alcohol-related nutritional syndromes
(i)   Wernicke-Korsakoff syndrome (Vitamin B_1, thiamine)
(ii) nicotinic acid deficiency disorders (Vitamin B_6, niacin)
(iii) polyneuropathy (Victor, 1984)
(iv) optic neuropathy (Victor *et al*, 1960)

Group V. Alcohol-related disorders of uncertain pathogenesis
(i)   alcoholic hallucinosis – chronic
(ii) alcohol-associated cerebral atrophy and dementia
(iii) central pontine myelinolysis
(iv) Marchiafava-Bignami disease
(v)   alcoholic personality change (Lishman, 1987)
(vi) cerebellar degeneration (Victor *et al*, 1989)

Group VI. Foetal alcohol syndromes (Barrison *et al*, 1985)

Group VII. Hepatocerebral disorders

Group VIII. Miscellaneous alcohol-related disorders
(i)   alcohol-induced hypoglycaemia
(ii) alcohol-related electrolyte and acid-base disturbance
(iii) alcohol-related stroke (Gorelick, 1989)

Note: disorders not discussed in the text are referenced.

After one or two drinks a non-tolerant occasional drinker will display mild changes in mood, behaviour, cognition and motor control. If more is consumed and the blood alcohol level rises above 100 mg/100 ml, lability of mood and disinhibited behaviour, accompanied by impairment of judgement, memory and attention, slurring of speech and incoordination will be manifested. Similar symptoms may occur after head injury, post-ictally and because of hypoglycaemia. Beyond 200 mg/100 ml these changes become markedly exacerbated. At around 300 mg/100 ml depression of medullary function occurs, with the attendant risk of cardiorespiratory failure and coma. High blood alcohol levels inhibit gluconeogenesis and may induce severe hypoglycaemia, especially in malnourished individuals – the usual signs may be missed if the individual is comatose and hypothermic; hypovolaemia, lactic acidosis and acute renal failure are additional risks. The median lethal blood alcohol level is 400–500 mg/100 ml (Reynolds, 1989).

Such patients require careful appraisal and management. The margin between narcosis and dangerous respiratory depression is narrower than with other central nervous system depressants such as anaesthetic agents. There is *great* danger attached to the practice of leaving a severely intoxicated person to "sleep it off". Coma due to alcohol is a medical emergency as death may occur through aspiration or respiratory depression. Careful consideration should be given to alternative explanations of coma in the alcoholic, particularly stroke, head injury, drug overdosage, subdural haematoma, hypoglycaemia, liver failure, circulatory failure and hypothermia. If a patient is comatose or close to coma, a decision will have to be taken as to whether intensive treatments such an intravenous fructose (which may increase the rate of fall of alcohol levels by approximately 25%) or dialysis are warranted (O'Neill *et al*, 1984).

Memory blackouts

Loss of memory for actions and events occurring when intoxicated with alcohol is termed a memory blackout. Normally the gap in memory is for a matter of hours, although it can be longer. Memory blackouts are widely experienced by dependent drinkers, but are also reported by occasional drinkers quite early in their drinking history.

Two distinctive types of memory loss have been delineated during a memory blackout, "en-bloc" and "fragmentary" memory loss. En-bloc memory loss has a discrete onset and terminates with a sense of lost time and apprehension. It is seldom followed by return of the lost memory (Goodwin *et al*, 1969*a,b*); large amounts of alcohol are required to induce en-bloc memory loss. Fragmentary memory loss is characterised by partial loss of memory in which islets of recollection remain. These islets of memory loss often coalesce to produce a somewhat imperfect record of the lost events. Memory blackouts are important because they are often referred to by drinkers and have to be distinguished from the memory impairment of thiamine deficiency and even fugue. They have considerable medico-legal significance (Sweeney, 1990).

Pathological intoxication

Unusual susceptibility to alcohol is a well-recognised sequel to brain insults, but the question as to whether there are individuals who undergo a 'pathological' reaction to alcohol (manie à potu; pathologische alkoholreaction) has been debated for over a century (Banay, 1944). The condition is not uncommon, particularly in medico-legal practice. The DSM–III–R term Alcohol Idiosyncratic Intoxication is no longer employed in DSM–IV. Both DSM–IV and ICD–10 define it as maladaptive behavioural change, usually aggressive, due to recent ingestion of alcohol insufficient to induce intoxication in most people, which is atypical of the person when not drinking, and not due to any other physical or mental disorder.

The four main components are:

(1) the condition follows the consumption of alcohol (possibly an unexpectedly small quantity);
(2) the occurrence of irrational violence with or without delirium or psychosis;
(3) the occurrence of terminal sleep;
(4) the presence of a degree of amnesia for the events which occurred (Coid, 1979).

Many authorities are sceptical about the validity of pathological intoxication as a clinical entity. May & Ebaugh (1953), for example, concluded "amnesia and violence are symptoms . . . indications for a careful diagnostic evaluation" – a contention which they justified with illustrative case histories. The controversy has been thoroughly reviewed by Coid (1979).

Traumatic head injury

Traumatic head injuries in the alcoholic are frequently an accompaniment of intoxication and not remembered. Of all the potential sequelae, bleeding into the subdural spaces presents particular diagnostic difficulties.

Subdural collections, which can be bilateral, can swell and exert pressure effects – sometimes without localising signs. Furthermore, the condition may be present for months before it manifests, only being suspected when the patient's mental state deteriorates and delirium or coma supervene. The clinical features may be subtle with the patient merely complaining of intermittent headache, or alternatively there might be a florid presentation with fluctuating consciousness (Adams & Victor, 1989). Skull percussion may reveal lateralised tenderness, sufficient to arouse deeply stuporous patients (Robinson & Stott, 1980). Dementia may emerge insidiously in long-standing cases and be mistaken for the effects of continuing inebriation and social decline. If suspected, the absence of a clear history of trauma should not deter further investigation. Radiological procedures, particularly computerised tomography or magnetic resonance imaging, will usually reveal

---

Box 24.3   The main elements of the alcohol dependence syndrome

1. Narrowing of the repertoire of drinking behaviour
2. Salience of drink-seeking behaviour
3. Increased tolerance to alcohol
4. Repeated withdrawal symptoms
5. Repeated relief or avoidance of withdrawal symptoms by further drinking
6. Subjective awareness of a compulsion to drink
7. Reinstatement of the syndrome after abstinence

---

the diagnosis, although a normal scan in a deteriorating patient should arouse suspicion that there could be bilateral haematomas with no mass effect.

Alcohol dependence syndrome

Physical dependence will inevitably follow the sustained intake of alcohol, although the exact quantity required varies between individuals. The alcohol dependence syndrome has seven principal components (Box 24.3) (Edwards & Gross, 1976); these are chiefly manifestations of physical dependency, but they are also affected by personality and cultural factors (Drummond, 1991).

The severity of alcohol dependence is measured using the Severity of Alcohol Dependence Questionnaire (SADQ), a self-rated questionnaire with good validity which can be completed in a few minutes (Stockwell *et al*, 1979). The criteria for alcohol dependency syndrome should be sought whenever an alcohol history is being taken. Patients, their families and their doctors are often unaware that the inability to respond to advice to "stop drinking" is due to established dependence, which causes aversive and potentially dangerous symptoms whenever abstinence is attempted. The presence of anorexia and/or night sweats is usually indicative of alcohol dependence.

Alcohol withdrawal syndromes

When a dependent drinker withdraws from alcohol, an extensive range of physical and mental changes are triggered, collectively termed the 'alcohol withdrawal syndrome'. These changes can be grouped into three major syndromes: simple alcohol withdrawal, alcoholic hallucinosis (acute/ subacute) and alcohol withdrawal delirium. There is usually considerable overlap between the three syndromes, and a patient experiencing alcohol withdrawal delirium will almost always have experienced the other two previously. Withdrawal features are precipitated by both complete *and* partial withdrawal, and if drinking has recommenced this will disguise the clinical presentation. The occurrence appears to be directly related to cessation of intake (Victor & Adams, 1953), the severity being linked to the quantity and duration of alcohol consumption (Isbell *et al*, 1953) and the pattern of recent drinking (Mello & Mendelson, 1970).

Simple alcohol withdrawal

This is known by a variety of broadly equivalent terms, notably the tremulousness syndrome, alcohol withdrawal (DSM–IV), and "withdrawal state – uncomplicated" or "withdrawal state – with convulsions" (ICD–10).

About 3–12 hours after cessation of drinking, a dependent drinker will experience tremulousness associated with one or more of a range of physical and mental changes (Table 24.1). Many of these symptoms are reported by patients who continue to drink because they regularly enter partial withdrawal (e.g. at night or at work). Tremulousness, which can range from mild to severe, is generalised but is typically most evident in the upper limbs; patients will mention embarrassed attempts to conceal their shaking hands.

The simple withdrawal features reach peak intensity at 24–36 hours into the withdrawal period, thereafter subsiding, although it is not uncommon for insomnia, anxiety, and depression to persist for 1–2 weeks or more. Appetite tends to return after 3–5 days. Epileptic seizures ("rum fits") can complicate this otherwise benign syndrome, typically 12–18 hours into withdrawal. These seizures are usually generalised and are thought to be more common in those with a pre-existing history of epilepsy. Hypoglycaemia,

Table 24.1 Clinical features associated with simple alcohol withdrawal (Victor & Adams, 1953; Salum, 1972)

Physical	Mental
Generalised tremor	Anxiety
Sweating	Depression
Nausea or vomiting	Insomnia
Fever	Irritability
Tachycardia	Anorexia[1]
Hypertension	Malaise
Brisk reflexes	Possible illusions
Epileptic seizures	Possible elemental hallucinations
Headache	
Visual disturbance	
Disturbance of gait	
Paraesthesia	

1. Anorexia is also a feature of established alcohol dependency.

Table 24.2 Differential diagnosis of delirium in the dependent drinker

Intoxication	Water/sodium imbalance
Alcohol withdrawal delirium	Endocrine disorders
Thiamine deficiency (Wernicke's disease)	Hypoglycaemia
Head trauma	Hyperglycaemia
Infection	Pancreatic dysfunction
Post-ictal states	Nicotinic acid deficiency
Liver failure	Hypophosphataemia

hyponatraemia and hypomagnesaemia are potential causes of seizures in the drinker and should be excluded. Post-ictal delirium should be distinguished from the other causes of delirium in the dependent drinker (Table 24.2).

Alcoholic hallucinosis – acute/subacute

Perceptual disturbance is a common accompaniment of alcohol withdrawal in the dependent drinker, and alcohol is almost certainly the commonest cause of hallucinosis in the general population. In dependent drinkers hallucinations can occur: (1) in partial withdrawal; (2) where drinking has recommenced but the features of withdrawal are incompletely suppressed; (3) in established withdrawal, with or without alcohol withdrawal delirium; (4) as a consequence of nutritional, traumatic, ictal, toxic, metabolic or biochemical disturbances; and (5) due to unknown mechanisms. In a small percentage of individuals hallucinations may become chronic, whether or not abstinence has been achieved. Careful history-taking is required to establish which type, or types, of alcohol hallucinosis a patient is describing. Withdrawal hallucinations are not usually associated with impaired cognition, but where this occurs it is more correct to use the term alcohol withdrawal delirium (delirium tremens).

Alcohol withdrawal hallucinations usually occur 12–48 hours into withdrawal. Characteristically, they are most pronounced during the first night of withdrawal – a practical point which must be borne in mind when prescribing medication for the first 24 hours of withdrawal. They are usually fleeting but may last for several minutes, thus holding the individual in a state of perplexity or terror. Insight is variable; full insight is often impeded by the potential threat of the perceived image. One patient likened the experience to watching a horror film alone; watching a horror film can be frightening, particularly if forced to do so. These experiences often affect the person's mood; Legrain (1892) observed: "The patient is gloomy, sad and restless. It seems as if the nocturnal tragedies at which he is present continue to impress him during the day, and that he seeks in his surroundings for their explanation." Patients report a range of phenomena: vivid dreams, dreams intruding into the waking periods of a broken night's sleep, illusions and misperceptions, simple elemental hallucinations (such as clicks and snatched glimpses of a form), and fully formed hallucinations (such as music and conversation, or of insects, birds, and people). In a survey of 50 consecutive cases, the distribution of affected perceptual modalities was: visual (58%), auditory (16%), and mixed auditory and visual (26%); hallucinations in other modalities were infrequent but certainly occurred (Victor & Hope, 1958). Alcohol withdrawal hallucinations, although usually acute or subacute, in a minority of individuals do become chronic.

Patients may be reluctant to disclose their experiences; some fear disclosing what they privately construe as madness. Such symptoms, however, are important clues to the level of a patient's consumption and should be specifically enquired about. The following case history was obtained by the author and is representative.

> *Case example*
> A 35-year-old man awoke after dozing in his chair some 16 hours after his last drink. He had earlier been out to buy new jeans and there on his jeans was a shiny spider. He brushed it away but to his horror it transformed into a teaming mass of spiders. In terror he ran downstairs, filled a bucket with a strong bleach solution and immersed his jeans. As he watched, dozens of spiders seemed to come to the surface. After his wife rebuked him he realised it must have been his "imagination".

It should be noted that third person auditory hallucinosis in clear consciousness is not unique to schizophrenia but also occurs in alcoholic hallucinosis (Sabot *et al*, 1968) and that the distinction may be difficult (Cohen & Johnson, 1988; Galfond, 1989). This is especially so when the patient conceals or disregards his drinking history, the drinking is accompanied by other substance abuse, secondary delusions arise, or the hallucinosis is long-lasting.

The disorder can be coded in DSM–IV under the heading substance-induced psychotic disorder, where "with onset during withdrawal" and "with hallucinations" should be added. In ICD–10 the disorder is classified in the alcohol section as psychotic disorder, either as "schizophrenia-like" or "predominantly hallucinatory".

Alcohol withdrawal delirium (delirium tremens)

This usually occurs within 18–36 hours of abstaining from alcohol, although it can occur later. In contrast to alcoholic hallucinosis there is usually cognitive impairment, although a mild degree of cognitive impairment can sometimes occur with alcohol withdrawal hallucinosis. In DSM–IV, alcohol withdrawal delirium is placed within the category of "substance withdrawal delirium" and alcohol is specified. In ICD–10, alcohol withdrawal delirium is qualified "without convulsions" or "with convulsions". A classic triad of symptoms occurs: clouding of consciousness and confusion; vivid hallucinations with illusions affecting any sensory modality; and marked tremor. Delusions, agitation, insomnia or sleep-cycle reversal, and autonomic over-activity are often present.

Literature is replete with accounts, the following one is by the great French novelist and observer of psychosocial pathology, Emile Zola (1876):

> Gervaise stayed with him until the evening. When the doctor came on his six o'clock round he made him hold up his hands. There was hardly a tremor left, just a slight trembling of the finger tips. But as darkness fell Coupeau gradually got more distressed. Twice he sat up in bed and searched the floor, into the dark corners. Suddenly he lashed out as though he were squashing some creature against the wall... 'The rats! The rats'. Then after a silence, as he was drowsing off he began to struggle a bit and talk disconnectedly. 'Oh Christ, they are digging holes in my skin!'... He aimed blows at the void...to protect himself from the bearded men he could not see.

While certainly encountered, more severe degrees of delirium are much rarer – most probably because it is now better recognised that it is potentially dangerous to leave a dependent drinker in withdrawal without some form of medication.

Severe alcohol withdrawal delirium presents abruptly and dramatically, but typically after prodromal simple withdrawal symptoms have occurred. Prodromal symptoms are easily overlooked, particularly when a dependent drinker is unexpectedly cut off from alcohol, as happens following admission to a medical or surgical unit a day or two earlier.

The individual is profoundly disorientated, and experiences vivid, often terrifying hallucinations with secondary delusions. Visual hallucinations are most common, but are usually accompanied by auditory and tactile hallucinations (Salum, 1972). Tremulousness is common, and pronounced agitation almost always occurs. The patient's mood is typically elevated but may become low in intervals of lucidity. Autonomic changes are usually striking – pupil dilatation, fever, tachycardia and profuse sweating are seen. The blood pressure may be high, but in an important minority hypotension is evident. Hypotension is an ominous development usually indicating dehydration and impending circulatory collapse. Thomas Sutton's account in 1813 was remarkable in that it pointed to the dangers of hypovolaemia (blood-letting) (Sutton, 1813). Subcutaneous haematomas are relatively common, and it is reported that in the severest cases pseudo-opisthotonus, which comprises retraction of the head and hyperextension of the back occurs (Salum, 1972). Epileptic seizures occur in approximately a third of cases, often preceding the onset of delirium. The delirium fluctuates in intensity and is usually worse at night or under conditions of minimal sensory stimulation. The delirious episode usually ends abruptly as the exhausted individual falls into a long terminal sleep. Memory for the preceding events is usually incomplete and can be absent altogether. Most episodes (80%) end within 72 hours or less. Ward staff should be warned that relapses can occur after apparent recovery, and that the condition may persist for a week or more with periods of lucidity between episodes.

Mortality from severe alcohol withdrawal delirium still occurs, figures of 5–15% are often quoted. Hyperthermia in combination with dehydration will precipitate circulatory collapse. Self-injury and infections also contribute to mortality. Dependent drinkers undoubtedly do die from delirium tremens when alone at home.

Two points deserve to be stressed. First, in clinical practice patients commonly present with symptoms from more than one type of withdrawal syndrome. Thus, symptoms such as drenching nocturnal sweats suggest the autonomic overactivity of nocturnal delirium, yet may not be accompanied by impairment of consciousness. Second, patients may or may not progress from a milder state to a more severe one. Detoxification regimens started early, and of sufficient dosage, will stem the progression to withdrawal delirium.

Table 24.3 The components of supportive care required for the nursing management of a patient in alcohol withdrawal (based on Naranjo & Sellers, 1986)

Requirements	Intervention
Control of environmental stimuli	Provide a quiet private room
	Control the lighting
	Only one staff member to be in contact
	Use a uniform, laboratory coat or name badge
Foods and fluids	Offer fluids every 60 minutes
	Normal, familiar diet at meal times
	Record the intake
Physical comfort	Support the patient's position with pillows
	Raise the bed-head if necessary
Body temperature	Apply or remove blankets
Rest and sleep	Allow rest and sleep between assessments
	Talk to the patient only if it is initiated
Elimination	Assist to the bathroom or commode
	Record the output
Reality orientation	Orientate with respect to time, place and person
Reassurance	Use positive encouragement
	Ensure hourly contact
Rehabilitation	Discuss only if it is raised by the patient
	Agree if the patient says he wants to stop drinking
Visitors	No visitors when intensive supportive care is under way
Smoking	Only if patient asks, and limit it due to the fire risk

Management of alcohol withdrawal states

Alcohol withdrawal presents in very many guises and clinicians should have a high index of suspicion in all newly referred psychiatric patients (Howells & Patrick, 1989). Ideally an informant should be spoken to, indicators of dependency should be sought, and specific enquiry should be made about withdrawal symptoms such as nocturnal sweats, morning shakes, nausea, anorexia and perceptual disturbance. Enquiry about the type of beverage being consumed is important; strong lagers are typically used by dependent drinkers as an inexpensive source of alcohol.

In order to plan treatment the severity of withdrawal needs to be gauged. The amount and duration of recent drinking appear to be linked to severity of withdrawal; the nature of past withdrawal symptoms, particularly the presence of fits, may also be helpful. The time of the last drinking episode should be recorded and, if available, a breath alcohol measurement should be made.

A minimum physical examination should assess the following: autonomic arousal (temperature, pulse, blood pressure, sweating), the severity of tremor and agitation, signs of liver disease and/or failure (cognitive impairment associated with restlessness, drowsiness, slurred speech, yawning, hiccups, liver flap, foetor hepaticus, various cutaneous signs and ascites), physical features of Wernicke's disease (ophthalmoplegia, nystagmus, ataxia, or neuropathy), dehydration (buccal dryness, reduced skin turgor, low JVP, postural drop in blood pressure and a fast, low amplitude pulse), and whether infection is present. Mental state examination should assess mood, anxiety, the presence or absence of abnormal perceptions and thoughts, cognition (especially orientation and memory) and the degree of insight.

In-patient management will be necessary if the patient has features of incipient delirium (particularly cognitive impairment, with autonomic over-activity or severe agitation), physical complications, a strong history of withdrawal seizures, or a history of poor compliance with out-patient detoxification regimes.

Simple withdrawal features of a mild degree may respond to structured in-patient nursing procedures (Table 24.2). Practical rating instruments are used such as the Selected Severity of Alcohol withdrawal (SSA; Gross *et al*, 1973) or its derivative, the Clinical Institute Withdrawal Assessment for Alcohol scale (CIWA-A; Shaw *et al*, 1981), thus allowing changes in autonomic and psychological indices to be easily monitored.

Patients in simple withdrawal or with uncomplicated alcohol withdrawal hallucinosis can undergo alcohol withdrawal as out-patients, attending daily to pick up a prescription and for clinical review. The medication of choice is a benzodiazepine drug such as chlordiazepoxide or diazepam. Benzodiazepines have cross-tolerance with alcohol, better efficacy and less toxicity than most other candidate drugs, and have excellent anticonvulsive properties. Chlordiazepoxide is used in the dose range 20–40 mg four times a day. Under-medicating patients receiving out-patient detoxification is dangerous. The prescription of one or two extra PRN doses of medication

---

Box 24.4 The principal clinical features of the Wernicke-Korsakoff syndrome (adapted from Victor *et al*, 1989)

Wernicke's disease

(1)*Disorders of cognition and consciousness* (three presentations are recognised)

        "Quiet" delirium (disorientation, apathy, drowsiness, impaired attention and memory)

        Stupor

        Coma

(2)*Ocular abnormalities*

        Nystagmus (horizontal and/or vertical)

        Lateral rectus palsy (bilaterally)

        Conjugate gaze palsy

(3)*Ataxia*

        Mild to severe gait ataxia

(4)*Polyneuropathy*

        The legs alone are affected in most cases

Korsakoff syndrome

(1)*Memory impairments*

        Preserved primary memory

        Impaired recent memory

        Extensive retrograde amnesia

(2)*Other criteria*

        These include relatively poor insight into the deficit, absence of impairment of consciousness, and the absence of global cognitive impairment

(3)*Other reported cognitive impairments*

        Frontal lobe dysfunction, visuoperceptive deficits and impairment on abstracting tasks

Note: confabulation, usually of the spontaneous type, occurs early as the Korsakoff state emerges, but does not persist. (Confabulation should not be regarded as a prerequisite for the diagnosis.)

---

for the first two nights is often helpful as symptoms are severest to begin with, at a time when the ideal dosage for symptom control is unknown. Decrements are made each day to enable the drug to be withdrawn after 7–14 days.

Since anorexia, poor diet and impaired absorption of vitamins occur in dependent drinkers, most authorities recommend a polyvitamin supplement. While parenteral administration overcomes the impairment of gut absorption that is thought to occur in alcoholic patients, it does carry the risk of causing an anaphylactic reaction. Precautionary arrangements should always be made.

Box 24.5 Circumstances in which thiamine deficiency may cause Wernicke's disease

Dietary deficiency
Alcoholism, anorexia nervosa, inadequately formulated total parenteral nutrition, starvation
Persistent vomiting
Hyperemesis gravidarum, alcoholism, bulimia nervosa or in any other context
States of impaired absorption
Alcoholism, pernicious anaemia, gastrointestinal carcinoma, chronic diarrhoea, gastroduodenal surgery
Increased metabolic demand in the context of deficiency
Through giving a glucose load to a thiamine deficient alcoholic. Hyperthyroidism
Others
Dialysis (haemodialysis or peritoneal), cancer, HIV syndromes

---

Patients with a history of recurring withdrawal seizures may warrant prophylactic treatment with an anticonvulsant, although the risks of prescribing anticonvulsants in this group are considerable. As alcohol withdrawal seizures are customarily generalised, partial seizures always warrant investigation.

Alcohol withdrawal delirium (delirium tremens) requires intensive nursing care as an in-patient. Minimum investigation comprises a full blood count and ESR, serum electrolytes and liver function tests, blood glucose analysis, chest and skull X-rays, and close observation of fluid balance.

Benzodiazepines are the drugs of choice. They are given either in divided doses throughout the day, or using a loading dose technique in which an oral dose of diazepam 20 mg (or equivalent benzodiazepine) is given hourly until the patient shows clinical improvement or becomes sedated. A minimum of 60 mg of diazepam is usually required (Naranjo & Sellers, 1986). It may be necessary to combine this loading dose technique with an initial stat dose of up to 50mg of diazepam, and an antipsychotic agent such as haloperidol may be required if unpleasant psychotic symptoms persist. *In extremis*, rapid control can be achieved with slow intravenous injection of diazepam or amylobarbitone, or with paraldehyde intra-muscularly. Alternative regimes have utilised drugs such as chlormethiazole, propranolol, phenothiazines (risk of precipitating hypotension and fits),chloral hydrate and even the reintroduction of alcohol. While they are generally effective they are not recommended – their associated complications have made benzodiazepines the first line agents (Naranjo & Sellers, 1986). Fluid and electrolyte problems are discussed separately below; details of the accompanying physical complications are available elsewhere (Saunders, 1991).

Wernicke-Korsakoff syndrome

Ophthalmoplegia, nystagmus, gait ataxia and mental confusion (delirium) constitute the cardinal features of Wernicke's disease (also known as Wernicke's encephalopathy), a disorder of abrupt onset first described in 1881 by Carl Wernicke in Germany. In 1887 Sergei Korsakoff, a prominent Russian psychiatrist, described an illness characterised by pronounced impairment of recent and retrograde memory – *cerebropathia psychica toxemica*. Korsakoff's "psychosis" was subsequently linked to Wernicke's disease. Wernicke-Korsakoff syndrome is a unitary disorder comprising acute Wernicke's disease, which proceeds in a proportion of cases to Korsakoff syndrome (Victor *et al*, 1989). In patients with both clinical presentations, post-mortem neuropathological examination reveals lesions in the following nuclei: medial dorsal, medial mamillary, dorsal hypothalamic, central grey, oculomotor, and medial vestibular, further confirming their unitary nature. The nucleus basalis of Meynert is also affected.

The cause of the Wernicke-Korsakoff syndrome was discovered to be thiamine deficiency. This appears to be due to poor appetite and malnutrition, as well as malabsorption and other factors (Bonjour, 1980; Ryle & Thomson, 1984).

The manifestations of Wernicke's disease and Korsakoff syndrome (Box 24.4) rarely present in their entirety, but the classical clinical triad indicative of Wernicke's disease (ophthalmoplegia/nystagmus, delirium and ataxia) should always be actively sought. Coincidental disorders such as alcohol withdrawal delirium can obscure the picture. While Korsakoff syndrome is usually the sequel, it can present without a preceding history of Wernicke's disease. In these cases, it seems likely that the preceding episode of Wernicke's disease may have occurred unnoticed outside hospital.

Wernicke's disease is mostly encountered in dependent drinkers, although psychiatrists must be well acquainted with the range of settings in which it can occur (Box 24.5).

It has been suggested that magnetic resonance imaging may be helpful in diagnosis of suspected cases. Gallucci *et al* (1990), who studied five acute cases of Wernicke's disease, reported hyperintense areas surrounding the third ventricle and aqueduct. Serum thiamine levels can be inferred indirectly from red cell transketolase and other enzymes, but the results are rarely available in time to influence management and, moreover, serum levels do not necessarily mirror central nervous system levels. If the diagnosis is suspected, treatment with parenteral thiamine should not be delayed. Wernicke's disease constitutes a medical emergency because, without rapid intervention, permanent brain damage (i.e. Korsakoff syndrome) is a likely consequence. In one series it was the sequel in 84% of cases (Victor *et al*, 1989). Without treatment patients face a significant risk of mortality; severely deficient patients can become stuporous, enter coma and die within 1–2 weeks, or develop 'beriberi' heart disease.

Most authorities recommend a regime of 50 mg thiamine intravenously and 50 mg intramuscularly as an immediate measure, followed by 50 mg intramuscularly each day thereafter until a normal diet is well established (Victor *et al*, 1989). As other vitamins are potentially deficient, it is customary to give thiamine within a polyvitamin preparation. There is a risk of inducing anaphylaxis with these injections. The ocular palsies which occur in Wernicke's disease are remarkably responsive to treatment, a helpful diagnostic point to note. Initially patients should have bed rest because of the small but significant risk of cardiovascular collapse from thiamine-induced 'beriberi' heart disease, a disorder in which there is peripheral vasodilatation and associated oedema, cardiac dilatation and ultimately high output cardiac failure. Supportive nursing measures are required (see Table 24.3). Nicotinic acid (niacin, nicotinamide) deficiency can coexist with thiamine deficiency and must be suspected if patients fail to respond to thiamine.

While the ophthalmoplegia, ataxia and delirium resolve rapidly with treatment, nystagmus can persist as a permanent marker of the episode. If significant brain damage has been incurred, the disorders of memory characteristic of Korsakoff syndrome come into sharper relief (Kopelman, 1987*a*), often heralded by spontaneous confabulation (Kopelman, 1987*b*). However, confabulation generally recedes and is not a feature of patients with established Korsakoff syndrome. Partial recovery of memory is usual, but the onset of this is delayed for several weeks or months, thereafter proceeding slowly over many months (Victor *et al*, 1989). Less than a quarter of patients recover their memory completely.

Nicotinic acid deficiency disorders

Deficiency of nicotinic acid (niacin, nicotinamide) is most commonly found among alcoholics and may have a significant mortality (Ishii & Nishihara, 1981). It appears to be due to poor dietary intake, decreased uptake, decreased conversion to the active coenzyme form, decreased storage and an increased requirement (Ryle & Thomson, 1984). It presents with the well-known triad of skin lesions, pellagra (which means rough skin), gastrointestinal disorder and mental changes. Some members of the triad may not be present or may go unrecognised. The skin lesions (erythema, pigmentation and hyperkeratosis) occur on parts of the body exposed to sunlight and are easily missed. The gastrointestinal disorders, such as diarrhoea, constipation and nausea, may be attributed to "gastritis" and dismissed. Furthermore, the mental changes of delirium, hallucinations, insomnia, anxiety and depression are indistinguishable from those of alcoholism. In less severe deficiency states, the clinical presentation is similar to neurasthenia (fatigue, loss of appetite, headache, disturbed sleep, anxiety, irritability and depression). Left untreated, a delirious state may arise (acute nicotinic acid encephalopathy) or dementia may develop insidiously.

The acute delirious state contrasts with that of Wernicke's disease in that it is usually accompanied by agitation and excitement. Stupor, coma and death may supervene before the diagnosis is made. The development of extrapyramidal rigidity is an important pointer to the presence of nicotinic acid deficiency rather than alcohol withdrawal delirium (Jolliffe *et al*, 1940; Ishii & Nishihara, 1981). Incontinence, spastic paralysis and hyper-reflexia have also been described. Post-mortem examination will reveal central chromatolysis in the Betz cells of the motor cortex, thalamic neurones, pontine neurones and anterior horn cells (Leigh, 1952). Administration of the deficient vitamin has a strikingly beneficial effect on the clinical course.

Alcohol-related disorders of uncertain pathogenesis

Alcoholic hallucinosis – chronic

Hallucinations occurring in cases of acute withdrawal hallucinosis, alcohol withdrawal delirium, and in other conditions in the alcoholic are commonly and erroneously grouped together under the term 'alcoholic hallucinosis'. The recorded drinking histories in such cases are often meagre, and it is not made clear whether other causes have been adequately excluded. Before making the diagnosis of chronic alcoholic hallucinosis, other cerebral disorders and substance misuse should be rigorously sought and excluded. Chronic hallucinosis presents a particular diagnostic problem when accompanied by changes in mental state, personality and behaviour resembling those seen in schizophrenia (such as downward social drift).

Management is straightforward; absolute abstinence should be enforced, and the misuse of other substances excluded by regular screening. A low starting dose of neuroleptics should be titrated against the symptoms. Periodically, attempts should be made to reduce or withdraw the medication.

Alcohol-associated cerebral atrophy and dementia

The issue as to whether or not alcohol toxicity itself causes a *primary* dementia remains unresolved. There are many complicating factors; firstly, any directly toxic effects are difficult to dissociate from other potential influences (i.e. nutritional deficiencies, hepato-cerebral disorder, misuse of other substances, head injury, Alzheimer's disease, arteriosclerotic disease and other dementing processes). Secondly, even the most elegant neuropsychometric protocols are affected by such problems as uncooperativeness, apathy and mood disturbance in the alcoholic subject. Thirdly, studies of the relationship between alcohol and cognitive function are influenced by the timing of cognitive testing in relation to periods of abstinence. Finally, gaining reliable drinking histories from alcoholics has proved to be notoriously difficult, although new methodologies do offer promise (Sobell, 1980).

There is compelling evidence that cortical atrophy, especially frontal atrophy, occurs in Wernicke-Korsakoff syndrome. This evidence comes from radiological studies (Jacobson & Lishman, 1990), morphological studies (Torvik *et al*, 1982; Harper & Kril, 1990) and cerebral blood flow studies (Hunter *et al*, 1989), but whether this is due to thiamine deficiency or the action of alcohol *directly* is unresolved.

Whether alcohol is the direct cause of some of the structural and functional deficits detectable in the brains of many chronic drinkers is far less certain. Such defects include the report by Ron (1983) of cerebral shrinkage in half to two-thirds of chronic alcoholics, often from quite early in their drinking careers, and reports of widespread cognitive deficits such as of memory, psychomotor speed, visuospatial and abstracting abilities and complex reasoning, which can persist after drying out. Four perspectives on this issue are provided for the interested reader (Thomas, 1986; Victor *et al*, 1989; Harper & Kril, 1990; Lishman, 1990).

Central pontine myelinolysis

Central pontine myelinolysis is an acute, usually fatal disorder first described by Adams *et al* (1959) in alcoholics and undernourished individuals. The aetiology is uncertain, but does not appear to be a direct result of alcohol toxicity or vitamin deficiency. The disorder typically occurs in conjunction with life-threatening illness, which may or may not be alcohol-related. Rapid correction of hyponatraemia may lead to central pontine myelinolysis, and disturbances of serum potassium levels have also been incriminated (Bahr *et al*, 1990). The presence of clinical features such as pseudobulbar palsy, quadriplegia, delirium and coma may lead to the diagnosis being made before death, but more usually it is made at post-mortem (Victor *et al*, 1989). Histological examination of the brain will show circumscribed areas of demyelination both in the pons and less commonly in certain extrapontine sites (Esiri & Oppenheimer, 1989).

Marchiafava-Bignami disease

This disorder is characterised by demyelination of parts of the corpus callosum, the anterior commissure, and other areas of the brain such as the third layer of the frontal and temporal cortices. While the majority of cases described have been chronic alcoholic patients, it is not exclusive to alcoholics. Nutritional factors are thought to be implicated.

The presentation can be very varied. Affected patients may exhibit neurological signs such as dysarthria, dysphasia, dyspraxias, ataxia and hemiparesis, typically accompanied by physical deterioration leading to stupor and coma. Marchiafava-Bignami disease may present as a frontal lobe syndrome, and as a progressive dementia evolving over 3–6 years. The diagnosis is notoriously difficult to make in life because of variability of the clinical picture; other complications of alcoholism can further obscure the presentation. A frontal lobe syndrome in an alcoholic should alert the clinician to the possibility of Marchiafava-Bignami disease, as should symptoms suggestive of a corpus callosal tumour (Adams & Victor, 1989). Magnetic resonance imaging is capable of detecting corpus callosal lesions early in the course of the disease (Ikeda *et al*, 1989).

Hepatocerebral disorder

The term "hepatic encephalopathy" has been used to describe the organic reactions of the brain to liver disease (Summerskill *et al*, 1956; Victor *et al*, 1965). Acute severe hepatic dysfunction, such as that caused by viruses and drugs, is relatively uncommon in the alcoholic (Sherlock & Dooley, 1993). Patients with acute severe hepatic dysfunction exhibit euphoria, depression, hypersomnia, posturing and behavioural change of a bizarre and socially inappropriate nature (Collis & Lloyd, 1992). Delirium is frequently accompanied by over-activity and hostility (Zacharski *et al*, 1970). The presence of psychiatric symptoms is almost always a grave prognostic indicator, as chemical and histological changes are severe and extensive by then (Lishman, 1987). Coma usually supervenes within a few days unless there is effective management of the many complications. Cerebral oedema is found at post-mortem, and histological changes are usually non-specific.

However, hepatocerebral disturbance in the alcoholic is more usually sub-acute, chronic, or acute on chronic, occurring as a consequence of the development of a shunt between the portal and systemic circulation (toxins from the portal system enter the cerebral circulation unchanged by the liver). Quite which toxic substance is responsible is unclear, but the regulation of nitrogenous compounds is undoubtedly the most effective management strategy (Fraser & Arieff, 1985).

Days to weeks before the onset of delirium, stupor or coma there may be an array of symptoms that are essentially reversible (Summerskill *et al*, 1956; Lipowski, 1990). These include changes in personality such as irritability, jocularity, neurotic symptoms, depressed or elated mood, restlessness and schizophreniform psychosis. Daytime hypersomnia with nocturnal wakefulness is usually present early on. It is often cautioned that hypersomnia, coupled with a fixed staring appearance and a reduction in spontaneous movement, is early evidence of clinical deterioration. Recent memory is often impaired and confabulation can be striking. Attention and orientation may be affected. Delirium is typically of the "quiet" type, but there may be episodes of irritability and over-activity. Hallucinations are usually simple or elemental, though complex visual hallucinations may occur. Catatonia and stupor are well-recognised developments, and deterioration into coma is a real risk. Hypoglycaemia, electrolyte imbalance, renal failure, infection, and cerebral oedema may all contribute to the altered mental state in hepatic failure. However, delirium in an alcoholic with liver disease should not be assumed to be always hepatocerebral.

As the patient deteriorates, extrapyramidal, cerebellar and pyramidal signs unfold. Initially there may be incoordination, impaired handwriting and constructional apraxia. Foetor hepaticus is typically present. In the course of time a flapping tremor (asterixis), dysarthria and muscle rigidity may develop (Adams & Foley, 1953). Pyramidal signs become increasingly pronounced, fits may occur and the patient becomes comatose, with flaccid tone, absent reflexes and extensor plantars (Lishman, 1987).

At post-mortem, protoplasmic astrocytes are typically increased in size and number in the cortex and many other brain regions. The astrocyte changes roughly parallel the severity and chronicity of the neurological and psychiatric disturbance (Victor *et al*, 1989). There is usually patchy necrosis and neuronal loss in the deep cerebral cortex (Esiri & Oppenheimer, 1989).

Some patients develop persistent global cognitive impairment, particularly where the acute episodes have been prolonged or frequent. This has been termed 'acquired hepatocerebral degeneration' (Victor *et al*, 1965). Attention is impaired but orientation in time and place is often intact. Memory is affected, particularly in the acquisition and retention of new material, but not disproportionately as in Korsakoff syndrome. Insight is generally lacking. A variety of neurological signs are usually present, particularly choreoathetosis, dysarthria, ataxia and pyramidal signs. These patients may periodically deteriorate as acute organic episodes are superimposed.

The assessment of the degree of cerebral disorder in a patient with liver failure is reviewed by Pappas & Jones (1983); they recommend that the mental state is staged and provide a scheme. It is important to note that verbal skills may be relatively well preserved, and thus mild degrees of cerebral disorder may go unnoticed unless psychometry is performed.

A normal EEG will usually exclude the diagnosis of hepatocerebral disorder (Parsons-Smith *et al*, 1957). EEG changes may antedate changes in mental state and persist after apparent clinical improvement.

The patient with hepatocerebral disorder should not drink alcohol. Dietary protein restriction and other measures are required (Fraser & Arieff, 1985). If sedation is required a benzodiazepine can be used cautiously; phenothiazines and butyrophenones are contraindicated. The patient should be made aware of the potential dangers of medications, particularly sedatives, whose absorption, protein-binding, metabolism and distribution will be altered (Collis & Lloyd, 1992). Renewed drinking, dietary indiscretion, a gastrointestinal bleed, inappropriate medication and infection are but a few of the potential causes of a resurgence of psychiatric disturbance in a previously well managed patient.

Miscellaneous alcohol-related disorders

Alcohol-induced hypoglycaemia

Hypoglycaemia is an often overlooked cause of morbidity in the alcoholic and should always be excluded. It is predominantly a disorder of more chronic, dependent drinkers who are malnourished. It has also been described in young people after first exposure to alcohol. The origin is thought to be a reduced hepatic output of glucose, due to reduced hepatic stores of glycogen and suppression of gluconeogenesis during metabolism of alcohol. This is a situation potentiated when there is anorexia, for then gluconeogenesis is the main source of glucose (Zilva & Pannall, 1979).

Hypoglycaemia typically occurs 2–16 hours after a large intake of alcohol. At a blood glucose level just under 2.0 mmol/l, autonomic symptoms appear and gradually intensify, heralding the onset of delirium. Hypoglycaemia may induce generalised seizures, which should not be mistaken for withdrawal seizures. Stupor may also occur. At a blood glucose level of around 0.6 mmol/l, life-threatening hypoglycaemic coma is usually evident and recovery will often be incomplete. The treatment is immediate administration of glucose intravenously, and thiamine should be given concurrently to avoid precipitating Wernicke's disease.

Alcohol-related electrolyte and acid-base disturbance

Fluid loss may be substantial in severe delirium, requiring close monitoring and prompt correction. As much as six litres of fluid a day may need to be given, of which no more than one litre of normal saline should be given. Conversely, hyponatraemia may complicate the consumption of large quantities of relatively dilute alcoholic drinks. It is a potential cause of convulsions and is managed by fluid restriction (Saunders, 1991). Hyponatraemia, hypokalaemia,

---

Box 24.6 Drugs with anticholinergic activity

Antispasmodic drugs
Antimotility (gastrointestinal) drugs
Antihistamines
Compound nasal decongestants
Antipsychotics
Antidepressants
Antiparkinsonian drugs
Antiemetics
Premedication agents
Drugs for urinary incontinence
Topical antipruritic drugs
Mydriatic and cycloplegic drugs

hypophosphataemia and hypomagnesaemia may all occur in alcoholics and have been associated with withdrawal delirium.

Medicinal drugs

Cerebral intoxication with medicines is a frequent cause of psychiatric morbidity. This can go unrecognised if there is ignorance of the adverse effects of a medication, or when patients overlook, deny or understate their usage. The young and elderly are especially vulnerable, as are those individuals with physical illness, alcohol dependency or a requirement for

---

Box 24.7   Management of anticholinergic intoxication (adapted from Heiser & Gillin, 1971; Lipowski, 1990)

Evaluate the patient paying particular attention to vital signs, anticholinergic effects and mental state. The patient should be attached to a cardiac monitor. Introduce nursing and supportive measures

If the aetiology is uncertain, physostigmine 1–2 mg intramuscularly (or subcutaneously) is given. If the patient has taken an anticholinergic substance, little or no change will occur. In the absence of such intake, cholinergic features such as lacrimation, miosis, salivation, bradycardia and sweating will occur within 30 minutes

Treatment begins with 1–2 mg of physostigmine intramuscularly or by slow intravenous infusion. If there is no clinical change within 15–30 minutes a further 1–2 mg is administered. If toxicity persists or the patient relapses, further doses are given every 30 minutes to 2 hours until the clinical state improves or cholinergic toxicity develops

In mild cases withdrawal of the offending drug and supportive reassurance may suffice. If sedation is required, diazepam is used. Phenothiazines and haloperidol should be avoided because of their anticholinergic properties

If cholinergic crisis is precipitated with physostigmine, 0.5–1.0 mg of atropine sulphate should be given intravenously

In children and the elderly, the dosage of physostigmine should be approximately half that of the adult dose

Contraindications to physostigmine include a history of allergy to the drug, renal hypertension, hyperthyroidism, coronary artery disease, certain cardiac dysrhythmias, peptic ulcer, obstructive airways disease, mechanical obstruction to the urogenital tract or bowel, glaucoma, pregnancy and myotonia congenita

---

more than one drug at a time. Drugs produce mental changes either by direct intoxication or, once physical tolerance has developed, as a consequence of withdrawal. Intoxication can occur at normal dosage, as an idiosyncratic reaction, or through interaction with other substances, but more usually it is due to excessive dosage, by accident or deliberately.

Delirium is a characteristic manifestation of drug intoxication, often with hallucinations. Other manifestations are dementia, psychosis in clear consciousness, mood change, lethargy, and anxiety. Predominantly physical adverse reactions, such as neuroleptic malignant syndrome, tardive dyskinesia and lithium intoxication, usually have accompanying mental changes.

A large range and number of drugs have the ability to cause delirium. Three types of drug intoxication have been selected for more detailed discussion: as a result of drugs with anticholinergic activity; from drugs with central stimulant properties; and intoxication from drugs available in over-the-counter medications. Information on the adverse psychiatric reactions of other drugs can be obtained from sources such as Jacobs (1987), Reynolds (1989) and Lipowski (1990).

Anticholinergic (antimuscarinic) intoxication

Anticholinergic poisoning from plants and medicines has been recognised since ancient times. The retreating troops of Mark Antony are said to have consumed *Datura stramonium* in 38 AD as they left Partia and developed confusion with many deaths. The same mistake was made by British troops in Jamestown, Virginia in 1676 (Goldfrank & Melinek, 1979). Drugs with antimuscarinic activity inhibit the actions of acetylcholine on autonomic effectors innervated by postganglionic cholinergic nerves, as well as having a direct effect on smooth muscles that lack cholinergic innervation (Weiner, 1980). Atropine is the best known of this class of drug, although there are very many others (Box 24.6). It should be noted that anticholinergic poisoning can occur as a result of ingestion of a number of plants, notably *Atropa belladonna* (deadly nightshade), *Datura stramonium* and *Hyoscyamus niger* (henbane).

The clinical picture has been described as "hot as a hare, blind as a bat, dry as a bone, red as beet and mad as a hatter". However, it should not be forgotten that intoxication commonly unfolds in an insidious fashion (Johnson *et al*, 1981). The symptoms of anticholinergic intoxication are essentially those of atropine intoxication. Small doses of atropine cause a dry mouth and reduce bronchial secretions. Inhibition of sweating is followed by fever. Larger doses impair pupillary accommodation, cause pupil dilatation and thus blurred vision. Tachycardia is common. Still larger doses inhibit parasympathetic control of the bowel and bladder resulting in difficulty passing urine and reduced bowel sounds. Doses as great as 5 mg of atropine produce difficulty in swallowing, restlessness, fatigue, and headache, together with dry, hot skin. Beyond this, the skin is hot, dry and scarlet in colour. Ataxia, restlessness and excitement occur. Delirium and hallucinations ensue and can be followed by coma. Impairment of recent memory is a prominent feature. The hallucinations may be auditory or visual. Without effective intervention there is a significant chance that the patient will die through brain-stem depression, hyperpyrexia or injury (while delirious).

Anticholinergic intoxication should not be confused with the neuroleptic malignant syndrome, which has certain features in common (notably tachycardia, labile blood pressure, hyperpyrexia and fluctuating levels of consciousness; Howells, 1994). The vital distinguishing features of anticholinergic intoxication are dilated pupils, with dry skin and mucous membranes.

Anticholinergic drug intoxication is managed with physostigmine, an anticholinesterase, in accordance with a management plan such as the one outlined in Box 24.7.

The importance of being aware of anticholinergic drug effects cannot be overemphasised. To illustrate this, two examples from everyday clinical practice might be considered. Firstly, tricyclic drug intoxication (due to anticholinergic effects) can produce agitation in a depressed patient. This agitation may then be treated with a sedative neuroleptic such as thioridazine, which itself has potent anticholinergic effects, so exacerbating

Table 24.4 Constituents of over-the-counter drugs available in the UK with the potential to cause cerebral intoxication and/or dependence

Group	Constituents
CNS stimulants with amphetamine-like effects	Ephedrine, methylephedrine, pseudoephedrine, phenylephrine, phenylpropanolamine, oxymetazoline (eye-drops)
Drugs with anticholinergic side-effects	Atropine, belladonna alkaloids, homatropine, hyoscine, chlorphenhydramine, diphenhydramine, promethazine, doxylamine
Alcohol	
Drugs with caffeine-like effects (xanthines)	Caffeine, theophylline
Opioids	Morphine, codeine, pholcodine, dextromethorphan
Miscellaneous drugs	Bismuth carbonate, menthol, chloroform

the problem. The second example concerns the treatment of schizophrenia. Excessive use of neuroleptics with anticholinergic properties can induce or exacerbate psychotic symptoms, which in turn are exacerbated by increasing the dose of the medication further.

Central nervous system stimulants and anoretics

In 1924 ephedrine, extracted from the ancient Chinese herb Ma Huang, was introduced into western medicine as a bronchodilator. Shortly afterwards ephedrine was synthesised chemically, and amphetamine was synthesised as a substitute for ephedrine (Alles, 1933). The structures of the two compounds are remarkably similar, as are their actions and those of the further synthetic derivatives which constitute this group of drugs.

Ephedrine, pseudoephedrine, phenylephrine and phenylpropanololamine are ingredients of cold remedies and constitute some of the most widely used over-the-counter drugs. An analysis of the non-proprietary drugs used in the UK (Reynolds, 1989) reveals some 12 compounds containing these ingredients.

In the UK the use of centrally acting stimulants (dexamphetamine sulphate or pemoline) is restricted principally to the treatment of narcolepsy, and hyperactivity in children. In the US, methylphenidate is prescribed very widely for school-age hyperactivity and attentional problems. A small range of drugs with amphetamine-like properties are available for use as anoretic pills.

The toxic effect of amphetamine is to induce a paranoid psychosis with ideas of reference, delusions of persecution, auditory and visual hallucinations, almost always in a setting of clear consciousness (Connell, 1958). Depression and somnolence are common in withdrawal. Intoxication with ephedrine produces a virtually identical clinical picture. First rank symptoms of schizophrenia are reported to be present in approximately 35%, delusions in 100%, and auditory hallucinations in 90% of cases (Whitehouse & Duncan, 1987). While children and the elderly are especially vulnerable, misuse and dependence also occur in other age groups. Similar effects are reported with anoretic agents and other centrally acting stimulants (Jacobs, 1987). A larger range of anoretics is available outside the UK, not uncommonly without prescription. Related compounds have been sold for indications such as "lack of drive", as in the following example:

> A middle aged Jamaican man with unstable paranoid schizophrenia and aggression was brought to England for clinical review. It transpired that he had been buying large quantities of fenethylline (Captagon Psychotonicum) which he had been able to purchase legally over the counter. A clear temporal relationship was demonstrated between the use of the drug and the occurrence of his symptoms. The patient understood and accepted the link but confessed an inability to change his habit.

These drugs achieve special significance when considering the differential diagnosis of schizophrenia – a diagnosis that, arguably, should only be made if symptoms are present when a person has been shown to be completely free of these substances. In the author's experience the clinical situation can be complicated by patients who conceal their drug use, volunteer symptoms that were present when they *were* taking the drug, and by misleading results from drug screening tests. Commonly used immunoassay techniques may fail to detect the presence of diethylpropion, phentermine and other drugs, while the more reliable (but less widely available) gas chromatographic assays can fail to detect pemoline.

Over-the-counter drugs

The misuse of over-the-counter drugs has long been recognised by pharmacists (Harrison, 1988). In the late 1980s, it was estimated that some 5 billion doses of phenylpropanolamine were taken annually in the US (Forman *et al*, 1989), revealing the extent of the problem.

Chronic affective disturbance, psychosis, delirium and personality change are the consequences of intoxication, dependence or withdrawal from these drugs (Jacobs, 1987). There are at least 80 over-the-counter products whose constituents have the potential to cause significant psychiatric symptomatology (Table 24.4). Intoxication has been reported from topical nasal compounds, eyedrops, inhalations, and even substances administered topically.

The hidden morbidity from these compounds is likely to be high, particularly in children who are commonly given cold remedies containing drugs with the potential to cause intoxication. Evidence for this can be adduced from Sweden, where in 1979 the Swedish adverse drug reaction committee received 61 reports of psychic disturbance from phenylpropanolamine – restlessness, irritability, aggression and sleep disturbance. The majority were in children, including three of the five individuals who had psychotic symptoms (Norvenius *et al*, 1979).

> *Case example*
> A physician gave his 2-year-old son 5 ml of a preparation of triprolidine and pseudoephedrine at bedtime because of an irritating cough and runny nose. The child awoke saying there were "ants crawling in his bed". This was assumed to be due to pyrexia. The next night the medicine was overlooked and the child had no sleep disturbance. On the third night the medicine was remembered and the hallucinations recurred. On reflection it was thought that these could have been induced a number of times over the preceding nine months, but the link had not been made (Drennan, 1984).

Dependence in adults is often concealed and is difficult to detect from drug screening. It may become extreme. Dependence does not always begin accidentally; some compounds, particularly phenylpropanolamine and ephedrine have long been regarded as convenient amphetamine substitutes (Blum, 1981; Loosemore & Armstrong, 1990).

Table 24.5 Plants with hallucinogenic potential (Emboden, 1972; Efron *et al*, 1979; Jacobs, 1987)

Latin name	Local name	Location
Amanita muscaria	Fly agaric	Temperate
Conocybe, Psilocybe	Magic mushrooms	Ubiquitous
Pancratium trianthum	Kwashi	West Africa
Catharanthus roseus	Madagascar periwinkle	Ubiquitous
Acorus calamus	Sweet flag	North America
Sarcostemma acidum	Soma	India
Lophophora williamsii	Peyote	Central America
Cannabis sativa	Pot, Ganja etc.	Ubiquitous
Catha edulis	Khat, Qat	Arabia/N.E.Africa
Argyreia nervosa	Silver morning glory	Tropics
Erythroxylon coca	Coca, Coke	S. America
Alcohornea floribunda	Niando	West Africa
Cytisus canariensis	Canary Island broom	Ubiquitous
Sophora secundiflora	Mescal bean	Central America
Claviceps purpura	Ergot	Temperate
Coleus blumei	El macho, El nene	Mexico, Asia
Lobelia inflata	Indian tobacco	North America
Heimia salicifolia	Sinicuichi	Central America
Mimosa hostilis	Vino de Jurema	Brazil
Myristica fragrans	Nutmeg	Tropics
Olmedioperebea sclerophylla	Rape dos indios	Brazil
Psychotria viridis		Equador
Atropa belladonna	Deadly nightshade	Ubiquitous
Datura innoxia	Thorn-apple	Central America
Datura stramonium	Jimson weed	Ubiquitous
Duboisia myoporoides	Pituri	Australia
Hyoscyamus niger	Henbane	Europe
Mandragora officinarum	Mandrake, Satan's apple	Southern Europe
Methysticodendrom amnesianum	Culebra-Borrachera	Columbia
Foeniculum vulgare	Fennel	Europe

Drugs of misuse

A detailed exposition of this group of drugs is beyond the remit of this chapter; however, many of these drugs represent important sources of brain intoxication. It should be noted that certain substances have prolonged effects that persist beyond the period during which an effect might reasonably be assumed to be operating. Flashbacks are a well-known example of this, but other effects include personality disorder, affective disorder, cognitive impairment and late-onset psychotic disorder. Interested readers are referred to *Seminars in Alcohol and Drug Misuse* (Chick & Cantwell, 1994).

Plants and plant-derived substances

Here the broad notion of intoxication from material derived from plants is introduced – the interested reader is encouraged to consult further sources such as Emboden (1972), Efron *et al* (1979) and Jacobs (1987). Intoxication from various plants occurs in at least four ways. Accidental exposure may occur through contamination, as in the instance of ergot-contaminated grain (*Claviceps purpurea*) or through accidental ingestion as with nutmeg (*Myristica fragrans*) and deadly nightshade (*Atropa belladonna*). Secondly, intoxication may occur as a result of traditional rites, rituals and practices. Examples range from the excessive use of caffeine-containing beverages, and the drinking and chewing of khat (*Catha edulis*) in Arabia and Somalia, to chewing a quid of pituri (*Duboisia hopwoodii*) (Australia) or drinking sinicuichi (*Heimia salicifolia*)(Central America). Thirdly, intoxication may be due to deliberate misuse of plant substances, either those available within one's culture, or by seeking out substances from other cultures or lands. The author had one patient who obtained peyote (*Lophophora williamsii*) from a south London herbalist shop and had regularly abused magic mushrooms (*Psilocybe*). Fourthly, intoxication may occur as a result of poisoning by another person.

The range of potential plant intoxicants is much wider than is often appreciated (Table 24.5 shows some of them). The chief relevance to the clinician is in differential diagnosis, particularly but not exclusively in transcultural practice; it should always be recalled that major psychiatric symptoms such as hallucinations can be caused by plant intoxicants.

Caffeine intoxication

Of the plant-derived substances with the potential to cause intoxication, caffeine (a xanthine) is surely the most popular and widely consumed. It is present in tea, coffee, soft drinks such as cola, and chocolate, and also

Table 24.6 Approximate caffeine content of beverages (Wells, 1984; Ashton, 1987; Greden & Walters, 1992)

Beverage	Caffeine content
Boiled coffee	100–500 mg/225 ml vessel
Roasted ground coffee	125 mg/225 ml vessel
Instant coffee	60–100 mg/225 ml vessel
Decaffeinated coffee	2–4 mg/225 ml vessel
Tea	30–100 mg/225 ml vessel
Cola drinks	25–50 mg/330 ml can
Chocolate drink	5–50 mg/225 ml vessel
(Chocolate bar)	(Approximately 30 mg/bar)

in some 27 or more over-the-counter compounds. Other xanthines are found in tea, coffee and chocolate, particularly theobromine and theophylline, the latter having a potent stimulant effect on the central nervous system (CNS).

Caffeine has a stimulant effect on the CNS, as well as wide-ranging systemic effects. The clinical features of intoxication include restlessness, nervousness, excitement, insomnia, flushed face, diuresis, gastrointestinal disturbance, muscle twitching, rambling flow of thought and speech, tachycardia or cardiac dysrhythmia, periods of inexhaustibility, and psychomotor agitation. After prolonged use, physical tolerance and dependence ensues (Greden & Walters, 1992). Withdrawal symptoms include headache, hypersomnia, irritability, lethargy, poor concentration and anxiety, all of which are countered by the inclusion of caffeine in many cold cures and over-the-counter compound analgesics. It is usual for the symptoms of intoxication and withdrawal, if recognised at all, to be attributed to other circumstances.

To gauge adequately the contribution of tea or coffee consumption to a patient's symptoms, consideration must be given to the individual's age and size, whether there is consumption of other caffeine-containing substances such as soft drinks, and whether other drugs which increase (oral contraceptive, cimetidine) or reduce (rifampicin, smoking) the half-life are being used. The nature of the beverage, size of the vessel, frequency of consumption and mode of preparation should be noted; boiling and percolating coffee dramatically increases the dosage, as does a long period of brewing tea. Merely asking about the number of cups of tea or coffee taken in a day is insufficient, although it does serve as a useful starting point (Table 24.6).

Caffeine consumption (and thus toxicity) has been shown to be increased in psychiatric patients with a dry mouth due to anticholinergic drug treatment. Furthermore, individual susceptibility to intoxication is variable; some individuals develop intoxication from as little as 250 mg of caffeine a day.

Caffeine may mimic or augment a range of neurotic disorders, such as panic disorder, generalised anxiety disorder, minor mood disturbance and neurasthenia. It may also aggravate stress reactions and affective disorder, impair personal effectiveness, and in exceptional circumstances following a sudden increase in consumption, even induce delirium (Bruce & Lader, 1986). The psychiatrist in family practice should be aware that caffeine enters breast milk and can cause babies to become restless, sleepless and "difficult".

Environmental elements and other chemical substances

One large group of brain intoxicants might be categorised together as the environmental intoxicants – metallic and non-metallic. The latter include solvents and vapours, herbicides and pesticides.

Metals and metal compounds

Aluminium

Aluminium accumulation can occur as a result of dialysis, industrial exposure, from parenteral nutrition, from certain foodstuffs, from the ingestion of aluminium-containing antacids and phosphate binding agents, and in other ways. Occupational exposure to aluminium has been associated with memory impairment and actual dementia, as well as a range of neurological disturbances. While aluminium is present in senile plaques and neurofibrillary tangles in the brains of cases of Alzheimer's disease, the relationship between aluminium exposure and Alzheimer's disease has yet to be clarified. It should be pointed out that anomalies in the levels of other metals such as iron and zinc are also found in Alzheimer's disease.

Arsenic

Arsenical compounds are widely employed as herbicides, insecticides and rodenticides, as well as within the metal, paint and dye industries. Acute poisoning can cause headache, nausea, vomiting, diarrhoea, burning of the mouth and throat, abdominal pain, delirium, coma, fits, peripheral neuropathy with profound paraesthesia, and heart failure. The actual clinical presentation reflects the dose received (Ghariani *et al*, 1991). Subacute intoxication is most likely to present to psychiatrists; this is characterised by fatigue, weakness, muscle aching, and anorexia. Schizophrenia-like psychoses occur, as also do cognitive impairments, particularly deficits in recent memory and new learning. Arsenic intoxication should be suspected if a significant number of these features are present in the context of possible poisoning or occupational exposure. Pronounced paraesthesia in the extremities along with scaly dermatitis and/or hyperpigmentation of the trunk and limbs provide additional evidence of exposure (Fuortes, 1988). Mees' lines are transverse white lines on the fingernails suggesting an earlier episode of exposure to arsenic. Arsenic can be identified in urine, hair and nails.

Bismuth

Intoxication with bismuth is quite commonly caused by the treatment of gastrointestinal complaints with bismuth compounds, particularly bismuth subgallate, bismuth subnitrate and tripotassium dicitratobismuthate. Bismuth subcitrate and bismuth subsalicylate appear to be safer. Intoxication is characterised by depression, anxiety, irritability, phobias, insomnia, and delusions. It may be associated with myoclonus, tremor, ataxia and other motor problems (Supino-Viterbo *et al*, 1977). The clinical resemblance to Creutzfeld-Jacob disease has been remarked upon (Von-Bose & Zaudig, 1991). Many of these clinical problems are reversible. Patients can develop hallucinations in the visual, auditory and/or gustatory modalities and delirium can occur. Memory impairment and progressive dementia is reported. Hyperdensities in the basal ganglia, cortex and cerebellum are sometimes evident on brain-imaging. Blood bismuth levels can be measured, as can the 24-hour urine bismuth level.

Gold

While gold has been used medicinally for centuries, it is mainly used now in the treatment of rheumatoid arthritis. Toxic symptoms include depression, hallucinations, delirium, ataxia, blurred vision, tremor and peripheral neuropathy.

Lead

Despite efforts to remove lead from our environment, intoxication by accumulation is still an occupational hazard, particularly for printers, painters, and workers manufacturing batteries. The main systemic features are gastrointestinal upset, mild anaemia, occasionally a "lead line" on the gingival margins, fatigue and muscle weakness. Acute brain intoxication results in irritability, auditory and visual hallucinations, memory difficulties, delirium and coma. It can manifest more insidiously with insomnia, headache, irritability and cognitive decline. Generalised seizures and raised intracranial pressure are reported complications (Jefferson & Marshall, 1981). The diagnosis can be confirmed by the presence of high blood and urine lead levels in association with a hypochromic anaemia with basophil stippling (Schroter *et al*, 1991). Antidotes for lead intoxication include sodium calciumedetate, penicallamine and dimercaprol. Recovery after severe poisoning is often incomplete, sequelae include mental handicap, seizures and neurological dysfunction.

Tetraethyl lead

Organic lead poisoning from tetraethyl or tetramethylead lead occurs either as a result of industrial exposure or, more usually, from sniffing petrol (Cullen *et al*, 1983). Typically it causes excitement, which progresses to delirium. Accidental exposure can lead to insidious accumulation of organic lead, in which case ataxia, peripheral nerve damage, anorexia, fatigue, nervousness, insomnia and memory loss precede the development of more acute symptoms. Chronic organic lead intoxication has been reported to simulate both schizophrenia and hypomania.

Manganese

Manganese intoxication is a particular hazard for manganese miners, battery and steel plant workers, welders, and glass workers. Three presentations of intoxication are identifiable. In the first few months after exposure, ataxia and speech problems occur in conjunction with fatigue, anorexia, insomnia, memory difficulties, hallucinations and mania. This state of "manganese madness" can closely resemble mania and schizophrenia. In the next phase, neurological symptoms such as incoordination, sleepiness and speech problems become more prominent. Finally, progressive parkinsonism, personality change and even dementia appear, a state referred to as "manganism" (Hartman, 1988).

Mercury

Mercury intoxication results from exposure to the elemental liquid or vapour, a mercury salt, or an organic mercury compound, the latter causing the most significant pathological changes in the brain (Vroom & Greer, 1972). Systemic features of chronic poisoning include gingivitis, loosening of the teeth, excessive salivation, a metallic taste, anorexia, renal damage, anaemia, hypertension, tremor, peripheral neuropathy and ataxia (Jefferson & Marshall, 1981). Psychiatric features include fatigue, lassitude, depression or irritability and insomnia. Certain individuals develop a curious behavioural syndrome termed "erythism". The remarkable feature is an inability to function in front of observers, coupled with timidity, nervousness and social anxiety. While memory difficulties and dementia are reported sequelae, delirium and psychosis are rare. Acute organic mercurial poisoning can produce a severe disorder characterised by paraesthesia, incoordination, blindness, parkinsonism and/or a clinical picture resembling amyotrophic lateral sclerosis. Intoxication in children can present with a combination of pruritic skin rashes and neurobehavioural disabilities, a syndrome which has been termed acrodynia (Dathan, 1954). To date there is no firm evidence of mercury intoxication resulting from dental fillings of amalgam containing mercury (Herrström & Högstedt, 1993), although dental staff may be exposed to unsafe levels of mercurial compounds in their daily work.

Nickel

Nickel carbonyl is a gas given off during the refining of nickel. It is said to have a toxicity five times that of carbon monoxide, and inhalation is reported to induce pulmonary oedema, delirium, fits and death (Hunter, 1978).

Thallium

Thallium salts are used in the manufacture of optical lenses, semiconductors, fireworks and jewellery, and also as catalysts in a range of chemical processes. There are regular reports of their use with murderous intent, which probably reflects the fact that thallium salts are odourless, colourless and tasteless (Moore *et al*, 1993). Acute thallium poisoning typically presents with prominent gastrointestinal and neuromuscular symptoms. Neurological and psychiatric features may be delayed for a few days; these include paraesthesia, hyperaesthesia, headaches, ptosis, optic atrophy, prominent myalgia, myopathy, fits, psychosis, delirium, and dementia. Sudden death may result from cardiac arrhythmias. The episode of poisoning is marked two to three weeks later by hair loss, parotid enlargement, skin lesions and sometimes Mees' lines on the nails. The impact of thallium poisoning can be alleviated with regular oral doses of Berlin blue and other measures (Moore *et al*, 1993). The differential diagnosis includes intoxication with lead, gold, carbon monoxide, organophosphates and such conditions as Guillain-Barré syndrome, diabetic polyneuritis and porphyria.

Organic tin compounds

Of the organic tin compounds, trimethyltin and triethyltin are especially toxic to the nervous system. Inhalation and transcutaneous exposure to trimethyltin has been associated with headache, fits, delirium, and impairment of recent memory, as well as anorexia, fatigue and personality change (Reiter & Ruppert, 1984). Triethyltin causes oedema of myelin and symptoms suggestive of raised intracranial pressure.

Other metals

Vanadium compounds have been shown to cause a range of respiratory complaints, depressed mood, anorexia, visual disturbance and tremor (Hunter, 1978). Zinc intoxication can cause fatigue, lethargy and delirium. Reports of the neuropsychiatric effects of intoxication with barium, boron, selenium, cadmium, platinum, silicon and tellurium are few.

Organic solvents, gases and vapours

Intoxication with this class of chemical is now chiefly encountered as a result of deliberate misuse. A large range of organic solvent-containing products are misused, notably lighter fuels, adhesives, typewriter correction fluid, dry cleaning fluids, aerosols, and nail polish remover. Pure solvents, antifreeze, petroleum, fire-extinguishers, whipped-cream aerosols and even asthma inhalers (fluorinated hydrocarbons) have also been similarly misused. In the UK, the majority of solvent misusers now employ butane; previously, adhesives containing toluene and acetone were most widely used. Fluorinated hydrocarbons (freons) and butane appear to be disproportionately associated with fatalities, possibly due to their cardiotoxicity. Intoxicated individuals can become sensitised to the effects of endogenous and exogenous catecholamines. Deaths also occur through asphyxiation, accidents, and liver failure.

Organic solvents have toxic effects on the central nervous system, liver, lungs, haemopoietic system, kidneys and heart. Teratogenic changes and a neonatal syndrome have been long suspected. Products often contain more than one solvent whose effects can be additive or synergistic with one another. The diagnosis and treatment of acute poisoning with volatile substances has been outlined by Meredith *et al* (1989).

Toluene usefully illustrates the general effects of solvent intoxication. As with other CNS depressants, toluene inhalation causes an initial excitatory effect, followed by a depressive phase that may result in narcosis and even loss of consciousness. The excitatory phase is characterised by euphoria, disinhibition, excitement, tinnitus, dizziness and diplopia. Sneezing and coughing, gastrointestinal disturbance, fits and paraesthesia, illusions, hallucinations (visual or auditory), delirium and coma are also reported (Ron, 1986). Regular use can cause physical tolerance and withdrawal phenomena (headache and lethargy), constituting a state of dependency (Westermeyer, 1987). While the evidence that toluene misuse routinely causes severe or lasting neuropsychological or psychiatric disorder is meagre, there are data suggesting that older, more severe misusers may have circumscribed cognitive impairments and cerebellar dysfunction (Fornazzari *et al*, 1983).

Solvent misuse should be suspected in the presence of an odour on the breath, freeze marks on the face, a perioral rash, glue on the hands or garments, and possession of solvent containers. Behavioural changes include social withdrawal and anorexia, as well as those of intoxication. Laboratory detection is difficult; blood levels of solvents are detectable for 12 hours to five days depending on the type of solvent. Toluene is detected in urine as increased hippuric acid levels, although if testing is delayed for more than two days it can be missed (King *et al*, 1981).

Straight chain aliphatic hydrocarbons

Small straight-chain aliphatic hydrocarbons such as methane and ethane are thought to cause a toxic effect by inducing hypoxia. Higher molecular weight aliphatic hydrocarbons, such as propane to octane, act as CNS depressants, thus producing intoxication in a manner generally similar to toluene. N-hexane deserves special mention. It is a widely used solvent which not only produces a peripheral nerve distal axonopathy, but also, with high level exposure, acute intoxication and CNS axonal degeneration. Like methyl butyl ketone (MBK), n-hexane is metabolised to 2,5,-hexanedione (2,5,-HD) which is reponsible for most of its neurotoxic effects (Sharp & Rosenberg, 1992). Butane abuse now exceeds toluene abuse, possibly reflecting the fact that it is conveniently packaged as lighter fuel.

Benzene

Acute intoxication with the aromatic hydrocarbon benzene produces features generally similar to toluene, though dyspnoea and impaired gait may persist for several weeks (Lipowski, 1990). Chronic exposure is linked to the subsequent development of aplastic anaemia and leukaemia.

Carbon tetrachloride

Carbon tetrachloride is a particularly toxic halogenated hydrocarbon solvent, but is now less commonly encountered. Transient exposure can cause irritation to the eyes, nose and throat, nausea and vomiting, dizziness, drowsiness, diplopia and headache. Continued higher level exposure leads to delirium, stupor, fits, coma and sudden death. Severe delayed systemic effects occur in the hepatic, renal and gastrointestinal systems (Ruprah *et al*, 1985).

Methyl bromide

Intoxication from methyl bromide, an insecticide, has been reported to induce persistent sequelae such as hallucinations, memory difficulties, aphasia and incoordination (Shield *et al*, 1977). In children it should be considered in the differential diagnosis of Reye's syndrome.

Methylene chloride

Methylene chloride is a ubiquitous solvent and refrigerant. It is metabolised to carbon monoxide and thus can have both narcotic and hypoxic effects on the brain (Sharp & Rosenberg, 1992). It causes permanent neurological effects after very high levels of acute exposure.

Trichloroethylene

Trichloroethylene exposure can cause cranial neuropathies, particularly trigeminal neuropathy. At higher levels of exposure the features are those of acute solvent intoxication. Alcohol potentiates the effects of trichloroethylene. The effects of chronic exposure are uncertain.

Trichloroethane

Trichloroethane was once a common aerosol propellent, but is now mainly used as an industrial degreasing solvent, in garment cleaners and in correction fluids. Acute low-level exposure (500 ppm) is thought to have only slight behavioural effects. However, permanent neurological sequelae have been associated with acute, massive exposure, probably as a result of cerebral hypoxia.

Methanol

Methanol poisoning is often due to the adulteration of alcoholic beverages. Initially a state of intoxication occurs which resembles that of ethanol. However, in the body it is oxidised to formaldehyde and formic acid, which can give rise to severe metabolic acidosis and retinal ganglion cell damage, resulting in scotomata and blindness. The onset of symptoms can be delayed for up to three days; these symptoms include visual changes, tiredness, delirium, stupor and coma. The three main components of treatment are intravenous sodium bicarbonate, ethanol and early haemodialysis.

Isopropanol

Intoxication with the alcohol isopropanol can result from either ingestion or exposure to the vapour. General features of intoxication are similar to ethanol, but more delayed and prolonged. Gastric symptoms can be severe; vomiting with aspiration is a recognised danger. Muscle spasms arise as a result of the chelation of calcium by the oxalate produced from the metabolism of isopropanol; this is a useful pointer to the diagnosis.

Ethylene glycol

Ethylene glycol is widely employed as a solvent and in antifreeze, and may be taken as an alcohol substitute. Inebriation can be rapidly followed by CNS depression, narcosis, coma and death. A severe metabolic acidosis usually arises and acute renal failure is a further complication. The emergency treatment is similar to that of methanol. The effects of diethylene glycol and propylene glycol resemble ethylene glycol, although propylene glycol is considerably less toxic.

Petroleum ethers

Petrol-sniffing results in acute exposure not only to a wide range of organic solvents (benzene, toluene, olefins, napthenes and paraffins) but also to tetraethyl lead, the symptoms of which are described in the section on metals.

Esters

Dimethyl sulphate, glyceryl trinitrate, amyl nitrate, butyl nitrite and isobutyl nitrite are esters which have all been known to cause delirium after intense exposure (Lipowski, 1990)

Chlorinated pesticide compounds

These chemicals cause CNS stimulation. Dichlorodiphenyltrichloroethane (DDT) now has major restrictions on its use because, being highly fat-soluble, it is biomagnified in the food chain of animals (Klaassen, 1990). Poisoning causes facial paralysis, dizziness, tremor, delirium and fits.

Chlorinated cyclodienes such as aldrin, dieldrin, heptachlor and chlordane produce the signs and symptoms of DDT poisoning but, being more potent CNS stimulants, often induce epileptic-type seizures before other symptoms. Compared with DDT, poisoning with these chemicals is more lethal.

Lindane, a commonly-used topical treatment for head lice, is the gamma isomer of benzene hexachloride. Acute poisoning results in tremors, ataxia, delirium and fits.

Organophosphate pesticides

Organophosphate compounds have replaced many chlorinated hydrocarbons as agricultural pesticides; exposure to these chemicals is a major cause of death and morbidity worldwide. Their use is not restricted to agriculture; they are also found in a range of occupational and domestic contexts, and are also constituents of chemical weapons. Malathion, diazinon and parathion are but three examples of many thousands of these chemicals. They act as irreversible acetylcholinesterase inhibitors, first stimulating and then blocking synaptic transmission in cholinergic neurones throughout the nervous system. Acute features include headache, vomiting, abdominal pains, sweating, excess salivation and lacrimation, wheezing, miosis and blurred vision, muscle weakness, cramps and fasciculations. Delirium and impaired memory are additional features. Hyperglycaemia, hypertension or hypotension may develop. After 1–4 days, weakness and/ or paralysis can develop in the proximal limb, neck and respiratory muscles. Cranial neuropathies, fatigue, irritability and memory difficulties are other features of this second phase, but tend to recede after two weeks. A third phase of delayed effects may occur, particularly the development of a distal sensorimotor neuropathy. Some organophospate compounds can also induce corticospinal damage in this phase. Lasting emotional and affective symptoms occur in individuals exposed to these chemicals, but it is not certain that discrete, persistent neuropsychological deficits occur (Minton & Murray, 1988). Treatment involves taking measures to stop further absorption, and the administration of atropine, with or without pralidoxime mesylate, a cholinesterase reactivator. It is only the initial effects which respond to these measures, so treatment must be rapidly instigated.

Carbamate insecticides such as carbyl are also cholinesterase inhibitors.

Miscellaneous chemicals

Carbon disulphide

Carbon disulphide (CS_2), an organic solvent, is a constituent of lacquers and varnishes and is used in the manufacture of rubber and plastics, notably rayon. It is peculiarly neurotoxic, causing both axon destruction and indirect damage by inducing arteriosclerosis. Acute psychiatric features of exposed chemical workers include fatigue, depression, irritability, insomnia, acute mania and delirium (Hanwinen, 1971). More chronic behavioural, motor and cognitive changes can develop (Wood, 1981).

Carbon monoxide

Carbon monoxide is a colourless, odourless, non-irritative gas formed by the incomplete combustion of organic material. Inadequately maintained gas appliances have become a notorious cause of carbon monoxide poisoning, as have suicide attempts in exhaust-filled cars. Carbon monoxide reduces the oxygen-carrying capacity of blood and causes hypoxia. Klaassen (1990) points out that a higher metabolic rate predisposes to carbon monoxide toxicity, hence children succumb earlier than adults. Exposure results in transient weakness, headache, nausea and vomiting, dimness of vision and syncope. However, there may be no prodromal warning before consciousness is lost. Delirium can be a presenting feature or occur as consciousness is regained, and can last as long as four weeks (Smith & Brandon, 1973). Approximately 10% of individuals who have experienced high levels of exposure develop a syndrome of delayed neurotoxicity (Min, 1986). Permanent sequelae include extrapyramidal and pyramidal motor disturbance, affective and personality disturbance, amnesic syndrome and other cognitive deficits, even dementia. The diagnosis is confirmed by high blood carboxyhaemoglobin levels. The initial management is to remove the person to fresh air, to administer 100% oxygen, and to give cardio-pulmonary support.

Hydrogen disulphide

Hydrogen disulphide is a product of decaying organic matter which contains sulphur, and is typically encountered in sewage works. Higher concentrations induce a rapid loss of consciousness, sometimes preceded by delirium.

Nitrous oxide

Nitrous oxide has been misused as a euphoriant for over a century. While acute exposure can cause delirium, prolonged exposure leads to the development of combined degeneration of the posterior and lateral columns of the spinal cord, akin to that found in vitamin B12 deficiency (Brodsky & Cohen, 1986).

Ketamine

Ketamine causes excitability, depersonalisation, hallucinations and delirium in a minority of patients in whom it is used for anaesthesia. It is a substance of misuse.

Metabolic and endocrine disorders

This section includes rarities that require listing along with more common conditions, to prevent underdiagnosis. Illustrative of this is the condition neuroacanthocytosis, a hitherto overlooked entity which is now recognised as an important differential diagnosis of Huntington's chorea. Multisystem disorder is a topic which requires a brief mention. Certain of the conditions to be discussed here have a significant chance of being associated with other disorders which will either precede their onset, coincide, or occur later after the presenting condition has been treated. The Multiple Endocrine Neoplasia (MEN) disorders and the polyglandular autoimmune syndrome Type II are examples of such linked conditions and are of considerable relevance to psychiatric practice. The MEN I disorders include adenomas and hyperplasias of the pituitary, parathyroid, pancreas as well as thymomas, schwannomas and skin lipomata. The MENIIa disorders include phaeochromocytoma, medullary thyroid carcinoma, and various brain tumours; and the final group MENIIb includes a variety of mucocutaneous lesions such as neuromas in various sites and Marfan's syndrome. The polyglandular autoimmune disorders include Addisons's disease, thyroiditis, hypoparathyroidism, diabetes mellitus, pernicious anaemia, vitiligo, myasthenia gravis, and other conditions. Patients with one of these disorders require investigations for associated conditions, sometimes indefinitely, and where conditions are inherited family members will require screening (Schmike, 1991).

Hyperthyroidism

Hyperthyroidism is a hypermetabolic state, typically of insidious onset. It was once a revered example of psychosomatic illness, but this notion is no longer accepted, although it is conceivable that premorbid psychological attributes may colour the presentation in some individuals (Weiner, 1977). Hyperthyroidism is more common in women, and usually presents between the second and fourth decades. The three commonest causes account for 99% of cases: diffuse toxic hyperplasia (Grave's disease); toxic solitary goitre (toxic adenoma); and toxic multinodular goitre (Robbins & Cotran, 1979). The commonest of these is Grave's disease, and it is in this type of hyperthyroidism that the distinctive eye signs are particularly identified.

Sustained hyperthyroidism is uncommon in psychiatric practice, occurring in 0.2–2.6% of psychiatric in-patients (White & Barraclough, 1988), approximately the same as the general population (McLarty *et al*, 1978). Psychiatric symptoms, however, are virtually universal when hyperthyroidism occurs, particularly overactivity, nervousness, anxiety, irritability and emotional lability (Lishman, 1987). A shortened sleep period and increased appetite are usually present. Depression can occur, but is not usually either sustained or severe, in contrast to hypothyroidism (Whybrow

Table 24.7 Disorders of metabolism with psychiatric manifestations (adapted from Lipowski, 1990). Disorders not discussed in the text are referenced.

1. Organ failure or dysfunction
   (a) Endocrinopathies
      i.   Hyperthyroidism
      ii.   Hypothryoidism
      iii. Cushing's syndrome
      iv.   Adrenocortical deficiency
      v.   Hyperparathyroidism
      vi.   Hypoparathyroidism
      vii. Acromegaly
      viii. Hypopituitarism
      ix.   Diabetes mellitus
      x.   Diabetes insipidus (Riggs, 1991)
      xi.   Insulinoma (see under 2b below)
      xii. Phaeochromocytoma
   (b) Hepatic dysfunction (Collis & Lloyd, 1992; see under Alcohol)
   (c) Pancreatic dysfunction (Estrada *et al*, 1979)
   (d) Renal dysfunction (Lishman, 1987)
   (e) Respiratory dysfunction (See under 3k and 3l below)

2. Deficiency of substrates of cerebral metabolism
   (a) Hypoxia
   (b) Hypoglycaemia (see under 1a and Alcohol)

3. Disorders of electrolyte, acid-base, and fluid balance
   (a) Hypernatraemia
   (b) Hyponatraemia (see also under 3m below)
   (c) Hyperkalaemia
   (d) Hypokalaemia
   (e) Hypercalcaemia (see under 1a above)
   (f) Hypocalcaemia (see under 1a above)
   (g) Hypermagnesaemia
   (h) Hypomagnesaemia
   (i) Hyper- and hypophosphataemia
   (j) Zinc deficiency
   (k) Acidosis
   (l) Alkalosis
   (m) Water intoxication
   (n) Water depletion (see under 3a,b above)
   (o) Uraemia

4. Disorders of vitamins
   (a) Vitamin deficiency (Carney, 1990)
   (b) Vitamin excess (Lipowski, 1990)

Table continues on next page.

Table 24.7 (continued)

---

5. Disorders of temperature regulation
    (a) Hypothermia
    (b) Hyperthermia
6. Miscellaneous disorders
    (a) Wilson's disease
    (b) Porphyria
    (c) Mitochondrial myopathy
    (d) Neuroacanthocytosis
    (e) Metachromatic leucodystrophy
    (f) Paraneoplastic syndromes (Cornelius *et al*, 1986)
    (g) Carcinoid syndrome (Major *et al*, 1973)
    (h) Kufs disease (Greenwood & Nelson, (1978)
    (i) Adrenoleucodystrophy (Eldridge *et al*, 1984)
    (j) Leigh disease (Kalimo *et al*, 1979)
    (k) Familial idiopathic calcification of the basal ganglia (Flint & Goldstein, 1992)
    (l) Cerebrotendinous xanthomatosis (Adams & Victor, 1989)
    (m) Hallervorden–Spatz syndrome (Dooling *et al*, 1974)
    (n) Gaucher disease (Winkelman *et al*, 1983)
    (o) Niemann–Pick disease (Adams & Victor, 1989)
    (p) GM2 gangliosidosis (Adams & Victor, 1989)
    [Whipple's disease (Adams *et al*, 1987). Almost certainly infective.]

---

et al, 1969). Checkley (1978) was unable to demonstrate a clear temporal relationship between hyperthyroid illness and manic episodes, suggesting that hyperthyroidism does not predispose to manic illness. Psychosis is well-recognised but uncommon (about 1%). Close examination of the mental state will often reveal a mixture of affective and psychotic disturbance in the context of mild global impairment of cognition (Lishman, 1987). Chorea, periodic paralysis, myopathy and myasthenia are recognised neurological accompaniments (Adams & Victor, 1989).

Fulminant episodes of delirium occur in some 3–4% of hyperthyroid patients (Lipowski, 1990). Such a state is usually accompanied by high fever, tachycardia, hypotension, vomiting and diarrhoea, and is termed a "thyroid crisis" or "thyroid storm". It can be precipitated by inadequate preparation for thyroidectomy, non-thyroidal surgery or infection, but often a precipitant is not found. Occasionally, the presentation is more subtle, with apathy, prostration, stupor and coma without a high temperature (Wartofsky & Ingbar, 1991). Thyroid crisis constitutes a medical emergency. Supportive measures include the administration of fluids, dexamethasone or hydrocortisone, glucose and B-vitamins. The patient may require cooling and digitalisation. Thyroid hormone synthesis should be blocked with propylthiouracil or carbimazole (by nasogastric tube) and release of thyroid hormone inhibited with iodine. Adrenergic antagonists have an important role in the absence of heart failure. Control is usually regained within 24 hours.

A small minority of hyperthyroid patients, more usually older patients, present with apathetic detachment without restless over-activity, a state termed "apathetic" hyperthyroidism by Lahey (1931) who contrasted it with the more normal presentation of "activated" hyperthyroidism. These patients usually have a masked hyperthyroid state without striking clinical signs. A goitre, if present, is usually small. Appetite is usually poor and weight loss considerable. These patients are at risk of developing cardiac complications, becoming stuporous, and sinking into terminal coma (Gambert & Escher, 1988).

The differentiation of anxiety and hyperthyroidism can be difficult. While physical signs of Grave's disease, particularly the eye signs, are strong evidence of hyperthyroidism, these may well be absent. Hyperthyroid patients are sensitive to higher temperatures, have increased appetite, and yet lose weight (Lishman, 1987). The onset of anxiety is often at an earlier age than is the case with hyperthyroidism. A 24-hour heart-rate chart is often helpful, as hyperthyroid patients tend to have a sleeping pulse rate above 90 beats per minute. Serum levels of free triiodothyronine (T3), free thyroxine (T4) and thyroid stimulating hormone (TSH) should be requested. It has been pointed out that in acute psychiatric admissions there is a high incidence of hyperthyroxinaemia. In these cases, serum TSH is generally high or normal, not low; it tends to normalise within two weeks and treatment is not indicated (Hein & Jackson, 1990). Elevation in the serum T3 without a raised T4 (T3 toxicosis) can occur, though this is usually an early phenomenon. T4 toxicosis is occasionally seen in particularly ill or elderly patients (Wartofsky & Ingbar, 1991).

The prognosis of psychiatric symptoms in hyperthyroidism is good, although it should be cautioned that psychotic symptoms and delirium can appear for the first time when treatment begins.

Hypothyroidism

Hypothyroidism is a hypometabolic state caused almost exclusively by inadequate thyroidal secretion of T3 and T4. Endemic or sporadic hypothyroidism present from birth is termed 'cretinism', and is usually accompanied by mental retardation (Hamilton, 1976a,b). It is noteworthy that milder cases may be missed at birth and, while usually recognised in childhood, they may present in adulthood. Myxoedema is the term applied to hypothyroidism in the child or adult. It is very much more common in women, and is most frequently a disorder of middle-life. On account of its insidious onset it is often overlooked. The commonest causes are over-treatment of hyperthyroidism, end-stage chronic thyroiditis or multinodular goitre. Inhibition of hormone synthesis or release by antithyroid drugs is another significant cause, lithium being the main culprit in psychiatric practice. Carbamazepine and phenytoin can also affect thyroid function.

As physical features accrue, the diagnosis becomes more obvious. Fatigue, poor appetite, slowed activity, aches and pains, constipation and cold intolerance are core features. Mucopolysaccharides infiltrate the dermis of the skin causing it to become characteristically thickened and doughy. The patient may develop a hoarse voice, an expressionless face and suffer hair-loss. Marked slowing of the recovery phase of the ankle jerk is a useful clinical sign. Patients may present with angina, impotence and hearing difficulties.

Psychiatric features occur early in virtually every case and were noted by both Sir William Gull in his original description of hypothyroidism, and by Ord, who coined the term myxoedema (Tonks, 1964). Fatigue accompanied by mental and physical slowing is a central psychiatric feature. Memory for recent events may be impaired (Hadden, 1882). Apathy and tranquillity are not always present – oppositional, explosive personality attributes are well-described, as also is paranoia. When depressed mood develops it can be severe and respond poorly to treatment. Insight is present to begin with, but fades as the disorder intensifies. Cognitive impairments range from quite subtle degrees of mental slowing, impaired concentration and impaired memory for recent events, to states of frank dementia (de Fine Olivarus & Röder, 1970).

Delusions (usually paranoid) and auditory or visual hallucinations, if present, are usually accompanied by impaired cognition and clouded consciousness. Such a presentation is well illustrated by the following case (Asher, 1949).

> *Case example*
> A housewife aged 60 was admitted with delusions of persecution and hallucinations. For 16 months she had noticed that her voice was croaking and she felt cold weather badly, but she had noted no other myxoedematous symptoms – no gain in weight, falling out of hair, or deafness. During the week before admission she had an idea that her landlord was trying to poison her "because she knew all about the shootings in the garden". She heard voices talking to her continuously, and locked herself in her room to protect herself from imaginary enemies. On examination she was completely confused and disorientated.

Hypothyroidism may be mistaken for depression, dementia, personality disorder and hypochondriacal neurosis. Serum TSH or free T4 are the initial investigations – a normal TSH will exclude primary hypothyroidism, but not hypothyroidism due to pituitary or hypothalamic disease (Zilva & Pannall, 1979). Thyroid antibodies should be requested and repeated in patients in whom clinical suspicions linger. In approximately a third of patients with hypothyroidism the EEG is abnormal, with a slowing of the dominant rhythm and a reduction of the background activity which corrects after treatment (Hooshmand & Sarhaddi, 1975).

Thyroid replacement treatment must be started cautiously as angina and heart failure can arise. Most of the psychiatric symptoms in hypothyroid patients can be expected to respond to treatment.

Lithium and the thyroid gland

Lithium treatment affects the thyroid gland directly by inhibiting release of iodine, T3 and T4, and indirectly by inducing thyroid autoantibodies. Hypothyroidism can occur at any time during the course of lithium treatment and, therefore, thyroid status must be checked prior to starting lithium and every six months thereafter. Weight gain and lethargy are useful clinical indices to monitor. Lithium-induced goitre is rarely of noticeable proportions. If lithium is stopped, the effects it has exerted on the thyroid reverse in 1–2 months. If it is necessary to continue treatment when there is evidence of hypothyroidism, treatment with thyroxine will restore euthyroid status. Other aspects of the effect of lithium treatment on the thyroid gland are described in accounts by Crowe *et al* (1973), Jefferson & Marshall (1981) and Lazarus *et al* (1981). The management of thyrotoxicosis in patients treated with lithium has been reviewed by Rosser (1976).

T3 and T4 supplementation for affective disorders

The role of the hypothalamic-pituitary-thyroid axis in the genesis and management of affective disorders is of considerable interest (Szabadi, 1991). For example, there is evidence that diurnal profiles of thyroid hormones are altered in depression (Wilson *et al*, 1992). There is hope that augmentation of thyroid function will not only be confirmed to accelerate the response to tricyclic antidepressants, but also be found to enhance the response in those showing treatment resistance (Chalmers & Cowen, 1990). The relative merits of different thyroid supplements are under investigation (Cooke *et al*, 1992), but presently lithium augmentation seems to be a more effective strategy (Thase *et al*, 1989). Some authorities favour the use of thyroid supplements in the treatment of "rapid cycling" manic–depressive patients – a group in which it has been reported that significant rates of hypothyroidism occur (Bauer & Whybrow, 1990; Bauer *et al*, 1990). The topic is also discussed on page 209.

Cushing's syndrome

Cushing's syndrome is due to excessive pituitary secretion of adreno-corticotrophic hormone (ACTH) in about 75% of cases. It is four times more common in women. It usually presents in the third or fourth decade but can occur at any age. Other causes include adrenal tumours, and ACTH-secreting tumours such as oat cell carcinoma of the lung. It may be confused with simple obesity, hirsutism, and functional ovarian tumours.

remediable psychiatric illness. Hypercalcaemia occurs for many reasons, including renal failure, carcinoma, immobilisation, bone disease, vitamin D excess, sarcoidosis and thyrotoxicosis. Fatigue, weakness, anorexia, constipation, thirst and polyuria are symptoms frequently associated with hypercalcaemia, and thus necessitate a serum calcium estimation when encountered. The nature and management of hyperparathyroidism has been reviewed by Potts (1991).

Primary hyperparathyroidism develops at any age, but mostly in middle life. Petersen (1968) reported that up to two-thirds of patients have mental changes, a third of these being severe. Psychiatric features can be divided into two main types. The most common is disturbed mood and drive; this may be the sole manifestation. Delirium is associated with higher calcium levels (Christie-Brown, 1968), and has been termed parathyroid crisis.

The earliest changes are subtle – personality change, depressed mood and insidiously progressive fatigue, listlessness and apathy. Impaired attention, mental slowing and impaired memory can develop, but actual dementia is a rare presentation. Schizophreniform psychosis is also rare, though persecutory delusions and hallucinations are not uncommon as calcium levels rise. Elevated calcium is a significant cause of stupor and catatonia. Depression can become very severe, profound psychotic features being accompanied by a significant risk of suicide. Antidepressants have a temporary role, but the depression is often resistant, and so the definitive treatment is to reverse the hypercalcaemia.

> *Case example*
> A 58-year-old woman was referred for an urgent psychiatric opinion as she had stated that she felt she could no longer carry on and she wished to die. At interview the patient sat in a languid, drooping fashion in an armchair. During the previous two months she had lost 7 kg in weight. Her mood was unaffected by external events. There was a considerable degree of psychomotor retardation, but no evidence of thought disorder, delusional thinking or hallucinations, or memory defect. Orientation was correct in all respects. The patient's level of consciousness was diminished, resembling that seen in pre-stuporous states. The most striking abnormality was that of an elevated serum calcium of 3.12 mmol/l and a lowered serum phosphate of 0.48 mmol/l. The disorder was revealed to be an extreme case of intoxication as a result of 15 years of therapy with vitamin D tablets and calcium tablets after thyroid surgery (Keddie, 1987).

Where the origin of the symptoms described above is in doubt, the EEG is a useful investigation. Slowing of the background rhythm and the appearance of bilateral high voltage delta episodes are suggestive of a metabolic cause (Cooper & Schapira, 1973).

The possibility of hypercalcaemia should be entertained in most psychiatric settings. In primary hyperparathyroidism, the psychiatric features usually, but not always, show a clear relationship to serum calcium levels, but not parathyroid hormone levels (Petersen, 1968). As calcium levels rise, affective disturbance, neurasthenic symptoms and personality change appear. At higher levels still, delirium, impaired cognition and/or delusions develop. At very high levels, somnolence and coma occur.

Correction of serum calcium usually results in reversal of psychiatric symptoms. Patients require careful observation after corrective treatment – even patients without prior mental changes can become psychotic in the week after surgical treatment, with or without rebound hypocalcaemia (Jefferson & Marshall, 1981).

Hypoparathyroidism

Hypoparathyroidism is most commonly secondary to damage or removal of the parathyroid glands, usually as a consequence of thyroid surgery. More rarely, there may be primary parathyroid disease, or end-organ unresponsiveness to circulating parathyroid hormone – pseudohypoparathyroidism. Patients with hypoparathyroidism are often female, have a history of surgery to the neck and may present with tetany, cramps, cataracts or generalised seizures. A skull X-ray may show symmetrical calcification within the basal ganglia in primary hypoparathyroidism, but extrapyramidal features such as chorea are relatively rare.

Cases of secondary hypoparathyroidism tend to present with more acute psychiatric disorders, such as delirium characterised by florid psychotic manifestations and irritability. Depression, manic–depression, schizophreniform psychosis, nervousness and irritability are all reported. Primary hypoparathyroidism, on the other hand, unfolds insidiously with symptoms such as emotional lability, impaired concentration and intellectual impairment (Denko & Kaelbling, 1962). The cause can be easily missed and slow progression over months or years may leave the patient demented.

Pseudohypoparathyroidism tends to be congenital and causes intellectual retardation, which is poorly responsive to medical intervention. The nature of familial calcification of the basal ganglia, its psychiatric presentations, and its relationship to pseudohypoparathyroidism have been reviewed by Flint & Goldstein (1992).

Patients who have low normal serum calcium levels are prone to develop intermittent psychiatric symptoms as their levels dip further. This can be alleviated with calcium supplements. The same mechanism may well operate in other borderline metabolic derangements.

The prognosis of psychiatric symptoms associated with secondary hypoparathyroidism is good, although some symptoms may take a few months to resolve once calcium levels are normal. The prognosis of dementia due to primary hypoparathryroidism is less certain, but cases which have reversed well are certainly described (Eraut, 1974; Mateo & Giménez-Roldan, 1982).

Acromegaly

This condition, also called Marie's disease, results from hypersecretion of growth hormone after puberty and is usually caused by a pituitary adenoma. Characteristic overgrowth of the head and extremities occurs (with need for increasing shoe size), often accompanied by headache, hypertension and glucose intolerance.

The psychiatric manifestations were extensively studied by Manfred Bleuler and colleagues at the Zürich Psychiatric Clinic (Bleuler, 1951). An "endocrine psychosyndrome" was proposed which was claimed to be common to many endocrine conditions. Apathy and lack of spontaneity were frequently present. Altered emotions were also common, including cheerfulness, self-satisfaction, elation, resentfulness coupled with anxiousness, tenseness and unpleasantness. Mood swings were noted, and libido was generally reduced. Psychosis was uncommon, except as a complication of the disease process. In the absence of raised intracranial pressure there were no striking cognitive deficits, other than those attributable to apathy and indifference. Patients were often regarded by others as egocentric, inconsiderate and touchy. It is likely that psychiatric changes reflect an amalgam of influences, consisting of metabolic changes, raised intracranial pressure, and the psychological reaction to illness and altered appearance (Avery, 1973; Margo, 1981).

Hypopituitarism

This disorder is most commonly due to a pituitary adenoma with a prolonged onset, rather than the result of infarction caused by postpartum haemorrhage (Sheehan's syndrome) as was once the case. Other causes include basal skull fracture or infection, sarcoidosis and craniophayngioma in children. Much of the information about the psychiatric effects of hypopituitarism is based on the studies of Hans Kind (1958) who worked with Manfred Bleuler in Zurich. The psychiatric effects reflect underfunctioning of the adrenal cortex, thyroid and other metabolic disturbances.

Most patients with hypopituitarism have psychiatric disturbance, usually an involutional state characterised by varying degrees of apathy, inertia, and insouciance (Kind, 1958; Michael & Gibbons, 1963). Impotence and impaired libido are early symptoms. The patient's mood is depressed and, in combination with apathy and memory impairment, resembles dementia. Delirium usually reflects actual or impending metabolic upset. Patients with hypopituitarism are peculiarly prone to coma, which is often lethal. Schizophreniform psychosis is rare.

The weight loss, impaired appetite, scanty axillary and pubic hair, and amenorrhoea of hypopituitarism should not be mistaken for anorexia nervosa. In hypopituitarism, the patient's attitude to food is less intense, drive is much less, the facial lanugo hair to be found in anorexia nervosa is absent, and the degree of weight loss is usually less.

Psychiatric symptoms typically respond well to hormone replacement, although long-standing apathy may not reverse completely. If vasopressin production and release has been disturbed, it may only come to light after steroid replacement has commenced, resulting in the polydipsia and polyuria characteristic of diabetes insipidus.

Diabetes mellitus

Diabetes mellitus is characterised by hyperglycaemia due to absolute or relative insulin deficiency. The UK prevalence is approximately 1%. Idiopathic (primary) diabetes, which is the commonest type, may or may not be insulin-dependent. Secondary diabetes has many causes, including excess growth hormone, thyroxine, cortisol or adrenalin (as in phaeochromocytoma), pregnancy, certain medications and liver disease (Foster, 1991).

Five types of coma may occur, hypoglycaemic, ketoacidotic, hyperosmolar non-ketotic, alcoholic ketoacidotic and that due to lactic acidosis. In diabetic ketoacidosis the level of consciousness correlates best with plasma osmolality (Alberti & Nattrass, 1978). Hyperosmolar coma is especially common in the elderly. The key signs and laboratory findings comprise lethargy, changes in cognition, profound dehydration, polydipsia and polyuria, shallow respiration, hypotension and tachycardia, hyperthermia, extreme hyperglycaemia, and minimal ketoacidosis (Braaten, 1987). Salicylate poisoning and stroke are two important differential diagnoses of diabetic coma.

Emotional upset is associated with poor diabetic control, and many mechanisms can be postulated, including altered diet, alcohol use, changes in routine and activity levels, carelessness and so forth. Occasionally, obvious manipulation occurs, which may respond well to an individual or family psychotherapeutic approach. The study of the role of life circumstances in diabetic control is complex because of the many confounding variables (Grant *et al*, 1974; Bradley, 1979; Rubin & Peyrot, 1992).

Diabetes can be accompanied by most forms of mental disorder. Fatigue and daytime somnolence are common. Delirium and dementia are due to metabolic disturbances, atherosclerosis and hypertension. Insulin and oral hypoglycaemic drugs are potentiated by alcohol, and monoamine oxidase inhibitors.

Insulinoma

Insulin-secreting tumours (insulinomata) of the beta-cells in the islets of Langerhans of the pancreas are rare but important sources of psychiatric morbidity – they are one of the "great mimics", such as syphilis and Wilson's disease. Approximately 10% are malignant. They affect all age groups, but are commonest after childhood and before 60. Two-thirds of patients also have adenomas of two or more endocrine systems, and a fifth have tumours of three or more systems; there can be many years between the presentations of each disorder (Schimke, 1991).

The effects usually unfold insidiously and comprise subacute and/or chronic hypoglycaemic symptoms, punctuated by acute hypoglycaemic episodes that increase in frequency. Diagnosis is made difficult by the changeability of the presenting phenomena in a given individual. They can present with the clinical picture of neurosis, personality disorder, mania, depression, schizophrenia, epilepsy, sleep disorder, delirium or dementia (Todd *et al*, 1962; Boyd & Cleveland, 1967; Service *et al*, 1976). Patients may experience memory blackouts. Careful questioning may elicit physical symptoms suggestive of hypoglycaemia, but only a minority notice a link with meals or exercise.

Investigation is best undertaken in a metabolic unit. While the ratio of plasma insulin to serum glucose is usually maintained at 0.3, in the presence of an insulinoma the ratio is usually >0.4 and rises with fasting.The diagnosis is made by demonstrating fasting hypoglycaemia in conjunction with normal or raised plasma insulin levels (Kaplan, 1991). Rising cortisol during fasting excludes hypothalamic-pituitary disorder as the cause of the hypoglycaemia. Th C-peptide of proinsulin normally varies in parallel with plasma insulin. If insulin has been administered surreptitiously, the level will be found to be suppressed (Kaplan,1991), thus allowing abuse of insulin to detected. Surgery is the definitive treatment for insulinoma, although medical treatments also have a place. First-degree relatives should be screened.

Phaeochromocytoma

Phaeochromocytomas are tumours derived from chromaffin cells which secrete catecholamines and other substances. About 10% of these tumours are malignant. In the US there are about 36 000 affected individuals (Melicow, 1977). Roughly 90% of the tumours are located in the adrenal medulla, 10% being bilateral (Robbins & Cotran, 1979). They occur at any age, but mostly in the fourth and fifth decades. They present in many clinical guises: as "turns"; as diabetes in which there is severe hypertension; as angina with normal coronary arteries; as pre-eclampsia in pregnancy; and in many more ways. The variability of the presentation is partly due to the variation in the nature and quantity of catecholamines released. In one study the majority of cases had presented with paroxysmal attacks of less than an hour, in which the four most prominent symptoms were headache, perspiration, palpitations and pallor (Thomas *et al*, 1966). Attacks usually progress in frequency and severity, although the form is fairly uniform for each individual. During attacks the blood pressure is usually high and accompanied by tachycardia. Glucose intolerance, elevated packed cell volume, polycythaemia, orthostatic hypotension, cardiac ischaemia and cardiomyopathy can all occur.

Psychological accompaniments include intense anxiety, fear, over-arousal, delirium, depression, psychosis and dementia. Epileptic fits can occur. Reported precipitants of attacks include bending, turning in bed, sexual intercourse, straining, excitement and physical exertion, but a precipitant may not be identified (Thomas *et al*, 1966; Melicow, 1977). Tricyclic antidepressants enhance the effects of circulating catecholamines, and indeed all drugs must be carefully considered before being used in a patient suspected of having a phaeochromocytoma (Landsberg & Young, 1991).

A high index of suspicion is required in psychiatric patients with anxiety disorders or depression, and in those who present with "turns". Work-up should include thorough blood pressure monitoring, retinoscopy, a blood glucose and three 24 hour urinary vanillymandelic acid (VMA) estimations using acidified containers which should be kept cold. Further investigations involve pharmacological tests, intravascular sampling and imaging techniques.

Suspected phaeochromocytoma is one of the few *absolute* contra-indications for electroconvulsive therapy (Drake & Ebaugh, 1956).

Hypoxia

Hypoxia of the brain causes psychological symptoms whose severity are related to the rate at which hypoxia occurs, its duration, the cause and the context (Gibson, 1985; Lishman, 1987). Four brain areas are thought to be especially vulnerable: the arterial boundary zones, the thalamus, Ammon's horns and the cerebellum. It can present with lethargy, mental slowing, impaired judgement, hallucinations and delirium. Permanent psychological sequelae include regional psychological deficits, amnesic syndrome and dementia. When evaluating a patient with chronic cognitive impairment, it should always be established if the patient could have been hypoxic at any time in the past. General anaesthesia, cardiovascular events, lung disease, carbon monoxide poisoning, hypoglycaemia, epilepsy, anaemia, cerebral malaria or activities such as climbing or diving are potential causes. Cyanide and carbon disulphide poisoning are but two examples of toxic causes. Acute mental changes at altitude tend to become apparent at 4000–5000 m, causing disturbance of mood, memory, judgement and orientation (Nelson, 1982).

Hypoglycaemia

The CNS has a single source of energy, glucose. Damage, sometimes permanent, results from hypoglycaemia. The damage is not uniform, but occurs in a rostrocaudal fashion – the middle layers of the cerebral cortex (but for the striate area), and the hippocampus are most affected, followed in turn by the basal ganglia and anterior thalamus. The brain-stem and spinal cord are most resistant (*Lancet*, 1985).

Hypoglycaemia may be extremely subtle in its presentation, with obscure causes (e.g. insulinoma, ingestion of the Caribbean ackee fruit, and deliberate poisoning with hypoglycaemic medicines). It is helpful to subdivide hypoglycaemia into acute, subacute and chronic forms (Marks & Rose, 1987).

In its acute form hypoglycaemia unfolds with a characteristic progression of symptoms – a feeling of emptiness, weakness, hunger, sweating, palpitations, tremor, faintness, headache and blurred vision, delirium, and coma. Seizures occur in 10–20% of adults (*Lancet*, 1985). The person's behaviour may be out of character, inappropriate and even violent. When hypoglycaemia is nocturnal, only sweats will be recalled, but in the daytime fatigue and under-performance occur (Gale & Tattersall, 1979). The triad of hypoglycaemia, CNS symptoms and prompt relief after intravenous glucose (Whipple's triad) forms the basis of diagnosis. For the emergency treatment of hypoglycaemia, 50 ml of 50% glucose is administered intravenously, followed by additional supplements until recovery has occurred.

Malouf & Brust (1985) studied 125 cases of hypoglycaemia presenting acutely during a 12-month period: 65 were obtunded, stuporous or in coma; 38 had acute focal or generalised cognitive impairments and/or psychiatric symptoms; ten were dizzy or tremulous; nine had seizures; and three had suffered sudden hemiparesis. Diabetes, alcohol (see alcoholic hypoglycaemia above) and/or sepsis accounted for 90% of the predisposing conditions. Only one patient died from hypoglycaemia, although four had residual neurological signs. There is evidence that several severe episodes of hypoglycaemia can cause permanent memory impairment (Sachon *et al*, 1992).

In subacute hypoglycaemia the symptoms of excess sympathetic activity are usually absent; the picture is more that of languor, apathy, and withdrawal. Cognitive impairment is often present and delirium can occur (Lishman, 1987).

Chronic hypoglycaemia may be punctuated by episodes of either of the two aforementioned presentations and is the rarest of the three. Personality change occurs, mirroring ongoing brain damage. Memory is often affected and, left untreated, dementia may result.

Hypernatraemia

Hypernatraemia, a serum sodium above 150 mmol/l, is present in the following four circumstances: excessive water loss (e.g. pyrexia, extensive burns, ventilator loss, hypercatabolism and diabetes insipidus); water loss exceeding sodium loss (e.g. sweating, vomiting, diarrhoea, and conditions in which there is osmotic diuresis); inadequate fluid intake (e.g. with impairment of consciousness); and after the excessive administration of sodium (e.g. salt poisoning, sodium in dialysate) (Jefferson & Marshall, 1981). Hypernatraemia causes brain shrinkage, and in extreme cases subdural, subarachnoid or intracerebral haemorrhages occur. The main symptoms are relatively non-specific irritability, lethargy, weakness, illusions and visual hallucinations, delirium, stupor and coma. The more rapid the development of hypernatraemia the more pronounced the symptoms; when the onset is insidious the diagnosis can be easily overlooked. Physical signs of dehydration are less marked than with salt depletion and may be delayed. These include tachycardia, low amplitude pulse, depressed jugular venous pressure, reduced skin turgor, sunken eyes and postural hypotension. Too rapid correction of the electrolyte imbalance may induce cerebral oedema and fits.

Hyponatraemia

Hyponatraemia commonly accompanies numerous systemic diseases and is due to depletion or dilution of sodium reserves (Arieff & Guisado, 1976). It is often iatrogenic, being due to incorrect intravenous infusion regimes, diuretic treatment, and can be induced by many drugs (e.g. carbamazepine, lithium, amitriptyline and phenothiazines). Hyponatraemia can be induced deliberately, but also accidentally through excessive beer drinking ('beer potomania'). Other causes include renal disorder, the syndrome of inappropriate secretion of antidiuretic hormone (SIADH), hepatic cirrhosis, congestive heart failure and Addison's disease.

The neurobehavioural symptoms of acute hyponatraemia are due to brain swelling, and are described in the section on water intoxication (see below). Chronic hyponatraemia may present with lethargy, muscle weakness and somnolence. Serum urea, electrolytes, creatinine and liver function tests should be assayed, serum and urinary osmolality measured, and the patient examined for the presence of oedema. The treatment of hyponatraemia is complex; it has been outlined by Sterns (1987). Rapid correction of hyponatraemia is hazardous as it can cause acute brain shrinkage and is implicated in the development of central pontine myelinolysis.

Hyperkalaemia

Hyperkalaemia is due to reduced renal excretion or transcellular potassium shifts (Andreoli, 1982). Diminished renal excretion is due to reduced glomerular filtration rate (acute oliguric renal failure or chronic renal failure) or reduced tubular secretion (potassium sparing diuretics or Addison's disease). Transcellular shifts occur with acidosis, cell destruction (trauma, burns, rhabdomyolysis and haemolysis), hyperkalaemic periodic paralysis and diabetic hyperglycaemia. Overzealous fist-clenching during venepuncture or an overnight delay in sending a sample to the laboratory can also cause hyperkalaemia, but this is artefactual.

Hyperkalaemia causes an organic brain syndrome characterised by weakness, dysarthria and a range of neuromuscular symptoms (Webb & Gehi, 1981) that can be mistaken for neurotic illness. In more severe disturbances, delirium and an ascending flaccid paralysis can occur.

Hyperkalaemic periodic paralysis is an autosomal dominant condition which may be mistaken for hysteria. Episodes of paralysis can occur spontaneously, after exercise or following excessive dietary potassium. The occurrence of myotonia suggests the diagnosis, and an electrocardiogram can confirm it.

There are three particular aspects to the treatment of hyperkalaemia – reduction of cardiac excitability (calcium gluconate therapy), the transfer of potassium into intracellular fluid (sodium bicarbonate or glucose and insulin therapy), and the elimination of potassium from the body (diuretic administration and renal dialysis).

Hypokalaemia

Hypokalaemia is due to inadequate intake of potassium, excessive renal loss (e.g. diuretics, mineralocorticoid excess, antibiotics and chronic renal failure), vomiting and diarrhoea, and shifts into the intracellular compartment (alkalosis, periodic hypokalaemic paralysis, and insulin therapy). Hypokalaemia produces neuromuscular symptoms (weakness and/or paralysis), lassitude and, more rarely, delirium.

Periodic hypokalaemic paralysis is a rare condition characterised by episodic weakness and/or paralysis following the ingestion of a high load of carbohydrate. The lack of an obvious precipitant may result in it being taken for a hysterical conversion disorder (Mitchell & Feldman, 1968).

Hypermagnesaemia

The effects of magnesium and calcium disturbances can be difficult to dissociate. Hypermagnesaemia may result from the use of magnesium-containing antacids and from renal failure. Among the symptoms reported by Randall *et al* (1964) were nausea, vomiting, malaise, drowsiness, dysarthria, gait ataxia, difficulty in voiding urine and defecating, hyporeflexia, and coma. Hypermagnesaemia from habitual antacid is a cause of reversible dementia in the elderly. Its recognition and management have been reviewed by Ratzan *et al* (1980).

Hypomagnesaemia

Isolated hypomagnesaemia is rare. While hypomagnesaemia has a large range of causes, alcoholism is one of the most common. Psychiatric manifestations include personality change, apathy, depression, agitation, anxiety, disorientation, hallucinations and delirium (Berkelhammer & Bear, 1985). Magnesium deficiency may aggravate Wernicke-Korsakoff syndrome (Flink, 1986), induce seizures and may be accompanied by myoclonus, chorea, and athetosis. Serum levels may be normal in the presence of whole body depletion – 99% of magnesium is in intracellular stores or bone. In order to make the diagnosis a 24-hour urine collection is also required.

Hyperphosphataemia and hypophosphataemia

Discrete psychiatric symptoms have not been linked to hyperphosphataemia. Hypophosphataemia is usually mild and of little consequence. It is most commonly encountered in severe alcohol withdrawal and during recovery from diabetic ketoacidosis. It has been associated with a range of neurobehavioural features ranging from irritability to delirium or coma (Knochel, 1977), but it is not clear whether these features are due to associated metabolic disturbances.

Zinc deficiency

Zinc deficiency causes anorexia and weight loss, impaired taste and olfaction, and altered mood and behaviour. Experimental studies indicate it can also cause a paranoid state, memory impairment, and cerebellar symptoms (Henkin *et al*, 1975). Zinc deficiency may present to the psychiatrist as fatigue states, depression, anorexia and progressive dementia. As patients with anorexia nervosa and low serum zinc levels have been reported to respond to zinc supplementation, it is reasonable to consider zinc supplementation in anorexia nervosa as an adjunct to psychological and other measures (Yamaguchi *et al*, 1992).

Serum zinc levels are subject to various factors – there is a pronounced diurnal variation with peak levels at 10 a.m., and large fluctuations occur following meals. Levels increase after prolonged fasting, and are low in hypoalbuminaemia, pregnancy, oestrogen therapy and in the presence of certain malignancies. Low activity of serum alkaline phosphatase, which is a zinc dependent enzyme, may indicate zinc deficiency.

Acidosis

Metabolic acidosis is caused by hyperglycaemia, salicylate overdosage, renal disease, and any condition causing alkali loss. Deep, fast breathing (Kussmaul breathing) is often a prominent clinical feature. Fatigue, progressive depression of consciousness and seizures occur. Salicylate poisoning constitutes a medical emergency. Restlessness, facial flushing, sweating, hyperventilation, tinnitus and an impaired sensorium are all features. Blood levels should always be measured and the patient is best managed in a medical unit.

Respiratory acidosis is associated with carbon dioxide retention and was studied in end-stage chronic obstructive airways disease by Westlake *et al* (1955). Delirium with hallucinations (auditory and visual) may occur, but some patients exhibit progressive impairment of consciousness alone. The nursing staff may report that an affected patient is becoming increasingly oversensitive, obstreperous and "difficult". Both acidosis and hypercapnia can independently cause coma. Hypercapnia is associated with headache, sweating, muscle twitching (particularly facial) and raised intracranial pressure (Westlake *et al*, 1955).

Alkalosis

The causes of metabolic alkalosis include chloride depletion, hyper-adrenocorticism, severe potassium depletion and excessive alkali intake (Jefferson & Marshall, 1981). As the arterial pH exceeds 7.55, irritability, muscle weakness, apathy, delirium and stupor occur.

Respiratory alkalosis as a result of hyperventilation is relatively common in psychiatric practice; typically it is due to anxiety or habit. Hyperventilation, however, has many causes – salicylate poisoning, metabolic acidosis, hypercapnia, pregnancy and many others should always be ruled out. In the anxious person, hyperventilation produces a range of symptoms that can reinforce any original anxiety, so creating a vicious circle of events. These include fatigue, general weakness, atypical chest pain, tachycardia, palpitations, dyspnoea, lightheadedness, faintness, impaired concentration and memory, derealisation, blurred vision, paraesthesia, tetany and mild delirium (Engel *et al*, 1947; Waites, 1978). Hallucinations have been described as a result of hyperventilation, and it may precipitate epilepsy. Hyperventilation is best managed by teaching the patient about how it arises, ideally in the company of a friend or relative. Voluntary hyperventilation is performed, and the patient is taught how to respond, emphasising diaphragmatic breathing (see also page 602). The classic remedy of breathing into a paper bag may be of value in acute situations, but understanding, rehearsal and prevention are most effective (Missri & Alexander (1978).

Water intoxication

The excessive drinking of water is a relatively common practice among psychiatric patients, particularly those with schizophrenia, and is a very important source of morbidity and mortality (Vieweg *et al*, 1985). The early features of water intoxication include headache, blurred vision, polyuria, vomiting, tremor, and exacerbation of psychosis. Eventually delirium, a generalised epileptic fit, muscle cramps, ataxia, stupor or even coma can also occur (Ferrier, 1985). Modelling the conduct of others may be part of the explanation for the activity. It seems that there is rarely a compulsion, the majority want to do it (Crammer, 1991), and state that they do it to feel better (Millson *et al*, 1992).

The diagnosis of water intoxication is made when a symptomatic patient has a plasma sodium of less than 120 mmol/l. To confirm that overdrinking of water has occurred, staff and other informants should be questioned about the patient's behaviour, and observations undertaken. Such observation tends to reveal a common pattern: drinking begins around breakfast time and continues through the day until the evening. Fluid retention is maximal late in the afternoon or in the early evening and then tends to reverse to normal, or near normal, overnight. It follows that the serum sodium level should be estimated in the late afternoon, and *not* in the morning as is more customary.

Other causes of polydipsia and polyuria should be excluded: these comprise diabetes mellitus, chronic renal failure, hypercalcaemia and diabetes insipidus (Illowsky & Kirch, 1988). The possibility of hypothalamic lesions and pituitary tumours should be borne in mind. The effects of drugs such as lithium, alcohol and diuretics must also be excluded. The syndrome of inappropriate antidiuretic hormone release (SIADH) is identified by the presence of a low serum sodium concentration in the presence of relatively concentrated urine, and confirmed by further tests. It should be noted that amitriptyline, desipramine, tranylcypromine, thioridazine, fluphenazine, trifluoperazine, haloperidol, and other psychotropic drugs can induce hyponatraemia (Sandifer, 1983).

Nursing approaches are reviewed by Davidhizar (1991). Water intoxication is best managed by stopping all fluid intake and awaiting the urinary excretion of excess water (Crammer, 1991).

Uraemia

Mental changes are a feature of both acute and chronic renal failure. The relationship between the level of urea and the nature and degree of mental changes is not necessarily causal, since patients with renal failure can have mental disturbances for a host of reasons. The range of symptoms covers a wide spectrum; apathy, detachment and fatigue are prominent early on, and may be misconstrued as a depressive episode. Other patients become expansive and irritable. Impaired concentration is complained of at an early stage, and more global cognitive problems develop subsequently. Activities become slowed and speech becomes slurred. Delirium is a feature of both acute and chronic renal failure, foreshadowed by higher urea levels and rapid fluctuations. Auditory and visual hallucinations occur and are accompanied by delusions, often persecutory in type. Epileptic seizures are an additional complication. Patients ultimately become stuporous and enter coma. Myoclonus, muscular twitches, asterixis, choreoathetosis and catatonia are all reported. EEG changes occur and these comprise background slowing, bouts of paroxysmal slow waves and reduced rapid eye movement (REM) and slow wave sleep. As renal function is being corrected, underlying medical complications should be actively sought.

If dialysis is too rapid, patients may develop any of the following constellation of symptoms – headache, cramps, lethargy or agitation, hallucinations, delusions and behavioural changes. This is sometimes referred to as the 'dialysis dysequilibrium syndrome'. 'Dialysis dementia' is the term given to a potentially more lethal condition which can develop abruptly or insidiously after months or years of dialysis with aluminium-containing dialysis fluids. Intoxication with aluminium in renal failure also occurs through the use of aluminium-containing phosphate buffers. It may be heralded by speech disorder ranging from hesitancy to frank dysphasia, delirium, progressive dementia and personality change. The dementia of chronic low-level aluminium overload in renal failure appears to resemble a slow-onset version of dialysis delirium, rather than Alzheimer's disease (Kerr *et al*, 1992).

Hypothermia and hyperthermia

Hypothermia is defined as a drop in the core temperature to 35°C or less. At less than 30°C consciousness is impaired, and coma is the rule at 26.7°C or less. Hypothermia causes delirium and other mental changes. It is most likely to be encountered among elderly patients with psychiatric illness, as a consequence of drug over-dosage or self-neglect.

Hyperthermia ("heat stroke") is defined as occurring at a core temperature of 40.6°C or more. It is classified as exertional or non-exertional in nature. In psychiatric patients, it is especially common in those taking medication with anticholinergic effects during hot weather (Bark, 1982). Hyperthermia is a feature of neuroleptic malignant syndrome and complicates overdosage with lithium, MAOI antidepressants and amphetamines.

Hyperthermia causes agitation, delirium and/or coma. Lethargy, hallucinations, stupor and seizures are other well-recognised features. Delirium appears to be the predominant presenting symptom (Carter, 1988). Affected individuals have hot, dry skin, tachycardia, and flaccid muscles with reduced or absent reflexes (Petersdorf, 1991). Hypotension and hypoventilation are usually present.

Hyperthermia is a medical emergency; patients can die within a few hours if left untreated. Hyperthermia must be anticipated during hot weather, particularly with in-patients receiving medication with strong anticholinergic properties.

Porphyria

The porphyrias are a set of metabolic disorders caused by a partial deficiency of enzymes responsible for haem synthesis. Excessive production of haem precursors results, and these precursors are readily oxidised to porphyrins. Characteristic clinical presentations include episodes of acute porphyria and/or photosensitive skin reactions. The porphyrias are of importance in psychiatry due to their ability to present with a range of major psychiatric manifestations, sometimes in the absence of physical symptoms. Furthermore, they may be precipitated or exacerbated by drugs used in psychiatry. The details of the biochemistry of porphyria were reviewed by Elder *et al* (1990).

Four types of porphyria are virtually indistinguishable clinically – as the liver is the main site of excess porphyrin production, these are called acute hepatic porphyrias. These are rare before puberty, more common in women, and are associated with fatality in about 5% of hospitalised cases. They present with three core features – abdominal pain, psychiatric disturbances and peripheral neuropathy. Skin lesions are found in most types of porphyria.

Fifty cases of acute intermittent porphyria (AIP) were evaluated by Goldberg (1959) who found that neurological or psychiatric symptoms were the predominant feature at presentation in about 25% of cases. However, more recent accounts agree that abdominal pain is even more common, occurring in over 90% of cases (Stein & Tschudy, 1970). Approximately 50–75% of cases exhibit psychiatric symptoms (Ackner *et al*, 1962), including personality change, neurotic disorders (minor depression, anxiety, hysteria), depression, schizophreniform psychosis, hallucinations, delirium and dementia. Epilepsy and coma may occur. Between episodes, few residual cognitive deficits were found in a sample of 25 cases of AIP (Wetterberg & Österberg, 1969). The initial neurological manifestation is usually a rapidly spreading, symmetrical, predominantly motor polyneuropathy. Cranial nerve lesions and a Guillian-Barré type syndrome can occur in more severe cases, ending with fatal cardiac or respiratory failure.

Drugs are probably the most important precipitants of porphyria, including tricyclic and MAOI antidepressants, barbiturates, most older anticonvulsants, sulpiride, zuclopenthixol, thioridazine and amphetamines. Other precipitants include fever, alcohol, menstrual change, starvation and pregnancy.

Porphyria has been mistaken for hysteria, affective disorder, schizophrenia and dementia. Physical examination may reveal neuropathy, hypertension or a laparotomy scar. Leucocytosis and fever can occur during acute attacks. In AIP, urine left to stand may turn to a purple-red colour.

Each enzyme deficiency has a characteristic pattern of plasma, erythrocyte and excretory (urinary and faecal) abnormalities that form the basis of biochemical diagnostic procedures. It should be noted that lead intoxication, gastrointestinal bleeding, liver disease and certain other conditions also cause the excretion of porphyrins to be increased. Biochemical diagnosis is best made during symptomatic illness as afterwards biochemical parameters may return to normal. Most laboratories will be able to identify porphyria with urinary and faecal tests which must include measurement of urinary porphobilinogen if acute porphyria is suspected. Urine, faecal and blood porphyrias should be determined to avoid errors in the identification of individual porphyrias. Screening of relatives for latent forms is best conducted by reference laboratories (Elder *et al*, 1990).

Much of the initial treatment is supportive. Exposure to sunlight and trauma to the skin should be avoided. Suspected drug precipitants should be removed, but chlorpromazine has been widely used to control mental disturbance, and diazepam can be used to control seizures. Paraldehyde is a safe and effective reserve agent. The prognosis for psychological symptoms is said to be good.

Mitochondrial myopathy

The mitochondrial myopathies are a rare group of metabolic disorders which are clinically and biochemically heterogeneous, but share the common feature of structural mitochondrial abnormalities on skeletal muscle biopsy (Morgan-Hughes, 1986). The majority of cases present before the age of 20. Three overlapping clinical groups are reported (Petty *et al*, 1986). The first is characterised by external ophthalmoplegia and limb weakness, the second by limb weakness alone, and the third by predominantly CNS manifestations – ataxia, dementia, deafness, involuntary movements, pigmented retinopathy and seizures. Mitochondrial myopathy may present as a chronic fatigue syndrome, hysteria or progressive dementia at a young age. The family history should be explored carefully. Presently there is no definitive treatment.

Neuroacanthocytosis

Neuroacanthocytosis refers to a constellation of metabolic disorders, often familial, characterised by neurological disorder in conjunction with acanthocytic red blood cells (red cells with spiky projections). Various other terms have been applied to these disorders, particularly choreo-acanthocytosis, which signals the frequent association of chorea with acanthocytosis. The clinical, haematological and pathological features of 19 cases have recently been described (Hardie *et al*, 1991). Orofacial dyskinesia, tongue and lip-biting, dysarthria, chorea, tics, dystonia, parkinsonism and muscle disorder are frequent features. Cases presenting with solely psychiatric features are not uncommon (Wyszynski *et al*, 1989). Personality change (of the frontal lobe type), depression, anxiety, paranoid delusions and obsessive–compulsive disorder are all described. Seizures occur and can be the presenting feature (Schwartz *et al*, 1992). While mild cognitive impairments occur, the occurrence of progressive dementia is well recognised (Medalia *et al*, 1989).

The diagnosis should be entertained in any patient presenting with movement disorder, personality change and progressive intellectual deterioration. It should be excluded in all suspected cases of Huntington's chorea, and in atypical cases of tic disorder. Screening and counselling are an important aspect of management.

Metachromatic leucodystrophy

Metachromatic leucodystrophy is a lysosomal storage disease. While rare, it warrants inclusion here as it exemplifies a recurring rule within this chapter, namely that a psychiatric disorder may have an unusual cause, one which may be readily overlooked or not even known about. Other lysosomal storage diseases with psychiatric manifestations include Gaucher disease, Niemann-Pick disease, GM2 gangliodiosis and neuronal ceroid lipofuscinosis (Kufs disease).

In metachromatic leucodystrophy, the enzyme aryl sulphatase is deficient and levels of lysosomal galactosyl sylphatide are high throughout the nervous system. The inheritance is autosomal recessive. Progressive impairment of motor function occurs, which in the adult form, may be preceded by a range of mental changes – personality change, affective disorder and schizophrenia-like psychosis. The prognosis is poor – progressive dementia accompanies a relentless deterioration in neurological function.

The diagnosis is strongly suggested by low or absent urinary aryl sulphatase A; in addition metachromatic material may be seen in Schwann cells obtained by sural nerve or rectal biopsy. CSF protein is usually raised and in established cases brain imaging will reveal cerebral atrophy and periventricular white matter changes.

References

Ackner, B., Cooper, J. E., Gray, C. H., *et al* (1962) Acute porphyria: a neuropsychiatric and biochemical study. *Journal of Psychosomatic Research*, **6**, 1–24.

Adams, R. D. & Foley, J. M. (1953) The neurological disorder associated with liver disease. In *Metabolic and Toxic Disease of the Nervous System* (eds H. H. Merritt & C. C. Hare), pp. 198–237. Research Publications of the Association for Research in Metabolic and Nervous Disease, Vol. 32. Baltimore: Williams & Wilkins.

——, Victor, M. & Mancall, E. L. (1959) Central pontine myelinolysis. *Archives of Neurology*, **81**, 154–172.

——, Rhyner, P. A., Day, J., *et al* (1987) Whipple's disease confined to the nervous system. *Annals of Neurology*, **21**, 104–108.

—— & Victor, M. (1989) *Principles of Neurology* (4th edn). New York: McGraw Hill.

Alberti, K. G. M. M. & Nattrass, M. (1978) Severe diabetic ketoacidosis. *Medical Clinics of North America*, **62**, 799–814.

Alles, G. A. (1933) The comparative physiological actions of *dl*-ß-phenyl-isopropylamines. I. Pressor effect and toxicity. *Journal of Pharmacology and Experimental Therapeutics*, **46**, 161–174.

Andreoli, T. E. (1982) Disorders of fluid volume, electrolyte, and acid-base balance. In *Cecil Textbook of Medicine* (16th edn) (eds J. B. Wyngaarden & L. H. Smith), pp. 468–481. Philadelphia: W. B. Saunders.

Arieff, A. I. & Guisado, R. (1976) Effects on the central nervous system of hypernatremic and hyponatremic states. *Kidney International*, **10**, 104–116.

Asher, R. (1949) Myxoedematous madness. *British Medical Journal*, **2**, 555–556.

Ashton, C. H. (1987) Caffeine and health. *British Medical Journal*, **295**, 1293–1294.

Avery, T. L. (1973) A case of acromegaly and gigantism with depression. *British Journal of Psychiatry*, **122**, 599–600.

Bahr, M., Sommer, N., Petersen, D., *et al* (1990) Central pontine myelinolysis associated with low potassium levels in alcoholism. *Journal of Neurology*, **237**, 275–276.

Banay, R. S. (1944) Pathological reaction to alcohol. I. Review of the literature and original case reports. *Quarterly Journal of Studies on Alcohol*, **4**, 580–605.

Bark, N. M. (1982) Heatstroke in psychiatric patients: two cases and a review. *Journal of Clinical Psychiatry*, **43**, 377–380.

Barrison, I. G., Waterson, E. J. & Murray Lyon, I. M. (1985) Adverse effects of alcohol in pregnancy. *British Journal of Addiction*, **80**, 11–22.

Bauer, M. S. & Whybrow, P. C. (1990) Rapid cycling bipolar affective disorder. II. Treatment of refractory rapid cycling with high-dose levothyroxine. *Archives of General Psychiatry*, **47**, 435–440.

——, —— & Winokur, A. (1990) Rapid cycling bipolar affective disorder. I. Association with grade I hypothyroidism. *Archives of General Psychiatry*, **47**, 427–432.

Berkelhammer, C. & Bear, R. A. (1985) A clinical approach to common electrolyte problems: 4. Hypomagnesemia. *Canadian Medical Association Journal*, **132**, 360–368.

Bleuler, M. (1951) The psychopathology of acromegaly. *Journal of Nervous and Mental Disease*, **113**, 497–511.

Blum, A. (1981) Phenylpropanolamine: an over-the-counter amphetamine? *Journal of the American Medical Association*, **245**, 1346–1347.

Bonjour, J. P. (1980) Vitamins and alcoholism. IV. Thiamin. *International Journal for Vitamin and Nutritional Research*, **50**, 321–338.

Boyd, I. H. & Cleveland, S. E. (1967) Psychiatric symptoms masking an insulinoma. A case report. *Diseases of the Nervous System*, **28**, 457–458.

Braaten, J. T. (1987) Hyperosmolar nonketotic diabetic coma: diagnosis and management. *Geriatrics*, **42**, 83–92.

Bradley, C. (1979) Life events and the control of diabetes mellitus. *Journal of Psychosomatic Research*, **23**, 159–162.

Brodsky, J. B. & Cohen, E. N. (1986) Adverse effects of nitrous oxide. *Medical Toxicology*, **1**, 362–374.

Bruce, M. S. & Lader, M. (1986) Caffeine: clinical and experimental effects in humans. *Human Psychopharmacology*, **1**, 63–82.

Carney, M. W. P. (1990) Vitamin deficiency and mental symptoms. *British Journal of Psychiatry*, **156**, 878–882.

Carter, B. J. (1988) A phenomenology of heat injury: the predominance of confusion. *Military Medicine*, **153**, 118–125.

Chalmers, J. S. & Cohen, P. J. (1990) Drug treatment of tricyclic resistant depression. *International Review of Psychiatry*, **2**, 239–248.

Checkley, S. A. (1978) Thyrotoxicosis and the course of manic–depressive illness. *British Journal of Psychiatry*, **133**, 418–424.

Chick, J. & Cantwell, R. (eds) (1994) *Seminars in Alcohol and Drug Misuse*. London: Gaskell.

Christie-Brown, J. R. W. (1968) Mood changes following parathyroidectomy. *Proceedings of the Royal Society of Medicine*, **61**, 1121–1123.

Cleghorn, R. A. (1951) Adrenocortical insufficiency: psychological and neurological observations. *Canadian Medical Association Journal*, **65**, 449–454.

Cohen, S. I. (1980) Cushing's syndrome: a psychiatric study of 29 patients. *British Journal of Psychiatry*, **136**, 120–124.

—— & Johnson, K. (1988) Psychosis from alcohol or drug abuse. *British Medical Journal*, **297**, 1270–1271.

Coid, J. (1979) Manie à potu: a critical review of pathological intoxication. *British Journal of Psychiatry*, **9**, 709–719.

Collis, I. & Lloyd, G. (1992) Psychiatric aspects of liver disease. *British Journal of Psychiatry*, **161**, 12–22.

Connell, P. H. (1958) *Amphetamine Psychosis*. Maudsley Monograph No. 5. London: Chapman & Hall.

Cooke, R. G., Joffe, R. T. & Levitt, A. J. (1992) T3 augmentation of antidepressant treatment in T4-replaced thyroid patients. *Journal of Clinical Psychiatry*, **53**, 16–18.

Cooper, A. F. & Schapira, K. (1973) Case report: depression, catatonic stupor, and EEG changes in hyperparathyroidism. *Psychological Medicine*, **3**, 509–515.

Cornelius, J. R., Soloff, P. H. & Miewald, B. K. (1986) Behavioral manifestations of paraneoplastic encephalopathy. *Biological Psychiatry*, **21**, 686–690.

Crammer, J. L. (1991) Drinking, thirst and water intoxication. *British Journal of Psychiatry*, **159**, 83–89.

Crowe, M. J., Lloyd, G. G., Bloch, S., *et al* (1973) Hypothyroidism in patients treated with lithium: a review and two case reports. *Psychological Medicine*, **3**, 337–342.

Cullen, M. R., Robins, J. M. & Eskenazi, B. (1983) Adult inorganic lead intoxication: presentation of 31 new cases and a review of recent advances in the literature. *Medicine*, **62**, 221–247.

Dathan, J. G. (1954) Acrodynia associated with excessive intake of mercury. *British Medical Journal*, **i**, 247–249.

Davidhazar, R. (1991) Understanding water intoxication. 2. Nursing care for the patient with self-induced water intoxication. *Advances in Clinical Care*, **6**, 30–31.

De Fine Olivarus, B. & Röder, E. (1970) Reversible psychosis and dementia in myxedema. *Acta Psychiatrica Scandinavica*, **46**, 1–13.

Denko, J. & Kaelbling, T. (1962) The psychiatric aspects of hypoparathyroidism. *Acta Psychiatrica Scandinavica*, **38**, 7–70.

Dixon, R. B. & Christy, N. P. (1980) On the various forms of corticosteroid withdrawal syndrome. *American Journal of Medicine*, **68**, 224–230.

Dooling, E. C., Schoene, W. C. & Richardson, E. P. (1974) Hallervorden–Spatz syndrome. *Archives of Neurology*, **30**, 70–83.

Drake, F. R. (1957) Neuropsychiatric-like symptomatology of Addison's disease: a review. *American Journal of Medical Sciences*, **234**, 106–113.

—— & Ebaugh, F. G. (1956) Phaeochromocytoma and electroconvulsive therapy. *American Journal of Psychiatry*, **113**, 295–301.

Drennan, P. C. (1984) Visual hallucinations in children receiving decongestants. *British Medical Journal*, **288**, 1688.

Drummond, D. C. (1991) Dependence on psychoactive drugs: finding a common language. In *International Handbook of Addiction Behaviour* (ed. I. B. Glass), pp. 1–14. London: Routledge.

Edwards, G. & Gross, M. M. (1976) Alcohol dependence: provisional description of a clinical syndrome. *British Medical Journal*, **i**, 1058–1061.

Efron, D. H., Holmstedt, B. & Kline, N. S. (1979) *Ethnopharmacological Search for Psychoactive Drugs*. New York: Raven.

Elder, G. H., Shith, S. G. & Smyth, S. J. (1990) Laboratory investigation of the porphyrias. *Annals of Clinical Biochemistry*, **27**, 395–412.

Eldridge, R., Anayiotos, C. P., Schelsinger, S., *et al* (1984) Hereditary adult-onset leukodystrophy simulating chronic progressive multiple sclerosis. *New England Journal of Medicine*, **311**, 948–953.

Emboden, W. (1972) *Narcotic Plants*. London: Studio Vista.

Engel, G. L., Ferris, E. B. & Logan, M. (1947) Hyperventilation: analysis of clinical symptomatology. *Annals of Internal Medicine*, **27**, 683–704.

Eraut, D. (1974) Idiopathic hypoparathyroidism presenting as dementia. *British Medical Journal*, **1**, 429–430.

Esiri, M. M. & Oppenheimer, D. R. (1989) *Diagnostic Neuropathology*. Oxford: Blackwell Scientific.

Estrada, R. V., Moreno, J., Martinez, E., *et al* (1979) Pancreatic encephalopathy. *Acta Neurologica Scandinavica*, **59**, 135–139.

Ferrier, I. N. (1985) Water intoxication in patients with psychiatric illness. *British Medical Journal*, **291**, 1594–1596.

—— (1987) Endocrinology and psychosis. *British Medical Bulletin*, **43**, 672–688.

Flink, E. B. (1986) Magnesium deficiency in alcoholics. *Alcoholism: Clinical and Experimental Research*, **10**, 590–594.

Flint, J. & Goldstein, L. H. (1992) Familial calcification of the basal ganglia: a case report and review of the literature. *Psychological Medicine*, **22**, 581–595.

Forman, H. P., Levin, S., Stewart, B., *et al* (1989) Cerebral vasculitis and hemorrhage in an adolescent taking diet pills containing phenylpropanolamine: case report and review of literature. *Pediatrics*, **83**, 737–741.

Fornazzari, L., Wilkinson, D. A., Kapur, B. M., *et al* (1983) Cerebellar, cortical and functional impairment in toluene abusers. *Acta Neurologica Scandinavica*, **67**, 319–329.

Foster, D. W. (1991) Diabetes mellitus. In *Harrison's Principles of Internal Medicine* (12th edn) (eds J. D. Wilson, E. Braunwald, K. J. Isselbacher, *et al*), pp. 1739–1759. New York: McGraw-Hill.

Fraser, C. L. & Arieff, A. I. (1985) Hepatic encephalopathy. *New England Journal of Medicine*, **313**, 865–873.

Fuortes, L. (1988) Arsenic poisoning. *Postgraduate Medicine*, **83**, 233–234.

Gale, E. A. M. & Tattersall, R. B. (1979) Unrecognized nocturnal hypoglycaemia in insulin-treated diabetics. *Lancet*, **i**, 1049–1052.

Galfond, D. (1989) Psychosis from alcohol or drug abuse. *British Medical Journal*, **298**, 524.

Gallucci, M., Bozzao, A., Spleniani, A., *et al* (1990) Wernicke encephalopathy: MR findings in five patients. *American Journal of Neuroradiology*, **11**, 887–892.

Gambert, S. R. & Escher, J. E. (1988) Atypical presentations of endocrine disorders in the elderly. *Geriatrics*, **43**, 69–78.

Ghariani, M., Adrien, M. L., Bayle, J., *et al* (1991) Intoxication suraigue a l'arsenic. *Annales Francaise D'Anesthesie et de Reanimation*, **10**, 304–307.

Gibson, G. E. (1985) Hypoxia. In *Cerebral Energy Metabolism and Metabolic Encephalopathy* (ed. D. W. McCandless), pp. 43–78. New York: Plenum.

Goldberg, A. (1959) Acute intermittent porphyria. A study of fifty cases. *Quarterly Journal of Medicine*, **28**, 183–209.

Goldfrank, L. & Melinek, M. (1979) Locoweed and other anticholinergics. *Hospital Physician*, **8**, 18–39.

Goodwin, D. W., Crane, B. & Guze, S. B. (1969*a*) Alcoholic "blackouts": a review and clinical study of 100 alcoholics. *American Journal of Psychiatry*, **126**, 191–198.

——, Crane, B. & Guze, S. B. (1969*b*) Phenomenological aspects of the alcoholic blackout. *British Journal of Psychiatry*, **115**, 1033–1038.

Gorelick, P. B. (1989) The status of alcohol as a risk factor for stroke. *Stroke*, **20**, 1607–1610.

Grant, I., Kyle, G. C., Teichman, A., *et al* (1974) Recent life events and diabetes in adults. *Psychosomatic Medicine*, **36**, 121–128.

Greden, J. F. & Walters, M. D. (1992) Caffeine. In *Substance Abuse: a Comprehensive Textbook* (eds J. C. Lowinson, P. Ruiz, R. B. Millman, *et al*), pp. 357–370. Baltimore: Williams & Wilkins.

Greenwood, R. S. & Nelson, J. S. (1978) Atypical neuronal ceroid-lipofuscinosis. *Neurology*, **28**, 710–717.

Gross, M. M., Lewis, E. & Nagarajan, M. (1973) An improved quantitative system for assessing the acute alcohol psychoses and related states (TSA and SSA). In *Alcohol Intoxication and Withdrawal Experimental Studies* (ed. M. M. Gross), pp. 365–376. New York: Plenum Press.

Hadden, W. B. (1882) The nervous symptoms of myxoedema. *Brain*, **5**, 188–196.

Hall, R. C. W., Popkin, M. K. & Kirkpatrick, B. (1978) Tricyclic exacerbation of steroid psychosis. *Journal of Nervous and Mental Disease*, **166**, 738–742.

——, ——, Stickney, R. N., *et al* (1979) Presentation of the steroid psychoses. *Journal of Nervous and Mental Disease*, **167**, 229–236.

Hamilton, W. (1976*a*) Sporadic cretinism. *Developmental Medicine and Child Neurology*, **18**, 384–386.

—— (1976*b*) Endemic cretinism. *Developmental Medicine and Child Neurology*, **18**, 386–391.

Hanwinen, H. (1971) Psychological picture of manifest and latent carbon disulphide poisoning. *British Journal of Industrial Medicine*, **28**, 374–381.

Hardie, R. J., Pullon, H. W. H., Harding, A. E., *et al* (1991) Neuroacanthocytosis. A clinical haematological and pathological study of 19 cases. *Brain*, **114**, 13–49.

Harper, C. G. & Kril, J. J. (1990) Neuropathology of alcoholism. *Alcohol and Alcoholism*, **25**, 207–216.

Harrison, I. (1988) Sale of medicines liable to abuse. *Pharmaceutical Journal*, **240**, 600.

Hartman, D. E. (1988) *Neuropsychological Toxicology*. New York: Pergamon.

Haskett, R. F. (1985) Diagnostic categorization of psychiatric disturbance in Cushing's syndrome. *American Journal of Psychiatry*, **142**, 911–916.

Hein, M. D. & Jackson, I. M. (1990) Review: thyroid function in psychiatric illness. *General Hospital Psychiatry*, **12**, 232–244.

Heiser, J. F. & Gillin, J. C. (1971) The reversal of anticholinergic drug-induced delirium and coma with physostigmine. *American Journal of Psychiatry*, **127**, 1050–1054.

Henkin, R. I., Patten, B. M., Re, P. K., *et al* (1975) A syndrome of acute zinc loss. Cerebellar dysfunction, mental changes, anorexia, and taste and smell dysfunction. *Archives of Neurology*, **32**, 745–751.

Herrström, P. & Högstedt, B. (1993) Clinical studies of oral galvanism: no evidence of toxic mercury exposure but anxiety disorder an important background factor. *Scandinavian Journal of Dental Research*, **101**, 232–237.

Hooshmand, H. & Sarhaddi, S. (1975) Hypothyroidism in adults and children. EEG findings. *Clinical Electroencephalography*, **6**, 61–67.

Howells, R. B. (1994) Neuroleptic malignant syndrome. Don't confuse with anticholinergic intoxication. *British Medical Journal*, **308**, 200–201.

—— & Patrick, M. (1989) Delirium tremens. *British Medical Journal*, **298**, 457.

Hunter, D. (1978) *The Diseases of Occupations*. London: Hodder & Stoughton.

Hunter, R., McLuskie, R., Wyper, D., *et al* (1989) The pattern of function-related regional blood flow investigated by single photon emission tomography with ^{99m}Tc-HMPAO in patients with presenile Alzheimer's disease and Korsakoff psychosis. *Psychological Medicine*, **19**, 847–855.

Ikeda, A., Antoku, Y., Abe, T., *et al* (1989) Marchiafava-Bignami disease: consecutive observation at acute stage by magnetic resonance imaging and computerized tomography. *Japanese Journal of Medicine*, **28**, 740–743.

Illowsky, B. P. & Kirch, D. G. (1988) Polydipsia and hyponatraemia in psychiatric patients. *American Journal of Psychiatry*, **145**, 675–683.

Isbell, H., Fraser, H. F., Wickler, A., *et al* (1953) An experimental study of the aetiology of 'rum fits' and delirium tremens. *Quarterly Journal of Studies on Alcohol*, **16**, 1–33.

Ishii, N. & Nishihara, Y. (1981) Pellagra among chronic alcoholics: clinical and pathological study of 20 necropsy cases. *Journal of Neurology, Neurosurgery and Psychiatry*, **44**, 209–215.

Jacobs, M. R. (1987) *Drugs and Drug Abuse*. Toronto: Alcoholism and Drug Addiction Research Foundation.

Jacobson, R. R. & Lishman, W. A. (1990) Cortical and diencephalic lesions in Korsakoff's syndrome: a clinical and CT scan study. *Psychological Medicine*, **20**, 63–75.

Jefferson, J. W. & Marshall, J. R. (1981) *Neuropsychiatric Features of Medical Disorders*. New York: Plenum.

Johnson, A. L., Hollister, L. E. & Berger, P. A. (1981) The anticholinergic intoxication syndrome: diagnosis and treatment. *Journal of Clinical Psychiatry*, **42**, 313–317.

Johnson, J. (1975) Schizophrenia and Cushing's syndrome cured by adrenalectomy. *Psychological Medicine*, **5**, 165–168.

Jolliffe, N., Bowman, K. M., Rosenblum, L. A., *et al* (1940) Nicotinic acid deficiency encephalopathy. *Journal of the American Medical Association*, **114**, 307–312.

Kalimo, H., Lundberg, P. O. & Olsson, Y. (1979) Familial subacute necrotising encephalomyelopathy of the adult form (adult Leigh syndrome). *Annals of Neurology*, **6**, 200–206.

Kaplan, L. M. (1991) Endocrine tumors of the gastrointestinal tract and pancreas. In *Harrison's Principles of Internal Medicine* (12th edn) (eds J. D. Wilson, E. Braunwald, K. J. Isselbacher, *et al*), pp. 1388–1393. New York: McGraw-Hill.

Keddie, K. M. G. (1987) Case report: severe depressive illness in the context of hypervitaminosis D. *British Journal of Psychiatry*, **150**, 394–396.

Kelly, W. F., Checkley, S. A., Bender, D. A., *et al* (1983) Cushing's syndrome and depression – a prospective study of 26 patients. *British Journal of Psychiatry*, **142**, 16–19.

Kerr, D. N., Ward, M. K., Ellis, H. A., *et al* (1992) Aluminium intoxication in renal disease. *Ciba Foundation Symposium*, **169**, 123–135.

Kind, H. (1958) Die psychiatrie der hypophyseninsuffizienz speziell der simmondsschen krankeit. *Fortschritte der Neurologie und Psychiatrie*, **26**, 501–563.

King, M. D., Day, R. E., Oliver, J. S., *et al* (1981) Solvent encephalopathy. *British Medical Journal*, **283**, 663–665.

Klaassen, C. D. (1990) Nonmetallic environmental toxicants: air pollutants, solvents and vapors, and pesticides. In *The Pharmacological Basis of Therapeutics* (8th edn)(eds I. Goodman, *et al*). New York: Pergamon Press.

Knochel, J. P. (1977) The pathophysiology and clinical characteristics of severe hypophosphatemia. *Archives of Internal Medicine*, **137**, 203–219.

Kopelman, M. D. (1987*a*) Amnesia: organic and psychogenic. *British Journal of Psychiatry*, **150**, 428–442.

—— (1987*b*) Two types of confabulation. *Journal of Neurology, Neurosurgery and Psychiatry*, **50**, 1482–1487.

Lahey, F. H. (1931) Non-activated (apathetic) type of hyperthyroidism. *New England Journal of Medicine*, **204**, 747–748.

Lancet (1985) Editorial. Hypoglycaemia and the nervous system. *Lancet*, **2**, 759–760.

Landsberg, L. L. & Young, J. B. (1991) Pheochromocytoma. In *Harrison's Principles of Internal Medicine* (12th edn) (eds J. D. Wilson, E. Braunwald, K. J. Isselbacher, *et al*). New York: McGraw-Hill.

Lazarus, J. H., John, R., Bennie, R. J., *et al* (1981) Lithium therapy and thyroid function: a long-term study. *Psychological Medicine*, **11**, 85–92.

Legrain, M. (1892) Alcoholism. In *A Dictionary of Psychological Medicine* (ed. D. H. Tuke), pp. 69. London: Churchill.

Leigh, D. (1952) Pellagra and the nutritional neuropathies: a neuropathological review. *Journal of Mental Science*, **98**, 130–142.

Ling, M. H., Perry, P. J. & Tsuang, M. T. (1981) Side effects of corticosteroid therapy. *Archives of General Psychiatry*, **38**, 471–477.

Lipowski, Z. J. (1990) *Delirium: Acute Confusional States* (2nd edn). Oxford: Oxford University Press.

Lishman, W. A. (1987) *Organic Psychiatry* (2nd edn). Oxford: Blackwell Scientific.

—— (1990) Alcohol and the brain. *British Journal of Psychiatry*, **156**, 635–644.

Loosemore, S. & Armstrong, D. (1990) Do-Do abuse. *British Journal of Psychiatry*, **157**, 278–281.

Major, L. F., Brown, L. & Wilson, W. P. (1973) Carcinoid syndrome and psychiatric symptoms. *Southern Medical Journal*, **66**, 787–789.

Malouf, R. & Brust, J. C. M. (1985) Hypoglycaemia: causes, neurological manifestations, and outcome. *Annals of Neurology*, **17**, 421–430.

Margo, A. (1981) Acromegaly and depression. *British Journal of Psychiatry*, **139**, 467–468.

Marks, V. & Rose, C. F. (1987) *Hypoglycaemia*. New York: Raven Press.

Mateo, D. & Giménez-Roldan, S. (1982) Dementia in idiopathic hypoparathyroidism. Rapid efficacy of alfacalcidol. *Archives of Neurology*, **39**, 424–425.

May, P. R. A. & Ebaugh, F. G. (1953) Pathological intoxication, alcoholic hallucinosis, and other reactions to alcohol: a clinical study. *Quarterly Journal of Studies on Alcohol*, **14**, 200–227.

McLarty, D. G., Ratcliffe, W. A., Ratcliffe, J. G., *et al* (1978) A study of thyroid function in psychiatric in-patients. *British Journal of Psychiatry*, **133**, 211–218.

Medalia, A., Merriam, A. & Sandberg, M. (1989) Neuropsychological deficits in choreoacanthocytosis. *Archives of Neurology*, **46**, 573–575.

Melicow, M. M. (1977) One hundred cases of pheochromocytoma (107 tumors) at the Columbia-Presbyterian medical center, 1926–1976. A clinicopathological analysis. *Cancer*, **40**, 1987–2004.

Mello, N. K. & Mendelson, J. H. (1970) Experimentally induced intoxication in alcoholics: a comparison between programmed and spontaneous drinking. *Journal of Pharmacology and Experimental Therapeutics*, **173**, 101–116.

Meredith, T. J., Ruprah, M., Liddle, A., *et al* (1989) Diagnosis and treatment of acute poisoning with volatile substances. *Human Toxicology*, **8**, 277–286.

Michael, R. P. & Gibbons, J. L. (1963) Interrelationships between the endocrine system and neuropsychiatry. *International Review of Neurobiology*, **5**, 243–302.

Milson, R. C., Koczapski, A. B., Cook, M. I., *et al* (1992) A survey of patient's attitudes towards self-induced water intoxication. *Canadian Journal of Psychiatry*, **37**, 46–47.

Min, S. K. (1986) A brain syndrome associated with delayed neuropsychiatric sequelae following carbon monoxide intoxication. *Acta Psychiatrica Scandinavica*, **73**, 80–86.

Minton, N. A. & Murray, V. S. G. (1988) A review of organophosphate poisoning. *Medical Toxicology*, **3**, 350–375.

Missri, J. C. & Alexander, S. (1978) Hyperventilation syndrome, a brief review. *Journal of the American Medical Association*, **240**, 2093–2096.

Mitchell, W. & Feldman, F. (1968) Neuropsychiatric aspects of hypokalemia. *Canadian Medical Association Journal*, **98**, 49–51.

Moore, D., House, I. & Dixon, A. (1993) Thallium poisoning. *British Medical Journal*, **306**, 1527–1529.

Morgan-Hughes, J. A. (1986) Mitochondrial diseases. *Trends in Neuroscience*, **9**, 15–19.

Murphree, H. B. (1971) The importance of congeners in the effects of alcoholic beverages. In *The Biological Basis of Alcoholism* (eds Y. Israel & J. Mardones), pp. 209–234. New York: John Wiley.

Naranjo, C. A. & Sellers, E. M. (1986) Clinical assessment and pharmacotherapy of the alcohol withdrawal syndrome. In *Recent Developments in Alcoholism* (ed. M. Galanter), pp. 265–280. New York: Plenum.

Nathan, P. E. & Hay, W. (1984) Alcoholism: psychopathology, etiology and treatment. In *Comprehensive Handbook of Psychopathology* (eds H. E. Adams & P. B. Sutker), pp. 549–583. New York: Plenum Press.

Nelson, M. (1982) Psychological testing at high altitude. *Aviation Space and Environmental Medicine*, **53**, 122–126.

Norvenius, G., Widerlöv, E. & Lönnerholm, G. (1979) Phenylpropanolamine and mental disturbances. *Lancet*, **ii**, 1367–1368.

O'Neill, S., Tipton, K. F., Prichard, J. S., *et al* (1984) Survival after high blood alcohol levels. *Archives of Internal Medicine*, **144**, 641–642.

Pappas, S. C. & Jones, E. A. (1983) Methods for assessing hepatic encephalopathy. *Seminars in Liver Disease*, **3**, 298–307.

Parsons-Smith, B. G., Summerskill, W. H. J., Dawson, A. M., *et al* (1957) The electroencephalograph in liver disease. *Lancet*, **2**, 867–871.

Petersdorf, R. G. (1991) Hypothermia and hyperthermia. In *Harrison's Principles of Internal Medicine* (12th edn) (eds J. D. Wilson, E. Braunwald, K. J. Isselbacher, *et al*). New York: McGraw-Hill.

Petersen, P. (1968) Psychiatric disorders in primary hyperparathyroidism. *Journal of Clinical Endocrinology and Metabolism*, **28**, 1491–1495.

Petty, R. K. H., Harding, A. E. & Morgan-Hughes, J. A. (1986) The clinical features of mitochondrial myopathy. *Brain*, **109**, 915–938.

Potts, J. T. (1991) Diseases of the parathyroid gland and other hyper- and hypocalcaemic disorders. In *Harrison's Principles of Internal Medicine* (12th edn) (eds J. D. Wilson, E. Braunwald, K. J. Isselbacher, *et al*). New York: McGraw-Hill.

Randall, R. E., Cohen, M. D., Spray, C. C., *et al* (1964) Hypermagnesemia in renal failure. *Annals of Internal Medicine*, **61**, 73–88.

Ratzan, R. M., Chapron, D. J., Mumford, D., *et al* (1980) Uncovering magnesium toxicity. *Geriatrics*, **35**, 75–86.

Reiter, L. W. & Ruppert, P. H. (1984) Behavioral toxicity of trialkyltin compounds: a review. *Neurotoxicology*, **5**, 177–186.

Reynolds, J. E. F. (ed.) (1989) *Martindale, the Extra Pharmacopoeia* (29th edn). London: The Pharmaceutical Press.

Robbins, S. L. & Cotran, R. S. (1979) *The Pathologic Basis of Disease* (2nd edn). Philadelphia: W. B. Saunders.

Robinson, R. & Stott, R. (1980) *Medical Emergencies, Diagnosis and Management*. London: Heinemann.

Ron, M. A. (1983) The alcoholic brain: CT scan and psychological findings. *Psychological Medicine*, Monograph Supplement 3.

—— (1986) Volatile substance abuse: a review of possible long-term neurological, intellectual and psychiatric sequelae. *British Journal of Psychiatry*, **148**, 235–246.

Rosser, R. (1976) Thyrotoxicosis and lithium. *British Journal of Psychiatry*, **128**, 61–66.

Rubin, R. R. & Peyrot, M. (1992) Psychosocial problems and interventions in diabetes. A review of the literature. *Diabetes Care*, **15**, 1640–1657.

Ruprah, M., Mant, T. G. K. & Flanagan, R. J. (1985) Acute carbon tetrachloride poisoning in 19 patients. Implications for diagnosis and treatment. *Lancet*, **i**, 1027–1029.

Ryle, P. R. & Thomson, A. D. (1984) Nutrition and vitamins in alcoholism. *Contemporary Issues in Clinical Biochemistry*, **1**, 188–224.

Sabot, L. M., Gross, M. M. & Halpert, E. (1968) A study of acute alcoholic psychoses in women. *British Journal of Addiction*, **63**, 29–49.

Sachon, C., Grimaldi, A., Digy, J. P., *et al* (1992) Cognitive function, insulin-dependent diabetes and hypoglycaemia. *Journal of Internal Medicine*, **231**, 471–475.

Salum, I. (1972) Delirium tremens and certain other acute sequels of alcohol abuse. *Acta Psychiatrica Scandinavica*, suppl. 234, 1–145.

Sandifer, M. G. (1983) Hyponatraemia due to psychotropic drugs. *Journal of Clinical Psychiatry*, **44**, 301–303.

Saunders, J. B. (1991) Physical complications of alcohol abuse. In *International Handbook of Addiction Behaviour* (ed. I. B. Glass), pp. 134–140. London: Routledge.

Schimke, R. N. (1991) Disorders affecting multiple endocrine systems. In *Harrison's Principles of Internal Medicine* (12th edn) (eds J. D. Wilson, E. Braunwald, K. J. Isselbacher, *et al*). New York: McGraw-Hill.

Schroter, C., Schroter, H. & Huffmann, G. (1991) Neurological and psychiatric manifestations of lead poisoning in adults (case report and literature review). *Fortschritte der Neurologie und Psychiatrie*, **59**, 413–424.

Schwartz, M. S., Monroe, P. S. & Leigh, P. N. (1992) Epilepsy as the presenting feature of neuroacanthocytosis in siblings. *Journal of Neurology*, **239**, 261–262.

Service, J. F., Dale, A. J. D., Eleveback, L. R., *et al* (1976) Insulinoma. Clinical and diagnostic features of 60 consecutive cases. *Mayo Clinic Proceedings*, **51**, 417–429.

Sharp, C. W. & Rosenberg, N. L. (1992) Volatile substances. In *Substance Abuse* (2nd edn) (eds J. H. Lowinson, *et al*). Baltimore: Williams & Wilkins.

Shaw, J. M., Kolesar, G. S., Sellers, E. M., *et al* (1981) Development of optimal treatment tactics for alcohol withdrawal. I. Assessment and effectiveness of supportive care. *Journal of Clinical Psychopharmacology*, **1**, 382–387.

Sherlock, S. & Dooley, J. (1993) *Diseases of the Liver and Biliary System* (9th edn). Oxford: Blackwell.

Shield, L. K., Coleman, T. L. & Marksbery, W. R. (1977) Methylbromide intoxication: neurological features, including simulation of Reye syndrome. *Neurology*, **27**, 959–962.

Smith, J. S. & Brandon, S. (1973) Morbidity from carbon monoxide poisoning at three-year follow-up. *British Medical Journal*, **i**, 318–321.

Sobell, L. C. (1980) *Evaluating Alcohol and Drug Abuse Treatment Effectiveness*. New York: Pergamon Press.

Starkman, M. N. & Schteingart, D. E. (1981) Neuropsychiatric manifestations of patients with Cushing's syndrome. Relationship to cortisol and adrenocorticotropic hormone. *Archives of Internal Medicine*, **141**, 215–219.

——, —— & Schork, M. A. (1986) Correlation of bedside cognitive and neuropsychological tests in patient's with Cushing's syndrome. *Psychosomatics*, **27**, 508–511.

Sterns, R. H. (1987) Severe symptomatic hyponatremia: treatment and outcome. *Annals of Internal Medicine*, **107**, 656–664.

Stockwell, T., Murphy, D. & Hodgson, R. (1979) The severity of alcohol dependence questionnaire: its use, reliability and validity. *British Journal of Addiction*, **78**, 145–155.

Summerskill, W. H. J., Davidson, E. A., Sherlock, S., *et al* (1956) The neuropsychiatric syndrome associated with hepatic cirrhosis and an extensive portal collateral circulation. *Quarterly Journal of Medicine*, **25**, 245–266.

Supino-Viterbo, V., Sicard, C., Risvegliato, G., *et al* (1977) Toxic encephalopathy due to ingestion of bismuth salts: clinical and EEG studies of 45 patients. *Journal of Neurology, Neurosurgery and Psychiatry*, **40**, 748–752.

Sweeney, D. F. (1990) Alcoholic blackouts: legal implications. *Journal of Substance Abuse Treatment*, **7**, 155–159.

Szabadi, E. (1991) Thyroid dysfunction and affective illness. *British Medical Journal*, **302**, 923–924.

Thase, M. E., Kupfer, D. J., Frank, E., *et al* (1989) Treatment of imipramine-resistant recurrent depression. II. An open trial of lithium augmentation. *Journal of Clinical Psychiatry*, **50**, 413–417.

Thomas, J. E., Rooke, E. D. & Kvale, W. F. (1966) The neurologist's experience with phaeochromocytoma. A review of 100 cases. *Journal of the American Medical Association*, **197**, 100–104.

Thomas, P. K. (1986) Brain atrophy and alcoholism. *British Medical Journal*, **292**, 787.

Todd, J., Collins, A. D., Martin, F. R. R., *et al* (1962) Mental symptoms due to insulinomata. Report on two cases. *British Medical Journal*, **2**, 828–831.

Tonks, C. M. (1964) Mental illness in hypothyroid patients. *British Journal of Psychiatry*, **110**, 706–710.

Torvik, A., Lindboe, C. E. & Rodge, S. (1982) Brain lesions in alcoholics. A neuropathological study with clinical correlations. *Journal of the Neurological Sciences*, **56**, 233–248.

Victor, M. (1984) Polyneuropathy due to nutritional deficiency and alcoholism. In *Peripheral Neuropathy* (2nd edn) (eds P. J. Dyck, P. K. Thomas, E. H. Lambert, *et al*), pp. 1899–1940. Philadelphia: W. B. Saunders.

—— & Adams, R. D. (1953) The effect of alcohol on the nervous system. In *Metabolic and Toxic Disease of the Nervous System* (eds H. H. Merritt & C. C. Hare).

Research Publications of the Association for Research in Metabolic and Nervous Disease, Vol 32. Baltimore: Williams & Wilkins.

—— & Hope, J. M. (1958) The phenomenon of auditory hallucinations in chronic alcoholism. A critical evaluation of the status of alcoholic hallucinosis. *Journal of Nervous and Mental Diseases*, **126**, 451–481.

——, Mancall, E. L. & Dreyfus, P. M. (1960) Deficiency amblyopia in the alcoholic patient. A clinicopathologic study. *Archives of Ophthalmology*, **64**, 1–33.

——, Adams, R. D. & Cole, M. (1965) The acquired (non-Wilsonian) type of chronic hepatocerebral degeneration. *Medicine*, **44**, 345–396.

——, —— & Collins, G. H. (1989) *The Wernicke–Korsakoff Syndrome and Related Neurological Disorders due to Alcoholism and Malnutrition* (2nd edn). Philadelphia: F. A. Davis.

Vieweg, W. V. R., David, J. J., Rowe, W. T., *et al* (1985) Death from self-induced water intoxication among patients with schizophrenic disorders. *Journal of Nervous and Mental Diseases*, **173**, 161–165.

Von Bose, M. J. & Zaudig, M. (1991) Encephalopathy resembling Creutzfeldt-Jakob disease following oral, prescribed doses of bismuth nitrate. *British Journal of Psychiatry*, **158**, 278–280.

Vroom, F. Q. & Greer, M. (1972) Mercury vapour intoxication. *Brain*, **95**, 305–318.

Waites, T. F. (1978) Hyperventilation – chronic and acute. *Archives of Internal Medicine*, **138**, 1700–1701.

Wartofsky, L. & Ingbar, S. H. (1991) Diseases of the thyroid. In *Harrison's Principles of Internal Medicine* (12th edn) (eds J. D. Wilson, E. Braunwald, K. J. Isselbacher, *et al*). New York: McGraw-Hill.

Webb, W. L. & Gehi, M. (1981) Electrolyte and fluid imbalance: neuropsychiatric manifestations. *Psychosomatics*, **22**, 199–203.

Weiner, H. (1977) *Psychobiology and Human Disease*. New York: Elsevier.

Weiner, N. (1980) Atropine, scopolamine, and related antimuscarinic drugs. In *The Pharmacological Basis of Therapeutics* (eds A. G. Gilman, L. S. Goodman & A. Gilman). New York: Pergamon.

Wells, S. J. (1984) Caffeine: implications of recent research for clinical practice. *American Journal of Orthopsychiatry*, **54**, 375–389.

Westermeyer, J. (1987) The psychiatrist and solvent-inhaler abuse: recognition, assessment, and treatment. *American Journal of Psychiatry*, **144**, 903–907.

Westlake, E. K., Simpson, T. & Kaye, M. (1955) Carbon dioxide narcosis in emphysema. *Quarterly Journal of Medicine*, **24**, 155–173.

Wetterberg, L. & Österberg, E. (1969) Acute intermittent porphyria: a psychometric study of twenty-five patients. *Journal of Psychosomatic Research*, **13**, 91–93.

White, A. J. & Barraclough, B. (1988) Thyroid disease and mental illness: a study of thyroid disease in psychiatric admissions. *Journal of Psychosomatic Research*, **32**, 99–106.

Whitehouse, A. M. & Duncan, J. M. (1987) Ephedrine psychosis revisited. *British Journal of Psychiatry*, **150**, 258–261.

Whybrow, P. C., Prange, A. J. & Treadway, C. R. (1969) Mental changes accompanying thyroid gland dysfunction: a reappraisal using objective measurement. *Archives of General Psychiatry*, **20**, 48–63.

Williams, G. H. & Dluhy, R. G. (1991) Diseases of the adrenal cortex. In *Harrison's Principles of Internal Medicine* (12th edn) (eds J. D. Wilson, E. Braunwald, K. J. Isselbacher, *et al*). New York: McGraw-Hill.

Wilson, D. A., Mulder, R. T. & Joyce, P. R. (1992) Diurnal profiles of thyroid hormones are altered in depression. *Journal of Affective Disorders*, **24**, 11–16.

Winkelman, M. D., Banker, B. Q., Victor, M., *et al* (1983) Non-infantile neuronopathic Gaucher's disease: a clinico-pathologic study. *Neurology*, **33**, 994–1008.

Wood, R. (1981) Neurobehavioral toxicity of carbon disulphide. *Neurobehavioral Toxicology and Teratology*, **3**, 397–405.

Wyszynski, B., Merriam, A., Medalia, A., *et al* (1989) Choreoacanthocytosis. Report of a case with psychiatric features. *Neuropsychiatry, Neuropathology and Behavioral Neurology*, **2**, 137–144.

Yamaguchi, H., Arita, Y., Hara, Y., *et al* (1992) Anorexia nervosa responding to zinc supplementation: a case report. *Gastroenterology Japan*, **27**, 554–558.

Zacharski, L. R., Litin, E. M., Mulder, D. W., *et al* (1970) Acute, fatal hepatic failure presenting with psychiatric symptoms. *American Journal of Psychiatry*, **127**, 382–386.

Zilva, J. F. & Pannall, P. R. (1979) *Clinical Chemistry in Diagnosis and Treatment*. London: Lloyd-Luke.

25 Sleep disorders

Mark Tattersall, Philip Sedgwick & Sharon Borrows

Neurophysiology of sleep ● Function of sleep ● Circadian rhythm ● Laboratory measurement ● Clinical assessment ● Sleep disorders ● Sleep disorders secondary to disorders of physical health ● Sleep disorders secondary to psychiatric disorders ● Substance induced sleep disorders ● Sleep and crime

---

Although we sleep for about a third of our lives, the purpose and nature of sleep remain obscure, and have fascinated and baffled man throughout recorded time. While the study of sleep has been to some extent neglected by modern medical education and practice, we all know from experience that poor sleep affects many aspects of our waking lives. Some sleep disorders also carry considerable risks of morbidity and mortality to the sufferer. Many sleep disorders have an additional impact on the sleep of the bed partner, and can result in conflict within a relationship. Some sleep disorders which result in excessive daytime tiredness also contribute significantly to road traffic accident and mortality statistics. As sleep disorders in general are common, the impact of these complications is considerable. Yet these are complaints for which there is a disproportionate lack of understanding, research or available treatment. This chapter aims to describe the underlying neurophysiology of sleep, its investigation in the sleep laboratory, and its clinical assessment, and then discusses the range of sleep disorders and their management.

Neurophysiology of sleep

The sleep-wake cycle

Adult humans undertake a rhythm of alternating wakefulness and sleep known as the sleep-wake cycle. This has a length of approximately 24 hours and is closely linked to the light-dark cycle. Most adult human sleep-wake cycles are monophasic in that only one episode of sleep is taken per light-dark cycle. In countries where an afternoon nap or *siesta* is commonplace it may be biphasic. With advancing age, naps are often taken during the day and the sleep-wake cycle is described as polyphasic.

Sleep architecture

Sleep was originally thought to be a simple and inactive process. This concept changed in 1937 when Loomis *et al* discovered unique patterns in the electrical activity of the brain characterising states of sleep. Sixteen years later, Aserinksy & Kleitman (1953) observed the periodic appearance of conjugate rapid eye movements, later linked to dreaming sleep by Dement & Kleitman (1957). Today, sleep is known to be an active and complex process consisting of a series of states known as stages, identified electrophysiologically according to the guidelines of Rechtschaffen & Kales (1968). The term 'sleep architecture' is used to describe these states and their interrelationships, and is widely documented (Hartmann, 1968; Brezinová, 1974; Horne, 1990; Hauri, 1992; Shapiro & Flanigan, 1993; Carskadon & Dement, 1994).

NREM and REM sleep

Two distinct electrophysiological states of sleep exist: non-rapid eye movement (NREM, pronounced non-REM) sleep, also known as orthodox sleep; and rapid-eye movement (REM) sleep, sometimes called paradoxical or dreaming sleep, or the D-state. NREM sleep is further subdivided into stages 1, 2, 3 and 4, forming a continuum of depth of sleep with arousal thresholds lowest in stage 1 and greatest in stage 4. Stage 1 sleep is a drowsy state; softly calling a person's name will be enough to arouse them. Stage 2 is a light sleep while stages 3 and 4, collectively known as slow wave sleep (SWS), are a deep sleep. REM sleep is variable in its range of arousal thresholds, but is generally considered to be a light sleep. There is a further stage known as movement time which represents gross body movements, for example turning over. Minor or transient arousals are also observed but do not represent a stage (Guilleminault, 1992).

Progression of sleep states across the night

Sleep is entered through NREM sleep in a normal healthy adult, with a transition from wakefulness to stage 1 sleep, followed within a few minutes by stage 2 sleep, which then continues for 10–25 minutes. Stage 3 sleep is then entered, lasting only for a few minutes, before a transition to stage 4 sleep which may continue for 20–40 minutes. The first episode of REM sleep then arises, approximately 70 minutes after sleep onset, and completes the first NREM-REM sleep cycle.

The NREM-REM sleep cycle will repeat some 4–6 times throughout the night with a periodicity of about 90 minutes. As the night progresses the proportion of SWS in each cycle will diminish, while the proportion of stage 2 and REM sleep will increase.

Stage 1 may reoccur during the night ephemerally interrupting stage 2, sometimes as a transition to brief awakenings which are often not recalled the following morning. Brief interludes of wakefulness or stages 1 and 2 may also intrude into episodes of REM throughout the night. Movement time may occur at anytime, although usually when moving into, and during the lighter stages of sleep and wakefulness. Minor arousals will also occur in the lighter stages of sleep.

In a young normal adult, stage 1 will occupy approximately 2–5% of the night's sleep; stage 2, 45–55%; stages 3 and 4, 15–25%; REM sleep, 20–25% and wakefulness less than 5%.

A single night's sleep can be represented diagrammatically in the form of a hypnograph, with that of a normal 20-year-old woman shown in Fig. 25.1 to illustrate the progression of sleep stages. The vertical axis indicates the sleep stage with time shown on the horizontal axis. Movement time and minor arousals are plotted as events in time.

Factors that modify the distribution of sleep states

The appearance of sleep stages and their progression across the night is influenced by many factors. Age is probably the strongest factor affecting the patterning of sleep (Williams *et al*, 1974). While the total amount of NREM sleep remains more or less constant throughout life, the SWS component is maximal in adolescence and declines with advancing years so that by the age of 60 it may no longer be present. REM sleep as a percentage of total sleep is maintained well into old age.

The total duration of sleep is at its greatest in babies, who sleep an average of 17 hours throughout the day. In childhood night-time sleep averages about 10 hours. By early adult life, an individuals sleep lasts a mean of 7.5 hours duration. With increasing age this falls gradually to a mean of 6.5 hours, with an increase in individual variability, and an increase in time spent in bed. In latter life, the nocturnal pattern of sleep can become fragmented, with an increase in daytime sleep.

Gender has little influence on the quantity and quality of sleep although SWS is more vulnerable to the effects of age in men.

Little is known about the effects of diet on sleep. Brezinová & Oswald (1972) showed that a hot milk drink at bedtime induced more restful and consolidated sleep. High-carbohydrate/low fat and low-carbohydrate/high fat diets have been found to significantly increase nocturnal REM sleep, whilst the former also comparably affected SWS (Phillips *et al*, 1975). L-tryptophan is an essential amino acid and a precursor of serotonin, an inhibitory neurotransmitter which has long been associated with sleep. The effects of tryptophan are reviewed by Gaillard *et al* (1994).

Mood states such as anxiety, and particularly anger, are largely incompatible with normal sleep, and are important aetiological factors in the development of various sleep disorders (most commonly insomnia). Depressed or elevated moods also have powerful effects on sleep initiation and maintenance. Waters *et al* (1993) showed that negative mood states are important in influencing insomnia, while Hauri (1970) found positive relationships between the subjective measure of a good night's sleep and

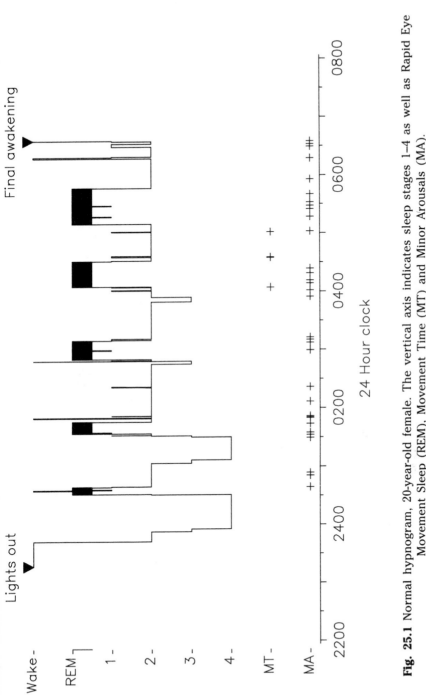

Fig. 25.1 Normal hypnogram, 20-year-old female. The vertical axis indicates sleep stages 1–4 as well as Rapid Eye Movement Sleep (REM), Movement Time (MT) and Minor Arousals (MA).

mood changes over night. Totterdell *et al* (1994) found that sleep was more strongly associated with subsequent rather than prior well-being.

Physical exercise may increase SWS, although possibly only in physically fit subjects, and the literature remains contradictory (Trinder *et al*, 1988). Extremes of ambient temperature result in a decrease in total sleep time, but transient deviations from a comfortable ambient temperature do not disturb sleep.

Humans lose much of their ability to thermoregulate during REM sleep (Glotzbach & Heller, 1994). Heat exposure also causes a reduction in REM sleep and SWS with an increase in wakefulness, while exposure to cold reduces REM and stage 2 sleep and increases wakefulness and sleep latency (Haskell *et al*, 1981).

Controversy exists as to the precise effects of noise on sleep. An individual's sensitivity to sound is influenced by the relevance of the sound, and by adaptation to it. For example a mother may be able to sleep through loud traffic noise, yet wake at the slightest cry of her baby. Varying types of surfaces on which people sleep appear to have little effect on sleep (Roehrs *et al*, 1994).

The effects that bed partners have on sleep has received little attention. Subjects whom habitually sleep alone have less movements than those who sleep regularly with a partner (Pankhurst & Horne, 1994). Movements are reduced when the bed partner is temporarily absent, although better sleep is reported when they are present.

Function of sleep

Despite the wealth of knowledge that has been acquired about sleep, its precise function is not known. The most acceptable theories of its function are that of restoration of both body and brain (Oswald, 1970; Zepelin, 1994). While sleep also conserves energy, it is unlikely that this is an important function in the human as the amount of energy saved by eight hours of uninterrupted sleep, compared to resting, would only be 120 calories (Zepelin, 1994).

Sleep fulfils a physiological need that builds up during the day for tissue repair and restoring other losses. It may be that this restoration is in part necessary for the immune response as sleep onset is associated with the secretion of interleukin 1 and interleukin 2. Additionally, as growth hormone is mainly released at night in association with SWS, such sleep may be necessary for adequate tissue growth.

The mental activity of dreams has been singled out as a restorative agent of the brain, fulfilling a psychological need that accumulates during wakefulness. There continues to be controversy surrounding their purpose, ranging from the theories of Freud, who interpreted dreams as disguised wish fulfilments, to Schatzman (1983), who viewed them as vehicles to solve waking problems. The most pragmatic, and least poetic perspective is that dreams are merely linguistic translations of waking concerns and already known solutions (Blagrove, 1992).

Circadian rhythm

Human body temperature displays a 24-hour rhythm which is roughly sinusoidal in shape, reaching its zenith at approximately 17.00 hours, and its nadir at 05.00 hours (Monk, 1991). The phase of this easily measurable rhythm is used as a marker for the phase of the human timekeeping system, the circadian clock (Latin, Circa=about, diem=a day).

Fatigue, which generally increases following sleep deprivation, displays a circadian rhythm more or less in phase with that of body temperature (Waterhouse, 1993). Lavie (1986) introduced the notion of 'sleep gates' when sleep onset is most likely to occur, primarily at night, but with a secondary mid-afternoon peak (determined by sleep latency tests). These are separated by a 'forbidden zone' for sleep centred at around 20.00 to 22.00 hours. This has led to the concept of 'sunday night insomnia' (Strogatz, 1986) which results from keeping later hours at weekends. This allows the circadian cycle and its forbidden zone to inadvertently advance to later hours and intrude on the regular weekday bedtime. It has also been hypothesised that a malfunction of the phasing of the circadian pacemaker in relation to the sleep-wake cycle underlies the insomnia associated with sleep-scheduling disorders (Strogatz *et al*, 1987).

Length of sleep is strongly influenced by the phase of the body temperature rhythm at which it is initiated, being shortest when body temperature is at its lowest and greatest when body temperature is at its highest (Czeisler *et al*, 1980).

REM sleep shows an underlying circadian rhythm with a peak at around 10.00 hours and a minimum at around 22.00 hours (Zulley, 1980), as evidenced by the increasing duration of REM episodes as the night progresses. By contrast, SWS does not display a circadian rhythm but is dependent on the duration of prior wakefulness (Webb & Agnew, 1971).

When temporally isolated from the light-dark cycle and all other time cues, both the body temperature rhythm and the sleep-wake cycle typically develop a length of approximately 25 hours (Wever, 1979), as shown in Fig. 25.2. They normally remain internally synchronised, with time of going to bed occurring on the falling limb of the body temperature curve. For a few individuals in such 'free running' experiments, the sleep-wake and body temperature rhythms spontaneously desynchronise after a period of several biological days. In such cases the sleep-wake cycle can lengthen to up to 35 hours, while the ratio of wakefulness to sleep remains around 2:1. In such instances body temperature rhythm remains stable at approximately 25 hours, and is therefore a more reliable marker for the body clock than the sleep-wake cycle.

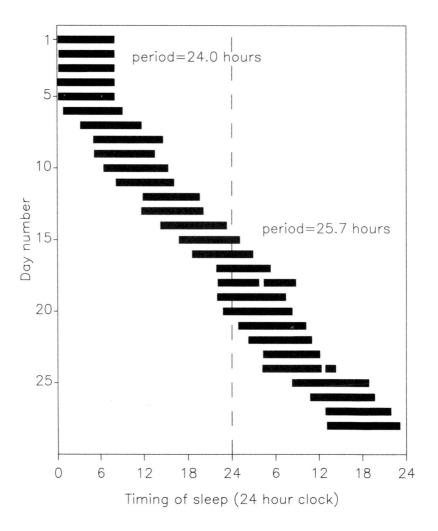

Fig. 25.2 24-hour entrained and free running sleep-wake cycles in a normal subject. The black bars represent episodes of sleep. The ordinate represents successive 24-hour days. The abscissa is "double-plotted" over 48 hours (top line, day 1 to day 2; next line day 2 to day 3; and so on) so as to allow the uninterrupted procession in the sleep-wake cycle. From day 1 through to 5, bedtimes and waking times were scheduled on a regular 24-hour cycle. Thereafter the subject was allowed to go to bed and arise at will. The sleep-wake cycle subsequently "free-runs" with a period of 25.7 hours.

When a regular 24 hour light-dark cycle, not necessarily coinciding with the natural light-dark cycle, is imposed upon internally synchronised individuals in 'free-running' experiments, it results in the sleep-wake cycle adjusting with sleep times coinciding with the hours of imposed darkness (Waterhouse, 1993). By entraining the sleep-wake cycle, the light-dark cycle is termed a zeitgeber (from the German: zeit=time, geber=to give). While light is undoubtedly the strongest zeitgeber in humans, in modern society time cues are also obtained from social influences, meal times and activity. The inherent instability of a 25 hour endogenous rhythm constantly being entrained by 24 hour zeitgebers probably facilitates adaptation to changes in seasons and time zones.

Laboratory measurement

The electrophysiological measurement of sleep is a complex and usually long process, described in detail by Carskadon & Rechtschaffen (1994). According to the standard criteria of Rechtschaffen & Kales (1968), in order to record adult human sleep electrophysiologically three basic systems need to be monitored. These are;
  (i)   the electroencephalogram (EEG),
  (ii) the electro-oculogram (EOG) which detects muscular movement of the eyes,
  (iii) the electromyogram (EMG), to record the activity of the mentalis/ submentalis muscles.
The recording of the central EEG is according to the international ten-twenty system of electrode placement (Jasper, 1958). Standard EOG electrode placements are half an inch from the right and left outer canthi. The EMG involves the placement of two electrodes under the chin, overlying the mentalis / submentalis muscles. A further electrode is placed on the forehead to act as an earth. Figures 25.3 and 25.4 show the facial electrodes in position.

After recording onto a suitable medium, the polysomnographic recording is staged. The recording is initially subdivided into units of real time termed 'epochs' of either 20 or 30 seconds. The stage of sleep within each epoch is then rated, this data being the basis for the hypnograph and descriptive statistics of the night's sleep.

The stages of sleep are distinguished by unique forms of electrical activity. Figures 25.5 – 25.12 illustrate how they manifest themselves in electro-physiological terms, with one epoch of 20 seconds shown in each case. When staging sleep it is the frequency, expressed in cycles per second (cps), and amplitude of the activity that is of greatest importance. Four EEG frequency bands are used, these being alpha (8–13 cps), beta (>14 cps), delta (<4 cps) and theta (4–7 cps).

The state of relaxed wakefulness with eyes closed is distinguished by the dominance of rhythmic alpha waves in the EEG and high muscle tone in

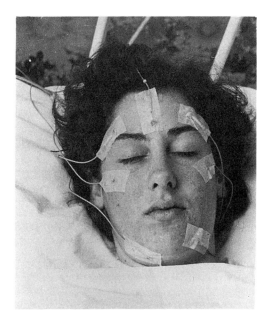

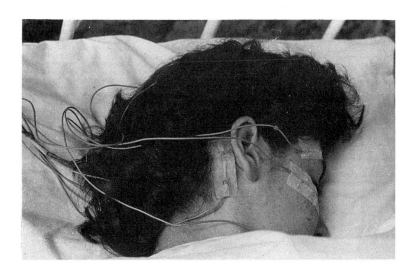

Figs 25.3 & 25.4 Positioning of electrodes for the EOG and EMG. Our thanks to the member of laboratory staff pictured.

the EMG. Large amplitude quick eye movements may also be seen in the EOG. NREM sleep is particularly distinguished by the EEG. Stage 1 is rather nondescript in that the EEG is of mixed frequency and has no real distinguishing features. At sleep onset, the EOG often takes on a slow, rolling appearance which is unique to this stage. The background activity of the EEG in stage 2 is relatively low-voltage mixed-frequency activity. However, it does have two notable features that occur sporadically, namely sleep spindles and k-complexes. The former are transient bursts of frequency 12–14 cps, while k-complexes consist of a well-delineated negative sharp wave followed by a positive component exceeding half a second.

SWS is characterised by the appearance of large amplitude delta waves in the EEG, which tend also to be seen in the EOG. When this slow wave activity comes to occupy between 20–50% of the epoch, it is classified as stage 3; above 50% it becomes stage 4. As the stages of sleep progress from stage 1 to stage 4 the EMG reduces in tone. However it is in stage REM that it is at its lowest. This, combined with phasic rapid eye movements in the EOG, are the cardinal signs of REM sleep.

Movement during sleep typically obscures and blocks the EEG and EOG while producing high activity in the EMG. When it lasts for more than 50% of the epoch, it is classified as movement time, and anything less as a minor arousal.

It is standard practice when monitoring sleep to undertake an adaptation night prior to polysomnographic recording, with the patient sleeping in the laboratory setting with electrodes applied in order to promote adaptation to the surroundings. Such stress and novel surroundings induces what is known as the 'first night effect' where the sleep architecture is disrupted. This results in a reduced amount of REM sleep due to a delayed onset and often the first REM sleep episode is missed (Agnew *et al*, 1966). In addition both sleep latency and the onset of stage 4 are delayed whilst wakefulness is increased. These effects rapidly disappear by the second night in the laboratory.

Recording of additional parameters may be necessary for the diagnosis of sleep disorders; these have been described by McGregor *et al* (1985) and McGregor (1989). To fully evaluate sleep apnoea, both respiratory effort and the actual movement of air to and from the lungs are recorded. Effort is monitored by strain gauges in elastic belts around the thorax and abdomen. Thermistors at the opening of the nostrils and over the mouth indicate the movement of air (cold in, warm out). The cessation of both respiratory effort and airflow is indicative of central apnoea, but the more common finding is that respiratory effort continues with no movement of air, signifying an episode of obstructive apnoea. Capillary blood oxygen saturation is monitored by a light absorption probe attached to either an ear lobe or finger.

Videotelemetry is advised in the assessment of those parasomnias in which motor activity and snoring is of interest. Further appropriately placed EMGs

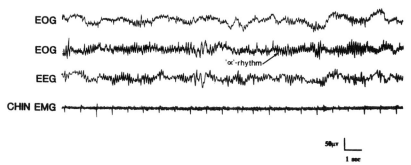

Fig. 25.5 Awake (eyes closed). See text for details.

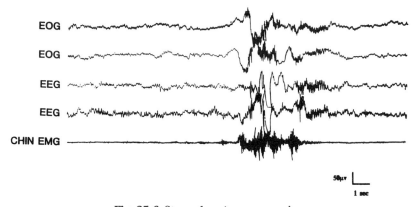

Fig 25.6 Stage 1, minor arousal.

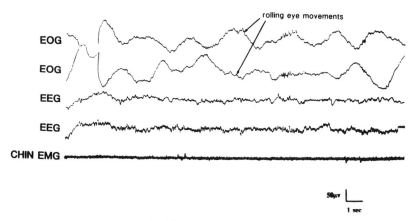

Fig 25.7 Stage 1 sleep.

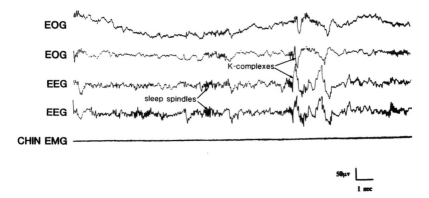

Fig. 25.8 Stage 2 sleep.

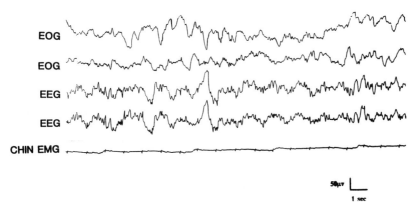

Fig. 25.9 Stage 3 (20–50% slow waves).

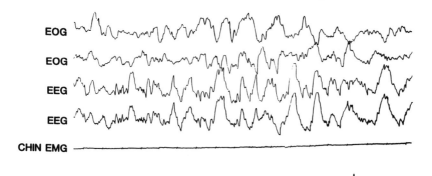

Fig. 25.10 Stage 4 (over 50% slow waves).

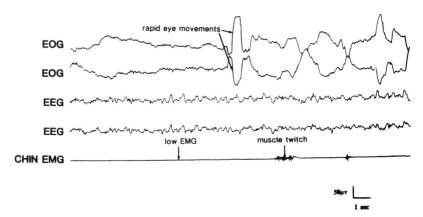

Fig. 25.11 Stage REM sleep.

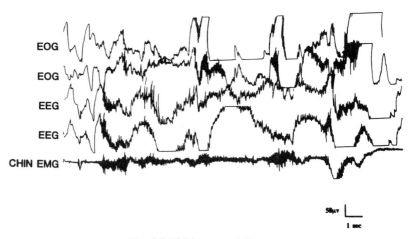

Fig. 25.12 Movement time.

may be used in order to assess periodic limb movement disorder or the restless legs syndrome (Montpaisir *et al*, 1994). Mercury strain gauges are used to monitor nocturnal penile tumescence in the assessment of either impaired or painful sleep-related penile erections (Catesby *et al*, 1994).

The original technology recorded directly onto paper, the polysomnographic recording being approximately two-thirds of a kilometre in length, which would then be staged manually. The recording can now be made straight onto magnetic media, with considerable improvement in reliability. It can still be staged manually but automatic sleep staging systems are available, although there is some lack of confidence in them, as discussed by Hirshkowitz & Moore (1994).

The last 15 years have seen the emergence of ambulatory monitoring systems for standard polysomnography, as well as for recording electrocardiograms (ECG), respiratory activity, oxygen saturation, body temperature, body position and movement. Ambulatory monitoring is either analogue or digital in its mode of data acquisition; various systems are discussed by Broughton (1994). Digital systems are not capable of recording the high frequency EEG and EMG of the polysomnograph whilst analogue systems are restricted by only being able to record eight channels. The major disadvantages of such systems are that they are not able to describe patient behaviour, and technical faults or failures can not be remedied at the time as they could be in the sleep laboratory. Despite these drawbacks they have become increasingly popular due to their cost effectiveness, the ability to record with little inconvenience to the patient, and the absence of any 'first night effect' (Sharpley *et al*, 1988).

Clinical assessment

The assessment interview should whenever possible include an interview with the patient and their bed partner and the appointment letter should explicitly invite the bed partner or most relevant informant. The information from the bed partner is particularly important in obtaining a sleep history, as the patient will be unable to report first hand what has occurred while they were asleep. Also, the change from a sleep behaviour into a sleep disorder may sometimes represent a shift in the relationship with the bed partner. Sleep disorders commonly place a greater burden on the bed partner than the patient, and certain aspects of management are best directed to the partner or to the couple.

The interview with the patient should cover a full psychiatric history. It is helpful to build up a picture of the patient's rhythms and routines. their personality structure and beliefs, and the various genetic and environmental threads that have contributed towards these. Specific sleep symptoms should also be elicited and the following information actively sought:

(1) Sleep pattern at the present time, including time of going to bed, time of going to sleep, times and durations of awakenings in the night, time of final awakening, and time of arising.

(2) A full 24 hour activity/behaviour chart, including times of meals, periods of rest, naps, intake of stimulants (including caffeine) and depressants (including alcohol).

(3) Specific details of the sleep complaint: what happens, when does it happen, what is the patient subjectively aware of, and what is reported by others, its significance to the patient and to others, and any associated fears.

(4) Sleep pattern throughout life, the sleep pattern of the bed partner, and any familial sleep problems or characteristics

The purpose of the interview is not only to attempt to delineate the sleep abnormality itself, but also to place it in a meaningful context in terms of the patient's life history.

While many sleep disorders can be diagnosed from the history, further investigations play an important role. They may be subdivided into:

(1)   General 'routine' tests, to screen for organic disorders and physical attributes that disrupt sleep. These should include measurement of height and weight, full blood count and erythrocyte sedimentation rate (ESR), urea and electrolytes, liver and thyroid function tests, and random blood glucose.

(2)   Tests to detect and provide further information about the nature of the sleep problem, including the use of a sleep diary, polysomnography at home, and overnight sleep laboratory polysomnographic investigations.

(3)   Psychometric questionnaires, such as the Eysenck Personality Questionnaire (Eysenck & Eysenck, 1975), Crown–Crisp Experiential Index (Crown & Crisp, 1979), and the Direction of Hostility Questionnaire (Caine *et al*, 1967), which help build up a psychological profile and expose possible aetiological factors.

Once the results of the investigations are available the patient and bed partner (or other informant) should be seen together again. The working hypotheses formulated at the assessment may then be adjusted as required in the light of these results, and a management plan agreed.

Sleep disorders

Most of the sleep disorders described in the section below are also included in the DSM–IV and ICD–10 schemes, but not all are included in both systems. Some of these disorders have different names in each scheme, and this is indicated in parenthesis following the titles of each disorder.

Insomnia (Non organic insomnia, ICD–10; Primary insomnia DSM–IV)

Insomnia is a symptom, not a disease, and is very common, with a one year prevalence rate of between 20 and 40% of adults, about 17% of whom consider the problem serious (Gillin & Byerley, 1990). A third of patients attending their GPs, and two-thirds of psychiatric patients complain of inadequately restorative sleep. As a symptom, it is commonly secondary to other sleep disorders. It may also be due to psychiatric or medical conditions, drug effects, life events and disruptions in life's rhythms, which are all described later in this chapter. Less commonly (15% of cases of insomnia investigated in sleep laboratories) the insomnia is primary. ICD–

10 non organic insominia is defined as "A condition of unsatisfactory quantity and/or quality of sleep, which persists for a considerable period of time" (ICD–10, 1992). DSM–IV primary insomnia diagnostic criteria are shown in Box 25.1.

Aetiology

Predisposing factors – Patterns of sleep are established in infancy, and are to some extent genetically determined, and are firmly established by the late teens. Factors that influence the underlying vulnerability to insomnia include age and sex, with an increase in prevalence with age and in women. The young tend to complain more of difficulty in initiating sleep, while the old complain more of difficulty in maintaining sleep, with frequent awakenings and early morning wakening.

Psychologically, subjects with insomnia tend to rely heavily on the defences of repression and denial, and also tend to score highly on questionnaires that rate hostility. As anger induces arousal, it is incompatible with sleep. If, due to repression and denial, this anger is not fully conscious, the individual may not be sufficiently aware of this mechanism to be able to attempt to defuse it.

Precipitating factors – A wide range of psychological, social or medical stressors can trigger the onset of insomnia, which in most cases is sudden. In primary insomnia the perpetuating factors are then unrelated to the precipitant.

Perpetuating factors – Disrupted sleep may be maintained by several different mechanisms. One of the commonest is a variant on performance anxiety, when after a night of poor sleep, there is a foreboding of a repeat experience and this anxiety then keeps the person awake once more. This

---

Box 25.1 Primary insomnia (DSM–IV)

The predominant complaint is difficulty initiating or maintaining sleep, or non-restorative sleep, for at least one month.

The sleep disturbance (or associated daytime fatigue) causes clinically significant distress or impairment in social, occupational, or other important areas of functioning.

The sleep disturbance does not occur exclusively during the course of narcolepsy, breathing related sleep disorder, circadian rhythm sleep disorder, or a parasomnia.

The disturbance does not occur exclusively during the course of another mental disorder (e.g. major depressive disorder, generalised anxiety disorder, a delirium).

The disturbance is not due to the direct physiological effects of a substance (e.g. a drug of abuse, a medication) or a general medical condition (DSM–IV, 1994).

Adapted with permission from DSM–IV. Copyright 1994 American Psychiatric Association.

results in an entrenched negative conditioning cycle, with negative associations for sleep and bed. This may cause high arousal in bed, with hostility and anger levels incompatible with sleep.

Negative beliefs such as that the insomnia might result in irreversible physical and mental damage may also heighten the anxiety.

Sleep laboratory investigation

Polysomnography may reveal poor sleep continuity, with increased sleep latency, increased intermittent wakefulness, and decreased sleep efficiency. Typically stage 1 sleep is increased, and stage 3 and 4 sleep are decreased. There may be increased muscle tension, or increased EEG alpha activity. A hypnogram of a man with onset insomnia and early morning wakening is shown in Fig. 25.13. Commonly individuals sleep for longer in total than they realise. In addition, some may sleep better in the sleep laboratory than at home (controls show the opposite pattern), suggesting elements of situation specific conditioning as an active aetiological factor.

Management

Treatment interventions will need to be sensitively matched to the individual and the response to treatment should be carefully monitored, using a sleep diary, and the treatment readjusted accordingly to ensure an optimal management strategy.

Acute insomnias are usually related to identifiable precipitating causes, such as a recent major life event, and counselling or brief psychotherapy may be helpful as well as giving advice about sleep hygiene (see below). Hypnotics may have a limited role in the short-term, although they should be used with caution. This is because they may interfere with the psychological processes involved in a satisfactory resolution of, for example, bereavement and this applies particularly to drugs with a long duration of action. Hypnotics that induce pronounced rebound insomnia should be avoided as the iatrogenic insomnia that follows their withdrawal may be more severe than the presenting insomnia and so result in chronic dependence.

In chronic insomnia the precipitating aetiological factor is rarely of continuing relevance, and may have been long forgotten. In such cases it is important to use interventions that are sustainable and do no further harm. Therefore hypnotic drugs, with their propensity to induce tolerance, dependence, and rebound withdrawal effects, have a limited role. They may be used when other treatments have failed and the individual's daytime functioning is sufficiently severely impaired to outweigh the risks of long-term hypnotic treatment. The development of tolerance may be reduced if the hypnotic is used on no more than two nights of the week. In certain cases, prescribing a hypnotic for a one night only may be helpful in breaking the cycle of insomnia as part of a multidimensional strategy.

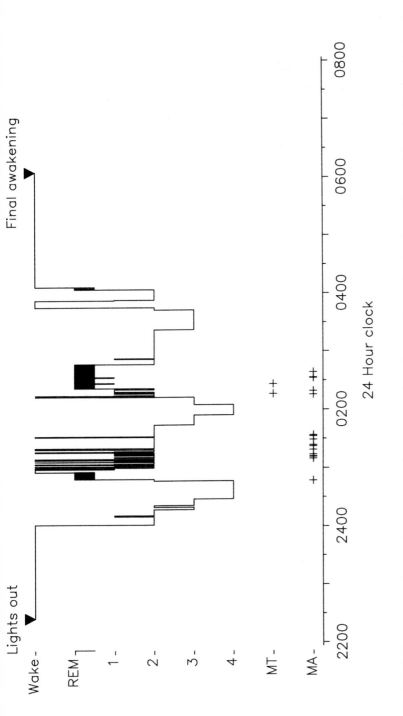

Fig 25.13 Hypnogram demonstrating onset insomnia and early morning wakening in a 49-year-old male. The vertical axis indicates sleep stages 1–4 as well as rapid eye movement sleep (REM), movement time (MT) and minor arousals (MA).

The mainstay of treatment for chronic insomnia is education about sleep, addressing any unfounded beliefs or expectations, and encouraging the use of behaviourial techniques aimed at improving either total sleep time or sleep efficiency (the proportion of time asleep compared with time spent in bed).

Many individuals believe that their physical health will be seriously and irreversibly damaged if they do not have eight hours sleep a night, and this may fuel the performance anxiety that then increases their insomnia. They should be advised sleep is a natural process that finds its own equilibrium, and that the need for sleep diminishes with age.

Sleep hygiene advice includes avoiding excessively long periods of time in bed, adopting a regular time of rising in the morning, avoiding daytime naps, engaging in moderate regular physical exercise, avoiding extremes of temperature in the bedroom, eating regular meals of sufficient quantity to avoid feeling hungry in the night, but avoiding snacks at bedtime. Caffeine should be avoided in the evening, as should excessive alcohol or tobacco use. A small hot milky and caffeine-free drink at bedtime may be helpful. If unable to fall asleep it may be preferable to get up and engage in a restful activity and only return to bed when sleepiness ensues, rather than continuing to lie awake in bed.

Most of the distress associated with insomnia relates to the duration of time spent each night trying to sleep, or by individuals wishing that they were asleep, rather than to the effects of sleep deprivation. Behavioural techniques therefore generally involve restricting the time spent in bed awake, and the avoidance of cues in the bedroom that exacerbate anxiety and anger (Sloan *et al*, 1993). Individuals should identify a consistent time when they want to wake up, and set their alarm for this time every day. The clock should be hidden from view and possibly lightly covered so the tick cannot be heard. Bed time should be set at this wake-up time minus the reported average subjective sleep duration but with a minimum of four hours. The bed should only be used for sleep or sex, and any other activities should be carried out in another room. If the proportion of time spent in bed and asleep rises above 90% for a week, then bedtime can be brought forward by 15 minutes, but if this proportion is less than 80%, then bedtime should be delayed by a further 15 minutes. This process should be continued until the patient has established a stable sleep pattern with a sleep efficiency of 80–90% (Spielman *et al*, 1987). Occasional follow-up sessions may help to sustain the improvement.

Problem solving techniques used prior to bed time, and relaxation techniques once in bed may also be helpful. These methods can be taught as part of an anxiety management course, and may block the intrusion of anxiety provoking ideas into the patient's mind as these prevent sleep.

Cognitive therapy may also help. The individual's specific dysfunctional sleep cognitions are identified and monitored. Education and experiment-ation are then used to explore their validity. The aims are to challenge a uni-dimensional explanation for the insomnia, and to open up new avenues for influencing it. The believed consequences of insomnia can be questioned and decatastrophised, and any unrealistic expectations concerning sleep may be challenged, and performance anxiety, issues of control and learned helplessness and other dysfunctional cognitions may be explored.

The educational, behavioural and cognitive strategies outlined above may be combined in a structured time-limited (typically eight sessions) group treatment. This can have a reinforcing effect particularly for individuals who engage well in the group process (Kupych-Woloshyn *et al*, 1993).

Hypersomnia

This term is commonly applied to both excessive sleep duration (primary hypersomnia), and to excessive daytime sleepiness. Daytime sleepiness is also a symptom of other sleep-related syndromes that compromise nocturnal sleep but in these cases the term hypersomnia is probably a misnomer. Idiopathic hypersomnia is comparatively rare and is diagnosed only after exclusion of the more common sleep problems associated with excessive daytime sleepiness described below.

Narcolepsy (ICD–10 & DSM–IV)

This syndrome was first described by Gelineau, and is sometimes known as Gelineau's syndrome. It is neither psychogenic, nor a form of epilepsy, but a distinct disorder. The cardinal characteristic is irresistible episodes of sleep at inappropriate times, even when the individual is engaged in an absorbing task. It may be accompanied by three important additional symptoms:

a) *Cataplexy* – sudden attacks of muscular weakness. This may involve a portion of the body and pass unnoticed by anyone except the patient. Rarely , they are extreme and result in complete physical collapse of the patient who still remains fully conscious. The attacks may be provoked by emotional stimuli that produce an urge to laugh, cry or feel angry. The event may last from a few seconds to many minutes.

b) *Sleep paralysis* – the experience of being suddenly unable to move, either at the point of waking, or of falling asleep. This may also last a few seconds or minutes. It resolves spontaneously but is usually very frightening while it lasts. Sleep paralysis can occur in the absence of narcolepsy, but is more common in this condition.

c) *Hypnagogic and hypnopompic hallucinations* – these are usually visual images, but can be auditory or tactile sensations that accompany sleep onset or waking whether it is at night or during the day. Hypnagogic (at sleep onset) or hypnopompic (at the point of waking) hallucinations are not exclusive to narcoleptics and their clinical significance must be assessed in the context of their frequency, severity, and presence or absence of other symptoms. In patients presenting with a prominent history of such hallucinations, especially if auditory, there is a risk of mistakenly diagnosing schizophrenia.

Sudden daytime sleeps of a refreshing nature, cataplexy, sleep paralysis and hypnagogic hallucinations form a tetrad of symptoms, that are identified with narcolepsy. Opinion is divided as to the number and configuration of the symptoms which are necessary to diagnose narcolepsy.

Additional symptoms of narcolepsy include the following; automatic behaviour, with episodes of amnesia associated with semi-purposeful activity, often monotonous or repetitive; disrupted nocturnal sleep, with frequent awakenings, increased body movements and apnoeic episodes; memory impairment related to reduced concentration, and blurred vision.

Narcolepsy appears to affect 1:10 000 in the population, with an equal sex distribution. Susceptibility is probably genetically determined as cases cluster in families, and 98–100% of cases are linked to the HLA-DR2 and HLA-DQw1 antigens. The mode of inheritance is probably dominant with variable penetrance, which would account for cases of discordance in monozygotic twins. The site of the gene responsible may be close to the HLA-DQ and HLA-DR subregions on the short arm of chromosome six (Aldrich, 1990).

The first symptoms, generally sudden daytime sleeps, typically appear between the ages of 15 and 35. They become more pronounced and may be accompanied by others in the tetrad with advancing years. The frequency of attacks varies from just a few episodes in a life-time, to several attacks each day. They may be exacerbated by environmental factors such as heat or heavy meals.

Narcolepsy often leads to considerable psychosocial problems. The individual may be regarded as slothful or at times drunk. Memory, concentration and performance socially and at work may be seriously impaired. Activities such as driving or operating machinery become hazardous, as 60–80% of subjects with narcolepsy fall asleep when driving or at work, or both.

The differential diagnoses include the other hypersomnias discussed in this chapter, as well as schizophrenia as described above. Other causes of daytime sleepiness should be excluded, most commonly drug treatment or alcohol and drug misuse, psychiatric disorders such as atypical depression, and medical conditions such as anaemia or carcinoma.

Clinical evaluation – The hallmark of narcolepsy is that the individual falls directly into REM sleep from wakefulness. This applies particularly to daytime sleeps, but the REM sleep latency of nocturnal sleep is typically also very short (Benca *et al*, 1992). A sleep laboratory investigation that focuses on both nocturnal and daytime sleep is essential for diagnosis. Daytime REM latency is tested by the Multiple Sleep Latency Test. The patient is instructed to try to sleep at two hour intervals throughout the day, while monitored with a polysomnograph. More than 80% of subjects with narcolepsy have a mean sleep latency of less than five minutes, and at least two episodes of sleep onset REM. This sleep onset REM does not occur in normal adult sleep, except when REM sleep is severely disrupted and curtailed, for example by sleep apnoeas, endogenous depression, disturbances of the sleep-wake cycle, drug and alcohol withdrawal, and some structural brain lesions. Nocturnal respiration and oxygen saturation should be examined in cases of suspected narcolepsy to exclude obstructive sleep apnoea.

Management – Narcolepsy cannot be cured, but the symptoms and their social impact may be reduced. For milder cases a behavioural approach advising the patient to take regular naps at times when there is no need to be alert may be helpful. It is also possible to capitalise on the refractory period of alertness that follows the sleep of the narcoleptic to accomplish tasks during which a sleep attack might be dangerous, such as cooking, ironing or short drives. Patients with narcolepsy who are symptomatic are not permitted to drive and other patients with sleep disorders should inform the driving authorities (Parkes, 1995).

Pharmacological interventions include central nervous system stimulants such as dexamphetamine 5–50mg, or methylphenidate 10–60mg, to reduce daytime sleepiness. Pemoline, a rather more slow acting stimulant, or protriptyline, the most stimulating tricyclic, are sometimes helpful in patients who are resistant to or intolerant of other stimulants. Tricyclic antidepressants increase muscle tone, and can help to control cataplexy and sleep paralysis. Less sedative, or alerting tricyclic antidepressants such as protriptyline and imipramine are usually effective. Specific serotonin re-uptake inhibitor antidepressants can be helpful if tricyclics have caused troublesome side-effects. Short to medium-term acting benzodiazepines may be useful if nocturnal sleep disturbance is a prominent symptom, but should be used no more than two nights a week, to avoid the development of tolerance. Severe narcolepsy with the full tetrad of symptoms may require a combination of approaches.

The socially disabling aspects of narcolepsy can be minimised by explaining the syndrome to the patient's family and to teachers or others where appropriate. In some instances, sufferers should be advised against driving or operating machinery. Contact with support groups may mitigate the psychological impact of the disorder.

Obstructive sleep apnoea (ICD–10 & DSM–IV)

This is a respiratory problem that manifests itself during sleep. It frequently presents with excessive daytime sleepiness as the dominant symptom. The upper airway in the region of the pharynx loses patency during sleep and partially or totally obstructs breathing despite frantic respiratory efforts. Oxygen desaturation and the concomitant rise in blood CO_2 induces sufficient arousal to restore airway patency and hence respiration, before the cycle repeats.

There may be a variety of reasons for the failure of airway patency, which will have evolved over a long period. However, the final precipitant is the reduction in muscle tone that accompanies sleep which, in vulnerable individuals, causes the increase in upper airway resistance, leading to apnoea or hypopnoea.

Sleep apnoea can occur at any age, and may be implicated in sudden infant death syndrome. It is rare in adolescents and young adults, but its prevalence increases with age. It affects 1–5% of the adult working population, men more than women. In addition, 28% of the over 65s may have in excess of 30 apnoeas a night, but without severe additional symptoms. This high prevalence in the elderly may contribute towards complaints of insomnia, daytime tiredness and napping, nocturnal confusion, and possibly depression.

Clinical features – Classically, patients complain of feeling overwhelmingly tired during the day with a commensurate propensity to fall asleep, particularly under sedentary circumstances. This sleepiness may be accompanied by brief lapses of consciousness, or 'microsleeps' that result in confusion, poor concentration, impaired memory and judgement. Some patients complain of insomnia and disturbed sleep, but generally feel they sleep soundly at night, although in the morning they wake up feeling unrefreshed and lethargic, sometimes with a headache. Some patients wake up with a choking sensation and complain that their tongue is in the back of their throat. Others complain of nocturnal hypersomnia, sleeping 12 or 14 hours each night. A few report parasomnia type symptoms, such as automatic behaviour while asleep, or apparent sleepwalking. Such episodes can be differentiated from partial complex temporal lobe seizures by the absence of abnormal or stereotypic movements. Enuresis can occur, usually during the longer apnoeas when brain anoxia is severe, and some patients report nocturia, oesophageal reflux, heavy sweating and confusion at night.

Partners and others will complain of excessively loud snoring that every so often ceases abruptly. Silences may last up to three minutes in extreme cases and terminate with loud snorts and snores as airway resistance yields. Sometimes this involves an abrupt movement to a semi-sitting position and then relaxation as respiration is restored. Irritability, aggression, anxiety and depression may also be noticed by those close to the patient. Commonly, but not inevitably, patients will be overweight, if not definitively obese, with short, thick necks.

Complications – Unchecked obstructive sleep apnoea has serious implications for physical health, and for the cardiovascular system in particular. During apnoeic episodes, blood oxygen saturation may fall to less than 40%, and both pulmonary and systemic hypertension occur. During these attacks, premature ventricular complexes and bradycardias are frequent, and occasionally severe arrhythmias such as asystole may occur, and may result in fatality. Although uncommon, chronic heart failure and more sustained hypertension may also develop.

The risk of accidents is high. Social, psychological and economic consequences may also be profound. Relationships can be strained by the primary symptoms as well as their psychosocial sequelae. Normal social interactions may become restricted or impossible as a result of daytime sleepiness and fatigue, and night-time noise due to loud snoring and snorting. Performance at work is likely to suffer to an extent that can lead to dismissal, especially in occupations that require sustained vigilance.

Diagnosis – Patients in whom obstructive sleep apnoea is suspected need to be investigated during sleep. Ideally they should have a full sleep recording with concurrent monitoring of airflow, respiration, oxygen saturation and the electrocardiogram (ECG) in a sleep laboratory, or with ambulatory equipment in the patient's home. The hypnograph in sleep apnoea is characterised by as many as hundreds of brief full or partial arousals despite the subjective impression of sound sleep (see Fig. 25.14). In severe cases the whole night is affected and some stages of sleep obliterated altogether. In other cases only certain sleep stages, or particular portions of the night are affected. REM sleep is especially vulnerable, because respiration is naturally shallower at this time and muscle tone lower. The fragments of sleep are associated with either a complete cessation or a diminution of airflow. The diaphragm struggles to effect inspiration, while oxygen saturation falls.

Management – Once diagnosis is confirmed the patient should be examined by an ENT surgeon to exclude an abnormality of the upper airway, which might respond to surgery. Such abnormalities include deviated nasal septum, large uvula, large tonsils and adenoids, narrow palatal pillars, long soft palate, micrognathia, and abnormal position of the mandible or hyoid bones. In severe cases, and in the absence of reversible anatomical abnormalities, mechanical support of the airway during sleep by continuous positive air pressure (CPAP) can provide immediate relief. The patient sleeps with a mask or nasal cannulae attached to a machine that generates a stream of air at an individually titrated pressure. This splints the airway open and enables the patient to breathe. It is usually well tolerated and the relief from daytime symptoms is generally worth the inconvenience of sleeping with such a device.

When sleep apnoea is combined with obesity, weight loss eases and can cure the problem. Weight reduction can be tackled in conjunction with CPAP therapy and may be more successful because the patient is able to concentrate more consistently.

Smoking, alcohol and central nervous system depressants, such as benzodiazepines, all exacerbate the symptoms of obstructive sleep apnoea and should be avoided. Treatment with androgens has been implicated as an aetiological factor in some cases. Apnoea patients on long-term diuretic therapy can be particularly vulnerable to alkalosis.

If the daytime sleepiness cannot be controlled, basic safety advice about avoiding driving or operating machinery must be given.

Primary hypersomnia (DSM–IV) or nonorganic hypersomnia (ICD–10)

Also known as central nervous system hypersomnia, this amounts to persistent daytime sleepiness and the intrusion of sleep into normal waking hours, in conjunction with at least a normal amount of nocturnal sleep.

Clinical features – These include undisturbed nocturnal sleep and daytime drowsiness that may lead to prolonged naps, none of which are refreshing. Patients are often difficult to wake and may respond abusively while in a semi-awakened state when aroused, with subsequent amnesia for their behaviour. Awakenings may be accompanied by 'sleep drunkenness', mental confusion, disorientation and uncoordinated motor-activity, behaviour which is reminiscent of alcohol-induced drunkenness. 'Automatic behaviour' i.e. speech or activity with no purposeful, cognitive input may also occur, again with amnesia for the event. Symptoms typically start in late adolescence and young adulthood. The condition establishes itself quickly and intractably, sometimes over just a few weeks. Once established it is debilitating, incurable and unremitting. There may be a family history of such symptoms, and some evidence of a genetic propensity for the condition exists. It may arise following viral infection, or spontaneously.

Diagnosis – Accurate diagnosis can be made only with polysomnographic evaluation, preferably in a sleep laboratory. Ideally two consecutive nights and sleep in the intervening day should be investigated. There must be a minimum of seven hours nocturnal sleep and demonstrable sleep during the day that bears no resemblance to the sleep of narcolepsy or obstructive sleep apnoea. Medical causes of excessive sleep such as head injuries and hydrocephalus need to be excluded.

Management – Recognition and acceptance of the problem; explanation that its underlying causes are not understood and support are perhaps the main components to management. It is sensible to advise plenty of sleep at night and avoidance of aggravating factors such as alcohol, sleep loss and heavy meals. Daytime napping is often not helpful, but a nap at a convenient time might be incorporated into daily routine. Stimulants have a limited effect that is usually outweighed by undesirable side-effects and the development of tolerance.

The Kleine–Levin syndrome (ICD–10)

This is a rare disorder, and in contrast to the other hypersomnias, is intermittent. It is more common in young males. The symptoms are of recurrent episodes of severe hypersomnia, with the individual spending up to 18–20 hours a day in bed, combined with compulsive overeating, hypersexuality and polydipsia. Episodes may begin gradually or abruptly, usually last for a few days, but may be as long as a month. They may recur regularly or spasmodically, on average twice a year. After an attack there

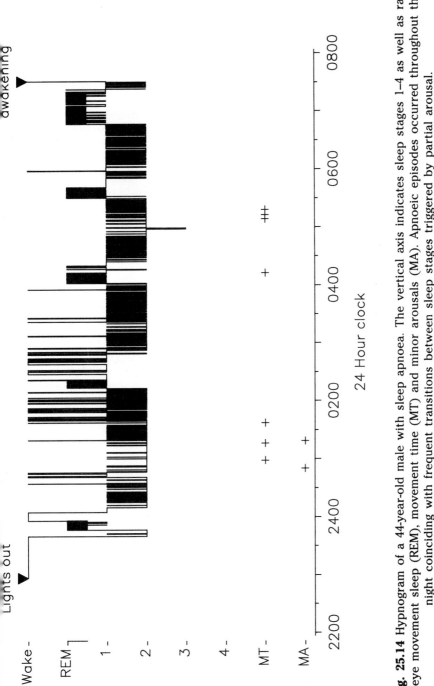

Fig. 25.14 Hypnogram of a 44-year-old male with sleep apnoea. The vertical axis indicates sleep stages 1–4 as well as rapid eye movement sleep (REM), movement time (MT) and minor arousals (MA). Apnoeic episodes occurred throughout the night coinciding with frequent transitions between sleep stages triggered by partial arousal.

may be a brief period of sleeplessness, with either elation or depression. Recurrences dissipate with time and eventually cease.

Aetiology is unknown, but is assumed to be organic, and may involve the hypothalamus. In contrast to the other hypersomnias it appears to be non-familial. The initial episode can follow minor infections or injury. The differential diagnosis includes atypical depression, and post-traumatic hypersomnia (a complication of head injury).

As the symptoms of the disorder are infrequent and resolve with time, active intervention may not be required. If it is, stimulants can be used to combat the somnolence and lithium therapy may modify the behavioural symptoms.

Menstrual hypersomnia

A disorder characterised by marked hypersomnia occurring episodically in phase with the menstrual cycle generally during the luteal phase, and which may respond to oestrogen therapy.

Parasomnias

These are a group of acute episodic partial arousal phenomena that occur in relation to sleep.

Sleep walking or somnambulism (ICD–10 and DSM–IV)

This is characterised by complex motor activity erupting abruptly from stage 4 SWS, usually early in the night. It is common in children, affecting about 15%, but tends not to be a major problem in the contained world of childhood. In about 2% of the population it persists into or begins in adulthood, and becomes a significant disorder.

Clinical features – The individual rises suddenly from complete quiescence, may leave the bed, and is able to perform complex tasks, and to talk. The eyes may be open, but the sufferer is in a state of detachment and may be unaware of, or misconstrue their surroundings, and either comes to "reality" during the episode, or may return to bed without reaching full wakefulness, and may remain unaware that the event took place.

Individuals commonly return to sleep quickly once the activity ceases, although on occasion they may become upset following an event. Mental ideation is not usually recalled, but if it is, it tends to be ephemeral and indefinable, more of a sensation than a narratable event.

Complications – In many cultures sleepwalking is equated with madness or demonic possession, and is the source of much anxiety for the sufferers, their bed partner and family. This anxiety may be heightened by the occasional cases of assault, and rarely murder, committed by such individuals.

The most common physical complication is accidental self-injury. This ranges from bruised shins from walking into the end of the bed, through lacerated arms from thrusting a limb through a closed window, to death from falling off a balcony. In winter there is a risk of walking out of the home in night attire and consequent hypothermia.

Aetiological factors – Sleepwalking runs in families, with a much higher concordance rate in monozygotic than dizygotic twins, suggesting an inherited aetiological factor. In predisposed individuals sleepwalking may be triggered by psychological stresses, lipid soluble beta-blockers, certain tricyclic antidepressants, and some benzodiazepines.

Diagnosis – With a clear history from the bed partner, it may be possible to reach a diagnosis from the clinical presentation alone. The diagnosis can be confirmed by polysomnography, particularly if an attack occurs during investigation, when the sleepwalking episode will be seen to arise directly from stage 4 sleep. If a sleepwalking episode is not captured in the sleep laboratory, the underlying susceptibility is often marked by a number of direct shifts from stage 4 sleep to brief wakefulness. A typical hypnogram of a male sufferer is shown in Fig. 25.15.

The differential diagnoses include nocturnal epilepsy, REM sleep behaviour disorder, obstructive sleep apnoea, and the effects of alcohol and other confusional states.

Management – Sleepwalking is unlikely to be cured, but the frequency and severity of its complications may be reduced. The risk of self-injury can be reduced by removing hazardous articles from the bedroom, where possible sleeping on the ground floor, and locating sources of light away from windows or other dangerous areas as many individuals seem drawn towards light during an event. Sleepwalkers who walk outside the home should be advised to wear pyjamas, which have a front door key sewn into the hem, should they lock themselves out. A variety of other manoeuvres tailored to the needs of the individual may also prove helpful.

In cases where there have been episodes of violence towards the bed partner during sleepwalking episodes, the partner should be advised to sleep in a separate locked room, or to keep a loud personal alarm within easy reach.

There is little basis to the popular belief that it is harmful to awaken someone who is sleepwalking, although it is usually simpler to gently guide the individual back to bed. Stress may influence the frequency of sleepwalking, and attempts should be made to modify any stresses identified at assessment. Other approaches include psychotherapy, hypnosis, and anxiety management techniques. Couple counselling may help if there are relationship problems.

Drug treatment is problematic. In individual cases benzodiazepines or SSRI antidepressants may be helpful, but in others they may make matters worse, and are not generally recommended.

Occasionally the history reveals a clear temporal association with alcohol intake, which should then be avoided, or moderated. Individuals should avoid becoming sleep deprived because this leads to an increase in both stage four sleep and sleepwalking.

Night terrors (ICD–10 and DSM–IV): Pavor nocturnus in children, Incubus in adults

These are similar to, and may occur together with sleepwalking. They are common in childhood, affecting about 30% of children at least once, but are much rarer in adults. Typically they arise in the first third of the night, erupting out of SWS, causing the individual to start suddenly with an expression of mortal terror, screaming or calling out loudly. The individual cannot be consoled, is temporarily unrousable, and will have signs of autonomic discharge including tachycardia, hypertension, sweating and pilo-erection. The parent or bed partner may be construed as a malevolent stranger about to attack, and the patient may act correspondingly defensively and aggressively. Each episode lasts from one to ten minutes, after which the individual often lapses back directly into normal sleep, leaving the parent or bed partner feeling traumatised and unable to sleep. The debilitating effect that this can have on the relationship between the sufferer and the bed partner is often the most serious complication. The disorder may also restrict the individual's lifestyle because attempts are made to avoid the social embarrassment of screaming at night while sleeping away from home. As with sleepwalking, there is usually complete amnesia for the event, or the patient may recall a fear, such as a sudden knowledge that the walls are about to close in on them. The aetiology, polysomnographic findings, and management are otherwise similar to sleepwalking, and the two conditions are frequently combined. The differential diagnoses are also similar, but in addition include nightmares, and nocturnal panic attacks.

Nightmares or dream anxiety attacks (ICD–10 & DSM–IV)

These are frightening dreams, technically different from night terrors, in that they emerge from REM sleep, which is associated with dreaming. There is usually a strong, readily recalled story content, from which the individual wakens fully in an anxious and highly aroused state. Nightmares tend to happen later in the night than night terrors (as does the REM sleep from which they arise), and the patient will always be aware of them. Sleep is then often difficult, or impossible, to resume. Nightmares, like night terrors, may be a response to stress and are particularly marked in some cases of post traumatic stress disorder. They can also be induced by various medications, such as lipid soluble beta blockers, other antihypertensive drugs and some anti-parkinsonian preparations. The withdrawal of drugs that suppress REM sleep such as benzodiazepines, monoamine oxidase

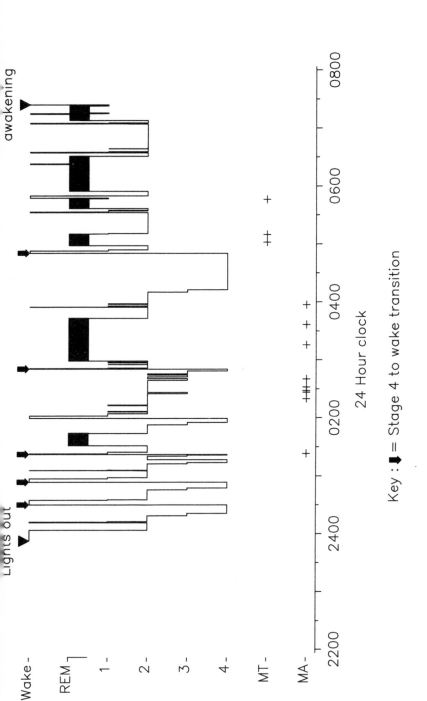

Fig 25.15 Hypnogram of a 27-year-old male with night terrors and sleepwalking. The vertical axis indicates sleep stages 1–4 as well as rapid eye movement sleep (REM), movement time (MT) and minor arousals (MA). Symptoms of night terrors occurred at the transitions from stage 4 sleep to wakefulness.

inhibitors and alcohol is associated with REM sleep rebound, and this may precipitate vivid dreams and nightmares.

Management – Psychotherapy may be helpful if the nightmare is thought to be of psychological origin. A behavioural technique to resolve a repetitive and unchanging nightmare is to consciously and frequently rehearse a benign outcome to the story (Blanes *et al*, 1993). Medication and drug use should be reviewed where these are implicated as precipitants.

REM sleep behaviour disorder

This arises in elderly patients, most often male. They lose the normal muscle atonia of REM sleep, and physically act out their dreams. Polysomnographic evaluation reveals sustained muscle tone during REM sleep, whilst video recordings show an unusual amount of movement during this stage of sleep. The condition can be controlled with clonazepam.

Nocturnal paroxysmal dystonia

This is a very debilitating disorder, in which sleep is interrupted by attacks, usually 15 seconds to two minutes in duration, of violent muscular discharge. The patient is awake, but unable to control the movements. Attacks may be frequent, throughout the night, every night. Typically, they emerge from stage 2, but so disrupt sleep that other stages, such as 3, 4 and REM sleep, may be completely absent. In severe cases the patient is chronically sleep deprived with a propensity to fall asleep in the day, when they are still vulnerable to the attacks. The syndrome can be readily treated with relatively low doses of carbamazepine, although there is no evidence of epilepsy or other neurological disorder in these patients.

Restless legs syndrome

This is primarily a sensory disorder, that occurs to some degree in up to 5% of the general population, increasing with age. The symptoms are of a deep seated creeping sensation, usually symmetrically in the lower half of the lower limbs. Attacks usually occur within 5–30 minutes of going to bed, but may also occur when sitting for long periods. The individual is compelled to flex his muscles, sometimes quite violently, and if in bed will typically get up, pace around, or swing and massage the legs, as constant movement brings some temporary relief . The symptoms may continue for between several minutes to several hours, and will prevent sleep onset. They may also arise later in the night, disrupting sleep continuity, and the bed partner's sleep will also be disturbed. The syndrome may start in or be exacerbated by pregnancy. Up to a quarter of women may be affected, especially in the second half of pregnancy, with rapid resolution following delivery. Most cases are mild, and require reassurance rather than treatment. Severe cases may respond to carbamazepine.

Nocturnal myoclonus

Periodic limb movements or myoclonus is primarily a motor rather than a sensory syndrome, and it commonly occurs together with restless legs syndrome. The lower limbs flex compulsively, usually with dorsiflexion of the big toe and ankle, and flexion at the knee and hip. These movements tend to recur every 20–40 seconds in protracted episodes throughout the night, and are associated with brief or more prolonged partial arousals. This leads to complaints of disturbed or non-restorative sleep, and/or of excessive daytime sleepiness, sometimes without recall or awareness of the sleep disruption. The symptoms may be aggravated by pregnancy, smoking, sleep deprivation, excessive heat or cold, and caffeine.

This syndrome is rare in childhood, but common in adults, and prevalence rises with age. Symptoms can be controlled by removal of precipitating factors, and may respond to benzodiazepines, notably clonazepam, and to dopaminergic drugs and some opiodes, although their usefulness is limited by their side-effects.

Rhythmic movement disorders

This term is applied to a range of repetitive movements that can occur either during sleep, or more frequently, during wakefulness immediately prior to sleep onset. Also known as *Jactatio capitis nocturna*, these movements range from a gentle rocking of the head and/or the trunk from side to side, to rapid and violent banging of the head and body backwards and forwards.

The activity tends to occur every night, rather than spasmodically. It nearly always begins in infancy and the affected children usually grow out of it. It is relatively more common in children with a significant learning disability, or brain damage, and in these patients is more likely to persist into adult life. There is evidence that psychological stress underlies the behaviour, and it may serve a self-comforting function. In some adolescents and adult cases it has been linked to sexual frustration.

Management – In cases where movement is violent and injurious, the child needs to be protected physically with appropriate padding round the bed. Precautions and reassurance for the parents form the best management approach. Care should be taken to ensure that children do not feel embarrassed by the symptoms as this may heighten stress and aggravate the situation. In older children and adults, where the social consequences of the behaviour become a concern (when staying away from home, or embarking on sexual relationships), it is advisable to explore, and if possible, to treat any underlying psychological difficulties. Symptoms may also be modified with behavioural treatment approaches, or as a last resort, judicious use of sedative drugs.

Enuresis

At the age of five enuresis occurs in 10% of girls and 15% of boys. By the age of 16 it is rare in girls, but still occurs in 1% of boys, and may persist as a primary enuresis throughout adult life. Secondary enuresis can arise as a complication of alcohol or drug misuse, or of a range of physical disorders that affect kidney excretion rates, bladder tone, sphincter function and depth of sleep or rousability. It may be the presenting symptom of nocturnal epilepsy, diabetes, urinary tract infection, or occasionally sleep apnoea. It may also result from psychological stress (including the impact of childhood sexual abuse), and in the absence of an organic aetiology this should be sensitively explored.

Enuresis usually occurs during SWS, when rousability is lowest, and is therefore most common in the early hours of the morning. Management of primary enuresis includes restriction of fluid intake before bedtime, and the use of a bell and pad that wakes the individual when incontinent. This can help condition a response of wakefulness to the stimulus of a full bladder. Every effort should be made not to increase the stress of the situation. If other methods fail, imipramine may be beneficial.

Bruxism

This is a fairly common problem, and involves violent repetitive grinding of the teeth for bursts of 4–5 seconds often repeatedly throughout the night. It can erupt in any stage of sleep. Individuals may be unaware of the activity, though some suffer with aching jaws. Partners may be disturbed by it, and dentists may notice damage to the teeth, which can be severe in some cases.

Bruxism tends to begin in adolescence, and may be related to psychological strain. It is aggravated by alcohol, but becomes less common after the age of 40. In cases of severe damage to the teeth a rubber guard should be worn. The condition sometimes improves with relaxation and stress management therapies.

Sleeptalking

Sleeptalking is a widespread phenomenon, that can erupt out of any stage of sleep, and it may disturb the bed partner. Occasionally it can be very pronounced, and it may also occur together with sleepwalking, night terrors, and nightmares. Sleeptalking can be an expression of psychological stress, and in such cases stress management may help.

Disorders of the sleep-wake cycle

The underlying problem in circadian rhythm sleep disorders is that the patient cannot sleep when sleep is desired, needed, and expected. As a result, episodes of sleep and periods of wakefulness occur at inappropriate times leading to complaints of insomnia or excessive sleepiness, although the overall duration of sleep throughout the day is unaffected.

Time zone change (jet lag) syndrome (ICD–10 and DSM–IV)

Jet lag or circadian dysrhythmia consists of a number of symptoms of varying degree. These include difficulty in initiating and maintaining sleep, excessive sleepiness, decrements in subjective daytime alertness and performance, and somatic symptoms mainly related to gastrointestinal function. They arise because of external desynchronisation; the individual's internal circadian rhythms and the external zeitgebers are no longer synchronised, the impact of which is maximal on arrival. Internal desynchronisation will then result as the different rhythms of the body adjust to the new environment at variable rates.

The severity and duration of these symptoms depend on the number of time zones crossed, the direction (east or west) of the travel, the time of take off and arrival, and individual susceptibility, some experimental evidence suggests that those over 50 are more vulnerable. Symptoms are worse after an eastward flight as this results in a shortening of the day whereas the natural tendency of the body clock is to run slow.

The symptoms of jet lag decline after a few days as the body clock and the body rhythms synchronise with the external influence of the zeitgebers in the new time zone. It has been estimated that recovery is at the rate of one and a half days for each time zone transition eastwards and one day for each one westwards. Countermeasures to jet lag are discussed by Graeber (1994). Travellers are encouraged to rest in a quiet, darkened room when it is bedtime even if they are not tired. Naps are not recommended. Currently interest is focused on melatonin because of the ability of the exogenous form to adjust the body clock in a time dependent way while also promoting sleep. Its production is suppressed by daylight levels of illumination, but stimulated during darkness. Melatonin has been shown to reduce fatigue and improve sleep in long distance travellers (Arendt *et al*, 1986).

Shift work sleep disorder (ICD–10 and DSM–IV)

Work scheduled during the habitual hours of sleep (shift work or night work) may cause similar symptoms to those of jet lag. A person who works every night for the same shift may adjust his circadian rhythm to a new one. However, the problem is exacerbated for shift workers who alternate a few days of night work (which is out of phase with the light-dark cycle) with a few days of rest (which is in phase with the light-dark cycle) and so find themselves in a continuous state of circadian realignment. A normal, full sleep episode during the daytime becomes more difficult with increasing age and chronic sleep disturbances may eventually develop.

Timed exposure to bright light during a night shift improves sleep and increases alertness, possibly by preventing a phase advance in the circadian pacemaker (Dawson & Campbell, 1991; Eastman *et al*, 1994). As such scheduling becomes more popular, strategies to cope with night and shift work (see Monk, 1994) are important not only to improve the health of the workforce but also to prevent human error due to circadian dysrhythmia (Lauber & Kayten, 1988).

Irregular sleep-wake pattern (ICD–10 and DSM–IV)

Although total 24 hour average sleep time is within normal limits for age, the sleep-wake pattern consists of temporally disorganised and variable length episodes of sleep and waking behaviour.

The disorder is rare in the general population, but is not uncommon in institutionalised patients with severe congenital, developmental, or degenerative brain dysfunction. Its cause is not known. In patients with diffuse brain disease the behaviour is probably due to a malfunction of the systems that govern sleep and wakefulness. Traditionally the treatment has been mainly behavioural directed at re-establishing a regular monophasic sleep-wake cycle.

Delayed sleep phase syndrome (ICD–10 and DSM–IV)

The major sleep episode is delayed in relation to conventional clock times with sleep onset and wake times that are intractably later than desired (Weitzman *et al*, 1981). The symptoms are therefore sleep onset insomnia and/or difficulty in awakening at the desired time. Actual sleep onset times are at nearly the same time each day and are typically between 2 and 6 a.m. Once sleep is initiated there is little difficulty in maintaining it. Attempts to move the sleep episode to more conventional times usually fail.

Patients with delayed sleep phase syndrome report that their difficulties began following a period of late night studying or shift work, subsequent to which they found it impossible to resume conventional sleep times. It is generally assumed that the circadian system of such patients is phase delayed and so therefore are their sleep gates and forbidden zones. Further they have a relatively weak ability to phase advance their circadian systems in response to normal environmental time cues. Although some form of psychopathology may be present in these individuals it is not the underlying cause. They typically state that they function best and feel most alert during the late evening and night hours. Usually they have a poor school or work record. While the general population prevalence of this syndrome is unknown, a prevalence of 7% has been reported in adolescents. Further it has been estimated that it represents between 5–10% of patients presenting to sleep disorders centres with the complaint of insomnia.

The treatment for delayed sleep phase syndrome is phase advance chronotherapy (Czeisler *et al*, 1981). This is a behavioural treatment based on the body clock's natural tendency to run slow in contrast to the 24 hour day. Bedtime is systematically delayed two or three hours each day until the desired bedtime is achieved. Subsequently the patient must rigidly adhere to the new scheduled bedtime. Since bright light has been shown to be capable of shifting the circadian system in normal subjects, with the magnitude and direction of the phase shift depending on the timing (Czeisler *et al*, 1989), it has been used as a treatment for this syndrome, sometimes in conjunction with chronotherapy (Rosenthal *et al*, 1990). Other treatments include oral melatonin (Dahlitz *et al*, 1991) and vitamin B_{12} treatment (Okawa *et al*, 1990). All treatments have been found to be successful, but results depend very much on motivation as well as the environment, and the advancement in sleep and wake timing tends not to be retained when treatment is stopped.

Advanced sleep phase syndrome (ICD–10 and DSM–IV)

The advanced sleep phase syndrome is the reciprocal of the delayed sleep phase syndrome; a persistent early evening sleep onset typically between 6 and 8 p.m., and early morning awakening insomnia occurring between 1 and 3 a.m. The symptoms are compelling evening sleepiness, an early sleep-onset, and an awakening that is earlier than desired. The sleep preceding the early morning awakening insomnia is otherwise undisturbed. Actual sleep-onset times are typically nearly the same time each day and attempts to move the sleep episode to more conventional times usually fail.

Too few patients have presented with this syndrome for a clear clinical picture to emerge. Prevalence is unknown and it is thought to be very rare. Given the apparent phase advance of the circadian timing that accompanies aging, advance sleep phase syndrome is theoretically more likely to occur in the elderly.

Chronotherapy has also been shown to be a successful behavioural treatment in the advanced sleep phase syndrome (Moldofsky *et al*, 1986). This involves a systematic advancement in bedtime by three hours each day until the desired bedtime is achieved. Subsequently the patient must rigidly adhere to the new scheduled bedtime. Bright light is being explored as a possible treatment.

Non 24 hour sleep-wake syndrome (ICD–10 and DSM–IV)

Also known as the *hypernyctohemeral syndrome,* it consists of a steady pattern comprising 1 to 2 hour daily delays in sleep onset and wake times.

The sleep-wake cycle of such an individual is free running, closely following the periodicity of the endogenous 25 hour circadian rhythm despite the presence of 24 hour time cues in the environment. The sleep-wake cycle regularly moves in and out of phase with the conventional social hours for sleep. When 'in phase' there may be no sleep complaint and daytime alertness is normal. As incremental phase delays occur, difficulties in initiating sleep at night will be coupled with oversleeping into the daytime hours or excessive daytime sleepiness. Any complications are related to impaired psychosocial functioning.

The majority of such patients described in the literature have been blind, due to either congenital or acquired cases (Miles *et al*, 1977; Klein *et al*, 1993). A survey revealed that 76% of blind individuals had sleep-wake complaints, with 40% of the respondents having recognised that their symptoms occurred in a cyclic fashion (Miles & Wilson, 1977).

Some blind individuals with the hypernyctohemeral syndrome have been successfully treated by the imposition of strict 24 hour scheduling consisting of strong social time cues. The administration of vitamin B_{12} has also helped individuals with this syndrome, although its mode of action is unknown (Okawa *et al*, 1990).

Sleep disorders secondary to disorders of physical health

Some disturbance of sleep is very common at times of physical ill health, and may even be a presenting symptom, or an indicator of illness severity. Excessive sleep, sleepiness and fatigue are symptoms of most infectious and chronic inflammatory disorders. In these conditions the duration of SWS is increased, and it is thought that the restorative and energy conservation effect of this increased SWS aids recovery.

In contrast to this adaptive mechanism, the severity of pain in many physical disorders can cause considerable sleep disruption, as can the hospital environment. This can result in decreased REM and SWS. The pain of peptic ulceration and of nocturnal angina are common causes of such sleep disruption.

Intensive care units, with their 24 hour noise, light, monitoring and invasive investigations can result in a sufficient degree of sleep deprivation to cause symptoms such as paranoia and pseudohallucinations and other mental state disturbance, and may delay physical recovery. A number of physical disorders have more specific associations with sleep problems, as described below.

Neurological disorders

Epilepsy has a particular relationship with sleep. In many cases of epilepsy, seizures occur at a regular time of day or night, and some may be exclusively nocturnal. Nocturnal sleep epilepsy denotes the occurrence of seizures wholly or mainly at night. This pattern is more common in children, and overall occurs in some 45% of people with epilepsy, with about half of these experiencing seizures exclusively during sleep. Detectable organic brain disease is more frequent in cases of sleep epilepsy than with waking epilepsy, although this is even more frequent in cases of epilepsy without a set pattern.

Epileptic events during sleep are usually generalised tonic-clonic seizures, often associated with incontinence, or focal psychomotor attacks. The latter can result in stereotyped dreams, half-waking confusion and simple automatisms, and polysomnography may be necessary to differentiate epileptic phenomena from true parasomnias.

Sleep seizures tend to occur at specific times in the night. Tonic-clonic seizures usually occur in the first two hours of sleep, or between four and six in the morning, or around the hour after awakening. Tonic generalised seizures, usually seen in children, occur in NREM sleep. Clonic generalised seizures are rare in sleep. Focal frontal lobe, supplementary motor and limbic seizures occur more often in REM sleep, while other focal attacks occur at random in all stages of sleep. Psychomotor seizures arise particularly from REM sleep, and in some individuals this relationship may be invariable. Arousal from sleep may precipitate both generalised and partial seizures (Parkes, 1985*a*).

Insomnia is commonly associated with many neurological disorders, such as head injury, parkinsonism, encephalitis and other infections, epilepsy, space occupying lesions, spinal cord damage, cerebrovascular disease and dementia (Parkes, 1985*b*). This insomnia can result from impairment of the sleep mechanisms, as in progressive supranuclear palsy, or from impaired sensory mechanisms, as with spinal cord injuries. It may also occur as a consequence of stress, discomfort and pain, or due to motor abnormalities, such as muscular twitches and jerks in parkinsonism, depression, or due to the effects of drugs. It may also be a symptom of depression arising as a complication of a physical disorder.

Endocrine disorders

Hyperthyroidism can cause short fragmented sleep, with increased EEG slow wave activity. Hypothyroidism causes excessive sleepiness with little or no EEG slow wave activity and disrupted REM sleep, as well as obstructive sleep apnoea. The sleep abnormalities may persist for a year or so following successful treatment of the thyroid disorder. Acromegaly is associated with obstructive sleep apnoea in 5–25% of cases. Insomnia may occur secondary to both hypogonadism and to the menopause (Parkes, 1985*b*).

Fibromyalgia and the chronic fatigue syndrome

These related disorders are associated with both daytime fatigue and non-restorative sleep. Polysomnography shows characteristic alpha wave intrusion into the sleep electroencephalogram, implying a light and fragile sleep.

End stage renal disease

Patients receiving dialysis commonly complain of insomnia and daytime fatigue. In end stage renal disease periodic involuntary limb movements can occur at 20–40 second intervals during sleep, leading to disruption in the continuity and quality of sleep. An increase in this type of insomnia often heralds a declining clinical state.

Rheumatoid arthritis

Exacerbations of rheumatoid arthritis are particularly associated with middle insomnia (frequent awakenings), the causal mechanism probably being the increase in night pain in affected joints. Treatment should focus more on pain relief than on hypnotics.

Nocturnal asthma and chronic obstructive airways disease

The discomfort and respiratory effort of these disorders disrupts sleep continuity. The use of hypnotics to correct this can be dangerous due to respiratory depression, except in cases where oxygen saturation remains normal ('pink puffers').

Sleep disorders secondary to psychiatric disorders

Depression

Sleep disturbance is a core symptom of major depression. This can take the form of early morning wakening, usually associated with a diurnal variation in mood, which is lowest on first awakening, and improves somewhat through the day. Alternatively there may be onset insomnia, sometimes associated with a reverse diurnal variation in mood, or middle insomnia, with awakenings that may be frequent, or fewer but prolonged. Complaints of hypersomnia, an atypical feature of depression, are relatively more common in younger depressed patients, particularly those with manic–depressive disorder. These patients complain of either difficulty in awakening in the morning, or of excessive sleepiness throughout the day.

Characteristic changes in sleep architecture are a disruption in sleep continuity, reduced SWS, shortened REM sleep latency, and an alteration in the temporal distribution of REM and SWS. Sleep continuity is impaired due to prolonged sleep latency, multiple awakenings, and early morning wakening. Total SWS is reduced, with a longer duration of SWS in the second sleep cycle compared with the first, a reversal of the normal pattern. As the first SWS episode is shortened, the subsequent first episode of REM sleep occurs sooner in the night (reduced REM latency). The normal pattern of increased REM sleep as the night progresses is reversed, with an increase in the amount of REM sleep in the first half of the night (Kupfer *et al*, 1990; Benca *et al*, 1992).

In cases of depressive hypersomnia, monitoring of daytime naps in the sleep laboratory has produced little objective evidence of pathological sleepiness (Nofzinger *et al*, 1991). The subjective complaint of daytime sleepiness in these patients probably relates to their lack of interest, anergy, retardation and withdrawal, rather than to true daytime hypersomnia.

Changes in the first NREM/REM sleep cycle in depressed patients tend to persist after symptomatic recovery. This is mirrored by changes in the pattern of growth hormone secretion. In normal subjects this is both pulsatile and follows a diurnal pattern, being maximal at around the time of sleep onset, while in depressed patients growth hormone secretion in sleep is significantly reduced. This is also persistent after recovery from a depressive episode, and both these sleep-related abnormalities may thus be trait markers for depression (Jarrett *et al*, 1990).

Most forms of treatment for depression, including antidepressants, lithium, carbamazepine and ECT induce suppression of REM sleep. Sleep deprivation itself can be an effective treatment for depression, especially where diurnal mood variation is pronounced, and is discussed in more detail later in this chapter.

Panic disorder

Panic attacks as a symptom of panic disorder can erupt out of sleep, awakening the sufferer, and is reported as occurring at least once by about one-third of patients with panic disorder. In about 5% of patients with panic disorder the attacks occur predominantly or exclusively during sleep. Panic disorder, whether the attacks are nocturnal or not, is associated with insomnia characterised by increased sleep latency. This correlates with, and may be due to increased levels of anxiety.

Nocturnal panic attacks occur at the time of transitions between stages 2 and 3 or 3 and 4 sleep (Mellman & Uhde, 1989). They can be distinguished from nightmares by their lack of recall of dream content, and from night terrors by the full wakefulness of the individual following the onset of an attack, and their difficulty in returning to sleep after it. In children panic attacks are rare compared with the high frequency of night terrors. Nocturnal asthma is a further differential diagnosis, and can be identified by measurement of respiratory peak flow during an attack. Treatment is the same as for panic disorder in general, and may include antidepressants and anxiety management therapy.

Schizophrenia

Schizophrenia is associated with reduced sleep efficiency, with increased sleep latency, more disrupted sleep, and a decline in REM sleep latency (Benca *et al*, 1992). These effects on sleep are compounded by antipsychotic medication as described below.

Eating disorders and malnutrition

Significant weight loss due to inadequate dietary intake, whether due to anorexia nervosa or famine, disrupts sleep continuity. The typical pattern is of middle insomnia or early morning wakening, which appears to be related to an enhanced drive towards food seeking behaviour. Hunger and food seeking behaviour has its own rhythmicity, which intrinsically follows an approximately four hourly pattern throughout the 24 hour day. With normal social entraining and adequate nutrition, food seeking behaviour during sleeping hours is suppressed during early infancy, but reemerges in response to malnutrition so long as hunger itself is not impaired as, for example, with some hypothalamic lesions.

In bulimia nervosa there is commonly a dietary pattern of daytime fasting with nocturnal bingeing and purging, usually in the early evening. In some cases the nocturnal binges occur when individuals wake hungry in the middle of the night, at a time when their will to sustain dietary restriction is low. As the process of bingeing and purging can be prolonged, this can lead to considerable disruption of sleep, resulting in complaints of excessive daytime tiredness.

Substance induced sleep disorders

Many prescribed, illicit and socially accepted recreational drugs can lead to the development of insomnia and, less commonly, to hypersomnias or parasomnias.

The effect that a drug has on sleep is influenced by its distribution across the blood–brain barrier, its central nervous system receptor binding profile, and its peripheral effects. Agonism at a specific neuroreceptor site has a characteristic effect on sleep architecture, as summarised in Table 25.1.

The rapidity of onset of any drug effect is related to its rate of absorption, while the duration of its action is related to its rate of elimination from the body, as well as its distribution rate into adipose tissue.

Clinically increased arousal manifests itself in complaints of insomnia, while increases in REM sleep lead to complaints of nightmares, and the exacerbation of other REM sleep disorders if present. Increases in SWS can lead to an exacerbation of the parasomnias associated with this sleep stage, such as sleep walking, night terrors or enuresis.

Effects of socially accepted recreational drugs on sleep

Alcohol

The most common sleep disorder associated with alcohol is insomnia. The immediate sedative effect of alcohol apparent with acute intoxication only lasts for 3–4 hours. Stage 3 and 4 sleep is increased, and REM sleep is diminished. In cases of sleep apnoea, the number of obstructive events is increased. Falling blood alcohol levels translate into a clinical picture of increased wakefulness, restless sleep, and disturbing dreams. During this phase, stage 3 and 4 sleep is reduced, and wakefulness and REM sleep is increased. The clinical presentation is then complaints of interrupted or non-restorative sleep, disturbing nightmares, or early morning wakening.

As the initial sedative effect of alcohol is preserved even with long-term use, patients often compound their problems by increasing their dose of alcohol in an attempt to prolong this effect. This can lead to dependence, and alcohol withdrawal symptoms emerging in the early morning hours.

In alcohol withdrawal there is gross disturbance of sleep architecture. Sleep continuity is disrupted, with an increase in REM sleep, and associated vivid and disturbing dreams, which can merge into the delirium of acute alcohol withdrawal.

When alcohol dependence is followed by successful withdrawal from alcohol, there may be continued long-term disturbance of sleep, with typically light and fragmented sleep often lasting for months or even years. Polysomnography in such cases reveals a persistent deficit in sleep continuity, and in the amount of stage 4 sleep. It is important to avoid treating this potentially long-term insomnia with hypnotics, as individuals who have been dependent on alcohol can rapidly switch to dependence on benzodiazepines and other minor tranquillisers.

Caffeine

Caffeine induces insomnia, while acute withdrawal can cause hypersomnia and daytime sleepiness. Effects on sleep are dose related, causing increased wakefulness, and decreased sleep continuity. There may be increased sleep latency, increased wakefulness, and reduced stage 3 and 4 sleep. Hypersomnia can emerge between daytime doses of caffeine, as fluctuating blood levels result in an oscillation between dose related stimulation, and withdrawal induced sedation.

Nicotine

The effects of nicotine are biphasic. At low concentrations it acts as a sedative and promotes sleep but at higher concentrations it functions as a stimulant. Both caffeine and nicotine have very long half-lives (Stradling, 1993).

Table 25.1 Effects on sleep of agonism at specific neuroreceptors

Receptor type	Effect of agonist binding
Histamine$_1$ receptors	Suppress REM and SWS
GABA receptors	Suppress REM and increase NREM sleep
Monoamine receptors and 5-HT receptors	Suppress REM sleep, can increase or reduce arousal according to receptor subtype
Alpha$_1$ adrenoceptors	Increase REM sleep, and arousal
Alpha$_2$ adrenoceptors	Suppress REM sleep, and sedate
Beta$_1$ adrenoceptors	Increase REM sleep, and arousal
Cholinergic receptors	Increase REM sleep, and arousal
Dopamine receptors	Decrease SWS, and increase arousal
Adenosine receptors	Increase slow wave and total sleep

Effects of illicit recreational drugs on sleep

Amphetamines, cocaine and related stimulants

These substances potentiate dopaminergic neurotransmisson, and induce insomnia during intoxication, and hypersomnia in withdrawal. Acute amphetamine intoxication is associated with increased sleep latency, and reduced total sleep time, continuity, REM and stage 3 and 4 sleep. During withdrawal from chronic use hypersomnia occurs, with prolonged nocturnal sleep as well as excessive daytime sleepiness, with REM and SWS rebound.

Opioids, cannabis and LSD

With short-term use of opioids, there is an associated increase in sleepiness and subjective depth of sleep, with a reduction in REM sleep but no change in total sleep time. With chronic use tolerance to the sedative effects develops and gives way to complaints of insomnia, with decreased sleep time and increased wakefulness. Opiate withdrawal is usually accompanied by hypersomnia. Cannabis use increases SWS duration. On first exposure to cannabis REM sleep duration is reduced, but returns to normal with regular use. On withdrawal from cannabis there is a rebound increase in REM duration, with a decreased REM latency. LSD use prolongs REM sleep duration, and SWS is disrupted by bursts of REM sleep, associated with increased body movements and arousals.

Effects of prescribed hypnotic drugs on sleep

Benzodiazepines

The benzodiazepines probably act on sleep by facilitating GABA neurotransmission. While they reduce sleep latency and increase total sleep time, they do not induce normal sleep architecture, but rather one characterised by reduced REM and stage 4 SWS duration, and increased stage 2 sleep duration (Borbély *et al*, 1991). Many individuals experience subjective relief from insomnia with brief or intermittent use of these drugs as hypnotics, but they do have a number of disadvantages, especially with long-term prescribing (over six weeks), which should therefore be avoided.

Benzodiazepines with a long half-life, such as diazepam, nitrazepam and flurazepam, have a significant hangover effect, impairing daytime psychomotor performance. The half-life of these compounds and their active metabolites is so long (up to several days) that their cumulative dose rises with continued treatment. This is a particular hazard for the elderly who are often prescribed them, to the point where confusion, oversedation and personality change can occur. By contrast, use of compounds with a short half-life such as triazolam (half life between two and three hours) avoids a hangover effect, but is associated with daytime withdrawal agitation and anxiety. Medium half-life (8–12 hours) benzodiazepines such as temazepam and oxazepam, are rather slowly absorbed, and so should be taken an hour before going to bed to avoid onset insomnia.

Tolerance is common after long-term use of all benzodiazepines, and rebound phenomena occur on discontinuation with increased REM sleep duration associated with vivid or frightening dreams, and rebound insomnia for 1–3 weeks (occasionally up to 2 months). This may be more severe than the original insomnia for which the drugs were initially prescribed, and may be misinterpreted by the sleepless patient as an indicator that they should resume their hypnotic use.

Benzodiazepine hypnotics have a number of other disadvantages, including disinhibition, which may lead to violence or other antisocial behaviours, and muscle weakness, which may lead to falls in the elderly. After regular use over several weeks or months, these drugs may all induce a state of physical dependence associated with symptoms of irritability, lethargy, anxiety, impaired concentration and personality change. Once dependent, sudden withdrawal from benzodiazepines will induce a withdrawal state, characterised by agitation, anxiety, insomnia, epileptic seizures and toxic confusion (see also page 608). Benzodiazepines are relatively safe in overdose alone, although they are commonly taken in combination with more dangerous substances, such as alcohol, whose effects are then potentiated.

Cyclopyrolones (Zopiclone)

Zopiclone apparently also acts on sleep by facilitating GABA neuro-transmission. Although sleep latency is reduced, the sleep that follows has a normal sleep architecture, or may demonstrate an increase in SWS duration. Although tolerance and a withdrawal syndrome have been described, this seems to be less common than with the benzodiazepines, as are rebound effects on sleep following discontinuation (Wadworth & McTavish, 1993).

Antidepressants

Tricyclic antidepressants have a sedative action, linked to their anticholinergic properties. For this reason they should be taken at bed time, to minimise adverse effects on daytime performance, as well as to reduce any insomnia. This prescribing strategy can be helpful but adverse effects on fine psychomotor tasks persist and are detectable the following day. Tricyclic induced sleep is also qualitatively different, with pronounced suppression of REM sleep, and increased slow wave and stage 1 sleep (these effects are particularly marked with clomipramine). Clinically this may give rise to complaints of difficulty in concentrating and performing fine motor and mental tasks during the day, and of non-restorative sleep. These symptoms may also reinforce the negative self-cognitions that form part of the perpetuating mechanism in depression. The REM sleep-suppressing properties of tricyclic antidepressants may be useful in the treatment of sleep disorders arising from REM sleep, such as severe nightmares, some apnoeas, and cataplexy in narcolepsy.

Selective serotonin reuptake inhibitor (SSRI) antidepressants are not clinically associated with sedation, or impaired psychomotor function. They suppress REM sleep, and tend to increase sleep fragmentation. As sleep disturbance in depression generally improves as the depression lifts, there is a clinical rationale for prescribing a three or four week course of a hypnotic when starting an SSRI antidepressant, particularly when insomnia forms an important part of the clinical presentation.

Monoamine oxidase inhibitor (MAOI) antidepressants also suppress REM sleep and there is a rebound increase in REM on discontinuation. ECT is associated with a temporary reduction in REM sleep duration. Lithium carbonate delays the onset and reduces the amount of REM sleep, and increases the amount of SWS. Severe sedation is a symptom of toxic overdose. Carbamazepine increases SWS, and suppresses REM sleep. Transient drowsiness is common at the start of treatment, or when the dosage is increased.

Neuroleptics

Although antipsychotic drugs have an affinity for a wide range of neuroreceptors, their sedative effects closely parallel their anticholinergic properties. Those with the least antipsychotic potency, such as thioridazine and chlorpromazine, are the most sedative, while the converse is true of potent antipsychotic drugs such as trifluoperazine or pimozide. H_1 (Histamine) receptor antagonism by phenothiazine antipsychotics accounts for most of the sedation they cause.

In general, these drugs increase SWS and decrease wakefulness. The effects on REM sleep are inconsistent. Relatively specific dopamine antagonists, such as pimozide or trifluoperazine, have little effect, while chlorpromazine increases REM sleep at low doses, and suppresses it at high doses, owing to a dose dependent shift in its relative antagonist effects at alpha$_1$ and alpha$_2$ adrenoceptor subtypes. Withdrawal from antipsychotic medication is followed by a pronounced suppression of REM sleep and a reduction in total sleep time.

Effects of some other non-psychotropic drugs on sleep

Phenytoin decreases REM sleep and increases Stage 4 sleep. Ethosuximide increases stage 1 sleep, and reduces slow wave and REM sleep, and patients may complain of sleeping less deeply. Valproic acid increases SWS in children, but decreases it in adults, along with suppression of awakenings and other sleep stage shifts, while total sleep time is increased.

As most appetite suppressants are stimulants, their effects on sleep are similar to the amphetamines as described above. Fenfluramine is an exception. Its action seems to be related to potentiation of serotonergic neurotransmission, and its use is associated with daytime sedation, disturbed sleep and reduced REM sleep duration.

Hyoscine reduces cholinergic neurotransmission, and its use leads to sedation and delay in the onset and reduction of REM sleep. Withdrawal is associated with a rebound increase in REM sleep.

Antihistamines affect a range of neuroreceptors in addition to the histamine receptor. They have sedative properties, and increase SWS, although sedative effects are less in some of the more recently developed antihistamines because of their reduced ability to cross the blood–brain barrier. Of the specific H$_2$ receptor subtype antagonists, cimetidine increases SWS while ranitidine (which has a higher H$_2$ receptor specificity) does not.

Antihypertensives

Hypertension is a common disorder, and anti-hypertensives frequently induce depression and sleep disturbances. Alpha methyldopa is metabolised to alpha-methylnoradrenaline, a potent alpha adrenoceptor agonist. It induces a reduction in SWS duration, and an increase in REM sleep duration. Clinically the patient may complain of increased daytime sedation, and nightmares. Reserpine blocks amine synthesis and leads to a reduction in REM sleep duration. Clinically the patient may complain of depression, drowsiness, lethargy, and nightmares.

Alpha blockers such as clonidine, and antagonists prazocin and indoramin, have complex effects on sleep which are dependent on their relative activity at different doses on the alpha$_1$ and alpha$_2$ receptor subtypes. Doxazocin causes somnolence. When these effects are problematic it is usually because they have induced sedation, or nightmares. Beta blockers have a similarly complex relationship with sleep mechanisms.

Clinically important effects occur with beta antagonists, which reduce both REM and SWS. This can cause both insomnia and nightmares, the latter occurring despite reduced REM sleep, perhaps due to improved recall with increased frequency of awakenings. The strength of these effects varies between the beta antagonists, increasing in direct proportion to their lipid solubility, and thus their ability to cross the blood–brain barrier, and is most pronounced with propranolol, and least so with atenolol. The polyuria induced by all diuretics may disrupt sleep, while spironolactone can cause sedation.

Sleep deprivation as a treatment for depression

Sleep deprivation has been used as a treatment for depression, either alone or as an adjunct to antidepressants. Sleep deprivation may be total, by keeping the patient awake for 36 hours, or partial, where the patient is awakened at 2 a.m., and kept awake until 10 p.m. This has a powerful short-term effect on mood in depressive disorder, particularly when diurnal variation in mood is present, with some 60% of patients reporting a significant improvement in mood the day following the sleep-deprived night. The effect seems to be the same for partial as for total sleep deprivation. The positive effect on mood is short lived, with a relapse rate in unmedicated patients of some 80% after one night of recovery (non-deprived) sleep.

The transitory nature of the response to sleep deprivation, along with the impossibility of maintaining continued sleep deprivation, limits its role as a single treatment for depression. Despite this, in individual cases intermittent sleep deprivation as a single treatment may be useful, particularly if other treatments are poorly tolerated. Due to the nature of the treatment double blind evaluations of this method are not possible. Open studies suggest that there may be a role for sleep deprivation combined with antidepressants in some cases of treatment resistant depression, or in order to hasten the onset of an antidepressant response in a suicidal or severely retarded patient, as an alternative to ECT.

Because there is a rapid and significant improvement in mood with sleep deprivation in depression, it may be used as a diagnostic tool, for example to distinguish depressive pseudodementia from an organic dementia. In this case performance on cognitive tests should improve on the post treatment day if the disorder is primarily depressive, but is likely to deteriorate if it is organic (Leibenluft & Wehr, 1992).

Sleep and crime

In cases that come to court, sleep related crimes usually involve violence to others, including murder. Such crimes committed while asleep used to be regarded in law as "non-insane automatisms", as would be the case if the individual were confused due to an extrinsic factor, such as concussion. If proven, this led to a complete acquittal, and there have been no recorded cases of a person committing further acts of violence after such a acquittal. More recently, following a series of cases culminating in the Court of Appeal's ruling in the case of *Quick and Paddison*, in 1991 there has been a clear transition in British law to viewing murder while asleep as an "insane automatism", due to an intrinsic abnormality or disorder of the mind. As such, if the case is proven, it leads to the finding of the special verdict of "not guilty by reason of insanity". At one time such a verdict used to result in detention in a special hospital at Her Majesty's pleasure, usually indefinitely. This situation was amended in the Criminal Procedure (Insanity and Unfitness to Plead) Act 1991, which in these circumstances gives courts the power to make a hospital order (with or without restriction), guardianship order, or a supervision and treatment order, or grant an absolute discharge (D'Orban *et al*, 1993).

In cases of sleepwalking accidental self-injury is common and injury to others is unusual. When it occurs it is most usually a poorly coordinated or coincidental injury from a flailing limb generally inflicted on the bed partner, who might be asleep, or attempting to prevent the individual from leaving the room. More rarely there may be a complex and highly coordinated assault, again usually on the bed partner. The nature of such assaults vary, but strangulation seems to be a common feature, as in the case of Boshears, an American airman who was acquitted in 1961 of strangling his girlfriend whilst asleep. We recently assessed one sleepwalker whose wife initiated the referral after surviving several somnambulant assaults so that there would be a prior record of her husband's disorder should he finally kill her. She hoped this would be an effective defence for him and so prevent her children from losing both parents.

In night terrors as with sleepwalking, most of the violence is inflicted on the self, usually accidentally while in a state of terror. Occasionally flailing limbs will make contact with a bed partner who may be injured, sometimes severely. Very rarely there may be a more coordinated assault, as in the 19th century Scottish law case of Fraser, a known sleepwalker who killed his baby son by throwing him against the wall while "dreaming" that he was struggling with a wild animal, during what was probably a night terror.

In patients with REM sleep behaviour disorder, violence to self or others occurs as a result of physical dream enactment during REM sleep, which is normally prevented by the flaccid paralysis that occurs in this sleep stage. Violence can sometimes occur in cases of confusion or sudden awakening; this state is known as sleep drunkenness and is characterised by confusion, disorientation and misinterpretation of reality on sudden arousal from SWS. The individual may act as though defending himself against attack, and lacks subsequent recall for the event. This may lead to injury to self or others, and occasionally to murder, as in the 19th century case of Fain, a guest who killed a hotel porter by shooting him three times with his pistol when the victim tried to awaken him.

Conclusions

Sleep disorders are common, and while their aetiology may be either psychological or organic, the end point is generally one of disturbed psychological wellbeing. The adverse effect of this can be considerable, and may be a powerful precipitating or perpetuating factor for psychiatric disorders such as anxiety and depression. Attempts to directly modify sleep disorders tend to be disappointing, as with the use of sedative drugs for insomnia, due to the re-emergence of symptoms after adaptation. By contrast, indirect treatments which address issues in the patient's conscious and waking hours, such as adopting a healthier and more regular daytime routine, and attempts to explore and defuse psychological stresses, often result in a more sustained improvement. Planning and implementing such interventions can result in considerable satisfaction for patient and clinician, but is dependent on the quality of the initial assessment. This requires time and interest, and where the diagnosis remains unclear, a full sleep laboratory investigation. If this can be achieved then much can be done to improve the mental and physical health, and the lives of the large number of people who suffer from sleep disorders.

References

Agnew, H. W., Webb, W. B. & Williams, R. L. (1966) The first night effect: An EEG study of sleep. *Psychophysiology*, **2**, 263–266.

Aldrich, M. S. (1990) Narcolepsy. *New England Journal of Medicine*, **323**, 389–394.

Arendt, J., Aldhous, M. & Marks, V. (1986) Alleviation of jet lag by melatonin: Preliminary results of a controlled double blind trial. *British Medical Journal*, **292**, 1170.

Aserinksy, E. & Kleitman, N. (1953) Regularly occurring periods of eye motility and concomitant phenomena during sleep. *Science*, **118**, 273–274.

Benca, R. M., Obermeyer, W. H., Thisted, R. A., *et al* (1992) Sleep and psychiatric disorders. *Archives of General Psychiatry*, **46**, 651–668.

Blagrove, M. (1992) Dreams as the reflection of our waking concerns and abilities: A critique of the problem-solving paradigm in dream research. *Dreaming*, **2**, 205–220.

Blanes, T., Burgess, M., Marks, I. M., et al (1993) Dream anxiety disorders (nightmares): a review. *Behavioural Psychotherapy*, **21**, 37–43.

Borbély, A. A., Akerstedt, T., Benoit, O., *et al* (1991) Hypnotics and sleep physiology: a consensus report. *European Archives of Psychiatry and Clinical Neuroscience*, **241**, 13–21.

Brezinová, V. (1974) Sleep cycle content and sleep cycle duration. *Electroencephalography and Clinical Neurophysiology*, **36**, 275–282.

—— & Oswald, I. (1972) Sleep after a bedtime beverage. *British Medical Journal,* **2**, 431–433.

Broughton, R. J. (1994) Ambulant home monitoring of sleep and its disorders. In *Principles and Practice of Sleep Medicine* (2nd edn)(eds M. H. Kryger, T. Roth & W. C. Dement), pp. 978–983. Philadelphia: W.B. Saunders.

Caine, T. M., Foulds, G. A. & Hope, K. (1967) *Manual of the Hostility and Direction of Hostility Questionnaire (HDHQ).* London: University of London Press.

Carskadon, M. A. & Dement, W. C. (1994) Normal human sleep: an overview. In *Principles and Practice of Sleep Medicine* (2nd edn) (eds M. H. Kryger, T. Roth & W. C. Dement), pp. 16–25. Philadelphia: W.B. Saunders.

—— & Rechtschaffen, A. (1994) Monitoring and staging human sleep. In *Principles and Practice of Sleep Medicine* (2nd edn) (eds M. H. Kryger, T. Roth & W. C. Dement), pp. 943–960. Philadelphia: W.B. Saunders.

Catesby Ware, J. & Hirshkowitz, M. (1994) Monitoring penile errections during sleep. In *Principles and Practice of Sleep Medicine* (2nd edn)(eds M. H. Kryger, T. Roth & W. C. Dement), pp. 967–977. Philadelphia: W.B. Saunders.

Crown, S. & Crisp, A. H. (1979) *Manual of the Crown–Crisp Experiential Index.* London: Hodder & Stoughton.

Czeisler, C. A., Weitzman, E. D., Moore-Ede, M. C., *et al* (1980) Human sleep: Its duration and organization depend on its circadian phase. *Science,* **210**, 1264–1267.

——, Richardson, G. S., Coleman, R. M., *et al* (1981) Chronotherapy: Resetting the circadian clocks of patients with delayed sleep phase insomnia. *Sleep,* **4**, 1–21.

——, Kronauer, R. E., Allan, J. S., *et al* (1989) Bright light induction of strong (type 0) resetting of the human circadian pacemaker. *Nature,* **244**, 1328–1333.

Dahlitz, M. J., Alvarez, B., Vignau, J., *et al* (1991) Delayed sleep phase syndrome response to melatonin. *Lancet,* **337**, 1121–1124.

Dawson, D. & Campbell, S. S. (1991) Timed exposure to bright light improves sleep and alertness during simulated night shifts. *Sleep,* **14**, 511–516.

Dement, W. C. & Kleitman, N. (1957) Cyclic variations in EEG during sleep and their relation to eye movements, body motility, and dreaming. *Electroencephalography and Clinical Neurophysiology,* **9**, 273–274.

D'Orban, P., Gunn, J., Holland, A., *et al* (1993) Organic disorder, mental handicap and offending. In *Forensic Psychiatry: clinical, legal and ethical issues* (ed J. Gunn & P. J. Taylor), pp. 286–327. Butterworth.

Eastman, C. I., Stewart, K. T., Mahoney, M. P., *et al* (1994) Dark goggles and bright light improve circadian rhythm adaptation to night-shift work. *Sleep,* **17**, 535–543.

Eysenck, H. J. & Eysenck, S. B. G. (1975) *Manual of the Eysenck Personality Questionnaire.* London: Hodder & Stoughton.

Gaillard, J.-M., Nicholson, A. N. & Pascoe, P. (1994) Neurotransmitter systems. In *Principles and Practice of Sleep Medicine,* (2nd edn)(eds M. H. Kryger, T. Roth & W. C. Dement), pp. 338–348. Philadelphia: W.B. Saunders.

Gillin, J. C. & Byerley, W. F. (1990) Diagnosis and management of insomnia. *New England Journal of Medicine,* **322**, 239–248.

Glotzbach, S. F. & Heller, H. C. (1994) Temperature regulation. In *Principles and Practice of Sleep Medicine,* (2nd edn) (eds M. H. Kryger, T. Roth, & W. C. Dement), pp. 260–275. Philadelphia: W.B. Saunders.

Graeber, R. C. (1994) Jet lag and sleep disruption. In *Principles and Practice of Sleep Medicine,* (2nd edn) (eds M. H. Kryger, T. Roth, & W. C. Dement), pp. 463–470. Philadelphia: W.B. Saunders.

Guilleminault, C. (1992) EEG arousals: Scoring rules and examples. *Sleep,* **15,** 173–184.

Hartmann, E. (1968) The 90-minute sleep dream cycle. *Archives of General Psychiatry,* **18,** 280–286.

Haskell, E. H., Palca, J.W., Walker, J. M., *et al* (1981) The effects of high and low ambient temperatures on human sleep stages. *Electroencephalography and Clinical Neurophysiology,* **51,** 494–501.

Hauri, P. (1970) What is good sleep? In *Sleep and Dreaming.*(ed E. Hartmann), pp. 56–59. Boston: Little Brown & Co.

—— (1992)*The Sleep Disorders,* Current concepts series. Michigan: Kalamazoo.

Horne, J. A. (1990) *Why We Sleep: The Functions of Sleep in Humans and Other Mammals.* Oxford: Oxford University Press.

Hirshkowitz, M. & Moore, C. A. (1994) Issues in computerized polysomnography. *Sleep,* **17,** 105–112.

Jarrett, D. B., Miewald, J. M. & Kupfer, D. J. (1990) Recurrent depression is associated with a persistent reduction in sleep-related growth hormone secretion. *Archives of General Psychiatry,* **47,** 113–118.

Jasper, H. H. (Committee chairman) (1958) The ten-twenty electrode system of the International Federation. *Electroencephalography and Clinical Neurophysiology,* **10,** 371–375.

Klein, T., Martens, H., Dijk, D. J., *et al* (1993) Circadian sleep regulation in the absence of light perception: Chronic non-24-hour circadian rhythm sleep disorder in a blind man with a regular 24-hour sleep-wake schedule. *Sleep,* **16,** 333–343.

Kupfer, D. J., Frank, E., McEachran, A. B., *et al* (1990) Delta sleep ratio. *Archives of General Psychiatry,* **47,** 1100–1105.

Kupych-Woloshyn, N., MacFarlane, J. & Shapiro, C. M. (1993) A group treatment approach for the management of insomnia. *Journal of Psychosomatic Research,* **37,** 39–44.

Lauber, J. K. & Kayten, P. J. (1988) Sleepiness, circadian dysrhythmia, and fatigue in transportation accidents. *Sleep,* **11,** 503–512.

Lavie, P. (1986) Ultrashort sleep-waking schedule III: 'Gates' and 'forbidden zones' for sleep. *Electroencephalography and Clinical Neurophysiology,* **63,** 414–425.

Leibenluft, E. & Wehr, T. A. (1992) Is sleep deprivation useful in the treatment of depression? *American Journal of Psychiatry,* **149,** 159–168.

Loomis, A. L., Harvey, E. N. & Hobart, G. (1937) Cerebral states during sleep as studied by human brain potentials. *Journal of Experimental Psychology,* **21,** 127–144.

McGregor, P. A. (1989) Updates in polysomnographic recording techniques used for the diagnosis of sleep disorders. *American Journal of EEG Technology,* **29,** 107–136.

——, Weitzman, E. D. & Pollak, C. P. (1985) Polysomnographic recording techniques used for the diagnosis of sleep disorders in a sleep disorders center. *American Journal of EEG Technology,* **21,** 1–13.

Mellman, T. A. & Uhde, T. W. (1989) Electroencephalographic sleep in panic disorder. *Archives of General Psychiatry,* **46,** 178–184.

Miles, L. E. M. & Wilson, M. A. (1977) High incidence of cyclic sleep/wake disorders in the blind. *Sleep Research,* **6,** 192.

——, Raynal, D. M. & Wilson, M. A. (1977) Blind man living in normal society has circadian rhythms of 24.9 hours. *Science,* **198,** 421–423.

Moldofsky, H., Musisi, S. & Phillipson, E. A. (1986) Treatment of a case of advanced sleep phase syndrome by phase advance chronotherapy. *Sleep*, **9**, 61–65.

Monk, T. H. (1991) Sleep and circadian rhythms. *Experimental Gerontology*, **26**, 233–243.

—— (1994) Shift work. In *Principles and Practice of Sleep Medicine* (2nd edn) (eds M. H. Kryger, T. Roth & W. C. Dement), pp. 471–476. Philadelphia: W.B. Saunders.

Montpaisir, J. Godbout, R., Pelletier, G., *et al* (1994) Restless legs syndrome and periodic limb movements during sleep. In *Principles and Practice of Sleep Medicine*, (2nd edn) (eds M. H. Kryger, T. Roth & W. C. Dement), pp. 589–597. Philadelphia: W.B. Saunders.

Nofzinger, E. A., Thase, M. E., Reynolds, C. F., *et al* (1991) Hypersomnia in bipolar depression: a comparison with narcolepsy using the multiple sleep latency test. *American Journal of Psychiatry*, **148**, 1177–1181.

Okawa, M., Mishima, K., Nanami, T., *et al* (1990) Vitamin B_{12} treatment for sleep-wake rhythm disorders. *Sleep*, **13**, 15–23.

Oswald, I. (1970) Sleep, the great restorer. *New Scientist*, **46**, 170–172.

Pankhurst, F. P. & Horne, J. A. (1994) The influence of bed partners on movement during sleep. *Sleep*, **17**, 308–315.

Parkes, J. D. (1985*a*) The parasomnias. In *Sleep and Its Disorders*, pp. 189–239, London: W. B. Saunders.

—— (1985*b*) Insomnia. In *Sleep and Its Disorders*, pp. 243–264. London: W. B. Saunders.

—— (1995) Sleep disorders. In *Medical Fitness to Drive* (ed. J. F. Taylor), pp. 94–95. London: Medical Commission on Accident Prevention.

Phillips, F., Chen, C. N., Crisp, A. H., *et al* (1975) Isocaloric diet changes and electroencephalographic sleep. *The Lancet*, *ii*, 723–725.

Rechtschaffen, A. & Kales, A.(1968) *A Manual of Standardized Terminology: Techniques and Scoring System for Sleep Stages of Human Subjects*. Los Angeles: UCLA Brain Information Service/Brain Research Institute.

Roehrs, T., Zorick, F. & Roth, T. (1994) Transient and short-term insomnia. In *Principles and Practice of Sleep Medicine*, (2nd edn) (eds M. H. Kryger, T. Roth & W. C. Dement), pp. 486–493. Philadelphia: W.B. Saunders.

Rosenthal, N. E., Joseph-Vanderpool, J. R., Levendosky, A. A., *et al* (1990) Phase-shifting effects of bright morning light as treatment for delayed sleep phase syndrome. *Sleep*, **13**, 354–361.

Schatzman, M. (1983) Sleeping on problems really can solve them. *New Scientist*, **99**, 416–417.

Shapiro, C. & Flanigan, M. J. (1993) Function of sleep: ABC of sleep disorders. *British Medical Journal*, **306**, 383–385.

Sharpley, A. L., Solomon, R. A. & Cowen, P. J. (1988) Evaluation of first night effect using ambulatory monitoring and automatic sleep stage analysis. *Sleep*, **11**, 273–276.

Sloan, E. P., Hauri, P., Bootzin, R., *et al* (1993) The nuts and bolts of behavioral therapy for insomnia. *Journal of Psychosomatic Research*, **37**, 19–37.

Spielman, A. J., Saskin, P. & Thorpy, M. J. (1987) Treatment of chronic insomnia by restriction of time in bed. *Sleep*, **10,** 45–56.

Stradling, J. R. (1993) Recreational drugs and sleep: ABC of sleep disorders. *British Medical Journal*, **306**, 573–575.

Strogatz, S. H. (1986) *Lecture Notes in Biomathematics: The Mathematical Structure of the Human Sleep-Wake Cycle*. Berlin: Springer-Verlag.

Strogatz, S. H., Kronauer, R. E. & Czeisler, C. A.(1987) Circadian pacemaker interferes with sleep onset at specific times each day: role in insomnia. *American Journal of Physiology,* **253**, R172–178.

Totterdell, P., Reynolds, S., Parkinson, B., *et al* (1994) Associations of sleep with everyday mood, minor symptoms and social interaction experience. *Sleep,* **17**, 466–475.

Trinder, J., Montgomery, I. & Paxton, S. J. (1988) The effect of exercise on sleep: The negative view. In: *Sleep and Exercise* (ed. C. M. Shapiro) *Acta Physiologica Scandinavica,* **133** (suppl. 574), 14–20.

Wadworth, A. N. & McTavish, D. (1993) Zopiclone: a review of its pharmacological properties and therapeutic efficacy as a hypnotic. *Drugs and Ageing,* **3**, 441–459.

Waters, W. F., Adams Jr., S. G., Binks, P., *et al* (1993) Attention, stress and negative emotion in persistent sleep-onset and sleep-maintenance insomnia. *Sleep,* **16**, 128–136.

Waterhouse, J. (1993) ABC of sleep disorders: Circadian rhythms. *British Medical Journal,* **306**, 448–451.

Webb, W. B. & Agnew, H. W. (1971) Stage 4 sleep: Influence of time course variables. *Science,* **174**, 1354–1356.

Weitzman, E. D. , Czeisler, C. A., Coleman, R. M., *et al* (1981) Delayed sleep phase syndrome: A chronobiological disorder with sleep-onset insomnia. *Archives of General Psychiatry,* **38**, 737–746.

Wever, R. A. (1979) *The Circadian System of Man.* New York: Springer-Verlag.

Williams, R. L., Karacan, I. & Hursch, C. J. (1974) *Electroencephalography (EEG) of Human Sleep: Clinical Applications.* New York: Wiley.

Zepelin, H. (1994) Mammalian sleep. In *Principles and Practice of Sleep Medicine* (2nd edn) (eds M. H. Kryger, T. Roth & W. C. Dement), pp. 69–80. Philadelphia: W.B. Saunders.

Zulley, J. (1980) Distribution of REM sleep in entrained 24 hour and free-running sleep-wake cycles. *Sleep,* **2**, 377–389.

26 Diagnosis, classification and measurement

Jeremy Pfeffer & George Stein

A brief history of psychiatric nosology • Uses and criticisms of diagnoses in psychiatry • Types of disorder definition • Hierarchies and comorbidity • Models of mental illness • Measurement • Structured clinical interviews • Screening • Devising a rating scale

---

The wit of man has rarely been more exercised than in the attempt to classify the morbid mental phenomena covered by the term insanity – the result has been disappointing... (Tuke, 1892).

A doctor's task is to diagnose and treat his or her patients. For the physician treating the physically ill, the suffering is generally obvious, there are often objective physical signs in addition to the presenting symptoms, and the diagnosis can usually be confirmed by special blood tests or X-rays. An appropriate physical remedy automatically follows on from the diagnosis. The physician is therefore less likely to worry about semantic issues concerning the nature of disease, or whether there are such entities as diseases, or whether he is merely treating a mild deviation from normality.

For the psychiatrist, because there are no physical signs or diagnostic tests, these issues assume greater importance yet are also more confusing. The diagnosis is based almost exclusively on the presenting symptoms, which may often blur imperceptibly into normality, and the constellation of presenting mental symptoms becomes almost synonymous with the disorder itself. Since aetiology is generally unknown psychiatrists have had to explore more deeply into the notions that underlie the concept of disease, how specific diseases should be defined, and the manner in which they are classified. These issues will be addressed in this chapter.

A brief history of psychiatric nosology

The ancient Greeks and Romans described five categories of mental disorder, these were distinguished on the basis of their phenomenology: phrenitis (delirium), mania, melancholia, hysteria and epilepsy. Hippocrates had even devised a system to describe Axis II disorders, i.e. the four temperaments; the choleric, sanguine, melancholic and phlegmatic (Frances *et al*, 1990). In the second century the Roman physician, Galen (circa 130–200 AD) switched the emphasis from phenomenology to aetiology. His system described three groups of disorders: the vesanias, which were caused by poisons; the lunacies caused by the phases of the moon, and the hereditary insanities. Whether classification should be based more on aetiology or phenomenology is an issue that has bedevilled classificatory schemes in psychiatry since the earliest of times.

Central to the problem of classification is the question of how diseases themselves are defined. There is little or no factual information about disease definition, and our understanding rests on the opinions of prominent physicians and philosophers. Both Kendell (1975) and Sartorius (1988) have traced the two main types of definition of disease back to the two ancient Greek schools of Plato and Aristotle. The School of Plato, the rationalists, maintained that disease entities had a real existence which was independent of the observer, and that these diseases could be described and classified. By contrast the school of Aristotle, and Hippocrates, maintained that the essence of medicine lay in careful clinical observation of the patient and that classification was of secondary importance. The abstract classes of the rationalists were only tools of the human mind, lacking in any independent existence (Sartorius, 1988). Even today the controversy continues, but the empiricists are now in the ascendent in most branches of medicine and psychiatry. This was not always the case and from the 17th to the first part of the 20th century Plato's school of rationalism was dominant. Sydenham believed that diseases were fixed entities comparable to plant species and could be classified in a similar way.

> Diseases are reduced to certain and determinate kinds with the same exactness as we see it done by botanic writers in their treatises on plants... Nature, in the production of disease is uniform and consistent, so much so, that for the same disease in different patients the symptoms are for the most part the same (Sydenham, quoted in Kendell, 1975).

Together with Willis (1682), Sydenham (1682) is credited with replacing the ancient 'humoral theory' with the concept of nervous disease.

An important influence in classification in the 18th century was the botanist Linnaeus who published *Systema Natura* in 1735; a system based on two principles. First, he proposed, species existed in nature, each constituting a finite stable category without continuity with others, and second, the discovery of the true categories could only be achieved by selecting the right criteria. Linnaeus tried to apply his method to medicine in *Genera Morborum* (1763) in which psychiatric cases were divided up into "Ideales", "Imaginari" and "Pathetici". However it was left to Boissier de Sauvages, the Professor of Botany at the Medical School in Montpelier, and William Cullen of Edinburgh to publish the first comprehensive medical nosologies. These adopted a botanical approach with classes, genera, and species. In his great textbook *Synopsis Nosologica Methodicae,* published in Latin in 1775, Cullen distinguished the local diseases (one class only) from the general diseases of which there were three classes. These were the pyrexias, neuroses, and "Cacquexias" (cachexias). The neuroses were general disorders but lacking fever, and there were four separate genera (subclasses), with each subclass having several different species. The subclasses of the neuroses were the Comata (Coma, apoplexy and paralysis); the adynamia (syncope, dyspepsia and hypochondriasis); the spasmii (tetanus, chorea, epilepsy and diabetes), and the vesaniae (the insanities).

Boissiers de Sauvages, writing at around the same time as Cullen, argued that symptoms rather than causes should form the basis of any classificatory scheme. In *Nosologica Methodica* (1768), he described over 2400 separate species of disease, most of which were little more than isolated symptoms (Temkin, 1968). This highly detailed scheme is mentioned because it represents an extreme example of another fundamental dilemma in psychiatric nosology. That is, is it better to have a large number of accurate descriptive categories, with the disadvantage of being more difficult to use and memorise; or is it preferable to rely on only a few categories and so make the scheme easier to use but less accurate. The trend in the more recent nosologies has been to favour greater descriptive accuracy with increasing numbers of categories even if this makes the schemes more complex; thus the DSM–I (American Psychiatric Association, 1952) had 106 categories, the DSM–II (1968) 182 categories, the DSM–III (1980) 265 categories and the DSM–III–R (1987) 292 categories (Frances *et al*, 1990).

The organic medical approach to psychiatry probably starts with Bayle (1822) who described general paralysis of the insane and "proved that insanity is sometimes the symptom of chronic inflammation of the arachnoid"; the concept that other brain lesions could cause insanity gradually took hold. Morel took a similar biological approach in writing about degeneracy in *Treatise on the Physical and Mental Degeneracies of Human Species* (1857). He classified mental disorders in a hierarchical way from the mildest, 'nervous temperament' to the most severe, 'idiocy'. These deviations were inherited, and he believed that degenerative influences tended to cumulate in successive generations, until they were finally extirpated by failure to reproduce. While the concept of 'degeneration' has been discarded, Jaspers (1913) points out that the current notion of endogeneity may originate from it.

With the discovery of the microscope and bacteria, the 'lesion' concept of disease came to greater prominence . Virchow, a German pathologist, emphasised the importance of an identifiable lesion or structural abnormality in the definition of disease.

> In my view the disease entity is an altered part of the body, in principal an altered cell or organ...that disease is a living entity, which has a parasitic relationship with the otherwise healthy body to which it belongs, and at the expense of which it lives (Virchow, 1895).

He used the word disease to apply to all those conditions which had a demonstrable lesion. If there was only altered function without any demonstrable abnormality the term 'disorder' was used. As no lesion has yet been identified for most psychiatric conditions, the DSM–IV (APA, 1994) describes only disorders, and not diseases. However, the lesion concept of disease remains very influential even today, for example, in modern biological psychiatry the search for the 'lesion' which causes schizophrenia, be it a gene, a pink spot in the urine, or some neuropathological abnormality in the temporal lobes, continues to have a dominant influence in research.

During the 19th century, eminent professors of psychiatry in the different European universities devised their own personal nosological schemes, in what Kendler (1991) has called 'the famous professor principle'. Boissier de Sauvages and Pinel in France tended to follow the Linnaean principle of disease species. Pinel's famous pupil, Esquirol (1838), emphasised the importance of clinical data such as age of onset or the course of illness as valuable additions to the cross-sectional description. In Germany, Griesinger (1845) put forward the principle of the *Einheit Psychose* or unitary psychosis, which proposed that all psychoses were simply different manifestations of the same single illness. In Munich, Kraepelin was the first to distinguish between manic depression and schizophrenia (which he called dementia praecox). He also devised an elaborate typology which lies at the basis of most modern psychiatric classificatory schemes.

Some of these 19th century schemes were better than others, notably that of Kraepelin (1896), but ultimately the authority of any scheme depended on the authority of its originator and was usually confined to one city or a region in one country. Different schemes held sway in different countries or even in different regions of the same country resulting in a balkanisation of psychiatric nosology. Many of the present day cross national differences in diagnostic practice can be traced back to the particular views of famous 19th century European professors.

In the 20th century there has been a huge proliferation of psychiatrists and according to Kendler (1990) the famous professor principle has been replaced by the 'committee of famous professors'. Thus, several hundred people were consulted in the drafting of the DSM–IV and ICD–10 systems (World Health Organization, 1992). Initially differences of opinion were settled either by consensus or by voting as in DSM–I (APA, 1952) and DSM–II (1968). A sweeping change of emphasis was made by the American Psychiatric Association when they sought to devise DSM–III (1980), to ensure that all the available scientific information was used to help frame the new nosology, rather than merely to rely on the views of important people.

The nature of disease: views of Scadding and Kraupl-Taylor

Recent psychiatric thinking on the nature of disease has been dominated by two contrasting definitions, that of Scadding in 1967 and Kraupl-Taylor in 1971. Scadding was a chest physician, who was primarily concerned with developing useful definitions of disease for chest medicine. Chest medicine, like psychiatry, has many non-specific symptoms such as cough, sputum, or shortness of breath, none of which are pathognomic of a single disease process, and may sometimes be quite normal. This makes the delineation of morbid disease processes more difficult. Scadding arrived at a definition of a 'particular disease' rather than 'disease in general' which he believed applied to all fields of medicine, including psychiatry as well as animal and plant diseases:

> A disease is the sum of all the abnormal phenomena displayed by a group of living organisms in association with a specified common characteristic by which they differ from the norm of their species in such a way as to place them at a biological disadvantage.

Essentially this definition implies the presence of a specific syndrome, which has harmful consequences. Scadding used the phrase 'abnormal phenomena' in two senses, first to describe qualitatively abnormal phenomena which do not occur in the healthy population, such as a shadow on the lung on chest x-ray, or in the case of psychiatry, persistent auditory hallucinations as occur in the psychoses. Abnormality in the second sense has a statistical meaning and refers to deviations from the norm, for example severe dyspnoea in the context of chest medicine or severe depression in psychiatry. These symptoms may occur mildly in normal populations, and it is only a quantitative difference that distinguishes the healthy normal population from those who are morbid and assigned a disease label (Goldberg, 1972).

The term 'biological disadvantage' was interpreted by Kendell (1975) to signify increased mortality and lowered fertility. However, for many of the milder neurotic illnesses or childhood psychiatric disorders there is little or no evidence indicating a change in either mortality or fertility and so, even though these disorders may cause concern, they fail to meet Scadding's criteria for disease.

The issue of 'causing concern' was first brought into the debate by Kraupl-Taylor, a psychiatrist who specialised in working with subjects with severe personality disorders, a group who are notoriously difficult to diagnose or treat. His definition of disease depended mainly on subjective criteria:

> The attributes of disease must be abnormal by the standards of the population or the norms of the individual and must be associated with at least three criteria: (a) therapeutic concern for the patient himself, experienced by the person (b) concern for him experienced by his social environment and (c) medical concern for him.

This definition was criticised by Kendell (1975) as amounting to almost a tautology "doctors treat diseases, therefore diseases are what doctors treat". Kendell also wrote that this definition of disease was far too flexible and so could alter with the fashion of the day and was at the whim of what patients, doctors or even what hospital administrators might consider to be worthy of treatment. Scadding (1990) was even more scathing in his criticism of this definition and believed that it was only possible to define a specific disease. Attempts at defining 'disease in general' were doomed to failure, rather like the problem faced by theologians who have tried without success for the last two thousand years to define the elusive concept of evil.

Despite these criticisms, Kraupl-Taylor's concept of 'concern' permeates most modern clinical definitions. For example, the definition of a 'disorder' in DSM–IV is:

> a clinically significant behavioural or psychological syndrome or pattern that occurs in a person and that is associated with present distress (painful symptoms) or disability (impairment in one or more important areas of functioning) or with a significant increased risk of suffering, pain, disability or important loss of freedom.

The judgement of whether a symptom is painful is made by the patient, and corresponds to criterion (a) in Kraupl-Taylor's definition. Also, although the phrase "impairment in one or more areas of function" is slightly different from Kraupl-Taylor's clause "concern for him, experienced by his social environment", the meaning is similar. Even a rigorous computer based diagnostic scheme such as the CATEGO relies ultimately on subjective criteria because many of the symptom definitions in the PSE Glossary (Wing *et al*, 1974) include the clause "and is distressing to the subject". Probably until more objective diagnostic tests are discovered, the definition of disease or disorder in psychiatry will continue to rely mainly on subjective criteria.

Uses and criticisms of diagnoses in psychiatry

The main uses of psychiatric diagnosis are listed in Box 26.1. A diagnosis may also have a therapeutic function. Many patients may like to have a diagnostic label as this gives meaning to their symptoms and it also verifies that they are suffering from an illness. There are, however, many criticisms of the value of diagnosis in psychiatry, and for routine clinical practice, its necessity can be questioned. Thus, a patient presents with depression and delusions and responds well to a neuroleptic and an antidepressant. A first doctor believes the diagnosis is schizophrenia, a second, psychotic depression, while a third elicits the features of schizoaffective disorder. Does it really matter what the actual diagnosis is? Kendell (1975) points out that because an accurate psychiatric diagnosis has relatively little bearing in determining treatment, and its power to predict the prognosis is poor, in psychiatry the diagnosis is relatively less useful than in other branches of medicine.

Psychotherapists, and particularly the depth psychologists, also criticise the use of psychiatric diagnoses on the grounds that they are far too reductionist and fail adequately to convey the essence of what may be a very complex human situation. Carl Jung, the Swiss psychoanalyst, even went so far as to declare that to talk of a science of individual psychology was a contradiction in terms (Akiskal, 1989). Those who follow Adolph Meyers' (1952) biographical approach believe that a patient's illness is but a single episode in the patient's life trajectory, which can only be understood in terms of his unique life history.

A further criticism is that having a psychiatric diagnosis may be a stigmatising process. Albee (1970) has pointed out that a diagnosis inevitably focuses on a patient's deficiencies rather than positive virtues, and most psychiatric diagnoses (some more than others) may have perjorative connotations. However, the stigma is usually more associated with being a psychiatric patient in the first place rather than the particular diagnostic label (Kendell, 1975). Also the degree of stigmatisation more fundamentally reflects the prevailing view of mental illness in society.

In busy clinical practice it is apparent that a diagnostic label is often used to justify a particular line of management. In this vein, Linder (1965) has argued that a diagnosis is not really a summary of the clinical information, nor an explanation of the condition, but rather a prescription for treatment. Thus, a patient presents with bizarre behaviour and hears voices. A psychiatrist makes a diagnosis of schizophrenia and this serves as a passport for immediate admission to hospital and the prescription of neuroleptics. If the same patient had also committed some crime the diagnosis of schizophrenia would save him from prison and punishment, and direct him to hospital and treatment. Linder (1965) argues that in most cases practical management considerations tend to dominate the diagnostic issue. Even though management based diagnosis can be observed in some busy clinical practices it leaves both the patient and the clinician open to exploitation and abuse. An extreme example of this occurred in the former Soviet Union where the government chose to silence political dissidents by locking them up in psychiatric institutions, and so psychiatrists were found, or coerced into supplying the necessary diagnostic label of schizophrenia to justify their actions (Bloch & Reddaway, 1984).

In addition, there are some psychiatrists, such as Szasz, who dislike diagnoses because they do not believe there is any such thing as mental illness. In *The Myth of Mental Illness* (1960), Szasz wrote:

Box 26.1. Important uses of psychiatric diagnosis

To plan treatment, management and other interventions for an individual patient

As a pre-requisite to understanding and therefore research

Epidemiological study of disease

As an approximate (though limited) guide to prognosis

To plan services

Accounting for the cost of psychiatric services (for particular categories) for both private insurance purposes and purchasing of services

---

Mental illness is a myth, psychiatrists are not concerned with mental illnesses and their treatment, in actual practice they deal with personal, social and ethical problems of living.

More recently he has restated the case that mental illness does not exist and in an oversimplistic manner argued;

if mental illnesses are diseases of the central nervous system, they are diseases of the brain, not the mind. While if mental illnesses are the names of misbehaviours they are behaviours and not diseases (Szasz, 1991).

Psychiatry, he maintains, is nothing more than the institutional denial of the tragic nature of life: "Individuals who want to reject the reality of free will and responsibility can medicalise life and thereby entrust its management to the health professionals". He believes that most psychiatric diagnoses are primarily driven by non-medical forces such as economic, personal, legal, social and political factors rather than being derived solely from clinical phenomena. There is some truth in this, particularly as recent research has demonstrated the importance of social factors. Mindham *et al* (1992) have rightly criticised Szasz, because he maligns psychiatrists by portraying them as the enemy of free will and personal responsibility. However, the main criticism of Szasz must be that by denying the existence of serious conditions such as schizophrenia or manic depression, by implication he denies the great suffering these illnesses inflict on patients and their families. On the other hand, Szasz may be right to draw attention to some of the more dubious areas of psychiatric practice in which a medical approach to many of society's ills such as juvenile delinquency, family problems or loneliness in old age may be quite inappropriate.

Why classify?

If psychiatric classification is so low in validity, so unreliable in quality, and of such little use in clinical situations, why should we bother to classify at all? The answer is quite clear: without some system of classification all psychiatric knowledge would be reduced to the memorisation of multiple single case histories, or as Cawley (in Mindham *et al*, 1992) put it "without categories or dimensions... We would be doomed to slosh around in impressionistic garbage". Classification is the mind's way of reducing the huge cognitive load of repetitive and broadly similar case histories. Classifying entails creating, defining or confining the boundaries of concepts. It is essentially a cognitive process, which can be found at every level of life, ranging from the early socialisation of a small child coping with everyday problems in life, all the way through to the development of a complex scientific theory (Jablensky, 1988). As well as having obvious logical advantages, Sokal (1974), one of the inventors of numerical taxonomy, believes that the ability to classify also confers some evolutionary advantage.

It may be appropriate here to provide some definitions of the terms used in describing classificatory systems. The term classification denotes "the activity of ordering or arranging objects into groups or sets on the basis of their relationships" (Sokal, 1974). The product of this process is called 'a classificatory system' while the act of assigning a particular object to one of the categories is known as identification. In medicine the process of identification is synonymous with diagnosis. According to Scadding (1992) diagnosis is:

> the process by which a patient's symptoms and signs are assessed and investigated with a view to the categorisation of his or her case with other cases of a similar sort which have been studied in the past, in order that the patient may benefit from the application of established knowledge to the problem.

The term 'taxonomy' refers to the studies of various strategies of classification, but in the medical domain, the word nosology is used instead. It denotes the system of concepts and theories that supports the strategy of classifying symptoms, signs, syndromes and diseases. Finally, nosography refers to the act of naming morbid conditions, and the names jointly constitute the nomenclature within a particular field of medicine (Jablensky, 1988).

What constitutes a good nosology?

Diagnostic criteria are used for two distinct yet related purposes, first to define mental disorders and, second, to diagnose individual cases. Werry (1992) has outlined what elements should go into a good nosology.

Reliability

This refers to the extent to which repeated measures of a relatively stable phenomenon fall closely to each other: repeatability and reproducability are alternative words which describe this property. The most common way to measure the reliability of a diagnostic definition is to assess the degree to which two raters can agree on the diagnosis in a series of cases. This is known as inter-rater reliability (see page 1255). In general, psychotic conditions such as hypomania have a high reliability while neurotic conditions which are rather harder to define have a lower interrater reliability. The authors of DSM–III took great pains to ensure that their definitions were written in a operational form and in a sufficiently clear language to ensure that reliability studies of the definitions could be undertaken.

Internal consistency

This is another type of reliability and refers to the degree of correlation that exists between the different elements of a definition. Not all symptoms need to be present at all times, but there should be some degree of what

Szatmari (1992) calls 'hanging together'. Modern polythetic diagnostic criteria often have a low internal consistency (see below).

Specificity

The separate elements in a good definition should tell not only what the diagnosis is, but also what it is not. For a physical illness such as lung cancer the boundary between the disorder and normality is obvious and even the distinction from a near neighbour, such as a benign tumour, is easily made. Boundaries between the severe psychoses and normality are also fairly clear but the boundaries separating the different psychoses, for example, between schizophrenia and schizoaffective disorder are more difficult to define. The boundaries between a neurotic condition and a personality disorder, and even normality, are less clearcut, because these conditions may lie on a continuum with normality at one end.

Kendell (1975) suggested that for an ideal discrimination, the phenomena that comprise diagnostic definitions for two separate disorders should be bimodally distributed in a population suffering from both disorders. There should also be a point of rarity in the middle establishing the boundary between the conditions (Fig. 26.1). If the distribution of the diagnostic elements of the two conditions shows a unimodal distribution, there is probably only one condition.

In his own well known studies of depression, Kendell (1968) tried to replicate the 'reactive/endogenous' dichotomy that had been described by the Newcastle School. However, he failed to establish a clear boundary between the two types of depression, as there was only a unimodal distribution of the clinical features, and so he concluded that while depression could vary in its severity, there was no support for the hypothesis of two separate disorders. Rosch (1976) has used the phrase "to carve nature at its joints" to describe an ideal situation in which disease categories are easily distinguished. Unfortunately, nature failed to give psychiatry many good joints, and among clinical populations a degree of overlap often occurs and comorbidity (making two or more diagnoses on the same subject) is a common finding.

More recently the authors of DSM–IV have acknowledged the problem of blurred boundaries between conditions and the difficulties in making diagnoses that fit exactly the definitions given in the manual:

> In DSM–IV, there is no assumption that each category of mental disorder is a completely discrete entity with absolute boundaries dividing it from other mental disorders or from no mental disorder. There is no assumption that all individuals described as having the same mental disorder are alike in all important ways. The clinician using the DSM–IV should consider that individuals sharing a diagnosis are likely to be heterogenous even in regard to the defining features of the diagnosis and that boundary cases will be difficult to diagnose in any but a probabilistic fashion (p. 22).

Validity (accuracy)

This refers to the degree to which the definition of an illness corresponds to the true state of affairs. Validity is straightforward to establish for a parameter that can be measured in the laboratory. For example, if a new technique for measuring serum lithium is discovered, it can be checked by calibrating the new technique against the old method with the same sample. Establishing valid definitions for the major mental disorders such as schizophrenia, has taxed the brains of many of the best psychiatrists for more than a century because there is no simple external calibration test for schizophrenia.

Validation for the definition of psychiatric disorders can only be demonstrated by several different and indirect avenues, for example, with epidemiological studies which show that cases fulfilling the criteria of the definition for the particular disorder can be found in the community; with prognostic studies, by showing that diagnoses tend to remain stable over time; and with treatment studies, to see if the response of groups defined in a particular way respond in a predictable manner to a given treatment.

Utility

This is a special and particularly important type of validity which poses the question "what use is the diagnosis in the real world?" Feinstein (1967) has pointed out that the end point of clinical medicine is the patient, and wrote "the care of the patient is the ultimate specific act that characterises the clinician". Any classificatory system that cannot assist a clinician to do that will fail to gain acceptance.

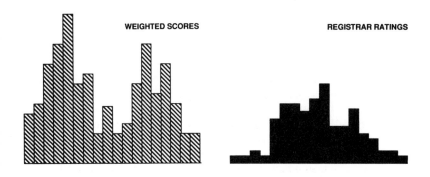

Fig. 26.1 Depression: one or two diseases? (*left*)Bimodal distribution of weighted depression scores from a series of Newcastle depressives (Carney *et al*, 1965). (*right*) Unimodal distribution of Maudsley registrar ratings of Kendell's depression index (Kendell, 1968, by permission of Oxford University Press).

Types of disorder definition

Operational definitions

The term 'operational definition' was originally coined by Bridgeman (1927), a physicist, and is defined as follows:

> An operational definition of a scientific term S, is a stipulation to the effect that S is to apply to all and only those cases for which performance of the test operation T, yields a specific outcome O.

The advantage of an operational definition is that provided operation T is described sufficiently clearly any person can apply it one or more times to confirm or refute the reliability of the definition S in a variety of different settings, or at different times.

Example

Operational definitions of psychiatric disorders are used in DSM–IV. They generally comprise three separate groups of items, although there may be any number of clauses. The first group of clauses usually gives a clinical description of the core features of the disorder, the second defines the severity or duration of the morbid phenomena which are required before it can be considered to be a significant clinical problem, while the final clauses describe the exclusion criteria, so that the condition can be more readily distinguished from its near neighbours. An example of such a modern operational definition for DSM–IV hypochondriasis is given in full below.

(1) Preoccupation with a fear of having, or the belief that one has, a serious disease, based on a person's misinterpretation of bodily symptoms. [This clause describes the core features of the disorder.]

(2) The preoccupation persists despite appropriate medical evaluation and reassurance. [This clause describes two specific operational tests, medical examination and reassurance, which should both be performed and found to be negative, to qualify for the diagnosis.]

(3) Belief in criterion (1) is not of delusional intensity (as in delusional disorder, somatic type), and is not restricted to a circumscribed concern about appearance (as in body dysmorphic disorder). [This is an exclusion clause and the two most important differential diagnoses, delusional disorder and body dysmorphic disorder are highlighted.]

(4) The preoccupation causes clinically significant distress or impairment in social, occupational or other important areas of functioning. [This clause describes the severity required for a significant clinical disorder. An identical clause is present in many DSM–IV definitions, particularly those where a milder version of the core feature of condition is common or may even be normal.]

(5) The duration of the disturbances is at least six months. [This clause describes the severity in terms of duration required for the diagnosis. Transient hypochondriacal feelings, particularly after an episode of flu or some other physical illness are relatively common, but these milder conditions are excluded by stipulating a six month period.]

(6) The preoccupation is not better accounted for by generalised anxiety disorder, obsessive–compulsive disorder, panic disorder, major depressive disorder, separation anxiety or another somatoform disorder. [This clause specifies what the condition is not, but might be confused with.]

Specify if with poor insight: if for most of the time during the present episode, the person does not recognise that the concern about having a serious illness is excessive or unreasonable.

[DSM–IV, more than ICD–10, has subtypes which are called specifiers for many of the disorders in the manual. In the case of hypochondriasis the specifiers are 'with poor insight' and 'with insight'.]

To qualify for a DSM–IV diagnosis of hypochondriasis, all the features 1–6 should be present.

Monothetic and polythetic diagnoses

The diagnosis of hypochondriasis is only made when all the criteria in the definition are present, i.e. a monothetic diagnosis. Monothetic criteria are easy to memorise and understand but their reliability will always depend on the reliability of the weakest item. A more serious disadvantage of monothetic criteria is that they fail to cope adequately with the varied presentation of many common psychiatric disorders. Thus, for many disorders only a few patients will have an identical clinical picture and fulfil the same diagnostic criteria, even though they probably suffer from the same underlying disorder.

To avoid this difficulty polythetic definitions may be used. According to Sokal (1974) a polythetic classification is one in which members of a class share a large proportion of their properties but do not necessarily agree on the presence of any one property. A typical polythetic definition comprises a list of all possible symptoms that a patient with a given disorder may have with the stipulation that a certain number of these items are required to make the diagnosis. For example, DSM–IV borderline personality disorder (see page 784) has nine items, of which five are required to make the diagnosis.

Polythetic diagnostic criteria have been likened to Chinese menus because in shorthand form they consist only of a set of numbers, and so making the diagnosis is rather like ordering a Chinese meal. Polythetic criteria are more robust and more reliable than monothetic criteria and they permit a considerably greater degree of diagnostic heterogeneity within a class. For example, there are 93 possible ways in which borderline personality disorder may present. For schizotypal disorder two patients may each satisfy diagnostic criteria yet fail to share a single clinical feature (Frances *et al*, 1990).

LEAD diagnosis

Because there is no ultimate criterion or 'gold standard' for making a diagnosis, Spitzer (1983) proposed a more modest standard, involving three components: Longitudinal, Expert and All Data. A more accurate diagnosis is made if longitudinal information is used and the information not confined to that obtained from a single cross-sectional interview. Experts are probably better than non-experts, and a consensus of experts may be better still in providing a more reliable diagnosis than a single expert. The use of All Data, from the patient, informants, and older case notes may further enhance diagnostic accuracy. LEAD diagnoses are probably the most accurate available, but apart from their use in nosological research they are too difficult and time consuming to adopt for routine clinical work.

Categories, dimensions and prototypes

A categorical approach assumes that all members of a class are relatively homogeneous in some chosen respect and that different classes are mutually exclusive. A nosological system should have sufficient categories to cover all possible disorders. A dimensional approach assigns positions on one or more axes (or dimensions), and it implies that index criteria are distributed in a continuum rather than in a binary, or all or none fashion. Assigning an item to a position on a dimension necessarily involves measurement, an operation that a busy clinician will rarely undertake.

Although the categorical approach is probably less accurate from the strictly scientific aspect, the bulk of clinical work involves making binary decisions, for example whether or not to admit to hospital, start treatment, discharge into the community, or support an insurance claim (Klerman, 1991). Clinicians therefore prefer diagnostic categories as these may be used to justify the many difficult decisions they must make. Kraepelin was the first to publish an extensive typology based on categories, but the DSM–IV and ICD–10 represent good modern examples of categorical schemes of classification.

Dimensions have the theoretical advantage that there is no loss of information and so maximum flexibility is preserved. There are no typical or atypical forms, rather most cases fall near the centre position, while the few outliers occupy the more extreme positions on the axis. Dimensions are favoured by psychologists as attributes such as intelligence, memory or personality traits are probably distributed in a continuum. Biostatisticians and psychopharmacologists conducting a drug trial also prefer a dimensional approach, because there is no loss of data. Psychotherapists use a dimensional approach because they view the psychopathology they uncover in their patients as being fundamentally similar in kind, though perhaps deviating in intensity or direction from the psychological processes present in normal people.

The third type of diagnostic definition is the prototypal categorisation. This classifies patients on the extent to which they resemble a prototypal description which includes the core features of the disorder. Descriptions found in textbooks of medicine adopt a prototypic approach and these are particularly useful in a training situation. A prototypic approach accepts that members of the class are heterogeneous and that border cases will be difficult to classify (Frances *et al*, 1990). Prototypic diagnoses resemble polythetic criteria but are less strict and accurate and are therefore less useful in research settings, for example in an epidemiological study there may be a genuine difficulty in deciding whether a case fulfils diagnostic criteria.

The International Classification of Diseases (ICD)

In 1853 at the International Statistical Congress in Paris, two medical statisticians, Jacques Bertillon from Paris, and William Farr from London, presented a list of the causes of death that became known as *Bertillon's Classification of the Cause of Death*. The International Statistical Institute revised this list every five years, and in 1899 the French Government took over this task, and published successive editions of the *International List of the Causes of Death*, which became the forerunner of the ICD. The World Health Organization (WHO) which came into being in 1948, revised this list, renaming it *The International Statistical Classification of Diseases, Injuries, and Causes of Death* (ICD–6) and this provided the first ever comprehensive nosology. Chapter V was entitled "Mental, Psychoneurotic and Personality Disorders" and covered psychiatric disorders. Approximately every 10 years since 1946 the ICD has been revised and the latest edition, ICD–10, was published by WHO in 1992.

ICD–10 represents a distillation of the efforts of some 700 psychiatrists in 52 countries. There has been cooperation with the American Psychiatric Association and many of the concepts which first appeared in DSM–III (1980), DSM–III–R (1987) and DSM–IV (1994) can be found in ICD–10. As with DSM–IV, the term 'disorder' is used throughout the text, to avoid the semantic issues associated with words like 'illness' or 'disease'. Similarly words with aetiological significance such as 'psychogenic' or 'psychosomatic' which were prominent in earlier classifications have been dropped from ICD–10. The main categories in ICD–10 are shown in Box 26.2. ICD–9 (WHO, 1978) and its predecessors made a firm distinction between neurosis and psychosis but this has been dropped in ICD–10. These words are still retained in the text but there is no attempt to define the two concepts.

An accompanying volume, the *Diagnostic Criteria for Research* (DCR–10), was published in 1993. This gives operational criteria for each condition described in ICD–10, written in such a way that they can be used for research. There was extensive collaboration with the APA Task Force so these definitions resemble those found in DSM–III–R and DSM–IV, although they are not always identical. This text also contains two annexes. The first annex describes five disorders whose clinical status it regards as presently uncertain, these being: seasonal affective disorder, bipolar II disorder, rapid cycling bipolar disorder, narcissistic personality disorder, and passive aggressive personality disorder. The second annex contains a fascinating and comprehensive account of the "culture bound syndromes" as they occur in different parts of the world.

Sartorius (1988) has spelled out the requirements of an international classification of disease. Apart from having acceptable validity and reliability it should be relatively simple, and easy to use by all those who deal with common psychiatric disorders. An international classification should never seek to displace a national or local scheme, but at the same time it should be sufficiently popular in a variety of countries on different continents. Because of this it should be written in a simple straightforward language as it will be translated into a multitude of different languages. In its content, it should be conservative, and both atheoretical and theoretically unenterprising so as to be acceptable to a wide variety of psychiatrists of different schools and cultures. Revisions should only be introduced when there is sufficient scientific evidence to justify the proposed changes, and successive revisions should occur infrequently, in order to preserve continuity for both scientific and economic reasons.

Box 26.2 The main categories in ICD–10

F.0 Organic mental disorders
F.1 Mental and behavioural disorders due to substance abuse.
F.2 Schizophrenic, schizotypal and delusional disorders
F.3 Mood (affective) disorders
F.4 Neurotic stress related and somatoform disorders
F.5 Behavioural syndromes and mental disorders associated with physiological dysfunction
F.6 Disorders of adult personality and behaviour
F.7 Mental retardation
F.8 Disorders of psychological development
F.9 Behavioural and emotional disorders with onset usually occurring in childhood or adolescence.

Diagnostic and Statistical Manual (DSM)

In contrast to the ICD, the DSM system is a national system and was developed by the American Psychiatric Association (APA) for use primarily in the USA. In 1917, the APA first adopted a classificatory scheme to obtain uniform statistics from American mental hospitals. This was replaced in 1934 by the American Medical Association's *Standard Classified Nomenclature of Disease* which contained 24 categories and was largely based on the sixth edition of Kraepelin's textbook. The first edition of the *Diagnostic and Statistical Manual of Mental Disorders* (DSM–I) was published by the APA in 1952, but it proved unsatisfactory. This was because it was heavily influenced by the then dominant American psychoanalytic movement and the description of reaction types of Adolf Meyer, and as a consequence was not widely adopted.

A reliability study of DSM–I concluded that two-thirds of all diagnostic disagreements between psychiatrists were the result of inadequacies in the classification itself (Ward *et al*, 1962). To remedy this situation the WHO commissioned a British psychiatrist, Stengel (1959), to examine the existing classificatory schemes, which he concluded were a "Tower of Babel". This review contained two important recommendations: first, since the widespread use of diagnostic terms with aetiological implications impeded agreement, there should be a set of neutral operational definitions which were primarily descriptive; second, these descriptive definitions should be incorporated in future editions of the ICD. The DSM–II was published in 1968 and represented a modest improvement, but the continued presence of both aetiological and phenomenological criteria in the definitions rendered it almost unusable.

A revolution in thinking on the definition of psychiatric disorders was initiated by Feighner and his colleagues at the Washington University in St. Louis, Missouri (Feighner *et al*, 1972). They published a set of diagnostic criteria for 15 major psychiatric disorders. These definitions were explicit, and were written in an unambiguous way, so that anyone could understand them and test their reliability. The Feighner criteria were the first modern operational criteria for psychiatric disorders. Around 75% of all psychiatric patients could be classified with these criteria, which were further refined in the Research Diagnostic Criteria (Spitzer *et al*, 1978). Around the same time the APA commissioned Spitzer and others to revise DSM–II with the stipulation that the new DSM–III should be atheoretical and adopt operational criteria to define psychiatric disorders. Some of these definitions proved unsatisfactory and were revised in DSM–III–R (1987). The preparation of the DSM–IV (1994) appears to have been a massive enterprise. A working group was designated for each clinical section and prepared 150 literature reviews on the clinical and diagnostic aspects of the various disorders. Data from published clinical studies were re-analysed, and field trials at 70 sites on more than 6000 subjects were conducted with the purpose of evaluating the proposed new diagnostic criteria. This huge quantity of data is presently in the process of being published in the five volume DSM–IV source book.

Multi-axial classification

Although the removal of any suggestion of aetiology from the definitions of psychiatric disorders helped to give more reliable definitions, it has led to an impoverishment in psychiatric diagnoses because of the loss of important clinical information which might explain why the patient had fallen ill at a particular point in time. A diagnosis based only on phenomenology is like an empty shell, and gives little clue about either cause, or future management. For example, a depression might be related to a marital breakdown, a longstanding personality problem, or the consequence of some serious medical condition. In order to ensure that this aetiological information could also be included in a nosological scheme, Essen-Moller & Wohlfahrt (1947) was the first to propose having a second axis, which described aetiology. Since then many different types of additional axes have been proposed and in a recent review Mezzick (1988) described 20 different diagnostic schemes, in which there were a total of 10 separate axes. DSM–IV has five axes:

Axis I – clinical syndromes
Axis II – developmental disorders and personality disorders
Axis III – general medical conditions
Axis IV – psychosocial and environmental problems
Axis V – global assessment or function.

ICD–10 is not officially designated as a multi-axial scheme. Thus the personality disorders are classified as mental disorders while the DSM system gives them a separate axis of their own.

However, the ICD–10 scheme also has an annex which it strongly recommends should be used. Within the annex are listed a wide variety of general medical conditions drawn from other sections of ICD–10 which may be relevant to psychiatric disorders, particularly endocrine, neurological and some cardiovascular and respiratory disorders. There are sections on "external causes of morbidity and mortality such as self-harm, poisoning, etc.," as well as a comprehensive list of social and psychosocial factors that might contribute to a psychiatric disorder. These items are not specified in the DSM–IV scheme.

ICD–10 also specifies that the severity and degree of handicap should be assessed according to *The International Classification of Impairments, Disabilities and Handicaps* (WHO, 1980). If all the separate categories in the main section of ICD–10, as well as the categories in the annexes are used, it effectively becomes a multi-axial scheme.

Hierarchies and comorbidity

It is a common clinical observation that some patients may have two or more psychiatric diagnoses. A patient with dementia develops delusions and then acts on them, behaving in a similar manner to a patient with schizophrenia. Are these two conditions independent or has one led on to another? Jaspers (1959) was the first to explicitly describe a diagnostic hierarchy that had probably been in use at the time of Kraepelin and possibly before. In this scheme, the more severe and pervasive disorder is regarded as primary and causal, and the less severe disorder as secondary. Organic disorder takes precedence over all other disorders, followed by schizophrenia, manic depression is at the third level, and finally at the fourth and lowest level are the neuroses and personality disorders. Thus, in a hierarchical system a patient with schizophrenia who also has affective features has a primary diagnosis of schizophrenia with the depression being considered secondary, and due to the schizophrenia.

In general, the rule of a hierarchy is that any given diagnosis excludes the presence of all diagnoses higher up in the hierarchy but may include any that are lower down (Kendell, 1975). Most psychiatrists use diagnostic hierarchies in their day to day work (often without realising it) and direct their therapeutic efforts towards the condition which they believe is the primary disorder. Thus, it would be a clinical error to offer only counselling or a course of anxiety management to a patient who had both anxiety and schizophrenia, without treating the underlying schizophrenia. Gruenberg (1969) believed that diagnostic hierarchies were primarily a defensive strategy employed by psychiatrists to preserve the treasured principle of a single diagnosis, particularly when confronted with a confusing mass of clinical information.

An interesting hierarchical classification scheme was developed by the clinical psychologist Foulds at a time when the existing psychiatric nosologies were less satisfactory than they are today. He proposed a continuum of the major classes of 'personal illness' arranged by "increasing degrees of failure to maintain or establish mutual personal relationships". In his system there were four classes of "increasing degrees of adverse change in the person" (Foulds, 1965). At the lowest level were the dysthymic states, which included states of elation, anxiety and depression and individuals falling into one of these states were "emotionally stirred up, but understandably so, and dysthymic states probably merge into normality". At the next level were the neurotic symptoms, dissociation, fear, compulsion and rumination. Using Foulds' terminology, "here the subject is in a state of distance in that he views a part of his behaviour and experiences as alien to himself". In the third level are integrated delusions which include delusions of grandeur, persecution or contrition (depressive delusions). This class refers to persons "who are distorted, warped or grossly changed from their normal selves". Finally, in the fourth and highest class are those with the "delusions of disintegration" as occur in schizophrenia when "the individual has lost the concept of himself as an agent of his own actions, feelings or thoughts".

To follow the rule of the hierarchy a patient has symptoms in his or her own class and may also have those at a lower level but not at a higher level. To test the validity of this model, Foulds & Bedford (1975) developed a questionnaire, *The Delusion, Symptoms and States Inventory,* incorporating the above symptoms, and found that 93% of 480 patients had a symptom pattern which conformed to the model. The scheme is rarely used in clinical practice, but it has attracted some research interest. Sturt (1985) in a study of the way in which PSE symptoms and syndromes aggregate together has shown that Foulds' hierarchy is an example of a very much more general principle of symptom association.

Symptoms do not aggregate randomly but rather into classes based on prevalence. The higher classes tend to have the rarer symptoms, but because each symptom is strongly associated with total symptom score, there is a tendency for the less frequent higher class symptoms to be associated with the symptoms of the lower classes as well. Sturt's (1985) observations that higher class symptoms tended to occur commonly with lower class symptoms, but the reverse pattern of lower class symptoms being rarely associated with higher class symptoms is similar to the pattern found in hierarchies, such as that described by Foulds. However Sturt points out there is no need to postulate a hierarchical model to explain this.

Comorbidity

Diagnostic hierarchies have the drawback that they make the unproven assumption that one disorder is more fundamental, pervasive or primary than another. Sometimes this may be true, but more often than not it is very difficult to make this distinction. For example, anxiety and depression commonly occur together and it is often impossible to decide which is primary and which secondary. Comorbidity makes no assumption as to cause and effect but merely documents that two or more disorders have been simultaneously diagnosed in the same individual. In contrast to hierarchies, comorbidity offers an atheoretical approach and this has found increasing favour in modern systems such as the ICD–10 and DSM–IV. A diagnostic approach which uses comorbidity is more reliable, and is associated with less loss of information, but on the other hand multiple diagnoses are more common, and an increased number of diagnostic categories are required to describe clinical phenomena.

In their comprehensive review, Caron & Rutter (1991) point out that as well as true comorbidity, there may be what they term 'false comorbidity' as a result of detection artefacts. The most common explanation for false comorbidity is that subjects with multiple diagnoses are more severely ill and are therefore more likely to be referred to a specialist centre. As a result true comorbidity cannot be studied in a clinic population but only in an epidemiological community survey.

A second reason for false comorbidity is that the definition of disorder may be so fundamentally flawed that only a few subjects fulfil the diagnostic criteria of just one disorder. An example of this may be the categorical definitions of personality disorder found in DSM–III–R and DSM–IV. Surveys have shown that perhaps a majority of subjects with personality disorders qualify for two or more different DSM–III–R personality disorder diagnoses. This does not imply there are two or more personalities but rather that the present definitions fail to adequately describe clinical reality. It may be that this can never be satisfactorily accomplished with a categorical system and a dimensional approach would be more satisfactory.

A third cause of false comorbidity is that the same item may appear in several different diagnostic categories. Anxiety and depressed mood are rather non-specific symptoms which occur widely. With increasing severity of disorder the more non-specific symptoms tend to occur together as noted by Sturt (1985) and this will also tend to increase the probability that a given patient will fulfil criteria for more than one disorder. A fourth cause of false comorbidity is an artificial subdivision of disorders, for example in the DSM–IV scheme, general anxiety disorder is separated from panic disorder but many individuals are comorbid for both conditions, indicating that there may not be a significant boundary between the two disorders in clinical populations.

True comorbidity

True comorbidity, which is established in an epidemiological survey, also has a variety of differing causes, apart from the simple hierarchical mechanism that a more pervasive or severe disorder is primary and has caused the less severe disorder. For example, different disorders may share common risk factors. Thus, depression and somatisation disorder occur more frequently than expected by chance. A possible explanation for this might be that life events are known to trigger both conditions and they may also share a common genetic predisposition. In other cases one disorder creates an increased risk for another through a variety of different mechanisms. An example of this is the increased incidence of schizophrenia among those with substance abuse which was demonstrated in the ECA study (Boyd *et al*, 1984).

A detailed clinical study of a group of individuals with both schizophrenia and substance misuse might reveal several different subgroups. Some subjects with schizophrenia may have found that substances such as cannabis or opium gave symptomatic relief. Another group drift into poor inner city areas where substance abuse is endemic, they mix with equally impoverished drug addicts and because they are susceptible, individuals begin to take drugs without becoming truly addicted and so the association is more coincidental than causal. A third group of subjects with apparent schizophrenia take amphetamines and it is only after admission to hospital that withdrawal of the amphetamines reveals an underlying personality disorder with drug abuse, and that the psychosis and schizophrenia-like picture is drug induced and secondary. If only a hierarchical explanation is applied then the schizophrenia would be regarded as the primary condition and substance abuse as the secondary disorder. A unitary explanation of this type fails to describe the complex situation found in clinical practice. Comorbidity makes no such assumptions and is therefore a much more flexible way of describing the association between disorders, particularly when the underlying mechanisms are complex or poorly understood.

Models of mental illness

Psychiatry is a broad discipline, encompassing many widely different schools of thought and philosophies. However, it has always been a clinical discipline and a branch of medicine and so the medical model, with its parallels to physical disorder, remains central. At the turn of the century, Freud discovered psychoanalysis, which at the time was a revolutionary way of treating psychological disorder, and with it came an elaborate theory of aetiology and the psychodynamic model of causation. In the early 20th century Watson discovered the principles of behavioural psychology and his ideas were further developed by Wolpe, Marks and others who showed that behavioural psychotherapy could rapidly cure conditions previously thought to be incurable. The behaviourists also developed their own behavioural model based on learning theory. More recently sociologists, such as Brown & Harris (1978) have convincingly demonstrated that most non-psychotic depression found in the community is caused more by recent life events and current external social factors than by psychodynamic or biological factors. A change in the social environment may often lead to a resolution of the disorder, and they have proposed a social model for causation.

The medical, psychodynamic, behavioural, and social models provide contrasting insights into the causation of mental illness and are all useful. No model can be completely true, and none are even verifiable, yet all survive mainly because each makes a valuable contribution to the management of individual patients. The following case example illustrates how the different models work in practice.

> *Case example*
> Jane was a pretty 29-year-old divorcee who lived with her two small children and a cat in a second floor council flat. She presented to the psychiatric clinic, saying she could no longer cope because she was feeling so depressed. Over the last six months she had had poor sleep, weight loss, poor appetite, difficulties in concentrating, panic attacks and recurrent thoughts of death. She was also very frightened to venture out of the flat, either to go to the supermarket, or to meet people socially. Her agoraphobia was sometimes so severe that the family occasionally went hungry, partly because there was no money, but also because she could not make it to the local supermarket.

Her early family life had not been happy, her father had been a difficult man who drank heavily and in his drunken state would sometimes beat her mother. He had never attacked the patient or sexually abused her but he could be verbally and emotionally abusive to her, particularly when drunk. His mother (the patient's grandmother) had committed suicide in late life. To escape from this unhappy home, when she was 17 years old Jane ran off with a man called Peter, who incidentally had the same name as her father. She had her first child by him but the marriage soon broke down and this was followed by a series of relationships with men characterised by violence and brutality. Her last relationship, which ended eight months previously, had been with a rather more gentle person who got on well with the children, and was also called Peter, but curiously while she was with this man she herself became aggressive and then ended the relationship.

The family lived in unsatisfactory housing conditions in a one bedroom flat on the third floor of a block of flats. There was a leak in the ceiling, so that whenever the old man in the flat upstairs took a bath, water would drip down on to the dining room table. Jane had financial difficulties and depended entirely on state benefits, and in a tearful state she produced a gas bill of £75 which threatened disconnection. Until one year previously she had worked as a legal secretary, however, a childminder had let her down badly with her younger child. As a result of this episode, and since the difference between her salary and state benefits was too small to make it worth her while to go out to work, she decided it made more sense for her to stop work and stay at home with the children.

The medical model

Clare (1986) has identified the particular characteristics of the medical model as follows: specific aetiology, predictable course, manifestations described in terms of symptom and signs, and a predictable outcome which can be modified by specific treatments. In Jane's case the psychiatrist, using a medical model, makes a diagnosis of depressive illness (she fulfils all the criteria for DSM–IV major depression, i.e. depressed mood with five out of nine key symptoms). Aetiology was mainly genetic, the father drank heavily probably as a result of depression, and the patient's grandmother had committed suicide suggesting an affective disorder in the family. Treatment should start with an antidepressant but if the depression fails to respond to a full course of this then another drug should be tried, and ECT might be considered. There are obvious psychosocial problems and so the patient is referred to the hospital social worker for counselling.

The behavioural model

Behavioural models look no further than the symptoms. Eliminating the symptoms will eliminate the neurosis. There is no underlying disease (Clare,

1986). The patient's symptoms have developed through a process of maladaptive learning and they persist because they have other beneficial effects or they may help avoid negative effects. Treatment will involve trying to reverse the faulty learning, by using behaviour therapy.

Jane has many problems, but the psychiatrist with a behavioural approach regards her agoraphobia as being of central importance. It handicaps her greatly because it impairs her ability to deal with day to day existence, such as dealing with the gas bill or shopping for food. Treatment involves a course of exposure *in vivo* with a nurse behaviour therapist. The nurse trains Jane in a series of tasks of increasing complexity, accompanying her initially to go out of the house, then to go to small shops, the supermarket and so forth. An antidepressant may be used in conjunction with the behaviour therapy because this sometimes helps. Cognitive therapy also proves helpful (see chapter 6) and through her own efforts Jane successfully overcomes her phobia. This gives her self-confidence a tremendous boost and she is then in a much better position to resolve all her other difficulties.

The social model

The social model highlights the manner in which an individual functions or rather fails to function in the social system. Patients become ill because bad things happen to them (adverse life events). They are even more likely to fall ill if they are in a lowly position in the social hierarchy, or are unable to share their difficulties in a close confiding relationship or suffer from some other specific vulnerabilities. Brown & Harris (1978) have specified more precisely what these vulnerabilities are (see page 131). The role of intangible biological predispositions or unobservable unconscious psychodynamic conflicts have little relevance in the social model.

Jane has many vulnerability factors: unemployment, poor housing, poverty and a lack of a close confiding relationship. The present episode was probably triggered by a cascade of recent life events which, in her case, were the loss of her job, disappointment with her childminder, and the break up of a recent relationship. Threats to daily existence such as having the gas supply disconnected and a leaky ceiling are much more potent causes of distress than long-term psychological difficulties. Neither an antidepressant, nor psychoanalysis will help settle the gas bill or stop the ceiling from leaking. Treatment involves trying to manipulate the social environment to the patient's advantage. Much of this can be done by a skilled social worker and the intervention of a medical practitioner is rarely required. Appropriate letters are sent to the gas board and housing authorities and the gas board makes an arrangement for her to pay off her bill at the rate of £1 a week. A few weeks later Jane is rehoused in an attractive two bedroomed ground floor maisonette. The children love the garden and she is elated. With her confidence restored she finds a job in the local supermarket and this has the twin beneficial effects of providing her with employment and helps her to conquer her agoraphobia.

Studies by Bebbington *et al* (1981) and others have demonstrated that the vast majority of depressive episodes in the community resolve because the patient has experienced positive life events, such as making new relationships, improved housing and so forth. Medical or psychiatric intervention only appear to have a marginal effect on the small minority of episodes which reach clinical attention and probably make little impact on the overall pattern of morbidity.

The psychodynamic model of causation

The psychodynamic model of causation places greatest emphasis on the experiences of early childhood. Early deprivation or distorted relationships during childhood particularly if combined with some biological vulnerability may result in developmental fixations. Later in life patients are unaware of the conflicts lurking within them, because these are largely unconscious. Conflicts are usually between the internal representations of the parents (or other important figures from early life) and the instinctual forces (the id) together with the pressing demands of the outside world and these conflicts provide a continual source of pressure on the patient's ego. For most of the time the patient's ego is able to withstand these pressures and conflicts, but sometimes the ego breaks down and this results in symptoms. These symptoms may have a particular symbolic meaning for the individual patient.

Perry *et al* (1987) suggests that a psychodynamic formulation aims to identify and understand the central conflicts which govern a patient's life and which under certain circumstances make the patient ill. A useful psychodynamic formulation should also try to make predictions with regard to therapy, particularly on the nature of the transference. Therapy consists of exploring the meaning of events, feelings, impulses, and present behaviours in the context of past or forgotten events or experiences, and this is done mainly through transference. Tyrer & Steinberg (1987) sum up the psychodynamic model: "how we feel and what we do are influenced powerfully by strongly competing forces which are largely unconscious and forged from past relationships as well as from our innate biology". It should be noted that there are many different psychodynamic models; some are based on ego psychology, others on object relations theory, and the reader is referred to psychoanalytic texts for more detailed accounts.

In Jane's case, the central conflict probably lies in her ambivalent relationship towards her father, and this extends to men in general. Her depressions serve as a defence against her tremendous but unconscious rage which is directed against her father for abusing both her and her mother during childhood. The phobia is also a defence against this rage as it prevents her going out into the street and screaming out about it. Beneath this more obvious anger, there is a suggestion possibly of some residual affection for her father because some of her lovers have the same name as her father. By continuing to consort with brutal men she is able through the mechanism of projective identification to only experience the violence as coming from men, and is thus not aware of her own aggressive and hostile impulses. When these do become manifest, in a relationship with a more caring person, it is all too much for her and the relationship has to be broken off. Although there is some superficial resemblance to sado-masochism, the pattern is more one of a repetitive fixation, and Jane is desperate to change the pattern which has brought her so little happiness.

The psychodynamically orientated psychiatrist postulates that unless Jane makes some attempt to grapple with her more fundamental relationship difficulties she will just continue to lurch from one unsatisfactory relationship to another, social crises and depression will inevitably follow on after each break-up repeating the pattern of the last decade. To focus solely on present day problems will help little in the long term and may even make matters worse by fostering dependency. Only psychodynamic psychotherapy which explores the previous relationship pattern and its links with her unhappy childhood has any chance of altering the maladaptive behaviour.

The eclectic model

The term 'eclectic' is derived from the Greek; according to the Oxford English Dictionary it was "the distinguishing epithet of a class of philosophers who neither attached themselves to any recognized school nor constructed independent systems, but selected such doctrines as pleased them in every school". Similarly eclectic psychiatrists have no particular theoretical model of their own, and do not adhere to any of the models described above, but use all the models of aetiology as the clinical situation demands.

Some eclectic psychiatrists believe in everything and others in nothing. Thus a young enthusiastic eclectic psychiatrist might believe that all the previously described models make a useful contribution in explaining Jane's illness. Treatment starts with antidepressants, and her agoraphobia is treated by a nurse therapist with behaviour therapy. Letters are sent to the housing authorities and the gas board on Jane's behalf, and once the depression and the immediate crises are resolved Jane is referred for more intensive psychodynamic psychotherapy. A rather older, and perhaps more nihilistic eclectic psychiatrist maintains that the cause of most psychiatric disorder is essentially unknown, and that there is little in the way of effective treatment. Most patients improve by virtue of their natural history – usually without any intervention. He thinks that Jane has an essentially good prognosis and so does little apart from offer her a follow up appointment in a few months time. Cox (1992) has recently suggested that part of the skill of a good general psychiatrist is to be able to move flexibly, during the treatment programme, between the different aetiological models in an individual case and between different cases, as well as knowing when it is wisest not to intervene at all.

Measurement

> When you can measure what you are speaking about, and express it in numbers you know something about it, but when you cannot measure it, when you cannot express it in numbers your knowledge is of a meagre unsatisfactory kind; it may be the beginning of knowledge but you have scarcely in your thoughts advanced to the stage of science whatever the matter might be (Sir William Thomson (Lord Kelvin), 1889).

Measurement is concerned with the process of assigning numbers to objects or observations so that these numbers can then be subjected to mathematical or statistical analysis with the aim of summarising a large quantity of information. It is then possible to make inferences and draw conclusions and in this way learn more about the original items or observations (Peck & Shapiro, 1990). In the practice of clinical psychiatry, measurement is a rather less useful tool than in other branches of medicine, but three important uses have been identified. Probably the most important application is in assessing the severity of mental symptoms so that any changes occurring as a result of treatment may be quantified. A second use has been in the development of screening instruments to help identify psychiatric cases in particular populations. This may help in service planning, for example, to detect the size of an alcohol problem in a community. Third, diagnostic instruments may help identify subjects with a particular disorder. Thus, even if a disorder has not been particularly well defined, a rating scale or diagnostic interview may help sharpen the accuracy of the diagnosis and so contribute to the debate surrounding the definition of a particular disorder (Murray & Mann, 1986).

While rating scales are most often used in research, all clinicians should be familiar with their content if only so they can interpret published drug trials and other treatment studies. This is because the outcome variable in almost all treatment studies is some sort of rating scale. Specific rating scales for each disorder are included in the relevant chapters in this book. The section below focuses on more theoretical aspects of rating scales, diagnostic interviews and screening instruments. Comprehensive accounts of psychiatric rating scales including descriptions of the individual scales are given in Thompson (1989), Peck & Shapiro (1990) and Bech *et al* (1993).

Theoretical aspects of rating scales

Reliability

Possibly the best way of assessing the reliability of an observer rating scale is by the inter-rater reliability. In this method, two or more observers examine the same material or events, for example, a video interview, and the degree of agreement between the ratings of the two observers on a range of items is calculated. Three types of statistical coefficients are used to measure inter-rater reliability. These are percentage agreement, Cohen's kappa (1960), and the intra-class correlation coefficient. Percentage agreement is the simplest but also the least satisfactory, because it ignores the possibility of chance agreements between observers, and for common conditions the possibility of a chance agreement is quite high. A rather better measure is Cohen's kappa which takes into account that some of the observed agreement might have happened by chance. It is a chance-corrected measure of agreement with a statistical base that takes into account the size of the population studied.

It is important to note that while some disagreements between two raters might be quite trivial, other types of disagreement may be more serious. To deal with this, it is possible to assign different weights to different types of disagreement, and a statistic known as weighted kappa (Cohen, 1968) may be used. Thus, for example, in a study of the reliability of the definitions of symptoms in the Present State Examination, Kendell *et al* (1968) assigned a weight of '4' to serious disagreements, for example, if the two raters disagreed on whether a symptom was present or not, but only '2' if the disagreement was less serious, for example, if the raters disagreed about the severity of the symptoms. Appropriate mathematical formulae for calculating kappa and weighted kappa are given in Bartko & Carpenter (1976). Kappa and weighted kappa are useful statistics for assessing the reliability of categorical information but cannot be used for dimensional data. For quantitative data, the degree of agreement is measured with the intraclass correlation coefficient.

A second method of testing reliability is the test-retest reliability. In this method an identical measure is applied to the same group of subjects under similar conditions but at two different times. There is no standard interval between the two measures but three weeks is generally taken as an acceptable time gap. This technique is helpful in assessing the reliability of instruments which measure relatively stable psychological characteristics, such as memory or intelligence, but is not so useful for gauging the reliability of psychiatric instruments, because mental disorder fluctuates over time.

Split-half reliability

The classical way of assessing split-half reliability is to divide the rating scale into two halves, either the upper half or the lower half, or by comparing odd-numbered items with even-numbered items. Both halves of the scale are administered to the same group of subjects under similar circumstances and a correlation between the scores of the two half scales is calculated. If the items are measuring the same characteristic then a high correlation between the two halves would be expected. There are many different ways of splitting a scale and theoretically there are many different split-half reliabilities. Cronbach's co-efficient α (Cronbach, 1951) reduces this problem by providing an estimate of the average correlation between all possible ways of splitting the items (Peck & Shapiro, 1990).

Validity

Establishing validity for a rating scale is a much greater problem than demonstrating reliability. This is because psychiatric disorders are not only difficult to define but they also lack any external validation criterion, such as blood glucose for diabetes. Several different types of validity are described, each of which makes some contribution to the general assessment of validity.

Face validity refers to whether on superficial examination the items in the scale appear to be covering the characteristic of interest. Face validity is of interest to a researcher who needs to select the most appropriate scale for the condition being studied. A study can best be interpreted with a working knowledge of the face validity of the scale in question and so it is useful to read papers on most of the commonly used scales.

Content validity is a similar but more detailed type of face validity. When a new scale is being devised, care is taken to ensure that all aspects of the phenomenon to be measured are sampled in a proportionate manner. Significant features should not be omitted, but nor should undue prominence be given to any one particular aspect of the disorder. Getting the balance or the content validity correct is a major preoccupation for those who devise rating scales. Later on, investigators using the scale may find that one or other aspect of the disorder has been given greater weight in a particular scale. For example, the Hamilton Scale (1960) tends to emphasise the biological symptoms of depression, while the Beck Scale (Beck *et al,* 1962) focuses more on depressive thoughts and cognitions. Face validity and content validity are important but cannot be measured.

Construct validity can be measured, and entails measuring concurrent validity and in a few instances predictive validity. Concurrent validity is the most commonly used method and provides the acid test of whether a new scale truly measures what it claims to measure. The scores on the new scale are correlated against the scores on some well established instrument which has also been given to the same population. Thus, a new depression scale might be correlated with the Hamilton rating scale. There are very few scales which have any predictive validity or even attempt prediction. One example is the Newcastle scale for predicting the outcome of ECT (Carney *et al,* 1965). Incremental validity refers to the question of whether a scale 'works' better than already existing or simpler measures, i.e. whether there is any advantage to the new more complicated method as compared to existing methods (Peck & Shapiro, 1990). As one can imagine, those who devise new scales rarely seek to assess incremental validity for fear of finding a negative result.

Validity and reliability are separate yet related concepts. To be valid a scale must always be reliable but the converse is not necessarily true. Thus, a perfectly reliable scale may not be valid as it might be measuring something quite different from the target disorder in question.

Individual items

Most scales are used to measure the severity of individual symptoms or disorders while a few observer rater interviews are primarily concerned with making psychiatric diagnoses. The core content of most of the individual items in a scale or interview are generally derived from familiar items in the mental state. Two methods are used for scoring, the most common being the Likert method (Likert, 1932), and the second, rather less commonly used, linear analogue scales.

Likert scales are categorical scales with which the respondent has to choose from a series of four or five statements and report exactly which statement is the best fit. Linear analogue scales consist of 10 cm lines with words describing the extremes placed at opposite ends, for example, happy/ sad, calm/tense. Subjects mark on the line how they currently feel. The method is useful for following rapid changes in mood and the assessment of pain.

Scoring on a Likert scale

Even though an item on a Likert scale may be strictly defined, for example, a symptom is present or absent, in practice most significant psychopathology is rather less clearly defined. For example, it may be quite difficult to assess whether a patient's feelings of guilt qualify as morbid guilt or not, and in practice such absolute or dichotomous decisions are difficult to make. Hamilton (1960) was one of the first to introduce an intermediate category of 'doubtful' for rating symptoms, suggesting a three point scale, 'absent, doubtful and present'. Most of the more recently devised interview schedules include a 'doubtful', 'possible' or 'probable' category which is always distinguished from the 'definitely present' category.

Although differences in severity occur in clinical populations, assigning a numerical value to different degrees of severity is quite arbitrary. A five point Likert scale based on adjectives is often used: 0 = absent; 1 = present, but mild; 2 = moderate; 3 = marked; 4 = severe. The very arbitrary nature of such a scale is obvious and there is no way of knowing whether the increment between 0 and 2 is half as much as the increment between 2 and 4 (Thompson, 1989). By contrast, in a physical disorder such as hypertension an increment of 5mm of blood pressure will have a similiar meaning regardless of the baseline level.

Another method of rating severity relies on a subjective estimate of the duration of symptoms but this method is also based on adjectives. For example, the Zung (1965) depression scale requires the subject to rate symptoms as 0 = never present; 1 = present some of the time; 2 = often present; 3 = always present. This method also makes unwarranted assumptions such as equating the difference between never and some of the time (0–1), with the difference between often and always (2–3). If there are too many rating points, even skilled raters cannot make a reliable distinction between the different points on the scale, while the presence of too few points renders the scale liable to errors of the central tendency. It is generally suggested that five to six points are optimal (Thompson, 1989).

How useful is an individual item?

This can be assessed in two ways.

Calibration – Does the item occur frequently enough in the population for which the scale is intended to warrant inclusion. An arbitrary cut-off of 10% has been suggested in the past.

Internal consistency – The item should correlate reasonably well with the total score. The item–total correlation provides a measure of internal consistency and to test for this each item is correlated with the total score. Items which correlate very poorly with the total score should probably be dropped from a scale designed to rate the severity of a disorder. On the other hand they should be retained in a more diagnostically orientated interview because an unusual symptom may have great diagnostic significance.

The paradox of internal consistency is that if the items are too highly inter-correlated they are redundant, that is they give no more information than one single item. On the other hand, a very low degree of item–total correlation indicates a lack of common dimension. In practice most items will have a moderate correlation with the total score.

Time frames

Psychiatric disorder is often transient, lasting for a few weeks or months, although for some conditions such as the personality disorders it may be lifelong. It is therefore essential for the instructions to specify the time frame that the scale refers to. A fluctuating condition such as anxiety might best be measured with a visual analogue scale requiring subjects to respond as they feel 'right now'. Daily ratings are commonly used in behavioural diaries or scales such as the Moos Menstrual Distress Questionnaire (Moos, 1968) in which the patient's feelings for each day are summarised. The time frame adopted for most rating scales is usually the previous three days, but some scales suggest a longer time frame, for example, the PSE rates symptoms over the last month.

Item bias

Different scales may all intend to measure the same condition but a more detailed scrutiny shows that they are actually measuring different facets of the disorder. Depression is a case in point; thus the Hamilton Rating Scale (1960) and Montgomery–Åsberg Scale (1979) are heavily weighted to the biological symptoms of depression. On the other hand, more than 50% of the score on the Beck Depression Inventory relates to cognitive items such as depressive thoughts of helplessness, hopelessness, guilt and indecisiveness, all of which may change during psychotherapy. All scales will have biases of one sort or another; in some cases the bias is deliberate and written in at the outset but in others the bias only becomes apparent after the scale itself has been the focus of several studies.

Modes of administration

Scales may be self-administered or administered by the doctor, or other trained personnel depending on the nature of the problem to be investigated. The simplest and most economical method is self-administration. It may be the best and only way of measuring subjective states such as anxiety. On the other hand, it requires a cooperative, well motivated, reasonably literate subject with adequate concentration who understands all the items in the scale (Paykel & Norton, 1986).

However, almost by definition, very few people with serious psychotic disturbance will have any of these attributes, so self-rating methods are probably invalid for subjects with more serious disorders. An observer-rated scale or a diagnostic interview can readily make allowance for any lack of insight as well as note the presence of any odd behaviour. Observer-rated scales and diagnostic interviews can be administered by doctors or any other trained personnel. For example, trained psychiatric nurses can measure the severity of psychopathology with a specific scale designed for nurses, the Nurses Observation Scale for In-patient Evaluation (NOSIE–30; Honigfield & Klett, 1965).

A few scales rely exclusively on information provided by an informant without there being any direct contact between the rater and the patient. These methods are particularly useful in personality disorder assessment. For example, the Standardised Assessment of Personality (Mann *et al*, 1981) requires a first observer (the doctor) to interview a second observer, (the informant, generally a close relative of the patient), while the patient is not actually examined.

Errors

A number of systematic errors may impair the reliability of a rating scale. Perhaps the most common bias found in almost all self-rating scales is the response set which refers to the tendency to either agree with all the statements made in the questionnaire, or for a few patients to disagree with every item without seriously considering their meaning. Related to this is the issue of social desirability. Most people tend to favour giving a positive answer to symptoms they regard as socially desirable, but become more defensive or may even deny the presence of socially undesirable symptoms. Errors of the central tendency refer to the reluctance of some respondents to use either the ends or extreme points of the scale in preference to the more central points. Thus in a five point scale there is an increased tendency to use the third point on the scale. A four point scale, however, forces a respondent to choose between either the first two or the last two items. The halo effect refers to the tendency to make a judgement early on in the process of rating and then apply this to all subsequent items. Proximity errors refer to the tendency to rate all adjacent items similarly. Interviews, particularly those which are used for diagnostic purposes, are subject to observer bias.

The meaning of the total score

Because the total score is the outcome variable most commonly used in published studies it is helpful to have some idea of what this might mean for any particular scale. While the meaning of any individual item on a rating scale is generally obvious, the meaning of the total score may be neither obvious nor represent what it was originally intended to measure. The logic of adding such diverse symptoms as weight loss together with suicidal thoughts is rather like adding chalk and cheese. Thompson (1989) justifies this by suggesting that under certain circumstances it is justifiable to add chalk and cheese together – if, for example, they are both on the same truck. Snaith (1981) also justifies the process of summation if it can be shown that all the items relate in the same way and in the same direction to the concept that is to be measured.

   A factor analysis may further help to clarify the meaning of the score in clinical populations or a group of subjects. In general, most items should load positively onto one factor related to severity. However, a factor analysis often reveals that the scale is measuring other aspects of the disorder in question, as well as its severity. Thus for the Hamilton depression scale the main factor relates to severity but there are also factors relating to anxiety and sleep (Berrios & Bulbena Villarasa, 1990). The GHQ appears to have four separate factors: somatic symptoms, anxiety, insomnia, social dysfunction and severe depression (Goldberg & Hillier, 1979). A study of eating behaviour in a private and state school using the Eating Attitudes Test (Garner *et al*, 1983) revealed that this questionnaire had five separate factors: (i) dieting, (ii) pre-occupation with food, (iii) vomiting, (iv) social pressure and (v) social eating. Most of the items loaded onto factor (i), indicating that a high total score indicated mainly dieting behaviour. Pupils in the state school were found to have higher total scores than those in the private school, but the factor structure of the scale was similar in both schools (Eisler & Szmukler, 1985).

Limitations of rating scales

There are many limitations to the use of psychiatric rating scales, perhaps most of all is the disappointment that they have little value in daily clinical practice. An exception is the therapeutic use of scales in behavioural and cognitive psychotherapy. Rating scales fail to provide an objective measure of a psychiatric disorder, in the same way as the blood sugar does for diabetes, or the peak flow for asthma, and so probably they add little more to the understanding of an individual patient's illness than can be gleaned from a simple clinical interview. Only symptoms can be measured reliably, and so many areas of important psychopathology are quite beyond the scope of present measurement techniques. How can one begin to assess the long-term impact of the death of a child upon a parent, or the harm done by an alcoholic father on the later relationships of his children – yet these may be far more important themes than the more easily measurable presenting symptoms of anxiety or depression.

A further problem associated with rating scales is their limited transferability. Thus a scale which may be shown to be valid in one population or in one age group may not necessarily be valid in a different culture or age group. For some disorders, there may be a shifting target as the concept of the disorder alters over the years. This particularly applies to the ever changing definitions of personality disorders and schizophrenia. New scales are constantly being devised to cope with the latest definitions, but this means that much of the information derived from scales based on the older definitions is either obsolete, or at least difficult to interpret in the light of the newer concepts. Hamilton (1968) advocated that scales should represent the end point of clinical description and therefore should only be devised when no further changes in the description of disease are to be made. Others have argued that descriptive perfection is irrelevant as a rating scale only represents an operationalised version of the most recent definition, and so applying a scale of this type to a clinical sample may help confirm (or refute) the validity of the most recent definition (Thompson, 1989).

Structured clinical interviews

According to Zubin, the first structured clinical interview was probably used in the Spanish Inquisition to ensure that all potential witches and heretics were systematically assessed (Spitzer, 1983). Given such a chilling ancestry there has been little enthusiasm in further tracing the history of such interviews. The modern era starts with the development of the Present State Examination in the UK (PSE; Wing *et al*, 1967) and in America, the Psychiatric Status Schedule (Spitzer *et al*, 1970).

A psychiatric diagnosis is usually made by clinical interview in clinical practice but this is a rough and ready procedure, and precisely what constitutes a diagnostic interview varies widely between individual practitioners. Some will enquire into the most remote detail of a patient's life history, while others will embark on therapy almost from the first moments of the encounter. An unstructured clinical interview is therefore a poorly defined and highly unreliable instrument. A structured clinical interview lays down exactly what questions should be asked, specifies their order and in some cases even lays down the precise wording as well. Most structured interviews usually also incorporate a glossary of the definitions of the relevant phenomenology so the interviewer only has to decide if the symptoms described by the patient fit the definition given in the manual. This helps to eliminate observer bias. A training programme may also help ensure the interview is used as it was originally intended.

To remove diagnostic bias the diagnostic process itself may be done by a computer program, and the diagnosis is then made according to a fixed algorithm. Some schedules, such as the PSE and the DIS, utilise computer programmes to make the diagnosis, but others, such as the SADS and SCID (see below), still require the clinician to make the diagnosis.

The PSE, which is probably the most reliable and valid of all the structured clinical interviews, is described more extensively on page 306. It has recently been updated and the PSE–10 is now part of a comprehensive instrument called the Schedule for Clinical Assessment in Neuropsychiatry (SCAN); the computer program for this (CATEGO–5) generates both an ICD–10 and DSM–III–R diagnosis. The interview is designed to give both a lifetime and a present state (last month) diagnosis.

The Schedule for Affective Disorders (SADS)

The SADS (Endicott & Spitzer, 1978) is a semi-structured interview which should be administered by those with clinical experience. The full SADS is a lengthy interview with a large number of detailed questions covering individual affective symptoms. Originally devised to yield RDC diagnoses it has been modfed to give DSM–III and DSM–III–R diagnoses. There are several other versions or modifications of the SADS: thus the SADS–L was devised to assess the life history, the SADS–C covers change in symptoms, the SADS–LA covers anxiety symptoms, and the SADS–LB covers bipolar disorder.

The Diagnostic Interview Schedule (DIS)

This interview was the first fully structured diagnostic interview designed for administration by non-clinicians. It was developed at Washington University, St. Louis (Robins *et al*, 1981) specifically for the National Institute of Mental Health (NIMH) in America as a relatively inexpensive method of making a diagnostic assessment on 15 000 subjects in the five separate sites in the Epidemiological Catchment Area study.

This interview derives its importance from being the basic tool of this huge study which provides the most comprehensive epidemiological data presently available.

It was originally derived from the Renard Diagnostic Interview (Helzer *et al*, 1981) to make diagnoses using the Feighner criteria. The interview is comprehensive and requires training but is rather rigid. Thus if the respondent does not understand the question the interviewer may repeat phrases or break the sentences down into shorter phrases but is not permitted to rephrase the original question. This is because a non-clinician, in the process of rephrasing the question, might subtly alter its original meaning. The DIS cannot be used for those with organic brain disease. Non-clinical subjects may take only 40 minutes, but for an overtalkative subject the DIS may take a long time to administer. The DIS is thought to be weak on psychosomatic conditions, organic disorders and personality disorders. The diagnosis is made by a computer program rather than by the interviewer.

The Structured Clinical Interview for DSM–III (SCID; Spitzer & Williams, 1983)

Spitzer & Williams (1983) raised several cogent criticisms of the DIS. They believed that clinicians were essential in making psychiatric diagnoses. This is because many severely ill subjects may present with complex mixtures of psychotic, affective and social pathology and clarifying the relevant phenomenology may be a taxing or difficult task even for an experienced clinician, and so may be impossible for a non-clinician. Second, the DIS does not permit interviewers to rephrase questions, yet quite often in routine practice a person may fail to grasp the meaning of a question, and suitable rephrasing is an integral part of the diagnostic process but rephrasing can only really be undertaken by someone with clinical knowledge.

The SCID is a rather more flexible clinical interview which has many open ended questions and is administered by someone with clinical experience taking advantage of the strengths of the traditional clinical interviews. For example, the opening question of the affective disorder section is "What has your mood been like?". There follows a series of detailed questions which focus on DSM–III–R items. Symptoms are rated at three levels: present and clinically relevant, marginally present but not relevant, and absent. The SCID focuses on the current clinical episode of illness which is assumed to have occurred in the last year. It has a number of screening questions and 'skip out' questions so that the interview can be shortened. The diagnosis is made according to DSM–III–R by the clinician. The SCID–2, used to assess personality disorders, is described on page 800.

Screening

The term 'screening' has been widely used in psychiatry. Sackett & Holland (1975) identify three separate but closely related procedures: epidemiological surveys, screening and case-finding.

Epidemiological surveys involve the measurement of a variety of health related and other characteristics in a given population sample. Here the aim of the survey is only to acquire new knowledge; no health benefit to the participant is implied.

By contrast, screening is a procedure in which a test is applied to apparently healthy volunteers in the general population with the aim of identifying those individuals who are at high risk of having some otherwise unrecognised disease. As in an epidemiological survey the testing is initiated by the investigator, but there is an important difference – those who take part in the screening programme should benefit, and receive appropriate diagnoses and treatment for any disorder that is discovered. Mammography and cervical smear testing are good examples of valid screening programmes.

Case-finding is a process in which patients who have already sought out health care are tested (with their consent) for disorders which may be unrelated to their presenting complaint. It differs from screening in that if a disorder is found treatment is not implied, and it differs from an epidemiological survey in that the encounter is initiated by the patient. An example of a case-finding exercise might be if a depression rating scale was administered to a group of subjects attending a gastro-enterological clinic, with the aim of estimating the prevalence of depression in this population.

Grant (1982) stipulated three important conditions for a screening programme: (i) the methods must be reliable; (ii) the number of positive findings must be sufficient to justify the cost of the programme; and (iii) evidence is needed that diagnosing the disease before symptoms appear improves the prognosis. On the basis of these criteria Eastwood (1971) concluded that it would be premature to advocate psychiatric screening in anything but a research setting since there was no evidence that early identification of psychiatric cases brought any benefit or improved the prognosis.

Strictly speaking the various psychiatric screening instruments should be referred to as 'case finding instruments', because they are used more to acquire knowledge rather than to help individual patients, but the term screening has come into common usage.

In psychiatry, perhaps most effort has gone into devising screening instruments which identify subjects with so called 'minor' psychiatric morbidity found in general practice settings. Well known scales include the Hopkins Symptom Checklist 90–R (HSCL–90; Derogatis, 1983) or the GHQ. The use of these instruments to find so-called 'cases' of psychiatric disorder has prompted considerable debate into precisely what constitutes a psychiatric case. Wing *et al* (1978) provide a flexible concept:

> the term case can be used in any way that the purposes of the clinician require; no single set of definitions is likely to be of universal value.

Devising a rating scale

In the preceding sections some of the many rating scales used in psychiatry have been described. It is also important to understand how a rating scale is developed and validated. Goldberg (1972) provides an excellent description of the many steps he took in devising the GHQ and a brief summary of this work is given below.

Background and aims

During World War II, doctors in the American Army were given the task of devising rapid screening methods for the millions of new recruits to the armed forces. To do this they developed the first ever comprehensive medical screening instrument, the Cornell Medical Index (CMI; Brodman *et al,* 1949). Some years later Shepherd *et al* (1966) applied the psychological section of this instrument to measure minor psychiatric morbidity in general practice populations. They found that many of the 51 psychological items in the CMI had little or no discriminatory value. There was therefore a need for a new screening instrument which could detect current episodes of neurotic and affective disturbance in community samples. At the time the GHQ was being devised there were no operational or scientific definitions for any mental disorders, but psychiatrists had a reasonable notion of the level of disturbance that might be found among patients attending out-patients.

Item selection

To select the best items for the new scale, Goldberg started with all the psychological items in the CMI, as well as the other scales which were available at the time; including the Taylor Manifest Anxiety Scale, Eysenck's Personality Inventory, and the MMPI, and he also added 30 of his own items, making a total of around 140 items. As the aim of the questionnaire was to detect current episodes of affective disturbance, those items with more obvious personality connotations were deleted. All items had to be rewritten in the present tense in order to detect current disturbance. Respondents were then asked to rate how they felt over the past few weeks and to compare their present state to how they usually felt.

The original 140 item questionnaire was far too long, for normal clinical purposes, and so studies were undertaken to select the more discriminating items. Three separate groups of patients, (i) a severely ill group (non-psychotic Maudsley in-patients); (ii) a less disturbed group from out-patients, and (iii) a group of normal subjects, were given the questionnaire. For an item to be a useful discriminator, it should show up frequently in the severely ill group, sometimes in the milder group, and rarely, if at all, in the normal group. Twenty-five items showed no difference at all between the three groups and a further 34 items were rejected because their discriminatory power was too poor. Another group of items, which appeared useful, such as "feeling easily upset over things" were eliminated because more than 10% of the normal group also responded positively. A final group of items were rejected because medically ill patients also gave a positive response, and in this way the total number of items was reduced from 140 to 60. Further statistical refinements were used to produce the 30, 28, 20 and 12 item GHQ scales.

Scoring

A new special method of scoring the GHQ was devised. The two grades of 'symptom present/mild' and 'symptom severe' were lumped together and given only a score of one point and the two statements which described absence of the symptom were also only given one point. Thus subjects thought they were completing a four point scale but were actually only completing a two point scale. This method used for scoring the GHQ leads to some loss of information but it eliminates the problems associated with middle users and end users. The four point scale also forces a response either to the left or right and this eliminates errors of the central tendency.

Reliability testing

To assess test-retest reliability a group of patients from the Maudsley Hospital with either chronic affective illness or longstanding personality disorders were selected as it was thought their state would change little over time. They were then given the GHQ on two separate occasions six months apart. In the second reliability study, 200 attenders at a general practice were given the GHQ and were simultaneously interviewed using the Clinical Interview Schedule (Goldberg *et al*, 1970) and the severity of disturbance was rated on two occasions six months apart. Around 20 of these subjects were found to have the same level of disturbance at the two interviews. The GHQs from these 20 subjects formed the basis of a test-retest reliability study, which showed a correlation of 0.9. The already completed questionnaires from other studies were used to assess the split-half reliability and this was found to be 0.95.

Validity, sensitivity and specificity

The GHQ was originally devised as a screening instrument and to test its usefulness a validity study was carried out in an urban general practice.

Under the guise of a family health survey, 200 patients who were attending their GPs completed the GHQ. This was then followed by an interview with a research psychiatrist using the Clinical Interview Schedule (Goldberg *et al*, 1970). On the basis of the interview patients were designated as cases or non-cases. Because a research psychiatrist using a standardised interview is more likely to make an accurate diagnosis than one based on a questionnaire, the interview data were taken as the standard and the results obtained with the GHQ were compared to obtain the following validity coefficients for the GHQ.

Specificity – this is the proportion of 'normals' who are true negatives, or correctly identified, and is therefore equal to GHQ negative cases/total number of non-cases at interview.

Sensitivity – this is the proportion of cases who are true positives or correctly identified, and is therefore equal to GHQ positive cases/total number of cases at interview.

Specificity and sensitivity are independent of the prevalence of cases in the sample, and are therefore widely used as measures of validity for rating scales. Three other measures are dependent upon the prevalence of cases, so that if they are to be used, the prevalence in the sample must be stated. The *positive predictive value* is the probability that someone with a high score will turn out to be a case. It is the characteristic of most interest to the clinician, but it is dramatically lowered if prevalence is low. The *negative predictive value* is the probability that someone with a low score will turn out to be a non-case. The *overall misclassification rate* is the proportion of individuals who are incorrectly classified, and is therefore (false positive + false negatives)/total number of cases seen. Formulae for calculating these coefficients are given in Goldberg & Williams (1988).

Meaning of the total score

The GHQ score has two meanings. It may signify a quantitative estimate of the degree of psychiatric disturbance, therefore the severity of an illness and, second, its score also provides a probability estimate of the likelihood of the subject being a psychiatric case. Thus, those scoring below the cut-off are unlikely to be a psychiatric case. Those at the cut-off have a 50% chance, while those above the cut-off have a much increased chance of being a psychiatric case.

Conclusion

Medicine, once an art, is now becoming a science, and psychiatry, perhaps its most inexact speciality, is itself also gradually acquiring a scientific mantle. Psychiatric diagnoses, in spite of much earlier criticism, have now become an essential component of clinical practice. Refining diagnostic criteria to make them accurate as well as easy to use is therefore a task of the greatest importance and has lead to the publication of comprehensive nosologies such as the ICD–10 and DSM–IV. New drugs and psychotherapeutic strategies appear almost every year and all require careful evaluation. Sound diagnoses and valid measuring instruments are at the heart of the evaluative process and for this reason alone it is important to understand the scientific principles underlying diagnosis and measurement in psychiatry.

Acknowledgements

We thank Dr John Cutting and Professor David Goldberg for helpful comments on an earlier draft of this chapter.

References

Akiskal, H. S. (1989) The classification of mental disorders. In *Comprehensive Textbook of Psychiatry* (5th edn) (eds H. I. Kaplan & B. J. Sadoch), pp. 583–598. Baltimore: Williams & Wilkins.

Albee, G. W. (1970) Notes towards a positive paper opposing psychiatric diagnoses. In *New Approaches to Personality Classification* (ed. A. R. Mahrer), pp. 385–395. New York: Columbia University Press.

American Psychiatric Association (1952) *Diagnostic and Statistical Manual* (1st edn) (DSM–I). Washington, DC: APA.

—— (1968) *Diagnostic and Statistical Manual* (2nd edn) (DSM–II).Washington, DC: APA.

—— (1980) *Diagnostic and Statistical Manual* (3rd edn) (DSM–III). Washington, DC: APA.

—— (1987) *Diagnostic and Statistical Manual of Mental Disorders* (3rd edn revised) (DSM–III–R).Washington, DC: APA.

—— (1994) *Diagnostic and Statistical Manual* (4th edn) (DSM–IV). Washington, DC: APA.

Bartko, J. J. & Carpenter, W. T. (1976) On the methods and theory of reliability. *Journal of Nervous and Mental Disorders*, **163**, 307–316.

Bayle, A. L. J. (1822) Recherches sur les maladies mentales (the-de Médecine, Paris). In *Centenaire de la These de Bayle*. Paris: Masson (1922).

Bebbington, P., Hurry, J., Tennant, C., *et al* (1981) Epidemiology of mental disorders in Camberwell. *Psychological Medicine*, **11**, 561–579.

Beck, A. T., Ward, C. H., Mendelson, M., *et al* (1962) An inventory for measuring depression. *Archives of General Psychiatry*, **4**, 561–571.

Bech, P., Malt, U. F., Dencker, S. J., *et al* (1993) Scales for assessment of diagnosis and severity of mental disorders. *Acta Psychiatrica Scandinavica*, **87** (suppl. 372).

Berrios, G. E. & Bulbena Villarasa, A. (1990) The Hamilton Depression Scale and the numerical description of the symptom of depression. In *The Hamilton Depression Scales* (eds P. Beck & A. Coppen), pp. 80–92. Berlin: Springer–Verlag.

Bloch, S. & Reddaway, P. (1984) *Soviet Psychiatric Abuse. The Shadow over World Psychiatry*. London: Gollancz.

Boissier De Sauvages, F. (1768) *Nosologia Methodica, Sistens Morborum Classes, Genera et Species Juxta Sydenhami Mentem et Botanicorum Ordinem*. Amsterdam: de Tournes.

Boyd, J. H., Burke, J. D. & Gruenberg, E. (1984) Exclusion Criteria of DSM–III. *Archives of General Psychiatry*, **41**, 983–989.

Bridgeman, P. W. (1927) *The Logic of Modern Physics*. New York: Macmillan.

Brodman, K., Erdman, A. J., Lorge, I., *et al* (1949) The Cornell Medical Index: an adjunct to medical interview. *Journal of the American Medical Association*, **140**, 530.

Brown, G. & Harris, T. (1978) *Social Origins of Depression: A Study of Psychiatric Disorder in Women*. London: Tavistock.

Carney, M. W. P., Roth, M. & Garside, R. F. (1965) The diagnosis of depressive syndromes and the prediction of ECT response. *British Journal of Psychiatry*, **111**, 659–674.

Caron, C. & Rutter, M (1991) Co-morbidity in child psychopathology, concepts, issues and research strategies. *Journal of Child Psychology and Psychiatry*, **32**, 1063–1080.

Clare, A. (1986) The disease concept in psychiatry. In *Essentials of Postgraduate Psychiatry* (eds P. Hill, R. Murray & A. Thorley), pp. 337–354. London: Grune and Stratton.

Cohen, J. (1960) A coefficient of agreement for nominal scales. *Educational Psychology Measurement*, **20**, 37–46.

—— (1968) Weighted kappa: nominal scale agreement with provision for scaled disagreement or partial credit. *Psychological Bulletin*, **70**, 213–220.

Cox, J. L. (1992) The general psychiatrist as specialist. *Psychiatric Bulletin*, **16**, 529–530.

Cronbach, L. J. (1951) Coefficient alpha and the internal structure of tests. *Psychometrika*, **16**, 297–334.

Cullen, W. (1775) *Synopsis Nosologicae Methodicae*. Amsterdam: de Tournes.

Derogatis, L. (1983) *HSCL–90–R Manual–II*. Towson, Maryland: Clinical Psychometric Research.

Eastwood, M. R. (1971) Screening for psychiatric disorder. *Psychological Medicine*, **1**, 107–208.

Eisler, I. & Szmukler, G. I. (1985) Social class as a confounding variable in the eating attitudes test. *Journal of Psychiatric Research*, **19**, 171–176.

Endicott, J. & —— (1978) A diagnostic interview: the Schedule for Affective Disorders and Schizophrenia. *Archives of General Psychiatry*, **35**, 837–844.

Esquirol, E. (1838) *Des Maladies Mentales Considérées sous les Rapports Médical, Hygiénique et Médico-Légal*. Paris: Baillière.

Essen-Moller, E. & Wohlfahrt, S. (1947) Suggestions for the amendment of the official classification of mental disorders. *Acta Psychiatrica Scandinavica*, **47** (suppl.), 551–555.

Feighner, J. P., Robins, E., Guze, S. B., *et al* (1972) Diagnostic criteria for use in psychiatric research. *Archives of General Psychiatry*, **26**, 57–63.

Feinstein, A. R. (1967) *Clinical Judgment*. Baltimore: Williams and Wilkins.

Foulds, G. A. (1965) *Personality and Personal Illness*. London: Tavistock.

—— & Bedford, A. (1975) Hierarchy of classes of personal illness. *Psychological Medicine*, **5**, 181–192.

Frances, A., Pincus, H. A., Widiger, T. A., *et al* (1990) DSM–IV: Work in Progress. *American Journal of Psychiatry*, **147**, 1439–1448.

Garner, D. M., Olmstead, M. P. & Polivy, J. (1983) Development and validation of a multidimensional eating disorder inventory for anorexia nervosa and bulimia. *International Journal of Eating Disorders*, **2**, 15–34.

Goldberg, D.P. (1972) *The Detection of Psychiatric Illness by Questionnaire.* Maudsley Monograph, No. 21, London: Oxford University Press.

——, Cooper, B., Eastwood, M. R., *et al* (1970) A standardised psychiatric interview suitable for use in community surveys. *British Journal of Preventive and Social Medicine*, **24**, 18.

—— & Hillier, V. F. (1979) A scaled version of the General Health Questionnaire. *Psychological Medicine*, **9**, 139–145.

—— & Williams (1988) A User's Guide to the GHQ. Windsor: NFER/Nelson.

Grant, I. W. (1982) Screening for lung cancer. *British Medical Journal*, **284**, 1209–1210.

Griesinger, W. (1845) *Mental Pathology and Therapeutics.* Translated 1867. London: New Sydenham Society.

Gruenberg, E. M. (1969) How can the new diagnostic manual help. *International Journal of Psychiatry*, **7**, 368–374.

Hamilton, M. (1960) A rating scale for depression. *Journal of Neurology, Neurosurgery and Psychiatry*, **23**, 56.

—— (1968) Some notes on rating scales. *Statistician*, **18**, 11–17.

Helzer, J. E., Robins, L. N., Croughan, J. L., *et al* (1981) Renard diagnostic interview; its reliability and procedural validity with physicians and lay interviewers. *Archives of General Psychiatry*, **38**, 393–398.

Honigfield, G. & Klett, C. J. (1965) The nurses observation scale for inpatient evaluation. *Journal of Clinical Psychology*, **21**, 65–71.

Jablensky, A. (1988) Methodological issues in psychiatric classification. *British Journal of Psychiatry*, **152** (suppl.1), 15–20.

Jaspers, K. (1913) *Allgemeine Psychopathologie.* Berlin: Springer.

Jaspers, M. K. (1959) *Allgemeine Psychopathologie* (7th edn) (Translation by J. Hoenig & M. W. Hamilton, 1962). Manchester: Manchester University Press.

Kendler, K. S. (1990) Towards a scientific nosology. *Archives of General Psychiatry*, **47**, 969–973.

Kendell, R. E. (1968) *The Classification of Depressive Illness.* Maudsley Monograph no. 18. London: Oxford University Press.

—— (1975) *The Role of Diagnosis in Psychiatry.* Oxford: Blackwell.

——, Everitt, B., Cooper, J. E., *et al* (1968) Reliability of the Present State Examination. *Social Psychiatry*, **3**, 123–129.

Klerman, G. L. (1991) An American perspective on the conceptual approaches to psychopathology. *In Concepts of Mental Disorder* (eds A. Kerr & H. McMelland) London: Gaskell.

Kraepelin, E. (1896) *Psychiatrie. Ein Lehrbuch für Studirende und Aerzte* (5th edn). Leipzig: J. A. Barth.

Kraupl-Taylor, F. (1971) A logical analysis of the medico-psychological concept of disease. *Psychological Medicine*, **1**, 356–364 and **2**, 7–16.

Likert, R. (1932) A technique for the measurement of attitudes. *Archives of Psychology*, **140**, 1–55.

Linder, R. (1965) Diagnosis: description or prescription? A case study in the psychology of diagnosis. *Perceptual and Motor Skills*, **20**, 1081–1092.

Linnaeus, C. Von (1735) *Systema Naturae Sive Regna tri-a Naturae Systematica Proposita per Clases, Ordines, Genera et Species.* Leyden: J. Haak.

Linnaeus, C. (1763) *Genera Morborum in Auditorum Usum.* Uppsale: C. E. Steinert.

Mann, A. H., Jenkins, R., Cutting, J. C. *et al* (1981) The development and use of a standardised assessment of abnormal personality. *Psychological Medicine*, 11, 839–847.

Meyer, A. (1952) *Collected Papers of Adolf Meyer (1948–52)* (ed. E. Winters). Baltimore: Johns Hopkins University Press.

Mezzick, J. E. (1988) On developing a psychiatric multi-axial scheme for ICD–10. *British Journal of Psychiatry*, 152 (suppl.1), 38–43.

Mindham, R. H. S., Scadding, J. G. & Cawley R. H. (1992) Diagnoses are not diseases. *British Journal of Psychiatry*, 161, 686–691.

Montgomery, S. A. & Åsberg, M. (1979) A new depression rating scale designed to be sensitive to change. *British Journal of Psychiatry*, 134, 382–389.

Moos, R. H. (1968) The development of a menstrual distress questionnaire. *Psychosomatic Medicine*, 30, 853–867.

Morel, B. A. (1857) *Traité des Dégénérescences Physiques, Intellectuelles et Morales de l'Espece Humaine et des Causes qui Produisent ces Varieétes Maladies.* Paris: Baillière.

Murray, R. M. & Mann, A. (1986) Measurement in psychiatry. In *Essentials of Postgraduate Psychiatry*, (eds P. Hill, R. Murray & T. Thorley), pp. 55–80. London: Grune & Stratton.

Paykel, E. S. & Norton, K. R. W. (1986) Self report and clinical interview. In *Assessment of Depression* (eds N. Sartorius & T. A. Ban) pp. 356–366. Berlin: Springer Verlag.

Peck, D. F. & Shapiro, C. (1990) *Measuring Human Problems.* Chichester: John Wiley.

Perry, S., Cooper, M. & Michels, R. (1987) The psychodynamic formulation: Its purpose, structure and clinical application. *American Journal of Psychiatry*, 144, 543–550.

Robins, L. N., Helzer, J. E., Croughan, J. *et al* (1981) National Institute of Mental Health Diagnostic Interview Schedule. *Archives of General Psychiatry*, 38, 381–389.

Rosch, E. (1976) Classification of real world objects; origins and representations in cognitions. In *La Memoire Semantique.* (eds S. Ehrich & E. Tislving). Paris: Bulletin de Psychologica.

Sackett, D. & Holland, W. (1975) Controversy in the detection of disease. *Lancet*, ii, 357–359.

Sartorius, N. (1988) International perspectives of psychiatric classification. *British Journal of Psychiatry*, 152 (suppl. 1), 9–14.

Scadding, J. G. (1967) Diagnosis: The clinician and the computer. *Lancet*, ii, 877–882.

—— (1990) The semantic problem of psychiatry. *Psychological Medicine*, 20, 243–248.

Shepherd, M., Cooper, A. B., Brown, A. C., *et al* (1966) *Psychiatric Illness in General Practice.* Oxford: Oxford University Press.

Snaith, R. P. (1981) Rating scales. *British Journal of Psychiatry*, 138, 512–514.

Sokal, R. R. (1974) Classification: purposes, principles, progress, prospects. *Science*, 185, 115–123.

Spitzer, R. L. (1983) Psychiatric diagnoses: are clinicians still necessary? *Comprehensive Psychiatry*, 24, 299–411.

——, Fleiss, J. L, Endicott, J., *et al* (1970) The Psychiatric Status Schedule: a technique for evaluating psychopathology and impairment in role functioning. *Archives of General Psychiatry*, 23, 41–55.

——, Endicott, J. L. & Robins, E. (1978) Research Diagnostic Criteria: rationale and reliability. *Archives of General Psychiatry*, **35**, 773–782.

Stengel, E. (1959) Classification of mental disorders. *Bulletin of the World Health Organization*, **21**, 601–603.

Sturt, E. (1985) Hierarchical patterns in the distribution of psychiatric symptoms. *Psychological Medicine*, **11**, 783–794.

Sydenham, T. (1682) *Dissertatio Epistolaris ad C. Cole de observationis Nuperis Circa Curationem Variolarum Confluentium, Necnam de Affectione Hysterica*. London: Kettelby.

Szasz, T. S. (1960) *The Myth of Mental Illness*. New York: Harper.

—— (1991) Diagnosis and not disease. *Lancet*, **338**, 1574–1576.

Szatmari, P. (1992) The validity of autistic spectrum disorders. A literature review. *Journal of Autism and Developmental Disorders*, **22**, 583–600.

Temkin, O. (1968) The history of classification in the medical sciences. In *The Role and Methodology in Psychiatry and Psychopathology* (eds M. M. Katz, J. O. Cole & W. E. Barton). Washington, DC: National Institute of Mental Health.

Thompson, C. (1989) Introduction. In *The Instruments of Psychiatric Research* (ed. C. Thompson). Chichester: John Wiley.

Thomson, W. (1889) *Popular Lectures and Addresses*. London: Macmillan.

Tuke, H. (1892) *Dictionary of Psychological Medicine. (Vol. II)*. London: J. & A. Churchill.

Tyrer, P. & Steinberg, D. (1987) *Models for Mental Disorder*. Chichester: John Wiley.

Virchow, R. (1895) *Hundert Jahre Allgemeiner Pathologie*. Hirschwald: Berlin.

Ward, C. H., Beck, A. T., Mendelson, M., *et al* (1962) The psychiatric nomenclature. *Archives of General Psychiatry*, **119**, 207–209.

Werry, J. S. (1992) Child psychiatric disorders: Are they classifiable? *British Journal of Psychiatry*, **161**, 472–480.

Willis, T. (1682) *Opera Omnia*. Amsterdam: Wetstenius.

Wing, J. K., Birley, J. L. T., Cooper, J. E., *et al* (1967) Reliability of a procedure for measuring and classifying 'Present Psychiatric State'. *British Journal of Psychiatry*, **113**, 499–515.

Wing, J. K., Cooper, J. E. & Sartorius, N. (1974) *The Measurement and Classification of Psychiatric Symptoms*. Cambridge University Press: Cambridge.

——, Mann, S. A., Left, J. P. *et al* (1978) The concept of "case" in psychiatric population surveys. *Psychological Medicine*, **8**, 203–217.

World Health Organization (1948) *Manual of the International Statistical Classification of Diseases, Injuries and Causes of Death* (ICD–6). *Bulletin of the World Health Organisation*, Suppl.1, Geneva: WHO.

—— (1980) *International Classification of Impairments, Disability and Handicaps* (ICIDH) Geneva: WHO.

—— (1992) *The Tenth Revision of the International Classification of Diseases and Related Health Problems* (ICD–10). Geneva: WHO.

—— (1993) *The ICD–10 Classification of Mental and Behavioural Disorders. Diagnostic Criteria for Research*. Geneva: WHO.

Zung, W. W. K. (1965) A self rating depression scale. *Archives of General Psychiatry*, **12**, 63–70.

27 Mental health services

Rosalind Ramsay & Frank Holloway

In-patient care • Day care • Out-patient services • Multidisciplinary teams • The profession of psychiatry • Access to services • Sectorisation • The voluntary sector • The private sector • User views and the user movement • Mental health policy in the UK • Residential services for the severely mentally ill • Hospital closure • Monitoring services • The future

---

This chapter examines the different settings used to deliver psychiatric care and the role played by the various professionals who make up the multidisciplinary team. Psychiatric services, like any other public service, essentially consist of people. The policies of a service reflect an underlying working philosophy which governs the interactions and tasks of the professionals, who will be drawn from a range of disciplines. A typical multidisciplinary team includes nurses, occupational therapists, psychiatrists, psychologists and social workers and will work closely with numerous non-specialists and untrained care workers.

In putting forward its vision for the future of mental health care in Britain the Royal College of Psychiatrists (1990) stated that a model service should be:

(a) comprehensive – able to meet the entire range of need of people with a mental illness in the community
(b) accessible – readily available and with a range of services at a reasonable distance from patients' homes
(c) acceptable to patients, relatives, professionals and the community
(d) integrated with other community agencies working with people with a mental disorder, notably primary care and social services authorities
(e) effective, with improved mental health as an outcome
(f) efficient, showing good value for the use of available resources.

A competent service should also have the capacity for teaching, research and public education. Good services do not come about by accident but are the fruit of long-term coherent planning. This should involve all the relevant local "stakeholders", including health and social services authorities (the purchasers), service providers, the voluntary sector and users and carers. Planning should be incremental and based on a sound understanding of local conditions and local need, a grasp of the epidemiology of mental illness and knowledge of what components make up an effective mental health service. Detailed discussion of the planning process is beyond the remit of this chapter; a number of relevant texts are available (Kingsley & Towell, 1988; Strathdee & Thornicroft, 1993; DoH, 1994).

To be comprehensive a local psychiatric service must be able to respond to the specialist health needs of anyone in the community diagnosed as suffering from a psychiatric disorder. This category includes mental illnesses such as schizophrenia, schizotypal and delusional disorders, mood disorders and the organic mental disorders. Services will also be required to provide effective treatments that have been developed for other mental illnesses, notably neurotic, stress-related and somatoform disorders and eating disorders. Specialist mental health teams play an important role in the overall management of people presenting with some forms of personality disorder. The care of people suffering from less severe psychological and emotional problems, psychosexual problems, personal distress and the abuse of alcohol and drugs is generally shared with other agencies, notably primary health care and specialist community teams.

A comprehensive mental health service will span the range of psychiatric disciplines. This chapter focuses on general adult psychiatric services and rehabilitation services.

Any service should address the range of needs of individuals with mental health disorders, and their carers. Services should incorporate a number of functions, as outlined in Box 27.1.

The core elements of a comprehensive local district psychiatric service were set out in the white paper *Better Services for the Mentally Ill* (DHSS, 1975). These included an NHS component, expected to be based around a district general hospital psychiatric unit; community services provided by the local social services department; liaison with primary care teams; and a network of voluntary services (Lavender & Holloway, 1992; Strathdee & Thornicroft, 1993; Department of Health, 1994) (See Box 27.2).

In some areas new models of service provision have been developed, for example, community mental health centres (Sayce *et al*, 1991), acute day

---

Box 27.1 Elements of a comprehensive service

Identification of people in need
Control of psychiatric symptoms and prevention of relapse
Intervention in crises
General health care
Provision of supportive accommodation, including hospital beds
Promotion of independent living skills
Advice on welfare rights
Opportunities for work and other structured activities
Opportunities for leisure activities
Development of social networks
Support and education of carers
Case management

Box 27.2 Key components of a district mental health service

Within the National Health Service:
(a) DGH psychiatric unit with out-patient and short-term in-patient facilities
(b) Rehabilitation facilities in hospital
(c) Arrangements for making and if necessary supervising an after-discharge plan for patients
(d) Day hospital places
(e) Community psychiatric nursing service
(f) Domiciliary visit team.

Within the Local Authority Social Services Department:
(a) Day centres, including facilities for occupational rehabilitation
(b) Social clubs and drop-in centres
(c) Hostels for those who need supervised living accommodation
(d) Group homes
(e) Domiciliary supervision
(f) Arrangements for social welfare benefits.

(After Wilkinson, 1991.)

---

care (Creed *et al*, 1990) and home based treatment teams (Dedman, 1993; Marks *et al*, 1994). The balance between hospital-based and community-based provision has slowly shifted over the past two decades (Raftery, 1991), accelerating as an increasing number of the large mental hospitals close. Recent policy developments (which are discussed in some detail later in the chapter) have identified local social services authorities as the lead agency in community care, with a key policy objective being the promotion of domiciliary, day and respite services that enable people with a disability to live in their own homes, if this is feasible and sensible (Thornicroft, 1994).

In-patient care

The traditional psychiatric hospital performed a bewildering array of functions (Bachrach, 1976). These included crisis intervention in an acute situation; assessment or reassessment of diagnosis and the development and institution of a treatment plan; respite (for patient and carer); removal of the patient from a stressful environment; long-term custodial care of patients with continuing disability; protection of the patient from exploitation; and protection of the public from dangerous or deviant behaviour, either in the long or short term (Bachrach, 1976; Talbott & Glick, 1986).

The mental hospital also provided for the basic needs of inmates for food, shelter, clothing and a minimal income and offered opportunities for occupation, leisure and social interaction. As experience has grown in the reprovision of long-stay hospitals and in community-based alternatives to acute admission, it has become clear that these functions can be satisfactorily fulfilled outside the hospital for the vast majority of patients who would previously have required a prolonged in-patient stay (Thornicroft & Bebbington, 1989; Muijen, 1992).

However, even in the era of deinstitutionalisation and community care, in-patient provision forms a vital component of the comprehensive mental health service. Admission is required to manage patients who are a danger to themselves or others or fail to comply with treatment (Stein & Test, 1980) and is also indicated when patients need assessment or treatment that cannot be provided on an out-patient or day patient basis. The respite function may more cheaply (and possibly more appropriately) be provided in alternative non-clinical settings (Strathdee & Thornicroft, 1992).

The acute unit

Three broad types of in-patient facility for the adult mentally ill may be identified: the acute unit; long-stay provision; and secure provision. The most familiar is the acute unit, which generally provides a comprehensive service to patients requiring in-patient admission within a catchment area. (Management of patients with schizophrenia during an acute in-patient episode is described on page 460.) Patients are usually admitted as a result of a psychiatric crisis; this may follow the involvement of the police or presentation to a general hospital after an act of deliberate self-harm (Moodley & Perkins, 1991). In some areas admissions may be accepted directly as a result of a GP referral; more usually patients will either already be in contact with a community mental health team or be assessed prior to admission by the team.

As acute bed numbers have declined over recent years an increasing proportion of admissions to acute units have been suffering from psychotic illness (Patrick *et al*, 1989), particularly in inner city areas where a "psychosis only" service has emerged. In some catchment areas the acute unit is supplemented by the psychiatric intensive care unit, a locked facility that admits patients who are too behaviourally disturbed to be managed on an open ward. In addition some services have wards carrying out specialist functions, for example, neuropsychiatry, the management of eating disorders and perinatal psychiatry. The majority of acute admissions are readmissions, a reflection of the 'revolving door' illness career of most psychiatric patients, which is characterised by more or less frequent relapses and readmissions rather than a single episode of illness or a prolonged hospital stay.

The principles of in-patient treatment are identical to those of any other form of psychiatric care. The effective management of an in-patient episode requires identification of the reasons for admission, thorough assessment of the problems presented by the patient (and to the patient by his or her home environment) and the early development of a set of treatment aims and objectives. This process should, as far as possible, involve the patient and the whole in-patient multidisciplinary team. Nursing staff, who have the primary responsibility for the maintenance of a safe and therapeutic environment within the ward, should produce a nursing care plan. Treatment will include specific interventions (for example, medication, occupational therapy, psychological therapies, addressing patients' practical problems) and the non-specific effect of removal from a stressful environment to one that is (hopefully) less stressful and more supportive. Patients identify the relationships that they build up with staff as the major therapeutic ingredient of hospital admission (Lieberman & Strauss, 1986).

One vital, and sometimes overlooked, element of in-patient treatment is discharge planning (Talbott & Glick, 1986). In Britain the need to provide adequate discharge planning and aftercare is codified in the Care Programme Approach (Kingdon, 1994), discussed in more detail below. Following a number of well-publicised tragedies in which the community care of seriously disturbed patients had broken down, British government policy insists that an assessment of dangerousness must now become part of pre-discharge planning for all patients (Fisher, 1994).

Long-stay patients

The average length of stay on the acute unit is steadily decreasing. Only a very small proportion of patients remain in hospital for prolonged periods, and it is generally agreed that such patients should not live within an acute ward (Bridges *et al*, 1994). A recent national survey of "new long-stay" patients (defined as those resident in hospital for between six months and three years) found that there were two main clinical groupings (Lelliott *et al*, 1994). First, there was a group of younger patients (aged 18 to 34 years) who were predominantly single men with schizophrenia, often with a history of serious violence, dangerous behaviour or admission to a special hospital. Second, there was a group of older patients (55 to 67 years), who were predominantly married or previously married women, often with a diagnosis of affective disorder or dementia and with poor social functioning (Table 27.1).

Traditionally long-stay patients were managed within the back wards of the large mental hospitals. They were mixed, with a much larger number of patients with long-term severe mental illnesses who are now known to be manageable within a spectrum of supported community facilities, ranging from supported group homes to community-based hospital-hostels (Morris, 1991; DoH, 1992*a*). Within contemporary hospital services long-stay patients will be found in acute wards, specialist long-term care units and secure units.

Secure provision

Patients who require treatment within a secure setting in the medium or long term will generally have committed serious offences, and be managed by forensic psychiatric services within medium secure facilities and the special hospitals under part III of the Mental Health Act (which relates to patients concerned in criminal proceedings or under sentence) (O'Grady, 1990). However, a significant number of psychotic patients are now placed in private sector secure units, usually because of severe and unremitting behavioural disturbance which has not resulted in an offence of sufficient severity to warrant the attention of forensic psychiatrists. The use of private sector placements reflects a shortfall identified by the "Reed" Committee of some 1500 places in secure or semi-secure settings (other than the special hospitals) in England and Wales (Department of Health and Home Office, 1992).

There is considerable overlap between patients treated by forensic psychiatry services, chronically handicapped and behaviourally disturbed patients rotating through the 'revolving door' and in and out of intensive care units, and those requiring long-stay hospital care in settings that do not offer a high degree of security.

Day care

The first recorded psychiatric day hospital started in Moscow in 1933, apparently as a result of a shortage of in-patient beds. In 1946 Cameron

Table 27.1. National audit of new long-stay psychiatric patients; selected data

Primary diagnosis	%
Schizophrenia	57.1
Affective psychosis (unipolar)	5.7
Affective psychosis (bipolar)	8.7
Paranoid state	1.9
Dementia	7.1
Other organic psychosis	4.5
Neurotic illness	5.5
Personality disorder	4.5
Other diagnosis	5.0
Gender	
Male	58
Female	42

(From Lelliott *et al*, 1994.)

opened the Allan Memorial Institute in Montreal, Canada, and Bierer opened the Paddington Social Psychotherapy Centre, later to become the Marlborough Day Hospital, in London (Holloway, 1988). The early rationale for day care was that it offered a less stigmatising and institutional alternative to traditional hospital care, with the added advantage that day treatment would be much cheaper than 24-hour hospital care. A variety of treatment models emerged. Some day units offered work-based rehabilitation while others adopted a psychotherapeutic model and ran along the lines of a therapeutic community, or they functioned essentially as traditional wards where the patients went home at night. Additionally the role of day care as a source of social support for people with long-term mental illnesses was quickly recognised (DHSS, 1975). Day care forms a vital component of any good quality community-oriented psychiatric service with a variety of functions (see Box 27.3).

Several controlled trials have shown that the day hospital can be an effective alternative to in-patient admission, even for patients with acute psychoses (Creed *et al*, 1989), although not all day hospitals can successfully provide acute day care (Creed *et al*, 1991).

A randomised controlled trial compared day patient versus in-patient treatment for patients with acute psychiatric illness in a small socially deprived inner city area of Manchester (Creed *et al*, 1990). Forty per cent of acutely ill patients presenting for admission to a teaching hospital psychiatric unit could be treated satisfactorily in a well staffed attached day hospital. Outcome of treatment at one year showed no significant differences between day patients and in-patients in terms of clinical symptoms or abnormal behaviour, level of social functioning, and burden on relatives. Costs were similar but patients with mania were withdrawn from the study and could not be managed in the day hospital.

A number of factors may make it impossible to manage a patient in an acute day hospital. For example, patients may be too disturbed or require

---

Box 27.3 Functions of day care

Acute day care: an alternative to admission on an acute ward.
Transitional day care: for patients being discharged after a brief in-patient stay.
Therapeutic day care: offering specific packages of treatment that cannot be provided on an out-patient basis.
Long-term supportive day care: includes structured and unstructured settings; drop-ins; sheltered work; sheltered leisure.
Generic day care: use of mainstream facilities open to the general public, for example adult education, training schemes.

detention under the Mental Health Act. There may be social reasons such as a lack of suitable accommodation, or patients or carers may refuse to accept day hospital treatment. The feasibility of day hospital treatment depends on adequate numbers of staff who have positive attitudes to managing acutely ill patients living in the community (Creed *et al*, 1991). Tantam (1985) suggests that day hospitals may offer an alternative to in-patient admission for between 20 and 30% of acute patients admitted to a conventional service.

In addition to a role as an alternative to in-patient admission day care can provide support, supervision and monitoring for patients just discharged after a period in hospital, and so help decrease the length of in-patient stays (Endicott *et al*, 1979). Brief intensive treatment can be provided within a day setting for patients whose needs cannot be met by out-patient or domiciliary services (Sims *et al*, 1993). Finally, and importantly, day treatment centres can act as a source of long-term structure and support for patients with chronic disabilities. In terms of preventing readmission of patients with schizophrenia, a controlled trial found that day centres with low readmission rates were characterised by an accepting low-key atmosphere, slower patient flows and an emphasis on recreation and occupation rather than "therapy" (Linn *et al*, 1979).

British government policy has traditionally identified two types of day unit: the day hospital, which should provide a short-term treatment-oriented service within a medical setting, and the day centre, which should provide longer term supportive and social care (DHSS, 1975). Unfortunately this neat distinction between the "health" and "social" components of day care cannot readily be identified in practice. Many day hospitals, particularly those located in inner city catchment areas or associated with a large psychiatric hospital, serve a mainly long-term clientele (Holloway, 1991). From the users' perspective long-term day care plays a psychological role akin to the "latent" functions of work. In addition to its obvious role in providing people with financial rewards (its "manifest" functions), work provides a structure to an individual's time, enforces activity, offers social relationships outside the home and produces external goals for achievement (Jahoda, 1981). Day care users stress the importance of having somewhere to go, the support of staff and fellow attenders and the availability of activities in favour of any therapeutic function (Holloway, 1989).

There is little empirical evidence regarding the activities offered in day settings. Although individual assessments, particularly of daily living skills, may be carried out within a day unit most activities involve groups of attenders. Groups should vary in the demands they make on members, but should foster the use of a range of social and functional skills. Practical activities, work assessment, social skills training, family therapy and other specific therapeutic interventions may all form part of a day care programme.

Patients often find evenings and weekends particularly difficult, and some services are now available out of working hours. Voluntary organisations can be particularly successful at providing informal 'drop-ins' which can complement the more formal statutory day care. Access to leisure activities is a major problem for some patients who may be restricted by lack of money, social anxiety, impaired social skills and lack of motivation. One important aspect of day care is that it provides users with a ready-made social network. A group of ex-psychiatric in-patients in New York started the Fountain House as a club, and the model with its emphasis on the equality of patients (members) and staff has been widely adopted and provides an opportunity for gainful employment within the clubhouse (Beard *et al*, 1982). It is important that this artificial social network encourages appropriately socially skilled behaviour. Ideally services should be encouraging patients to maintain or develop social networks unconnected with the mental health system. Professional support systems can make use of 'generic' resources which are open to members of the public. Adult education courses and local leisure centres are particularly valuable forms of generic provision.

Work was always an essential and effective element of rehabilitation within the traditional mental hospital (Wing & Brown, 1970). Until recently interest in sheltered work within mental health services was waning but it is now generally recognised that work is in itself potentially highly therapeutic, as well as bringing financial benefits and access to wider social networks (Pilling, 1988; Warner, 1994). A range of provision is required. This will include work assessment and training, careers counselling, sheltered work, sheltered placements in ordinary firms and access to open employment (Harding *et al*, 1987).

Community mental health centres (CMHCs)

The CMHC movement, which originated in the 1960s in the USA, is relatively new to the UK. It has been growing rapidly, with a fourfold increase reported in the 1980s (Bennett & Freeman, 1991; Sayce *et al*, 1991). The movement is highly diverse in its objectives and structures (McAusland, 1985) although consistently CMHCs work in parallel with rather than in tandem with primary care. They may be based on day services or specifically exclude the provision of day activities in favour of a service offering assessment and therapy only. Other CMHCs resemble small local psychiatric in-patient units with beds and 24-hour nursing cover. The management of a CMHC may come under the health service or local authority or it may be a joint venture (Ovretveit, 1994). Staff in CMHCs are often enthusiastic about preventive work and the promotion of positive mental health and may aim to be accessible by taking self-referrals as well as referrals from professionals.

An example is the Mental Health Advice Centre (MHAC) in Lewisham, London, an ordinary house in a pleasant residential area, run by a multiprofessional psychiatric team. At first, it offered a daily walk-in clinic, and later a crisis intervention team was formed. After the opening of the

MHAC, there was a decrease in the number of first admissions to hospital, new referrals to out-patients and consultant domiciliary visits. However the MHAC did not reduce admissions to the local psychiatric hospital, possibly because patients with severe chronic illness were not being seen, and because the service was only available during working hours (Boardman *et al*, 1987). Most of the referrals were from local GPs, with a higher number of patients attending than was expected, suggesting that the MHAC was treating a patient group that had not previously had access to a specialist service, and it was therefore meeting a previously unmet need.

The direct access function of CMHCs is potentially in conflict with the crucial role of primary medical care services. There is concern that CMHCs may attract patients who constitute the 'worried well' rather than the seriously mentally ill, resulting in a diversion of resources from the most severely mentally ill (Mollica, 1980). In Britain the role of the CMHC in providing comprehensive community care to people with a long-term mental illness is compromised by the introduction of 'care management' and the 'care package' (Peck, 1994). These are discussed in more detail below.

Out-patient services

One consequence of the well developed system of primary care in Britain is that the vast majority of patients come to out-patient care following referral by a GP or after episodes of acute in-patient treatment (Goldberg & Huxley, 1992). In many other countries, patients can refer themselves directly to any medical specialist. Out-patient clinics are held on the in-patient unit site or increasingly are locally based, for example, in health centres (Strathdee & Williams, 1984), in other hospitals within the catchment area or in locality team bases. Moving clinics into the community increases their accessibility and removes the stigma of attending a hospital psychiatric clinic, as well as allowing contact between psychiatric and primary care staff which may improve sharing of information. A disadvantage for psychiatrists, especially in rural areas, is the increased time spent travelling (Tyrer, 1984).

More than three-quarters of psychiatric out-patient attendances are for follow-up. The largest diagnostic group among new referrals to psychiatric clinics are patients with neurotic illness, including adverse reactions to stress such as bereavement. Among these patients factors which decrease the chance of being offered continuing psychiatric treatment are a short duration of illness, a history of alcohol misuse and/or deliberate self-harm, age over 50, being widowed, and (in rural catchment areas) living more than 20 miles from the main hospital base (Eagles & Alexander, 1988).

A study comparing the outcome of new psychiatric out-patients with neurotic disorders randomly allocated to out-patient or day hospital treatment found no appreciable difference between the short or medium-term outcome of the two groups (Tyrer *et al*, 1987). This indicates that out-patient treatment can be a cheap and effective form of management which could be further improved by developing a greater range of treatments.

The majority of out-patient attenders have chronic psychiatric disorders. Traditionally patients with schizophrenia were seen by a psychiatrist, often a trainee, every 3–6 months for a brief assessment of their mental state and monitoring of drug side-effects, in the interim attending a depot clinic run by community psychiatric nurses. Contemporary management, particularly for those with more serious illnesses, follows the principles of the Care Programme Approach (Kingdon, 1994), and involves regular multi-disciplinary review encompassing the whole range of needs of the patient and carers. In some services patients attend a specialised lithium clinic, which allows review of their mental state as well as the regular monitoring of lithium levels and thyroid and renal function.

General psychiatrists may offer in an out-patient setting a variety of specialist therapies such as individual psychodynamic, cognitive or behavioural therapy, group therapy or marital or family therapy. Psychiatrists with a special interest may run specialist clinics, for example, for those with post traumatic stress disorder, an eating disorder or behavioural problems. Others provide a liaison service to medical specialists within the general hospital. Psychologists and psychotherapists also run out-patient clinics for the assessment of new patients, and offer individual and sometimes couple, family or group treatment, generally for a limited number of sessions. These specialists may take referrals directly from primary care or other agencies as well as seeing patients referred by psychiatric services.

Patients may attend a follow-up clinic for no apparent reason, the purpose of continued attendance having become unclear and unquestioned by both doctor and patient. Kessel (1963) suggested that some of these difficulties might be overcome by greater use of the single consultation. In around a half of all cases referred by GPs, the expectation was that the GP would have continuing responsibility for patients but be given advice on how to manage them (Gask, 1986). Another alternative model to the traditional out-patient clinic is a service that provides initial assessments of patients at home as a matter of routine. A controlled study of home-based care found outcomes to be equivalent to standard care (Burns *et al*, 1993*a*) with a significant decrease in costs for home-based care consequent on a reduction in admissions (Burns *et al*, 1993*b*).

The traditional pattern of out-patient care is for a GP to refer to a named consultant psychiatrist. A recent development in some services has been to seek referrals to the catchment area treatment team as a whole and then for the team to allocate the assessment of the patient to the most appropriate member, but for more complex cases a number of team members may become involved.

Multidisciplinary teams

The most precious assets for a psychiatric service are its staff rather than its facilities (Jenkins & Griffiths, 1991). Psychiatric patients have multidimensional problems and therapeutic work is likely to require the intervention of a number of health and social care professionals with different skills. The needs of the mentally ill are so complex and demanding that long-term continuity of care can only realistically be provided by a team. Close structured collaboration between members of different disciplines ensures coordination of special skills and the development of comprehensive management plans for patients both in hospital and community settings (Soni *et al*, 1989). Care in the community is most effectively provided when professionals from all mental health disciplines (psychiatrists, psychiatric nurses, occupational therapists, clinical psychologists and social workers) work closely together within multi-disciplinary teams (MDTs) (Ovretveit, 1994).

Scientific research into the functioning of community mental health teams is in its infancy (Moss, 1994; Onyett *et al*, 1994). Practical experience has revealed many advantages to working within a MDT compared with a system in which professionals work in isolation. These include the capacity to offer more comprehensive service provision; easier access to the service for referrers and service users, who do not have to deal with many different professionals and agencies; better planning for new developments; the availability of support from colleagues or peers; protection from the burden of sole responsibility for patients with challenging and at times intractable problems; and more effective management of the workload, with opportunities for cross-cover during the inevitable absence of staff because of leave and sickness (Ovretveit, 1986, 1994; Pilling, 1991).

Effective MDTs require leadership (Watts & Bennett, 1983; Onyett *et al*, 1994). Leadership functions include the structuring of team tasks; demonstrating effective involvement with patients; communicating high expectations of other staff and showing that these expectations can be met; defining and articulating the goals of the team; offering supervision, which involves monitoring of performance, workload and sickness and attending to team members' needs for career development; and taking responsibility for the team's relationships with other elements of the system of care (including local management and the purchasers). In relation to clinical decisions team members will be responsible either to their own line manager or to their colleagues in the MDT. In practice effective decision-making within teams requires the participation of staff members who will be required to implement the team's decisions (Watts & Bennett, 1983).

Sims (1991) has argued that the psychiatrist should be the "leader" of the MDT. In Britain consultant psychiatrists, unlike other mental health professionals, have been independent of any form of line management. Traditionally consultant psychiatrists have had a "direct responsibility to see that the variety of disciplines caring for patients are coordinated" which "implies leadership of the MDT" (Royal College of Psychiatrists, 1984). The *Mental Health of the Nation* (Royal College of Psychiatrists, 1992) reinforced this position, identifying consultant psychiatrists as the fundamental unit of service delivery with responsibility to lead the MDT, and a role in management, as well as functioning as the patient's personal physician. The clinical responsibility of the psychiatrist as responsible medical officer (RMO) has a legal basis which cannot be abdicated, although other health care professionals have their own professional responsibilities. The RMO role, traditionally only relevant to in-patient care, now also carries responsibility for the development of an appropriate discharge plan (under section 117 of the 1983 Mental Health Act and the Care Programme Approach (Kingdon, 1994)) and the decision to include discharged patients on the Supervision Register (Holloway, 1994*a*). As the only team members to be free of management hierarchies consultant psychiatrists have in the past been in a strong position to act as advocates for their patients. There is also an expectation among patients and other organisations that the doctor is the person in charge, responsible for making decisions about treatment. In addition consultant psychiatrists receive a longer training than other mental health care professionals.

Few consultant psychiatrists have the skill, or the time, to carry out effectively all the leadership tasks set out above. Many MDTs have challenged the traditional leadership role of doctors among mental health professionals (which was in any case always a fiction within the mental hospital, where the nurses had almost absolute effective power over their patients' lives). Teams have instead chosen to work through collective decision making or have functioned with a non-medical member as team leader or coordinator (Ovretveit, 1994). In other teams there are different leaders for different functions; this 'distributive' model of leadership can be practical and effective (Watts & Bennett, 1983; Pilling, 1991).

The profession of psychiatry

"Absolutely central to the nature and traditions of the NHS is the particular nature of the doctor–patient relationship" (Reed, 1991). This underpins the principal role for the consultant psychiatrist, which is the "medical treatment of psychiatric illness, emotional disturbance and abnormal behaviour" (New Shorter Oxford English Dictionary).

The profession probably owes its origin to the urbanisation and industrialisation of the 18th century which resulted in the rapid growth of private "mad houses" and the emergence of a group of doctors known as the "mad doctors" or "mad house doctors", probably the first full time specialists. The mad houses were sometimes in large rectories and were sometimes run by the clergy, or doctors, but more often by lay businessmen for profit. A flourishing trade in lunacy developed as described by Parry-Jones (1972).

The increasing degree of medical involvement in the mad houses during the 18th century can be inferred from the various acts of parliament passed during this period (Jones, 1972, see also page 454). In the 1714 Vagrancy Act, lunatics only received a brief mention as one type of vagrant who could be detained or restrained; two or more justices of the peace could apprehend "lunatics who were furiously mad and dangerous". There was little advance in the 1744 Vagrancy Act which permitted any person to apprehend a lunatic, and provided two justices of the peace assented, the lunatic could be locked up in "some secure place", with no requirement for anyone to ascertain the person's insanity.

Over the next 30 years, following a series of scandals in the mad houses, and a parliamentary enquiry, there was a major shift in public opinion regarding the role of the doctor. The 1774 Act for Regulating Private Madhouses stipulated that "no person could be admitted to a mad house without having an order in writing under the hand and seal of some physician, surgeon or apothecary" (Hunter & MacAlpine, 1963, p.452). This Act also stated that all private mad houses had to be licensed by Commissioners appointed by the President of the Royal College of Physicians from among its Fellows. Although the Commissioners could visit the mad houses, their powers were limited, and they could not revoke or refuse a licence however adverse their report might be.

The 1808 Asylums Act for the first time recognised the role of the state in providing care for the insane, and each county was required to build an asylum. More importantly this act stipulated that the new asylums should have a medical superintendent. The speciality grew as more asylums were built, increasing numbers of patients were admitted and more medical superintendents and their assistants were appointed.

Similar changes took place in Europe. For example, in Paris the mentally ill were admitted to hospitals such as Salpetrière and the Bicêtre and so they became segregated and alienated from society. The patients were said to suffer from "mental alienation" and the doctors who cared for them became known as 'alienists'.

Professional associations

A profession comes of age when it forms its own professional society, publishes its own journal, permits entry only after a period of specialised training and has its own qualifications, gained by passing the professional examinations.

In this context the foundation of the Association of Medical Officers of Asylums and Hospitals for the Insane was a major landmark in the development of the profession in Great Britain. The first meeting of the asylum doctors was convened by Dr Samuel Hitch at the Gloucester General

Lunatic Asylum in 1843. The profession was quite small as Dr Hitch wrote to only 83 asylum doctors, and it could not be considered enthusiastic as only 10 doctors attended (Renvoize, 1991). Annual meetings continued to be poorly attended but the society picked up after 1853 when the *Asylum Journal of Mental Science* was first published. In 1858 this became the *Journal of Mental Science* and in 1963, the *British Journal of Psychiatry*. The Association gradually prospered becoming the Medico-Psychological Association in 1865, the Royal Medico-Psychological Association in 1926, finally receiving assent to become a Royal College in 1972 when it became the Royal College of Psychiatrists.

A profession's control over its standards lies in its examinations which monitor the national standards achieved by the training programme. The first examination, the Certificate of Efficiency in Psychological Medicine, was started by the Medico-Psychological Association in 1885 (Howells, 1991). This was replaced by a Diploma in Psychological Medicine in 1948 which was subsequently run by the conjoint board of the Royal Colleges of Physicians and Surgeons. Only in 1972, with the formation of the Royal College of Psychiatrists, was the present qualifying examination (Membership of the Royal College of Psychiatrists: MRCPsych) introduced.

The training presently consists of a rotation through several adult psychiatry placements and a variety of psychiatric subspecialities, as well as some psychotherapy training, and should last for at least three years before the MRCPsych examination can be taken. There is considerable debate within the profession in trying to obtain an optimum balance between adult psychiatry and the subspecialities, the basic sciences and the clinical disciplines, and hospital versus community approaches, but the general aim is to ensure that both the training and examination reflect current practice. Reviewing psychiatric training in relation to developments within mental health care, Cawley (1990) recommended that psychiatrists should consider what they do in their practice that other professionals such as the GP, clinical psychologist or psychiatric nurse cannot do either individually or collectively.

The number of consultant psychiatrists in the UK has been increasing, and current provision for the 16–65 age group is approximately one consultant psychiatrist per 50 000 in non-teaching hospital districts and one per 25 000 for teaching hospital populations (Sims, 1992). Sims has recommended doubling this number. The Calman report (DoH, 1993) has introduced further changes in psychiatric training. There is now a unified training grade and the number of consultant posts may be increased to promote a more consultant-based service, in line with the rest of Europe.

Clinical psychology

Clinical psychology involves the application of the principles and procedures of psychology to health care. There are approximately 1500 full-time equivalent clinical psychologists working in the NHS in England, one per

33 000 of the population (Manpower Planning Advisory Group, 1990). A formal role for clinical psychologists first emerged during the Second World War when they were used to assist in personnel recruitment and training, and later to work with soldiers or civilians with psychological trauma due to the war. In the immediate post-war years the role of psychologists was essentially that of laboratory scientists providing an ancillary service to the psychiatric profession. Increased psychological knowledge accompanied by the development of new techniques such as psychometric measurement, the application of learning theory in behaviour therapy and the increasing popularity of psychotherapy expanded the scope of clinical psychology.

The Trethowan Committee, which reported in 1977, was established to examine the role of clinical psychologists in the NHS. The committee ratified the independent status of the profession and formalised the organisation of services, proposing larger departments providing a comprehensive range of clinical psychology services in an area. After the 1982 NHS reforms, district managed psychology services headed by a district psychologist and taking referrals from primary care and specialist psychiatric services were set up. As a result of the latest NHS reforms these services are now located within provider units.

Clinical psychologists must obtain a good first degree in psychology, which is then followed by postgraduate academic and practical training in clinical psychology. Training schemes devote little attention to such psychiatric concepts as the diagnosis and phenomenology of mental illness, focusing instead on a variety of psychological approaches to distress or disorder. Competition for places on training schemes is intense, and most trainees will have obtained additional experience as assistant psychologists. The responsibilities of a clinical psychologist include assessment, therapy, teaching, training and research. Consultancy to staff teams, both about team functioning and the management of problematic patients, is a prominent activity within some psychology departments. Psychologists work in hospital, primary care and community settings. They offer psychological treatments for a broad range of psychological difficulties: these include emotional problems (for example, anxiety, depression, obsessions, grief); addictions and habit problems; psychosexual problems; social and interpersonal problems (including loneliness, shyness, aggressive behaviour, marital problems); and psychosomatic and medical problems (Hall & Marzillier, 1992).

Psychiatric nursing

Psychiatric nurses form the core staff group within mental health services. Nurses are by far the most numerous group of staff, and tend to have the greatest direct contact with patients and relatives, both in hospital and community settings.

With the rise of the asylums in the 19th century there was a corresponding increase in the numbers of staff, the attendants or keepers. In the self-contained community of an asylum, attendants were based in the wards, the infirmary, the laundry and the farm assisting the patients to maintain the asylum community. Life for the attendants was far from comfortable: they often worked 15 hours a day for low wages. In the middle of the century, with an improvement in attitudes towards the insane and a greater spirit of humanity in their treatment, there was an expectation that attendants would set an example for patients. However, as the asylums became more overcrowded the attendants resumed their traditional more custodial roles and were relied on for 'strength and intimidation, rather than friendliness and common sense' (Connolly, 1992).

In 1890 the Medico-Psychological Association of Medical Superintendents introduced a two year training programme for attendants, later extended to three years. The newly founded British Nursing Association for general nurses did not recognise this as a qualification and excluded attendants from its register. The attendants were more concerned about their poor working conditions than their status or professional development and founded the radical National Asylum Workers Union to campaign for better conditions of service and pay. With the Mental Treatment Act (1930) changes started to occur for staff as well as patients, and male and female attendants were now known as nurses. The Royal Medico-Psychological Association remained in control of psychiatric nurse training until after the Second World War when the General Nursing Council assumed responsibility for it.

Over the next 30 years the emphasis in the syllabus for psychiatric nurses changed in line with developments in services, and with the need for continuing education to include self-directed learning. More recently Project 2000 (UKCC, 1987) proposed a radical change in the structure of nurse education, leading to a new type of practitioner. The project involves a three year course with a first half common to all nurses. In the second half of the course the trainee nurse may specialise in one of four areas, including mental illness. In theory a 'practitioner' would be competent to provide care in both institutional and non-institutional settings, and with further specialist training can become a specialist practitioner. Specialist nurse therapists trained to offer behavioural treatment already practise in hospital and community settings, and post-basic training courses also exist for community psychiatric nurses. Different grades of registered mental nurse (RMNs) are recognised, including staff nurses (grades D and E), clinical charge nurses (grade F), and senior nurses (grade G and above). To retain their registration nurses must now attend continuing education courses throughout their career. There are also less qualified health care assistants who receive more limited vocational training.

The contemporary role of psychiatric nurses has been described as unclear (Connolly, 1992). There is a discrepancy between the nursing literature and the actual experience of hospital-based nurses. In 1968 a report on psychiatric nursing stated that the aim of work with patients and relatives was to carry out medical instructions and report objectively to the psychiatrist: "Information must be conveyed to other members of the team accurately and precisely and free from subjective bias as far as possible" (HMSO, 1968). In practice psychiatric nurses still largely play a formal therapeutic role, supporting and monitoring the treatment prescribed by the medical staff (Cormack, 1983). However, the recent introduction of the nursing process has given nurses a problem solving method for identifying the health needs of patients and providing care. Within the in-patient setting, nurses play a crucial role in determining the culture of the ward; the charge nurse is particularly important in ensuring that the ward environment is safe and therapeutic. The in-patient primary nurse has an important role in coordinating and integrating the contributions of other team members (Cormack, 1983), a role that is assumed by the key worker (often a nurse) within community teams.

Community psychiatric nursing

Community psychiatric nursing appeared in Britain in the mid 1950s at Warlingham Park Hospital, Surrey (Bennett, 1991a). The main impetus for the establishment of the service was the introduction of phenothiazine drugs and depot preparations which established a new demand for the follow-up and aftercare of patients with schizophrenia in the community (Simmons & Brooker, 1986). With the loss of specialised local authority mental health departments and mental welfare officers, nurses were quick to rise to the challenge of undertaking the social rehabilitative roles previously seen as the function of the social worker. Development of the CPN service occurred in parallel with falling bed occupancy and more use of short-term admissions.

Since the early 1970s the number and availability of CPNs has increased dramatically, and by the second half of the 1970s the role of CPNs in the long term care of patients with schizophrenia was well established. The early clinical work of CPNs involved observing patients for clinical signs and advising on nursing management, as well as administering and monitoring prescribed medication, observing side-effects and regulating treatment regimens (Sladden, 1979).

In the 1980s the role of CPNs diversified as different models of service developed. Some CPNs continued to work within specialist multidisciplinary teams while others were independent practitioners who worked in primary care settings. At the same time the proportion of referrals from psychiatrists to CPNs fell and referrals from GPs increased (White, 1990). Goldberg (1985) expressed concern that CPNs were drifting away from the hospital base, with the consequent risk that the care of chronic psychiatric patients would take second place. Work with patients with schizophrenia became characterised by short contact times, the administration of medication and referral for a consultant opinion if symptoms worsened. A national survey of CPNs confirmed that those with a diagnosis of schizophrenia accounted for only a quarter of all CPN caseloads throughout the UK and that a quarter of CPNs had no patients with schizophrenia (White, 1990). This reflected the changing pattern of referrals to CPNs. An additional problem was a lack of training in the specific skills required to deliver psychosocial interventions to patients with schizophrenia living at home with relatives (Brooker *et al*, 1992, 1994). While GPs greatly value the CPN role in primary care, a controlled study of CPN intervention in primary care showed that both CPN and control patients improved significantly and equally (Gournay & Brooking, 1994). Drop-out rates from CPN care were high: although the drop-outs were more disabled than those who completed CPN treatment they did as well as those who completed CPN treatment. There was no evidence that CPN treatment saved GP time.

In addition to generic CPNs there are also specialist CPNs who work with specific groups such as the elderly or substance misusers or have particular therapeutic skills, for example in behaviour therapy. Health authority manpower targets recommend one CPN per 10 000 population, although in contemporary services the CPN is increasingly been drawn into the multidisciplinary community team.

Social work

The emergence of the separate and paid profession of social work (as distinct from voluntary work or religious duty) with the specific aim of helping the poor arose from the chaos and destitution which followed in the wake of the industrial revolution. Charities sprang up to alleviate poverty but they and their benefactors were only willing to help the "deserving" poor – widows, orphans, the thrifty elderly or those who had fallen upon hard times. Their generosity failed to extend to the so-called "undeserving" poor – unmarried mothers, the unemployed, drinkers and others who were consigned to the vagaries of the Poor Law. To ensure that this distinction was properly made, and that their money was spent wisely, the Charities Organisation Service (COS) was formed in 1869 with officers appointed who were dedicated to this task. These officers developed their own specific form of enquiry into individuals' social circumstances and the causes of their poverty which was probably the first type of social case history. Gradually the officers of the COS became acknowledged experts on poverty, wrote articles and gave lectures on social issues of the day, provided evidence to parliamentary committees, and started the School of Sociology in 1903 to provide training. They were the predecessors of the present day social workers (Irvine, 1979). Medical social work derives from the hospital almoner, whose main task was to assess an individual's entitlement to charitable treatment in hospital. This role ceased with the advent of the NHS in 1948.

Social work involvement in psychiatry derives from two quite separate professions. The position of duty authorised relieving officer was introduced in the Lunacy Act (1890) as "an expert in the legal aspect of admission and discharge from the hospital as well as being protector of the public". This post became the duty authorised officer in the 1930 Mental Treatment Act, and the mental welfare officer in the 1959 Mental Health Act, with little change in role. In the 1983 Mental Health Act the mental welfare officer became the approved social worker (ASW), who in addition to a role as "protector of the public" was also an advocate of the patient, with a requirement to consider alternatives to hospitalisation during assessment of an application for compulsory admission (Olsen, 1984).

A quite different type of professional involvement was derived from the child guidance movement. In 1929 the Commonwealth Fund of America provided grants to train social workers to work in the new London Child Guidance Clinic (later to become the Child Guidance Training Centre). These workers soon embraced current psychoanalytic methods and started case work initially with the parents of disturbed children, later extending their role into the adult psychiatric domain.

Psychiatric social work became a flourishing profession until the early 1970s when it was effectively abolished following the 1968 Seebhom Report and the Social Services Act (1970). A consequence of the act, which introduced the current structure of local authority social services departments, was the replacement of specialists by generic social workers who were perhaps unrealistically expected to be competent at managing anyone presenting with a social problem, including disturbed children, blind people, the elderly, the mentally ill and the mentally handicapped (Martin, 1984). These changes had serious consequences for patients with mental illness. Case work ceased and the loss of expertise within the new social services departments was accompanied by a lack of investment in community facilities for the mentally ill during the 1970s and 1980s. The case work role of the psychiatric social worker was gradually taken over by CPNs.

Contemporary policy has once more placed social services authorities at the heart of community care for the mentally ill (Holloway, 1990). The statutory ASW role requires localities to have access to social workers with special mental health expertise (Olsen, 1994). More recently social workers have begun to function as care managers, with a requirement to contribute to the development of care packages under the Care Programme Approach (Kingdon, 1994; Thornicroft, 1994). Social workers are therefore central to the planning and provision of the "social care" element of the management of people with long-term mental illnesses, including day care, sheltered work and non-hospital supported accommodation, and they frequently function as key workers.

When working within a multidisciplinary mental health team the social worker plays a crucial role. This is likely to involve practical advice, advocacy and counselling and, occasionally, psychotherapy. Family or marital therapy may be required, or clients may be referred to specialist agencies such as

Relate, or in cases of more serious marital breakdown clients may be directed to appropriate legal representatives. Financial problems are also common among psychiatric patients, requiring intervention with housing authorities or housing associations, public utilities or other commercial companies. More complex cases of debt may require referral to a welfare advice agency, while if patients are unable to manage their financial affairs the social worker may need to call on the services of the Court of Protection. Referring clients to other agencies or liaising with them is an important part of the social work role.

Issues of child care and child abuse may dominate social work in child psychiatry, but are also relevant in adult psychiatry. (When children are at potential risk all mental health professionals will be required to follow the local child protection policy.) A social worker may also have to make emergency child fostering arrangements, for the short term care of older children whose mothers have been admitted to hospital, particularly when there is no other family back up. Longer term child care issues are now generally dealt with by specialist child and family sections within the social services departments.

Occupational therapy

The treatment of mental disorder by occupation probably goes back to ancient times (McDonald, 1976). Aesculapius, in ancient Greece is said to have "quietened delirium with songs, farces and music." Celsus, the 1st century anatomist, recommended occupational exercise for maintaining health: this included sailing, hunting, ball games, running and walking as well as reading aloud as treatment for a weak stomach. Aurelianus, a neurologist in the 5th century, prescribed passive and active exercise, massage, graded exercises and speech therapy for various types of paralysis. Although Philippe Pinel in France and William Tuke in England are generally credited with the invention in the 1790s of "moral treatment" and "occupation" as the principal methods of treating the mentally ill, psychological approaches towards the treatment of "consequential madness" were being advocated by Battie in the 1750s (Porter, 1990).

In the 19th century within the asylums responsibility for administering the new moral treatment fell upon the attendants. Some attendants specialised and became instructors teaching patients occupational skills, but at the same time remained responsible for nursing care. It was these treatment orientated attendants who became the first occupational therapists (OTs), but it was not until the turn of the century that George Barton of Clifton Springs first coined the term 'occupational therapist'.

The College of Occupational Therapists defines occupational therapy as "the treatment of physical and psychiatric conditions through specific activities in order to help people reach their maximum level of functioning and independence in all aspects of daily life." Most OT departments offer a wide range of therapies. Creative therapies derived from the arts have led to art therapy, pottery, sculpture or music therapy. Art therapy is not about acquiring the skills of painting but rather using art as a medium to describe inner feelings and so provide an opening into a person's inner world. Story writing and poetry groups may be helpful in a similar way, as is psychodrama. Many patients also benefit from more practical occupations such as woodwork or pottery. Some OT departments offer more specific types of psychotherapy, for example, anxiety management courses, relaxation classes, assertiveness training or stress management groups. For many patients with acute illnesses time spent in the OT department may be the main form of therapy they receive during their admission, and any of the above activities may serve to elevate self-esteem and promote symptom relief.

The OT approach to the long-term mentally ill is rather different and focuses more on rehabilitation and acquiring, or more usually re-acquiring, the skills of daily living which are often lost in chronic mental illness. These include personal hygiene, cooking, household cleaning, laundry, budgeting, and adequate nutrition and shopping. For a patient with chronic schizophrenia these activities may represent the major stumbling block to an independent existence.

A major OT skill is the development of structured programmes of daily activities which can prevent chronically disabled in-patients from losing more skills. Most in-patient OT departments have special kitchens or even whole flats designed to help patients learn these skills, while in other hospitals patients are taught these basic skills in groups before moving out into hostels or group homes. Industrial therapy units, once an integral part of the asylums, have been largely replaced by community-based work projects.

Occupational therapists frequently make home visits with patients prior to discharge, assessing their capacity for independent living *in vivo*. Safety assessments are particularly relevant in the assessment of elderly and cognitively impaired patients. Functional assessments are also required if discharge to supported accommodation is contemplated, as part of the needs-led care management assessment coordinated by social services. OT has long been an essential element of day hospital treatment. Increasingly OTs are working within multidisciplinary community mental health teams.

To work in the NHS an OT must be officially registered with the Council for Professions Supplementary to Medicine, which was set up following the Professions Supplementary to Medicine Act (1960). A report into the state of OT in the UK (Blom-Cooper, 1990) recommended that there should be 0.27 full-time equivalents of OTs per 1000 of the population. In addition to qualified OTs there are 77 unqualified OTs, known as OT helpers, per 100 qualified posts, providing a valuable additional practical resource. Mental health is the largest employer of OTs (31%), followed by care of the elderly (20%) and learning difficulties (11%). OTs are much in demand, and the profession is expanding, with an increase from 3500 qualified OTs in 1971 to 9300 in 1987 (Blom-Cooper, 1990). There is a national shortage of OTs and vacancies, when they occur, may remain unfilled for many months.

Burnout

The effects of stress in the helping professions are well documented (Freudenberger, 1974; Maslach, 1979). Stress occurs as environmental or internal demands on an individual exceed the resources of that person's coping mechanisms. For health care professionals job stress occurs when one or more factors at work make demands on individuals that disrupt their psychological or physical homeostasis. Failure to maintain homeostasis may lead to the condition of "burnout". Freudenberger (1974) coined the term when he recognised the symptoms of exhaustion in his staff of social workers. Burnout has subsequently been defined as "a syndrome of emotional exhaustion, depersonalisation and reduced personal accomplishment that can occur among individuals who do people work of some kind" (Maslach & Jackson, 1981) or more broadly as "negative changes in work related attitudes and behaviour in response to job stress" (Cherniss, 1980). Sufferers develop a negative self-concept, negative job attitudes and exhibit loss of concern and feelings for patients or clients (Maslach, 1979). There may also be changes in motivation including loss of enthusiasm and sense of purpose in work.

One of the difficulties in working with psychiatric patients can be the chronic nature of their disorders, which may mean that staff get little positive feedback about their work, so reducing their job satisfaction. Working in a multidisciplinary team can lead to role conflict or role ambiguity. Lack of clarity over tasks and lack of formal and informal support from within the team can increase staff stress. Individual risk factors that have been identified as increasing susceptibility to stress include neurotic anxiety, type A personality, an external locus of control, and introversion (Cherniss, 1980).

Burnout has far reaching effects on patient care. It is important to prevent and reduce the effects of stress at work (Carson *et al*, 1994). Possible interventions include ensuring adequate staff/patient ratios since high case loads are known to contribute, improved education about stress, adequate peer support and supervision at work, offering staff opportunities for career development and the acquisition of new skills, the encouragement of increased personal resources and relaxation, the provision of specific support services for those who are not coping and, if necessary, allowing for breaks from work.

Access to services

The role of primary care in the psychiatric services is described in chapter 28. Direct access to specialist medical services has traditionally been discouraged in the UK, since it could be seen to erode the position of the GP within the health care system. GPs act as an important filter with a crucial role in prioritising who has access to what are limited specialist resources.

However, studies of the views of mental health service users and carers have consistently shown that lack of access to effective help, particularly at times of crisis, is a major source of complaint and concern (Shepherd *et al*, 1994). As a response some specialist psychiatric services encourage self-referrals as an alternative to referrals from a professional such as a GP or hospital doctor. CMHCs may offer an open access service, which tends to attract people with neurotic conditions and psychosocial crises (Hutton, 1985). By contrast psychiatric emergency clinics, either located within an accident and emergency department (A&E) or in psychiatric hospitals, cater for the whole range of psychiatric disorder including patients with drug and alcohol problems (Lim, 1983; Haw & Lanceley, 1987). Specialist services also run outreach programmes, most notably in the network of court diversion schemes in which mentally disordered people appearing before a court can receive a rapid psychiatric assessment (Joseph & Potter, 1993).

Emergency services

People present to services urgently and in a manner that demands the bypassing of an appointments system for a wide range of reasons. These include the acute onset of severe mental illness, decompensation in a patient with a chronic disorder, and in situations of personal distress following a life crisis such as an unexpected severe loss. Acute behavioural disturbance, including dangerous behaviour to self or others, is a common cause of emergency presentation, as are the behavioural effects of acute intoxication by alcohol or illicit drugs.

One of the consequences of the development of district general hospital psychiatric units has been the increasing integration of psychiatric emergency services with general medical services. Advantages of integration include the ready availability of the service for both patients and other doctors, with increased opportunity for liaison between specialities. Patients and carers in crisis are more likely to attend an A&E than visit a large mental hospital, although a specialised emergency clinic within the local mental health unit has significant advantages over a crowded A&E (Lim, 1983). From a medical point of view the automatic inclusion of checks on physical health is especially relevant if the diagnosis is unclear and there is a possibility of an underlying organic condition (Katschnig & Cooper, 1991).

Primary care services including GPs and attached CPNs have continued to manage the more minor psychiatric emergencies in the community. In order to obtain an urgent specialist assessment for a disturbed patient, the GP may request a home visit by a consultant or medical member of the community psychiatric team. Home assessment may be incorporated as a routine aspect of a local psychiatric service (Burns *et al*, 1993*a*) or be provided as part of a rapid-intervention service when patients are presented as emergencies but do not require immediate hospital admission (Merson *et al*, 1992).

An example of this approach is the early intervention service, a rapid-response service to requests for psychiatric intervention from GPs, A&E departments and other agencies, based in Paddington, London. It consists of a multi-disciplinary team offering home-based assessments, treatment planning and follow-up using an identified key worker. This service has been shown to be more acceptable (in terms of patient satisfaction) and effective (in terms of symptom resolution and the use of in-patient bed days) than standard hospital-based care (Merson *et al*, 1992).

Alternatively the GP can refer the patient to the psychiatrist on call for the local psychiatric service for an emergency assessment. The psychiatrist on call (usually a junior doctor) will also deal with self-referrals and referrals by casualty officers, doctors in other specialities, and from social services and the police, who have powers under section 136 of the 1983 Mental Health Act to convey a mentally disordered person to a place of safety.

Domiciliary visits and urgent home assessments

The domiciliary consultation service was established with the introduction of the NHS in 1948. Although a domiciliary visit (DV) is defined as 'a visit to the patient's home, at the request of the general practitioner (GP), and normally in his company to advise on the diagnosis or treatment of a patient who cannot on medical grounds attend hospital' many consultants undertake DVs alone. Consultants receive a fee for carrying out a DV, which serves as an incentive to give DVs a priority.

In the 1950s DVs were one of the few forms of community provision available. Since then DVs have been used by GPs for a variety of purposes, most commonly to obtain an urgent assessment as an alternative to a hospital out-patient appointment which may involve a considerable delay. The traditional DV should be distinguished from the request for home assessment with a view to compulsory admission to hospital. It is the responsibility of the local mental health provider to ensure that senior on call doctors are available to carry out Mental Health Act duties at the request of GPs or social services departments.

DVs help to ensure the patient is assessed by the named consultant and not another member of the psychiatric team. They also allow evaluation of the home situation which can be particularly helpful with older patients. Home visiting is useful for assessing psychotic patients with impaired insight who may be unwilling to attend hospital, neurotic patients who deny they have an illness, for example patients with severe anorexia, or those who have difficulty leaving home either because of their mental state, for example, patients who have agoraphobia, or because they are physically unable to do so. If there is a shortage of in-patient beds DVs can assist in preadmission screening.

Critics of the current arrangements over DVs suggest that they are time consuming and clinically inefficient. The movement towards community care for psychiatric patients has encouraged the expansion of a range of alternative assessment services, including crisis intervention teams, CMHCs, out-patient clinics held in primary care settings and the incorporation of home assessment as part of routine clinical practice by community mental health teams. In any district the role of the DV is likely to depend on the availability of alternative or complementary emergency or community assessment facilities (Sutherby *et al*, 1992).

Crisis intervention

The development of specific crisis intervention teams owes much to Caplan's theory that in a crisis people's traditional patterns of coping break down (Caplan, 1964). Caplan hypothesised that in their response to an adverse event there is a critical period during which people are extremely responsive to therapeutic intervention, the disequilibrium of the crisis providing an opportunity for more adaptive coping skills to emerge. Scott & Seccombe (1976) saw the first crisis interview as being of supreme importance to the patient and as the beginning of treatment. Consideration of the crisis as affecting more than the presenting individual leads to a family approach to assessment and management.

Another influence on the development of crisis intervention teams comes from the development of community care, and the steady reduction in in-patient beds that has accompanied this policy which has stimulated interest in the management of people with acute psychiatric illness at home. Twenty years ago, as a first move out of their hospital base, some specialist psychiatric units established crisis intervention teams to respond to urgent calls for assistance (Waldron, 1983). Some teams are mobile, providing an outreach service, while others have an ambulatory or walk-in service. Teams may be based in a DGH unit or CMHC (Katschnig & Cooper, 1991). Services deal with all forms of psychiatric crisis or focus on particular patient groups, for example, specifically excluding patients with a psychotic illness while targeting those in an acute psychosocial crisis.

Home treatment for the acutely mentally ill

Although crisis theory remains fashionable there is a dearth of research to support the adoption of the crisis intervention model for most cases of acute personal distress; the empirical research literature has focused on the community management of people with major mental illnesses (Dedman, 1993). In the best resourced services members of the multidisciplinary team are available to patients in their homes up to 24 hours seven days a week, enabling the management of even the most disturbed psychiatric patients to be largely carried out within the community (Dean & Gadd, 1990; Marks *et al*, 1994). In addition to crisis teams some services offer a non-hospital residential facility (the "crisis house") as an alternative to in-patient admission, with the opportunity of admission to a "respite bed" for psychotic patients in long-term contact with services who are having problems coping at home (Strathdee & Thornicroft, 1993).

A series of papers have reported a study of intensive community care as an alternative to standard hospital-based care for people from the catchment area presenting acutely for admission to the Maudsley Hospital, London (Muijen *et al*, 1992*a,b*; Audini *et al*, 1994; Knapp *et al*, 1994; Marks *et al*, 1994). The daily living programme (DLP) followed a service model developed and successfully utilised in a classic study carried out by Stein & Test (1980) in Madison, Wisconsin. Patients allocated to the DLP spent much less time in hospital than those receiving standard care: 83% of the DLP sample were admitted to hospital (for a mean of 14 days) compared with 100% of the control group (for a mean of 72 days). (The control group length of stay is considerably longer than the current mean length of stay of the catchment area wards at the Maudsley Hospital, which is now 26 days; i.e. part of the success of the DLP reflected the prolonged duration of admissions, particularly for neurotic patients, then the norm within the Maudsley (Holloway, 1995).) Up to month 20 of the study the DLP improved the symptoms and social functioning of its patients, although these gains were subsequently lost during long-term follow-up. Patients and relatives were consistently more satisfied with DLP than standard hospital care. DLP staff experienced high levels of stress.

Within the first 18 months of the study there were three deaths from self-harm in the experimental group and one homicide compared with two deaths from self-harm in the control group out of a total sample of 187 patients and controls. The homicide occurred seven weeks after a five day admission of a previously unknown patient, apparently in response to well concealed persecutory delusions which were only elicited after the murder.

Compulsory admission

All developed countries have a legal framework governing the compulsory admission and detention of psychiatric patients. The Mental Health Act (1983) provides this framework for England and Wales: separate legislation which utilises similar principles applies in Scotland and Northern Ireland. Until the 1930 Mental Treatment Act all admissions to hospital in England and Wales were on a compulsory basis, although the notion of informal admissions had been previously suggested by many psychiatrists including Samuel Gaskell[1]. The spirit of the Mental Health Acts of 1959 and 1983 was to encourage informal admission if possible with compulsory admission being reserved as a last resort.

Local psychiatric units should produce policy documents which summarise the use of the Mental Health Act and provide training for staff. The act itself is readily available from HMSO and should be in the possession of all psychiatrists practising in England. It is supplemented by a Code of Practice, produced by the Mental Health Act Commission and regularly updated. There are a number of textbooks devoted specifically to mental health legislation (Bluglass, 1983; Jones, 1994). An excellent summary is given in *College Seminars in Forensic Psychiatry* (Chiswick & Cope, 1995; Cope, 1995).

In Britain the use of compulsory admission and treatment orders occurs largely in the context of emergency admission. In spite of guidance about the application of the Mental Health Act (1983) some variation remains in the interpretation of the legislation, resulting in variations in practice between local services (Hatfield *et al*, 1992). One generally accepted aim is to minimise the use of compulsory admission by encouraging people to accept in-patient treatment on an informal basis and it is the duty of the ASW to explore alternatives to admission for patients who are unwilling to come into hospital. Psychiatrists seem to be more inclined than non-psychiatric professionals to use compulsory orders, and inexperienced doctors generally produce higher compulsory admission rates than those with more experience (Marson *et al*, 1988).

Characteristics of detained patients

A comparison of the social and clinical characteristics of patients admitted formally and informally in the London borough of Camden was conducted by Szmukler *et al* (1981). This showed that patients admitted compulsorily were a socially handicapped group with high rates of unemployment, transient accommodation and frequently of no fixed abode. In many cases they had also lost contact with their relatives for long periods. High rates

---

Footnote 1: Samuel Gaskell (1807–1879) was an energetic and reforming Lunacy Commissioner of the 19th century. He came from a strongly religious unitarian family, the son of a successful sailcloth manufacturer in Warrington. After qualifying in Edinburgh he took up a position as Resident Surgeon in the Lancaster County Asylum where he spent most of his professional life and was later appointed as a Lunacy Commissioner. Even though the publishers of the Royal College of Psychiatrists bear his name Gaskell himself was not a prolific writer and published only one paper, which pleaded the case for informal admission "On the want of better provision for the labouring and middle classes when attacked or threatened with insanity" (1860). In 1865 he was run over by a vehicle and thereafter became a recluse and died in 1879. He never married, but his sister who married a wealthy banker left a bequeath in his memory to the Royal Medico-Psychological Association to fund an annual medal and prize (Freeman & Tantam, 1991).

of chronic mental illness were found among both formal and informal admissions, but among the formal patients there were higher rates of schizophrenia and mania while depression was under-represented. The formally detained patients had higher symptom ratings and were more ill on admission and, as expected, had less insight: 56% believed they did not need to be in hospital in comparison with only 14% in the informal group.

Although most of the above findings were in the expected direction the follow-up study of Szmukler *et al* (1981) was more revealing. This showed that fewer compulsorily admitted patients attended for psychiatric follow-up, saw their GP or took psychotropic medication. Their social and psychiatric handicaps persisted after discharge and the admissions appeared to serve only as brief interludes protecting the patients from more severe states of self-neglect, at the same time shielding society from the consequences of more florid disturbances.

A number of sociodemographic variables related to the patient may increase the chance of a compulsory admission, including higher age, male sex, low socioeconomic status and previous in-patient treatment (Marson *et al*, 1988) as well as being a member of an ethnic minority (Moodley, 1993). However, a recent study of admissions to hospital from two inner London catchment areas concluded that ethnicity was not a major factor in the use of the Mental Health Act. The major determining factors that could be identified were clinical: diagnosis of schizophrenia and the presence of challenging behaviours (Bebbington *et al*, 1994). Once patients are identified as requiring in-patient admission ethnicity is not a major factor in the application of the Mental Health Act (Holloway *et al*, 1992).

The 1959 and 1983 Mental Health Acts contained identical powers for the police to convey patients to hospital for assessment (section 136 of both acts). Patients admitted on police orders were more often male and had higher symptom ratings on admission, with higher rates of social handicap and social isolation than those admitted compulsorily via their GPs (Szmukler *et al*, 1981). The use of section 136 is controversial and varies markedly across England and Wales. Police involvement is particularly common in the admission of Afro-Caribbean patients with a functional psychosis (Ineichen *et al*, 1984; Harrison *et al*, 1989; Fahy *et al*, 1987; Dunn & Fahy, 1990; Lloyd & Moodley, 1992). In a study of the use of section 136, common reasons recorded by the police for instituting the admission included assault (non-domestic), suicidal gestures, drink and drug offences, clothing removed in public places and other bizarre episodes which were categorised under "offences against public order", while among women "wandering" was frequent (Sims & Symonds, 1975). Schizophrenia comprised 40% of the cases, manic–depression 12%, alcohol misuse 8%. A more recent study based in an inner London Borough (Fahy *et al*, 1987) found rather lower rates for schizophrenia (27%), but more alcohol and substance misuse (18%) and personality disorder, but these differences probably reflect the different populations studied. It strikingly uncommon for inappropriate patients to be brought to hospital by the police (Moodley & Perkins, 1991). More common is the inappropriate release of such patients after a hasty assessment.

Szmukler *et al* (1981) found that the majority of the readmissions of those previously compulsorily admitted on a section were again on a compulsory basis. They cautioned that it was naive to assume these patients acquired insight or changed during an admission so that they became compliant with treatment. These considerations, fuelled by widespread concern over isolated incidents of dangerous behaviour by psychiatric patients, have led to the introduction of the Supervision Register for monitoring vulnerable patients in the community (Holloway, 1994*a*), and amendment of the 1983 Mental Health Act to include a power of Supervised Discharge in the Mental Health (Patients in the Community) Act 1995, which came into effect in April 1996 (Holloway, 1996).

Sectorisation

In Britain local psychiatric services are managed by providers (NHS Trusts) which have contracts with purchasing Health Authorities or Health Commissions. The providers serve catchment area populations of 100 000 to 600 000, and the majority of catchment areas are further subdivided into sectors of between 25 000 and 100 000 people. Within the sector one or more clinical teams provides a comprehensive community service which usually has close links with an in-patient unit.

There are many potential advantages to a sectorised mental health service (see Box 27.4), of which the most obvious is the existence of clear-cut lines of responsibility for the care of patients. However, there are also potential disadvantages, notably in reducing the therapeutic choices open to patients and GPs (who may themselves be acting as purchasers of care). Another potential problem is the provision of care to rootless patients with psychotic disorder who drift from one catchment area to another, as in the notorious case of Christopher Clunis (Coid, 1994; Ritchie *et al*, 1994).

Sectorisation is also a feature of mental health services in a number of European countries, being particularly well developed in France and Italy (Bennett, 1991*b*). Countries that rely on insurance-based systems of care, for example the USA, Germany and Belgium, have generally less well developed sectorisation policies and poorer integration between hospital and community services (which may be in direct competition for resources or may have little incentive to work together) (Bennett, 1991*b*). There is some evidence that the introduction of a sectorised service can result in a decrease in the use of acute in-patient beds (Tyrer *et al*, 1989; Hansson, 1989; Thornicroft & Strathdee, 1994).

The voluntary sector

Since the foundation of the Mental Aftercare Association in 1879 voluntary organisations have had a key role in community services for the mentally ill (Bennett, 1983). Recent government policy has further encouraged the development of voluntary agencies as providers of mental health services (Groves, 1990), and social services authorities are specifically encouraged to purchase social care from private and voluntary sector providers. Non-statutory agencies are particularly involved in running day centres, drop-ins and sheltered work projects, in the provision of supported housing and residential care and in offering counselling services. A strength of the voluntary sector is its capacity to target a specific client group, for example offering specialist counselling for women or people from an ethnic minority.

Voluntary agencies range from large national organisations with a professional management structure to purely local bodies that run single projects. MIND (the National Association for Mental Health) combines a central office that serves as a pressure group campaigning on behalf of people who have a "mental health problem" with some 200 affiliated local groups which run a plethora of projects offering direct services. The Richmond Fellowship is a charity based in London which has 30 hostels throughout the country offering both short-term and long-term care for people with severe mental illness, as well as a range of unsupervised group homes. In total it caters for around 500 residents. There are many other smaller less publicised organisations, such as the Psychiatric Rehabilitation Association and the Mental After Care Association which have, day centres and hostels. They have often been started as an attempt to meet local needs, intending to fill a temporary gap in statutory services.

Supporting carers

There is an increasingly recognised role of professionals in the support and education of carers. Voluntary agencies also focus on offering support to the family or other informal carers of people with mental illness. The National Schizophrenia Fellowship (NSF) is a voluntary organisation for people with schizophrenia and their relatives. It has over 6000 members and 150 local groups, and receives over 5000 appeals for help and advice each year. Relatives of people with schizophrenia may themselves become anxious or depressed, or feel shunned by embarrassed friends. They may derive comfort from meeting other relatives of patients with schizophrenia who are in a similar position. Supporting and educating relatives may decrease their sense of isolation and encourage them to monitor a sufferer's mental health and recognise the early signs of a relapse. More generally NSF groups help families to cope with the disorder.

Helplines

Over the last 10 years there has been a rapid increase in the range of helplines in response to the expression of a need for such support and information. Helplines give callers quick and easy access to independent and confidential help, and anonymity if desired. The Telephone Helplines

---

Box 27.4 Reported advantages of sectorisation

Defined responsibility for each patient requiring a service
"Economies of small scale": the development of close working
links between agencies
Clarity of functions of local teams
Manageable scale for local needs assessments
Minimises patients lost to follow-up
Allows comparative research and evaluation between different
service models across sectors
Improves identity of staff with locality
Greater budgetary clarity
Potential for improved liaison with primary care
Allows inter-agency assessment, treatment and care
Enables integration of health, social and voluntary services
Facilitates home treatment and day care services
Preferred by patients and families

(From Strathdee & Thornicroft, 1993)

Group has published guidelines for good practice which cover the selection, training and supervision of staff and evaluation of services. Statutory support for helplines increased in 1993 when the Department of Health launched its Regional Health Information Services (Crone, 1993).

Helplines may play a particular therapeutic role for people in acute distress. The Samaritans helpline was founded by a clergyman, Chad Varah, in 1953 (Varah, 1973) and local branches are still run by trained volunteers. Although the Samaritans cannot claim to reduce the suicide rate they do offer easily made contact with someone who gives a sympathetic ear yet remains at a distance, allowing the caller to end the call at any time. In some cases Samaritans offer direct personal contact after the call.

Other helplines focus more on providing information to callers. Recently the campaigning charity Schizophrenia – A National Emergency (SANE) established a hotline, Saneline, to share information about psychiatric disorders and available services for people with mental illness and their carers. Saneline received 50 000 calls in its first year, over half of which were from people with a serious illness and who felt desperately in need of help.

Self-help groups

Marks (1992) argues that self-help methods can enhance care delivery. Therapeutic self-help groups such as those run by 'Triumph over Phobia' or 'Overeaters Anonymous' try to reduce a person's problems in a lasting way, while palliative groups have the more limited aim of offering information and support. Other self-help approaches involve books, computers, videotapes and audiotapes, and have been shown to be effective in the treatment of, for example, depression, anxiety, phobias and bulimia with therapeutic gains being maintained at two year follow-up. Sufferers understand their problems better, learning to cope with or reduce them and to cooperate better with clinicians. Self-help methods are also cost effective and in line with recommendations that 'users should be empowered to master their own illness and problems' (King's Fund Report, 1992). Patients vary in their capability to use self-help material.

The private sector

The growth in private in-patient care over the last three decades is largely related to the growth in private health insurance policies. Today around 11% of the UK population have private health cover (more in the wealthier suburbs of the southeast, and rather less in inner city or rural areas). In most instances the private insurance is purchased by employers, generally large companies, although there is a growing number of individuals who take out private cover for themselves and their families. Not all policies cover psychiatric care, and even when there is cover there are fairly tight restrictions, particularly for in-patient care with few companies paying for an admission of more than three months duration.

Although private in-patient care is essentially similar to NHS care there are a few important differences. First, private hospitals are not sectorised and so the pattern of care does not follow the closed model of having one consultant looking after one ward or one team but rather there may be a relatively large number of consultants (30–40) with admitting rights to a private hospital with each consultant having only a very few admissions. Second, the 1983 Mental Health Act specifies that neither the admitting consultant (the RMO) nor any doctor who is employed as a director of the private hospital is able to make a medical recommendation under the Mental Health Act. To ensure that financial considerations do not enter into the clinical decision an independent opinion is therefore required to assess cases for compulsory admission. Third, the insurance companies will only pay for relatively brief admissions, so most of those admitted tend to have affective or substance misuse disorders, and the contribution of the private sector in treating patients with schizophrenia, particularly chronic schizophrenia is relatively small.

Traditionally out-patient treatment by psychoanalysis and the other depth psychotherapies, which are both lengthy and expensive, has also been within the private sector and the act of payment is seen as an integral part of the therapy. Private hospitals have often catered for what are seen as market niches, such as eating disorders, impotence, substance misuse, stress reactions, and the behavioural treatment of head injuries. Although the evidence is not available, private sector providers claim to offer greater comfort, convenience and privacy, reduced waiting times, more intensive treatment and greater respect for the patient. There is also a greater degree of direct contact with the consultant, as all the out-patient work is done by the consultant, with rather less involvement of the multidisciplinary team, the latter only being involved during an in-patient episode.

The NHS and Community Care Act (1990) encourages pluralism in the provision of services and with the development of the free market certain deficiencies in the NHS have become apparent. For example, health authorities are purchasing large numbers of medium secure beds, while in London an imbalance in the supply of acute beds and the demand for admission have resulted in an overflow of acute admissions into purchased private hospital beds. Marks & Thornicroft (1990) have expressed concern that further growth in private psychiatric care could potentially threaten the catchment area concept, which might ultimately lead to a two tier system of psychiatric care in this country. Business analysts have identified growth opportunities for an expanding private sector both in tendering for NHS contracts as well as in providing services for people with private health insurance.

Social care and the private sector

Private sector providers are of crucial importance in the mixed economy of social care that has developed in the past decade. The majority of residential and nursing home care in Britain is now run on a for-profit basis and private providers are beginning to bid successfully with social services authorities for contracts for other forms of social care, notably home care provision. Private hospitals and nursing homes must be registered and regularly inspected by the local health authority, while residential care homes are inspected by social services departments.

User views and the user movement

There has been an enormous increase in interest in the views of users of mental health services over recent years (Leiper & Field, 1993; DoH, 1991). In part this derives from the psychiatric patients' rights movement, which originated in North America, focusing on the "abuses the [users] suffered at the hands of a system that couldn't understand their particular life crises, but could only warehouse them and give them the seclusion room, the chemical straitjacket and other harsh treatment" (Brown, 1981). From a very different perspective the Griffiths Report, which ushered general management into the NHS, and was the precursor of the internal market reforms that have led to providers competing for contracts with health service purchasers, recommended the use of "consumer" feedback as a measure of service quality (Jones *et al*, 1987). Subsequently the Department of Health has encouraged purchasers to include sampling of "consumer" opinion in contracts with providers.

A variety of approaches have been adopted towards advocacy for, and by, psychiatric patients: these include legal advocacy (routinely provided for patients who appeal against compulsory detention); "citizen" advocacy, which involves a concerned citizen seeking to act in the interests of a person who is severely disabled; and self-advocacy, which encourages current patients and "survivors" of the mental health system to speak out about their treatment (Royal College of Psychiatrists, 1989*b*). In some places user groups have started to assist in the planning of mental health services (Anderson, 1989; Beeforth, 1993). Users' charters have been developed which emphasise the rights of patients to privacy, consultation, information about services and treatment options and choice (Beeforth *et al*, 1991).

More pragmatically there is evidence that patient attitudes influence compliance with treatment, attendance at appointments, and willingness to accept admission, with increased patient participation leading to improved clinical outcomes (Slater *et al*, 1982; Corrigan *et al*, 1990). Health professionals can learn from the feedback patients provide about a service. Consumer opinion can be adopted as an outcome measure in studies of service efficacy; examples of this are found in a number of studies cited in this chapter.

In a survey of attitudes to care on acute admission in-patient wards, although patients found nursing and medical staff understanding and helpful, patients also felt that they spent long periods of time on the ward doing nothing. The main criticism of medical staff was their failure to discuss side-effects of medication, and a substantial number of patients singled out ward rounds as a distressing experience. In general patients perceived an apparent lack of emphasis on their social needs (Ballard & McDowell, 1990).

Mental health policy in the UK

Throughout the 19th and 20th century psychiatric services in Britain were dominated by the rise and fall of the asylum, as described in chapter 10. Mental health policy and practice have been evolving steadily away from a traditional asylum-based model of care since the end of the Second World War (Bennett, 1991*a*). The mental hospital population in Britain reached a peak in 1954 and then declined. As early as 1961 the Minister of Health, Enoch Powell, was envisaging the closure of the "isolated, majestic, imperious" asylums. The government white paper, *Better Services for the Mentally Ill* (HMSO, 1975), proposed a new model for comprehensive local mental health services, based on contemporary best practice. At the centre of the model was the psychiatric unit, usually but not invariably within the local district general hospital. The DGH unit would provide out-patient, in-patient and day hospital care and relate to a range of voluntary sector and social services provision. The white paper provided norms for the number of hospital beds, day places and hostel places that should be available within a district.

This model had two clear implications: first that the majority of mental hospitals would close, being replaced by more local and accessible DGH-based services; and second that local authority social services departments would take on an increasing role in the community support of the mentally ill. A variety of administrative measures were taken during the 1970s and 1980s to encourage a shift in the pattern of care from institutionally-based NHS funded services towards community-based local authority funded services for the so-called "priority groups" (elderly people, the mentally ill, people with a mental handicap, and physically and sensorially handicapped people) (Audit Commission, 1986). These measures included the setting up of joint care planning teams involving health and local authorities, the allocation of joint finance (health authority money that would pump-prime jointly agreed community projects) and the elaboration of a "dowry" system by which health authority money could be transferred to social services as patients moved out of long-stay hospitals into the community (Audit Commission, 1986). By the mid 1980s it had become clear that these measures had substantially failed, particularly for mental illness services. In 1986/7 84% of direct expenditure on the mentally ill went to in-patient services while local authority expenditure accounted for 3.7% of the total (Taylor & Taylor, 1989). At the same time there was an explosion in the costs of providing residential and nursing home care for elderly people and people with a mental illness through the social security budget (Audit Commission, 1986).

The failures of community care

From the outset of the community care movement concern had been expressed that there was a lack of appropriate community services and unacceptably heavy burdens were being born by families and other informal carers.

In the United States, which went through a rapid period of deinstitution-alisation in the 1960s and 1970s, a very visible problem developed of homeless mentally ill people living rough in the major cities (Bhugra, 1993). More recently similar problems have been experienced in Britain, although no clearcut causal link has been established between the increasing visibility of the homeless mentally ill and hospital rundown and closure (Hamid *et al*, 1993; Scott, 1993). There are also concerns that mentally ill people are being inappropriately diverted from psychiatric services into the criminal justice system. This has led to the development of court diversion schemes which involve psychiatrists and community nurses working within magistrates courts to identify mentally disordered offenders and, if necessary, rapidly diverting them to hospital rather than prison (Joseph & Potter, 1993). One recurring critical theme has been that too many patients receiving community care have fallen through the cracks of the system, resulting either in unnecessary clinical deterioration or in patients becoming a danger to themselves or others. The potential danger of patients evading the service was dramatically revealed in the case of Christopher Clunis, a man with schizophrenia who stabbed a stranger in an underground station while unmedicated and psychotic (Ritchie *et al*, 1994). He had been in contact with a large number of services over the six years before the offence, including a spell in prison and in hospital following a previous stabbing. The report of the subsequent inquiry spells out the failure of a whole range of services to provide Clunis with effective aftercare (Coid, 1994). The Clunis case, and other recent tragedies, have had a profound impact on policy makers and professional practices.

Health and social care in the '90s and beyond

The pace of change within British health and social care services since the end of the 1980s has been extremely rapid. A white paper *Working for Patients* (Secretaries of State, 1989*a*) has led to radical reform of the NHS, which is now dominated by the purchaser/provider split (between purchasing health authorities and NHS trust provider units), the internal market and the development of GP fundholding. More recently health authorities and family health service authorities (responsible for primary care) have been consolidating into joint bodies commissioning all NHS provision within large geographical areas.

A series of discussion documents identifying the problems of community care was produced during the 1980s (Social Services Committee, 1985; Audit Commission, 1986; Griffiths, 1988) culminating in the publication of the white paper *Caring for People* and its subsequent supporting documents (Secretaries of State, 1989*b*; HMSO, 1990; Social Services Inspectorate, 1991). *Caring for People* set out to provide a framework for community care in Britain for the 1990s and beyond. The key objectives of the policy are presented in Box 27.5. The two white papers were given legislative form in the 1990 NHS and Community Care Act (Thornicroft, 1994).

The community care reforms share significant similarities with the NHS reforms, notably a reliance on market-place mechanisms, which it is claimed will drive down the costs of care while improving its quality. Local social service authorities are identified as the lead agency for the implementation of community care; they now purchase services from a variety of providers (private sector, voluntary sector and local authority) within the so-called "mixed economy of care". There is a theoretical divide in responsibility for the "health" aspects of community care (which remain with the health authority) and "social" care, although this divide has proven difficult to make in practice (Thornicroft, 1994).

The community care reforms deprive both health and local authorities of the previous easy option of supporting vulnerable people in residential care at the expense of the social security budget. Instead local authorities have a duty to carry out a comprehensive needs assessment on vulnerable people in the community prior to any placement. The aim is that the needs assessment will result in a package of care that if possible avoids residential care in favour of domiciliary support (Secretaries of State, 1989*b*). The success of the reforms is yet to be evaluated definitively (Thornicroft, 1994).

Implementing community care

Caring for People (Secretaries of State, 1989*b*) contained a number of specific initiatives to improve the quality of community care. These include the requirement on each social services authority to set out, after consultation with the health authority and voluntary agencies, a community care plan; the development of the Care Programme Approach (CPA) for the mentally ill; the introduction of "care management"; and the provision of a Mental Illness Specific Grant.

The responsibility placed on local authorities to prepare a community care plan (including a mental health plan) has provided a focus for the work of joint planning teams, which bring together local authority representatives (including housing department staff), the local non-statutory services and representatives from health service purchasers and providers.

The Care Programme Approach (CPA)

The CPA is an initiative designed to improve the delivery of services to people with a severe mental illness and "it applies to all patients accepted by mental health services" (Kingdon, 1994). It stems from a recommendation made by the Spokes Inquiry into the *Care and After-care of Sharon Campbell* (DHSS, 1988). The inquiry identified that a breakdown of community services had resulted in the killing of Ms Campbell's social worker. It recommended that the duties of health and local authorities to provide effective aftercare be clarified so that vulnerable and potentially dangerous patients could no longer fall through the cracks of the service system (a conclusion that was echoed in the Clunis Inquiry). Key principles of the CPA are outlined in Box 27.6.

Under the CPA service providers (i.e. community psychiatric teams and staff working on in-patient units planning a patient's discharge) have a responsibility to carry out an assessment of service users' health and social care needs. In addition there should be an allocated key worker to coordinate and monitor care who works to a written care plan. Arrangements are required for regular reviews of progress, appropriate interprofessional collaboration and consultation with users and carers (Kingdon, 1994). Initially under the CPA a register of "vulnerable" patients was to be set up by local services. Subsequently health authorities have been required to ensure that service providers set up supervision registers of those patients who are "most at risk" of harming themselves and/or others (Holloway, 1994*a*).

Care management

If a patient has particularly complex needs for (expensive) community support or residential care there should, in addition to action under the CPA, be a care management assessment. This is carried out by or on behalf of the local authority. The care manager who holds a budget is responsible for purchasing, coordinating and monitoring the delivery of a package of care to meet the person's social care needs. The term care management should be distinguished from the broader and related term case management. The care manager is expected to act independently of direct service providers, who actually implement the service plans agreed by the care manager. This brokerage system is only one form of case management: the majority of successful case management systems in psychiatry combine brokerage with direct service provision (Holloway *et al*, 1991). Case management is discussed in more detail below.

The bulk of the resources allocated to care management comes from funds previously allocated to the Department of Social Security for spending on residential and nursing home care. Predictably most of the money expended by local authority care managers goes towards purchasing residential care for elderly people (Thornicroft, 1994). However, the intention remains that care management will result in a steadily increasing role for local authorities in purchasing community care services. This has to some extent been pump-primed by the Mental Illness Specific Grant to local authorities to fund community mental health schemes.

Case management for the mentally ill

Community care has resulted in a fragmentation of mental health services, and the need for some form of coordinating mechanism is now recognised. Case management systems are intended to provide this coordination and offer vulnerable patients long-term flexible support (Holloway *et al*, 1991). The core case management activities are: the assessment of need, the development of a comprehensive service plan, the arrangement of service delivery, and the monitoring and assessment of what is provided.

Case management has evolved during the 1980s to become a major element of the mental health care system in the USA. Two contrasting models may be distinguished. Paraprofessional case managers may act as service brokers, responsible for but not necessarily providing the assessment and implementation of a package of care. This model is closely akin to the role of a British local authority social services department care manager who is responsible for purchasing the social component of community care. Alternatively, in clinical case management a skilled psychiatric professional is "directly concerned with all aspects of the patient's physical and social environment" (Kanter, 1989). The clinical case manager not only arranges access to appropriate services but also works directly with the patient offering a range of interventions. These include supportive psychotherapy, training in community living skills, family and patient psychoeducation and support during crises (Kanter, 1989). With severely disabled patients staff–patient ratios may have to be very high (in the region of one staff member to 10 patients). Ideally clinical case managers should be anticipating impending crises and taking appropriate action; success in dealing effectively with relapses and other difficulties can give both client and carers a sense of confidence and control over events (Harris & Bergman, 1987). Clinical case management is similar to the traditional case work approach in social work, but involves a more active approach than solely focusing on psychotherapy.

Residential services for the severely mentally ill

Most people with long-term mental illness now either live independently or with their families. A minority, because of the disabilities associated with their illness or lack of help from their family, require temporary or permanent supported housing (Carling, 1993). In Britain accommodation for the mentally ill is provided by health authorities, the local authority social services and housing departments, housing associations and private and voluntary sector providers of residential and nursing home care. As the number of hospital beds has decreased there has been an increasing emphasis on the use of non-statutory services and care for people in their own homes. Table 27.2 provides a classification of residential provision for the mentally ill on a continuum from independent living to maximum support.

How many beds?

Wing (1992) has provided estimates of the need for specialist residential provision for patients aged 16 to 65 years. He suggests that the "average" district will require 66 in-patient beds per 100 000 total population (including acute wards and crisis units, intensive care beds, regional secure and special hospital places and hostel ward places for long-stay patients). Few, if any, districts can boast of having such a generous provision. This provision should be matched by staffed community housing. Wing recommends 30 places per 100 000 in high staffed hostels, 20 per 100 000 in day staffed provision

---

Box 27.5 Key objectives of British government community care policy

To promote the development of domiciliary, day and respite services to enable people to live in their own homes wherever feasible and sensible

To ensure that service providers make practical support for carers a high priority

To make proper assessment of need and good case management the cornerstone of high quality care

To promote the development of a flourishing independent sector alongside good quality public services

To clarify the responsibilities of agencies and so make it easier to hold them to account for their performance

To secure better value for taxpayers' money by introducing a new funding structure for social care

(Secretaries of State, 1989*b*)

---

and 18 per 100 000 in group homes with visiting staff only. Supported bed-sits (12 per 100 000) and direct access facilities (12 per 100 000) may be required to complete the spectrum of provision. These figures must be treated with caution, since evidence suggests an extremely wide range in need for residential care, with a strong association between need and indices of social deprivation both for acute and long-stay beds (Thornicroft, 1991; Thornicroft *et al*, 1992). A study in 20 districts in the North West Thames Region showed a correlation between admission rates and Jarman indices of social deprivation of 0.8, although in the same study the correlation with discharge rates was rather lower at 0.41 suggesting that illness variables rather than simply social factors may be most relevant to discharge rates (Hirsch, 1988).

There is considerable controversy over the number of acute in-patient beds required by an effective local psychiatric service (Thornicroft & Strathdee, 1994), but clear evidence of a significant shortfall in the provision of medium secure beds (Coid, 1994). In recent years the pressure on acute beds in London has been intense, with unacceptably high levels of bed occupancy and overflow of NHS patients into the private sector. The vast majority of patients admitted to units serving inner urban areas suffer from psychotic illnesses (Holloway *et al*, 1992; Flannigan *et al*, 1994), with an associated higher level of compulsory admission under the Mental Health Act and an increase in the general level of disturbance on the ward (Patrick *et al*, 1989).

Box 27.6 Key principles of the care programme approach

Applies to all patients accepted by the mental health services
Assessment of health and social care need
Nominated key worker to coordinate care
Regular reviews
Monitoring compliance
Collaboration with other professionals and agencies
Care programme register for "vulnerable" patients

The pattern of residential services

In the past many long-stay patients were discharged from the large British psychiatric hospitals to a room in a boarding house in a seaside resort but this practice has now stopped. More recently surveys have demonstrated considerable unmet housing need among patients discharged from acute psychiatric wards (Melzer *et al*, 1991). Many patients leave inner city hospitals for temporary bed and breakfast accommodation, and a few soon end up sleeping on the streets. There is a lack of accommodation that provides any form of support, and the shortage of highly supported provision is acute.

Residential services should be based on a number of principles (Carling, 1993). The degree of support should match the level of disability. Services should as far as possible be non-stigmatising, offer a homely environment and promote choice and independence for residents. Institutional practices initially described by Goffman (1961) such as block treatment, lack of personal possessions for residents and social distance between care staff and residents should be avoided. There should be flexibility to cope with changing needs, either by altering the level of support or by offering a more appropriate alternative. One constant dilemma in residential care is balancing the rights of the individual and the promotion of independence against the need to provide a safe and structured environment for people with very severe disabilities. Another common difficulty is the unrealistic aspirations of patients who may be unwilling to recognise that they cannot cope independently. Residential facilities should be backed up by a multidisciplinary team that is able to respond to psychiatric crises and regularly provides consultation about mental health issues.

The traditional forms of residential care available were the group home (a minimally staffed shared house); the more highly staffed hostel, which could either offer "rehabilitation" with an expectation that the resident would move on into less supported accommodation or provide a permanent home; and for the most disabled a long-stay hospital bed.

Patients now demand more independent accommodation than the traditional hostels can provide with adequate supervision and support

(Carling, 1993). One way of providing this is the 'core and cluster' model within which a central highly staffed unit (possibly offering day care) supports residents who live in a cluster of surrounding independent properties. An alternative is the extension of the sheltered housing model into the mental illness sector. Some residents require only occasional visits from a housing worker or social work aide to ensure that minimum standards are being met and the rent is paid. In adult fostering and boarding out schemes landladies offer patients considerable practical assistance with daily living and monitor their mental state within their homes. Foster care for the mentally ill has been practised in the Belgian town of Gheel for at least 700 years. Studies of foster care in Gheel suggest it is best if patients are discharged into small family homes with few other residents (Linn *et al*, 1980).

Even highly disabled long-stay patients can live successfully in ordinary housing with the support of non-professional care staff (Pickard *et al*, 1992). Patients no longer requiring continuing hospital care may also be discharged into elderly persons residential care homes and nursing homes, often far from their local area. (This is now the responsibility of the social services authority, which will fund placements following a needs led care management assessment.) Although the physical environment of such homes is often excellent levels of activity among residents are often very low. Close follow-up of private sector placements is essential (Holloway *et al*, 1994).

Hospital-hostels

The most thoroughly evaluated form of residential provision is the 'hospital-hostel' or 'ward-in-a-house', which was developed as an alternative to the long-stay hospital ward (Shepherd *et al*, 1994). The first to open was 111 Denmark Hill, which is in the grounds of the Maudsley Hospital (Garety & Morris, 1984). Subsequently units have been opened either adjacent to or some miles from district general hospital psychiatric units (Gibbons, 1986; Goldberg *et al*, 1985; Allen *et al*, 1993). These units, which have varied in size from 10 to 20 places, can offer individually planned (often behaviourally oriented) interventions in an intensively staffed setting that is also a homely environment. The units have varied in their approach, in particular in the expectations placed on residents to contribute to the daily chores within the hostel and the use made of day care and other facilities on the hospital campus. Improved functioning and quality of life have been demonstrated for patients who would otherwise have been on hospital back wards or inappropriately placed in acute units (Wykes & Wing, 1982; Gibbons & Butler, 1987). Despite the high staffing levels hospital-hostels can be cost-effective compared with hospital wards (Hyde *et al*, 1987).

Long-stay hospital provision

However, there are some patients who cannot even be managed within the highly supported environment of a hospital-hostel. This small residual group of patients who exhibit "challenging behaviours" as a result of their severe mental illnesses went almost unnoticed in the large mental hospitals as their disturbance was easily contained. No generally agreed service model has emerged in the era of deinstitutionalisation. Some of these patients will improve after intensive rehabilitation and aggressive pharmacological management over a period of years. Others appear to have intractable problems that may not improve significantly. A proportion of this group are managed within the special hospitals and regional secure units, although the latter were not designed or resourced to provide long-term care. One suggestion has been the 'haven' concept (Wing & Furlong, 1986), which seeks to recapture the positive aspects of the asylum without recourse to institutional care practices.

Hospital closure

Psychiatric services were historically based around large mental hospitals, often remote from the catchment area that they served. In both the UK and the USA the psychiatric hospital population has been declining steadily since the mid 1950s and the traditional asylum system has been replaced by an increasingly diverse service. Even if local services did develop, a substantial number of long-stay patients remained within the area mental hospitals, which continued to provide a silent service for the most disabled psychiatric patients (the 'old long-stay').

In 1962 there were 130 mental hospitals with over 100 beds in England (Davidge *et al*, 1993). Although a number of smaller hospitals closed or changed function in the next 25 years it was not until 1986 that the first large British public mental hospital, Banstead Hospital in Surrey, closed. Closing more of the remaining psychiatric hospitals is a mental health policy target of the British government. By 1993 only 89 of the 130 mental hospitals remained open, of which the majority were planned to close by the year 2000 (Davidge *et al*, 1993).

In spite of the scale of the task of reproviding these institutions relatively little is known about the process and outcome of mental hospital closure (O'Driscoll, 1993). The characteristics of the patients to be discharged are, however, well-documented. Clifford *et al* (1991) studied the long-stay population of five large mental hospitals. Patients were predominantly elderly (two-thirds being over 60 years old) and had spent a mean of 25 years in hospital. The overwhelming majority of patients suffered from schizophrenia (70%) with bipolar affective disorder (12%) the second commonest diagnosis. Physical disability, notably incontinence (30%) and impaired mobility (25%), was common. More than half of the patients needed supervision with basic activities of daily living such as dressing and personal hygiene while very few could shop and cook for themselves or use public transport unaided.

Table 27.2 A classification of residential services. Costs of care increase down this list.

Facility	Comments
Independent living	Own house, flat, bedsit
Independent living with support	Domiciliary support from home care team etc.
Living with family/supported lodgings	May involve considerable support from informal carers
Independent group home	Group living setting with minimal support
Supported group home	Group living setting with regular domiciliary support
Staffed home (low staffing) team	Daily contact from members of staff
Staffed home (high staffing)	24-hour staff cover (sleep-in staff)
Staffed home (very high staffing)	24-hour cover (night waking) May provide 'rehabilitation' or long-term care
(a) Residential home	Includes Part III homes for the elderly
(b) Nursing home	Includes elderly and mental illness provision; nursing staff team
Hospital care	Multiple potential providers now in competition
(a) Acute in-patient ward	
(b) Rehabilitation ward	
(c) On site hospital/hostel	
(d) Intensive care unit	
(e) Regional secure unit	
(f) Special hospital	

Long-stay patients also have significant active psychiatric symptomatology. In a detailed psychiatric assessment of the long-stay population at Horton Hospital, Curson *et al* (1988) found that even with energetic psychopharmacological treatment almost half the patients continued to exhibit florid delusions and/or hallucinations and a sizeable minority had obviously bizarre behaviours.

Apart from the large-scale and continuing study of the Friern/Claybury reprovision being carried out by the Team for the Assessment of Psychiatric Services (TAPS) (see, for example, Leff, 1993) the existing literature includes anecdotal accounts of closure from a managerial perspective (King, 1991); empirical analyses of the managerial issues involved in the closure process (McKee, 1988); and studies of particular reprovision projects (Chanfreau *et al*, 1990; Kingdon *et al*, 1991; Holloway & Faulkner, 1994).

There is no doubt that large mental hospitals can be closed, with the vast majority of the long-stay residents moving out to residential facilities in the community, often into provision that offers a high degree of support (Leff, 1993; Holloway, 1994*b*). The social functioning of patients relocated to community settings during hospital closure improves in line with the positive environmental changes that occur but to date no systematic changes in symptoms have been observed (Anderson *et al*, 1993; Holloway, 1994*b*). Very few patients involved in a British closure programme lose contact with services (Dayson, 1993), although this does not seem to have been the case in the USA where deinstitutionalised patients have joined the ranks of the homeless (Lamb, 1993). However, a small number of patients cannot be successfully discharged into community settings (Dayson *et al*, 1992) and 'new long-stay' patients continue to accumulate (Clifford *et al*, 1991; Thornicroft *et al*, 1992; Lelliott *et al*, 1994).

Monitoring services

Mental health services research can be difficult to design and perform and evaluative studies must be subject to critical scrutiny. Government policies and the development of community care have led to a wide variety of new types of care. Are these new systems any better than the older traditional hospital-based services which they seek to replace? Evaluation of a new service, like the evaluation of a new drug, must be scientifically based and requires a proper trial. Braun (1981) has detailed some of the specific requirements of the design and conduct of a trial of a service. These include:

(1) A clear method of allocating patients to the experimental and control groups (preferably random allocation).
(2) Adequate characterisation of the patients entering the study so that the case mix of patients is apparent.
(3) Good description of the treatment programme or the specific intervention, as well as information on other key treatment variables that might alter outcome such as medication. This will enable the study to be replicated by others. An important example of this is the study of the Daily Living Programme first described by Stein & Test (1980) and replicated more than a decade later by Muijen *et al* (1992*a*).
(4) A wide variety of different clinical outcome measures should be used. In a drug trial only symptoms are monitored, but a service trial would also monitor behaviour, social functioning, quality of life, the burden on carers, economic cost of the service to the community, and the occurence of rare but severely adverse events such as suicide or homicide.
(5) Follow-up should be for an adequate period of time because many gains made in the short term will often disappear over time.
(6) Differences between two types of service are often small and so sample size should be sufficiently large to ensure a Type II error does not

occur (failure to identify a difference between the experimental groups when one exists.

Research projects into novel treatment approaches may involve a specially selected and committed staff group who work within the project over a limited time period. An important issue is therefore the sustainability of the service model adopted when it is applied over decades by staff of average competence and enthusiasm. It is also important to locate these studies within a broader epidemiological context and assess the impact of model programmes on the total mental health system (Bachrach, 1982). Epidemiological studies of the prevalence of mental illness (for example, the NIMH epidemiological catchment area programme (Regier *et al*, 1984, 1988)) provide a foundation for service planning and evaluation (Goldberg & Huxley, 1992; Strathdee & Thornicroft, 1993).

Service quality can be defined and assessed from three different perspectives: "structure" (or "input"); "process" ; and "outcome" (or "output") (Donabedian, 1966). The "structural" or "input" approach to defining service quality relates to the physical resources available to the service (beds, day places) and its human resources (numbers, training and experience of its staff) (Lalonde, 1982). The "process" approach involves assessing the interaction between staff and patients and the extent to which standards of treatment and care match those expected of the service: standards might include the quality of record keeping, average length of stay and the appropriateness of the clinical management of a case. The methodological guidelines set out by Braun *et al* (1981) give the standard for controlled evaluations of the outcome of services: increasingly services are being pressed to incorporate monitoring of outcome into routine clinical practice (Department of Health, 1994).

Monitoring of services can be carried out within the clinical team (for example, by regular review of the process or outcome of treatment episodes), between teams (for example, peer review of randomly selected case-notes) or external to the team (for example, in an external review of serious untoward incidents, such as the suicide of a patient). Routinely gathered statistics can be used by management to compare the activity of clinical teams, and are increasingly used by purchasers to monitor their contract with the provider. Contracts uniformly contain 'quality standards' which, for example, set out waiting times for patients and minimum times for GPs to receive information on patients who have been discharged. The purchaser or provider must then monitor these standards, which change from year to year. Accurate activity monitoring also allows elements of a service (for example, an out-patient appointment; an in-patient bed day; a community assessment) to be costed.

In addition to the purchaser a number of external bodies have a role in monitoring the performance of mental health services. These include bodies responsible for educational standards (for example, Royal College of Psychiatrists visiting approval teams); the Mental Health Act Commission (which has a statutory role in the oversight of the welfare of detained patients in England and Wales) and the Scottish Mental Welfare Commission (which has a broader remit); the NHS Health Advisory Service (Seager, 1992; Williams & Travers, 1994); and more recently the Audit Commission (Renshaw, 1994). In the USA elaborate systems of accreditation of services are in place, with an explicit aim of the accreditation process being that services are not only of adequate quality but have in place mechanisms that minimise costs (Fauman, 1989).

One method for the monitoring of psychiatric services is the case register, which at its most comprehensive provides a local information system that records all contacts that individuals from a defined geographical area have with designated social and medical services (Fryers & Wooff, 1989). Case registers have been a powerful research tool in psychiatric epidemiology, enabling the analysis of patterns of service contact in respect to diagnosis, social class and geographic mobility and comparisons, both national and international, of psychiatric morbidity between catchment areas of differing social deprivation (Strathdee & Thornicroft, 1993). With the advent of new technology, and the demands on providers to report as accurately as possible their activity to purchasers, it becomes both feasible and desirable to develop case registers as a practical management and clinical tool. At their most sophisticated systems can identify when patients have dropped out of contact with a service, prompting the relevant key worker or clinician to take action.

Clinical audit

The results of research can be used to evaluate the efficacy of new treatments and innovative patterns of service provision. Research should be distinguished from audit, which has been defined as "the systematic critical analysis of the quality of medical care, including the procedures used for diagnosis and treatment, the use of resources, and the resulting outcome and quality of life for the patients" (Royal College of Psychiatrists, 1989b). Medical audit refers only to medical interventions. In a psychiatric context, clinical audit (which may involve other members of the team) should be seen as a cyclical process (Shaw & Costain, 1989).

Audit, like other forms of quality assurance, tends to focus on the "process" level but can investigate "inputs" and "outcomes". Ideally audit involves the selection of an area of activity for review (for example antidepressant prescribing practices); the setting of agreed standards relating to that activity (clear recording of the indications for initiating a prescription, ensuring that patients receive an adequate dose of an effective antidepressant for an adequate period before concluding that treatment is ineffective). This should be followed by observation of what happens in practice; comparison of current practice with the standards, and identification of need for change should current practice deviate from the standard. The next stage is the implementation of change (for example, education sessions for all medical staff, use of standardised rating scales in patient management, development of a system of feedback of prescribing from pharmacy) and the final phase is a review of practice following the change. Guidelines about the conduct of audit studies which emphasise the importance of the feedback loop in audit have been published by the Royal College of Psychiatrists (1994).

The future

The Government's commitment to the community care policy has been underlined by the identification of mental health as one of the five key target areas within its public health strategy, *Health of the Nation* (Secretary of State for Health, 1992). The mental health targets set out are to improve significantly the health and social functioning of mentally ill people; to reduce the overall suicide rate by at least 15% by the year 2000 (1990 baseline); and to reduce the suicide rate of severely mentally ill people by at least 33% by the year 2000 (1990 baseline).

In spite of more than three decades of development of community psychiatric care, public, professional and political concern over the move towards community-based services continues. There are persistent demands that the monitoring of potentially vulnerable or dangerous psychiatric patients be improved. The possibility of a swing of the pendulum back towards custodial care cannot be discounted.

References

Allen, H. Baigent, B., Kent, A., *et al* (1993) Rehabilitation and staffing levels in a "new look" hospital-hostel. *Psychological Medicine*, **23**, 203–211.

Anderson, J. (1989) Patient power in mental health. *British Medical Journal*, **299**, 1477–1478.

—, Dayson, D., Wills, W., *et al* (1993) The TAPS project 13: Clinical and social outcomes of long-stay psychiatric patients after one year in the community. *British Journal of Psychiatry*, suppl. 19, 45–46.

Audini, B., Marks, I. M., Lawrence, R. E., *et al* (1994) Home-based versus out-patient/in-patient care for people with serious mental illness. Phase II of a controlled study. *British Journal of Psychiatry*, **165**, 204–210.

Audit Commission (1986) *Making a Reality of Community Care*. London: HMSO.

Bachrach, L. L. (1976) *Deinstitutionalisation: An Analytical Review and Sociological Perspective*. Rockville, Maryland: US Department of Health, Education and Welfare, NIMH.

— (1982) Assessment of outcome in community support systems: results, problems and limitations. *Schizophrenia Bulletin*, **8**, 39–51.

Ballard, C.G. & McDowell, A. W. T. (1990) Psychiatric in-patient audit – the patient's perspective. *Psychiatric Bulletin*, **14**, 674–675.

Beard, J. H. Propst, R. & Malamud, T. J. (1982) The Fountain House model of psychiatric rehabilitation. *Psychosocial Rehabilitation Journal*, **5**, 47–53.

Bebbington, P. E., Feeney, S., Flannigan, C.B., *et al* (1994) Inner London collaborative audit of admissions. II: Ethnicity and the use of the Mental Health act. *British Journal of Psychiatry*, **165**, 743–749.

Beeforth, M. (1993) What does it mean to have effective user participation in planning? In *Counting for Something in Mental Health Services* (eds R. Leiper & V. Field). Aldershot: Avebury.

——, Conlon, E., Field, V., *et al* (1991) Whose service is it anyway? London: RDP.

Bennett, D. H. (1983) The historical development of rehabilitation services. In *Theory and Practice of Psychiatric Rehabilitation* (eds F. N. Watts & D. H. Bennett), pp. 15–42. Chichester: Wiley.

—— (1991a) The drive towards the community. In *150 Years of British Psychiatry 1841–1991.* (eds G. E. Berrios & H. Freeman), pp. 321–332. London: Gaskell.

—— (1991b) The international perspective. In *Community Psychiatry* (eds D. H. Bennett & H. L. Freeman), pp. 626–649. Edinburgh: Churchill Livingstone.

—— & Freeman, H. L. (1991) Principles and prospects. In *Community Psychiatry* (eds D. H. Bennett & H. L. Freeman), pp. 1–39. Edinburgh: Churchill Livingstone.

Bhugra, D. (1993) Unemployment, poverty and homelessness. In *Principles of Social Psychiatry* (eds D. Bhugra & J. Leff), pp. 355–382. Oxford: Blackwell.

Bland, R. C. (1988) Investigations of the prevalence of psychiatric disorders. *Acta Psychiatrica Scandinavica*, **77** (suppl. 338), 7–16.

Blom-Cooper, L. (1990) *Occupational Therapy, an Emerging Profession in Health Care. Report of a Commision of Inquiry.* London: Duckworth.

Bluglass, R. (1983) *Guide to the Mental Health Act 1983.* Edinburgh: Churchill Livingstone.

Boardman, A. P., Bouras, N. & Cundy, J. (1987) *The Mental Health Advice Centre in Lewisham. Service Usage: Trends from 1978–1984.* London: NUPRD.

Braun, P., Kochansky, G., Shapiro, R., *et al* (1981) Overview: Deinstitutionalisation of psychiatric patients. A critical review of outcome studies. *American Journal of Psychiatry*, **138**, 736–749.

Bridges, K., Davenport, S. & Goldberg, D. (1994) The need for hospital-based rehabilitation services. *Journal of Mental Health*, **3**, 205–212.

Brooker, C., Tarrier, N., Barrowclough, C., *et al* (1992) Training CPNs for psychosocial intervention. *British Journal of Psychiatry*, **160**, 836–844.

——, Falloon, I., Butterworth, A., *et al* (1994) The outcome of training community psychiatric nurses to deliver psychosocial intervention. *British Journal of Psychiatry*, **165**, 222–230.

Brown, P. (1981) The mental patients' rights movement and mental health institutional change. *International Journal of Health Services*, **11**, 523–540.

Brown, G. W., Bone, M., Dalison, B., *et al* (1966) *Schizophrenia and Social Care.* London: Oxford University Press.

Burns, T., Beardsmore, A., Bhat, A., *et al* (1993a) A controlled trial of home-based acute psychiatric services. I: Clinical and social outcome. *British Journal of Psychiatry*, **163**, 49–54.

——, Raferty, J., Beardsmore, A., *et al* (1993b) A controlled trial of home-based acute psychiatric service. II: Treatment patterns and costs. *British Journal of Psychiatry*, **163**, 55–61.

Caplan, G. (1964) *Principles of Preventive Psychiatry.* New York: Basic Books.

Carling, P. J. (1993) Housing and supports for persons with mental illness: emerging approaches to research and practice. *Hospital and Community Psychiatry*, **44**, 439–449.

Carson, J., Fagin, L. & Ritter, S. (1994) *Stress and Coping in Mental Health Nursing*. London: Chapman and Hall.

Cawley, R. H. (1990) Educating the psychiatrist of the 1st century. *British Journal of Psychiatry*, **157**, 174–181.

Chanfreau, D., Deadman, J. M., George, H., *et al* (1990) Transfer of long-stay psychiatric patients: A preliminary report of interinstitutional relocation. *British Journal of Clinical Psychology*, **29**, 59–69.

Cherniss, C. (1980) *Staff Burnout: Job Stress in the Human Services*. London: Sage.

Chiswick, D. & Cope, R. (eds) (1995) *College Seminars in Practical Forensic Psychiatry*. London: Gaskell.

Clifford, P., Charman, A., Webb, Y., *et al* (1991) Planning for community care. Long-stay populations of hospitals scheduled for rundown or closure. *British Journal of Psychiatry*, **158**, 190–196.

Coid, J. W. (1994) The Christopher Clunis enquiry. *Psychiatric Bulletin*, **18**, 449–452.

Connolly, M. J. (1992) History. In *Textbook of Psychiatric and Mental Health Nursing* (eds J. I. Brooking, S. A. H. Ritter & B. L. Thomas), pp. 5–13. Edinburgh: Churchill Livingstone.

Cope, R. (1995) Mental Health Legislation. In *College Seminars in Practical Forensic Psychiatry* (eds D. Chiswick & R. Cope), pp. 272–309. London: Gaskell.

Cormack, D. (1983) *Psychiatric Nursing Described*. Edinburgh: Churchill Livingstone.

Corrigan, P. W., Lieberman, R. P. & Engel, J. D. (1990) From non-compliance to collaboration in the treatment of schizophrenia. *Hospital and Community Psychiatry*, **41**, 1203–1211.

Creed, F., Black, D. & Anthony, P. (1989) Day hospital and community treatment for acute psychiatric illness: a critical appraisal. *British Journal of Psychiatry*, **129**, 452–456.

——, ——, ——, *et al* (1990) Randomised controlled trial of day patient versus inpatient psychiatric treatment. *British Medical Journal*, **300**, 1033–1037.

——, ——, ——, *et al* (1991) Randomised controlled trial of day patient versus inpatient psychiatric treatment. 2: Comparison of two hospitals. *British Journal of Psychiatry*, **158**, 183–189.

Crone, S. (1993) Why we need helplines. *British Journal of Hospital Medicine*, **49**, 685–686.

Curson, D., Pate, M., Liddle, P. F., *et al* (1988) Psychiatric morbidity of a long-stay hospital population with chronic schizophrenia and implications for future community care. *British Medical Journal*, **297**, 819–822.

Davidge, M., Elias, S., Jayes, B., *et al* (1993) *Survey of English Mental Illness Hospitals*. Inter-Authority Comparisons and Consultancy, Health Services Management Centre, University of Birmingham.

Dayson, D. (1993) The TAPS project 12: Crime, vagrancy, death and readmission of the long-term mentally ill during their first year of local reprovision. *British Journal of Psychiatry*, **162** (suppl. 19), 40–44.

——, Gooch, C. & Thornicroft, G. (1992) The TAPS Project 16: Difficult to place, long-term psychiatric patients: risk factors for failure to resettle long stay patients in community facilities. *British Medical Journal*, **305**, 993–995.

Dean, C. & Gadd, E. M. (1990) Home treatment for acute psychiatric illness. *British Medical Journal*, **301**, 1021–1023.

Dedman, P. (1993) Home treatment for acute psychiatric disorder. *British Medical Journal*, **306**, 1359–1360.

Department of Health and Social Security (1975) Better Services for the Mentally Ill. Cmnd 623. London: HMSO.

—— (1988) *Report of the Committee of Inquiry into the Care and Aftercare of Sharon Campbell*. London: HMSO.

Department of Health (1991) *The Patient's Charter: Raising the Standard*. London: HMSO.

—— (1992*a*) *Residential Needs of Severely Disabled Psychiatric Patients. The Case for Hospital Hostels*. London: HMSO.

—— (1992*b*) *The Health of the Nation. A Strategy for Health in England*. London: HMSO.

—— (1993) *Hospital Doctors: Training for the Future*. London: HMSO.

—— (1994) *Mental Illness Key Area Handbook, 2nd Edition*. London: HMSO.

Department of Health and Home Office (1992) *Review of Health and Social Services for Mentally Disordered Offenders and Others Requiring Similar Services. Final Summary Report*. Cmnd. 2088. London: HMSO.

Donabedian, A. (1966) Evaluating the quality of medical care. *Milbank Memorial Quarterly*, **4**, 166–206.

Dunn, J. & Fahy, T. A. (1990) Police admissions to a psychiatric hospital. Demographic and clinical differences between ethnic groups. *British Journal of Psychiatry*, **156**, 373–378.

Eagles, J. M. & Alexander, D. A. (1988) Which neurotic patients do psychiatrists treat? *British Journal of Psychiatry*, **152**, 222–228.

Endicott, J., Cohen, J., Nee, J., *et al* (1979) Brief vs standard hospitalisation. For whom? *Archives of General Psychiatry*, **36**, 706–712.

Fahy, T. A., Birmingham, D. & Dunn, J. (1987) Police admissions to psychiatric hospitals, a challenge to community psychiatry? *Medicine, Science and the Law*, **27**, 363–268.

Fauman, M. A. (1989) Quality assurance monitoring in psychiatry. *American Journal of Psychiatry*, **146**, 1121–1130.

Fisher, N. (1994) The discharge of mentally disordered people and their continuing care in the community. *Psychiatric Bulletin*, **18**, 453–456.

Flannigan, C. B., Glover, G. R., Feeney, S. T., *et al* (1994) Inner London collaborative audit of admissions in two health districts. I: Introduction, methods and preliminary findings. *British Journal of Psychiatry*, **165**, 734–742.

Freeman, H. F. & Tantam, D. (1991) Samuel Gaskell. In *150 Years of British Psychiatry 1841–1991* (eds. G. E. Berrios & H. F. Freeman), pp. 445–451. London: Gaskell.

Freudenberger, H. J. (1974) Staff burnout. *Journal of Social Issues*, **30**, 159–166.

Fryers, T. & Wooff, K. (1989) A decade of mental health care in an English urban community: patterns and trends in Salford, 1976–87. In *Health Services Planning and Research. Contributions from Psychiatric Case Registers* (ed. J. K. Wing), pp. 31–52. London: Gaskell.

Garety, P. & Morris, I. (1984) A new unit for long-stay patients: organisation, attitude and quality of care. *Psychological Medicine*, **14**, 183–192.

Gask, L. (1986) What happens when psychiatric out-patients are seen once only? *British Journal of Psychiatry*, **148**, 663–666.

Gibbons, J. (1986) Care of new long stay patients in a district general hospital psychiatric unit. The first two years of a hospital-hostel. *Acta Psychiatrica Scandinavica*, **73**, 582–588.

Gibbons, J. S. & Butler, J. P. (1987) Quality of life for new long stay psychiatric inpatients: the effects of moving to a hostel. *British Journal of Psychiatry*, **147**, 383–388.

Goffman, E. (1961) *Asylums: Essays on the Social Conditions of Mental Patients and Other Inmates*. New York: Doubleday.

Goldberg, D. (1985) Implementation of mental health policies in the north west of England. In *The Provision of Mental Health Services in Britain: The Way Ahead* (eds G. Wilkinson & H. Freeman). London: Gaskell.

——, Bridges, K., Cooper, W., *et al* (1985) Douglas House: A new type of hostel for chronic psychiatric patients. *British Journal of Psychiatry*, **147**, 383–388.

—— & Huxley, P. (1992) *Common Mental Disorders*. London: Routledge.

Gournay, K. & Brooking, J. (1994) Community psychiatric nurses in primary health care. *British Journal of Psychiatry*, **165**, 231–238.

Griffiths, R. (1988) *Community Care: An Agenda for Action*. London: HMSO.

Groves, T. (1990) What does community care mean now? *British Medical Journal*, **300**, 1060–1062.

Hamid, W. A., Wykes, T. & Stansfield, S. (1993) The homeless mentally ill: myths and realities. *International Journal of Social Psychiatry*, **39**, 237–254.

Hansson, L. (1989) Utilisation of psychiatric in-patient care. *Acta Psychiatrica Scandinavica*, **79**, 571–578.

Harding, C. M., Strauss, J. S., Hafez, H., *et al* (1987) Work and mental illness I. Toward an integration of the rehabilitation process. *Journal of Nervous and Mental Disease*, **175**, 317–325.

Harris, M. & Bergman, H. C. (1987) Case management with the chronically mentally ill: a clinical perspective. *American Journal of Orthopsychiatry*, **57**, 296–302.

Harrison, G., Holton, A., Neilson, D., *et al* (1989) Severe mental disorder in Afro-Caribbean patients: some social, demographic and service factors. *Psychological Medicine*, **19**, 683–696.

Hatfield, B., Mohamad, H. & Huxley, P. (1992) The 1983 Mental Health Act in five local authorities: a study of the practice of approved social workers. *International Journal of Social Psychiatry*, **38**, 189–207.

Haw, C. & Lanceley, C. (1987) Patients at a psychiatric walk in clinic: who, how, why and when. *Bulletin of the Royal College of Psychiatrists*, **11**, 329–332.

HMSO (1968) *Psychiatric Nursing: Today and Tomorrow*. London: HMSO.

—— (1975) *Better Services for the Mentally Ill*. Cmnd. 6233. London: HMSO.

—— (1990) *Community Care in the Next Decade and Beyond: Policy Guidance*. London: HMSO.

Hirsch, S. (1988) Psychiatric Beds as Resources: Factors influencing Bed use and Service Planning. Report of the Working Party of the Section for Social and Community Psychiatry of the Royal College of Psychiatrists. London: RCPsych.

Holloway, F. (1988) Day care and community support. In *Community Care in Practice* (eds A. Lavender & F. Holloway). Chichester: Wiley.

—— (1989) Psychiatric day care: the users' perspective. *International Journal of Social Psychiatry*, **35**, 252–264.

—— (1990) Caring for People. A critical review of British Government policy for the mentally ill. *Psychiatric Bulletin*, **14**, 641–645.

—— (1991) Day care in an inner city. I. Characteristics of attenders. *British Journal of Psychiatry*, **158**, 805–810.

—— (1994a) Supervision registers. *Psychiatric Bulletin*, **18**, 593–596.

—— (1994b) The RDP Cane Hill closure research project: an overview. *Journal of Mental Health*, **3**, 401–412.

—— (1995) Home treatment as an alternative to acute inpatient admission: a discussion. In *Community Psychiatry in Action* (eds P. Tyrer & F. Creed). Cambridge: Cambridge University Press.

—— (1996) Supervised discharge – paper tiger? *Psychiatric Bulletin*, **20**, 193–194.

——, McLean, E. & Robertson, J. A. (1991) Case management. *British Journal of Psychiatry*, **159**, 142–148.

——, Silverman, M. & Wainwright, T. (1992) "Not waving but drowning": Psychiatric services in East Lambeth 1990. *International Journal of Social Psychiatry*, 131–137.

—— & Faulkner, A. (1994) Psychiatric hospital reprovision and the long-stay patient: clinical outcome and the user perspective. *Journal of Mental Health*, **3**, 241–248.

——, Rutherford, J., Carson, J., *et al* (1994) Elderly graduates and a hospital closure programme: a five year follow-up study. *Psychiatric Bulletin*, **18**, 534–537.

Howells, J. (1991) The establishment of the Royal College of Psychiatrists. In *150 Years of British Psychiatry 1841–1991* (eds G. E. Berrios & H. Freeman). London: Gaskell.

Hunter, R. & McCalpine, I. (1963) *Three Hundred Years of Psychiatry*. London: Oxford University Press.

Hutton, F. (1985) Self referrals to a community mental health centre: a three year study. *British Journal of Psychiatry*, **147**, 540–544.

Hyde, C., Bridges, K., Goldberg, D., *et al* (1987) The evaluation of a hostel ward. A controlled study using modified cost-benefit analysis. *British Journal of Psychiatry*, **151**, 805–812.

Ineichen, B., Harrison, G. & Morgan, H. G. (1984) Psychiatric hospital admissions in Bristol. I. Geographical and ethnic factors. *British Journal of Psychiatry*, **145**, 600–604.

Irvine, E. (1979) *Social Work and Human Problems*. Oxford: Pergamon Press.

Jahoda, M. (1981) Work, employment and unemployment: values, theories and approaches in social research. *American Psychologist*, **36**, 184–191.

Jenkins, R. & Griffiths, S. (1991) *Setting Standards: A Service Blueprint in Indicators for Mental Health in the Population*. London: HMSO.

Jones, K. (1972) The Growth of Concern. In *A History of the Mental Health Services 1785–1794*, pp. 25–39. London: Routledge and Kegan Paul.

Jones, L., Leneman, L. & Maclean, U. (1987) *Consumer Feedback for the NHS. A Literature Review*. London: Kings Fund.

Jones, R. (1994) *Mental Health Act Manual*. London: Sweet and Maxwell.

Joseph, P. L. A. & Potter, M. (1993) Diversion from custody. I: Psychiatric assessment at the magistrates' court. *British Journal of Psychiatry*, **162**, 325–330.

Kanter, J. (1989) Case management: Definition, principles and components. *Hospital and Community Psychiatry*, **40**, 361–368.

Katschnig, H. & Cooper, J. (1991) Psychiatric emergency and crisis intervention services. In *Community Psychiatry* (eds D. H. Bennett & H. L. Freeman), pp. 517–542. Edinburgh: Churchill Livingstone.

Kessel, N. (1963) Who ought to see a psychiatrist? *Lancet, i,* 1092–1094.

King, D. (1991) *Moving on from Mental Hospitals to Community Care.* London: Nuffield Provincial Hospitals Trust.

King's Fund Report (1992) *London Health Care 2010.* London: King's Fund.

Kingdon, D. (1994) Care programme approach. Recent Government policy and legislation. *Psychiatric Bulletin,* **18,** 68–70.

——, Turkington, D., Malcolm, K., *et al* (1991) Replacing the mental hospital. Community provision for a district's chronically psychiatrically disabled in domestic environments? *British Journal of Psychiatry,* **158,** 113–117.

Kingsley, S. & Towell, D. (1988) Planning for high quality local services. In *Community Care in Practice* (eds A. Lavender & F. Holloway), pp. 51–74. Chichester: Wiley.

Knapp, M., Beecham, J., Koutsogeorgopoulou, V. *et al* (1994) Service use and costs of home-based versus hospital-based care for people with serious mental illness. *British Journal of Psychiatry,* **165,** 195–203.

Lalonde, B. I. D. (1982) Quality assurance. In *Handbook of Mental Health Administration* (eds M. J. Austin & W. E. Hershey) San Fransciso: Josey Bass.

Lamb, H. R. (1993) Lessons learned from deinstitutionalisation in the US. *British Journal of Psychiatry,* **162,** 587–592.

Lavender, T. & Holloway, F. (1992) Models of continuing care. In *Innovations in the Psychological Management of Schizophrenia* (eds M. Birchwood & N. Tarrier), pp. 207–234. Chichester: Wiley.

Leff, J. (ed) (1993) The TAPS project: Evaluating community placement of long-stay psychiatric patients. *British Journal of Psychiatry,* **162,** suppl. 19.

Leiper, R. & Field, V. (eds) (1993) *Counting for Something in Mental Health Services.* Aldershot: Avebury.

Lelliott, P., Wing, J. K. & Clifford, P. (1994) A national audit of new long-stay psychiatric patients. I: Method and description of the cohort. *British Journal of Psychiatry,* **165,** 160–169.

Lieberman, P. B. & Strauss, J. S. (1986) Brief hospitalization: what are its effects? *American Journal of Psychiatry,* **143,** 1557–1562.

Lim, M. H. (1983) A psychiatric emergency clinic: a study of attendances over six months. *British Journal of Psychiatry,* **143,** 460–466.

Linn, M. W., Caffey, E. M., Klett, J., *et al* (1979) Day treatment and psychotropic drugs in the aftercare of schizophrenic patients. *Archives of General Psychiatry,* **36,** 1055–1066.

——, Klett, K. & Caffey, E. (1980) Foster home characteristics and psychiatric patient outcome: The wisdom of Gheel confirmed. *Archives of General Psychiatry,* **37,** 129–132.

Lloyd, K. & Moodley, P. (1992) Psychotropic medication and ethnicity: an inpatient survey. *Social Psychiatry and Psychiatric Epidemiology,* **27,** 95–101.

Macdonald, E. M. (1976) *Occupational therapy in Rehabilitation.* 4th edn. London: Ballière Tindall.

McAusland, T. (ed) (1985) *Planning and Monitoring Community Mental Health.* London: King's Fund Centre.

McKee, L. (1988) Conflicts and context in managing the closure of a large psychiatric hospital. *Bulletin of the Royal College of Psychiatrists,* **12,** 310–319.

Manpower Planning Advisory Group (1990) *Clinical Psychology Project: Full Report.* London: Department of Health

Marks, I. (1992) Innovations in mental health care delivery. *British Journal of Psychiatry*, **160**, 589–597.

——, Connolly, J., Muijen, M., *et al* (1994) Home-based versus hospital care for people with serious mental illness. *British Journal of Psychiatry*, **165**, 179–194.

—— & Thornicroft, G. (1990) Private inpatient psychiatric care. *British Medical Journal*, **300**, 892.

Marson, D. C., McGovern, M. P. & Pomp, H. C. (1988) Psychiatric decision-making in the emergency room: a research overview. *American Journal of Psychiatry*, **145**, 918–925.

Martin, F. M. (1984) *Between the Acts*. London: Nuffield Provincial Hospitals Trust.

Marzillier, J. & Hall, J. (eds) (1992) The psychological treatment of adults. In *What is Clinical Psychology?*, pp. 1–32. Oxford: Oxford University Press.

Maslach, C. (1979) The burnout syndrome and patient care. In *Stress and Survival – the Emotional Realities of Life-Threatening Illness* (ed. C. A. Garfield). St Louis: CV Mosby.

—— & Jackson, S. (1981) The measurement of experienced burnout. *Journal of Occupational Behaviour*, **2**, 99–113.

Melzer, D., Hale, A. S., Malik, S. J., *et al* (1991) Community care for patients with schizophrenia one year after hospital discharge. *British Medical Journal*, **303**, 1023–1026.

Merson, S., Tyrer, P., Onyett, S., *et al* (1992) Early intervention in psychiatric emergencies: a controlled clinical trial. *Lancet*, **339**, 1311–1318.

Mollica, R. F. (1980) Community mental health centres. *Journal of the Royal Society of Medicine*, **73**, 863–870.

Moodley, P. (1993) Services for ethnic minorities. In *Principles of Social Psychiatry* (eds J. Leff & D. Bhugra), pp. 490–501. Oxford: Blackwell Scientific.

—— & Perkins, R. E. (1991) Routes to psychiatric inpatient care. *Social Psychiatry and Psychiatric Epidemiology*, **26**, 47–51.

Morris, I. (1991) Residential care. In *Community Psychiatry* (eds D. H. Bennett & H. L. Freeman), pp. 415–443. Edinburgh: Churchill Livingstone.

Moss, R. (1994) Community mental health teams: A developing culture. *Journal of Mental Health*, **3**, 167–174.

Muijen, M. (1992) The balance of care. In *Innovations in the Psychological Management of Schizophrenia* (eds M. Birchwood & N. Tarrier), pp. 253–276. Chichester: Wiley.

——, Marks, I., Connolly, J., *et al* (1992*a*) Home based care and standard hospital care for patients with severe mental illness: a randomised controlled trial. *British Medical Journal*, **304**, 749–754.

——, ——, ——, *et al* (1992*b*) The Daily Living Programme. Preliminary comparison of community versus hospital-based treatment for the seriously mentally ill facing emergency admission. *British Journal of Psychiatry*, **160**, 379–384.

O'Driscoll, C. (1993) The TAPS project 7: Mental hospital closure. A literature review of outcome studies and evaluative techniques. *British Journal of Psychiatry*, **162** (suppl. 19), 7–17.

O'Grady, J. C. (1990) The complementary role of regional and local secure provision for psychiatric patients: three years experience in Leeds. *Health Trends*, **22**, 14–16.

Olsen, M. R. (ed) (1984) The role of duties of social services/departments and the Approved Social Worker. In *Social Work and Mental Health, A Guide for the Approved Social Worker*, pp. 41–49. London: Tavistock.

Onyett, S., Heppleston, T. & Bushell, D. (1994) A national survey of community mental health teams: Team structures and processes. *Journal of Mental Health,* **3**, 175–194.

Ovretveit, J. (1986) Organisation of multidisciplinary community teams. Uxbridge: Brunel Institute of Organisation and Social Services (BIOSS).

—— (1994) *Coordinating Community Care. Multidisciplinary teams and Care Management.* Buckingham: Open University Press.

Parry Jones, W. L. (1972) *The Trade in Lunacy.* London: Routledge and Kegan Paul.

Peck, E. (1994) Community Mental Health Centres: Introduction. *Journal of Mental Health,* **3**, 151–156.

Patrick, M., Higgitt, A. & Holloway, F. (1989) Changes in an inner city psychiatric service following bed losses. *Health Trends,* **21**, 121–123.

Pickard, L., Proudfoot, R., Wolfson, P., *et al* (1992) *Evaluating the Closure of Cane Hill Hospital. Final Report of the Cane Hill Research Team.* RDP, London.

Pilling, S. (1988) Work and the continuing care client. In *Community Care in Practice* (eds A. Lavender & F. Holloway), pp. 187–205. Chichester: Wiley.

—— (1991) *Rehabilitation and Community Care.* London: Routledge.

Porter, R. (1990) *Mind-Forg'd Manacles.* Harmondsworth: Penguin.

Raftery, J. (1991) Social policy and community psychiatry. In *Community Psychiatry* (eds D. H. Bennett & H. L. Freeman),pp. 595–625. Edinburgh: Churchill Livingstone.

Reed, J. (1991) The future for psychiatry. *Psychiatric Bulletin,* **15**, 396–401.

Regier, D. A., Myers, J. K., Kramer, M., *et al* (1984) The NIMH epidemiologic catchment area program. *Archives of General Psychiatry,* **41**, 934–941.

——, Boyd, J. H., Burke, J. D. Jr. (1988) One month prevalence of mental disorders in the United States. *Archives of General Psychiatry,* **45**, 977–986.

Renshaw, J. (1994) The Audit Commission's review of mental health services. *Psychiatric Bulletin,* **18**, 421–422.

Renvoize, E. (1991) The Association of Medical Officers of Asylums and Hospitals for the Insane. In *150 Years of British Psychiatry 1841–1991* (eds G. E. Berrios & H. Freeman), pp. 29–78. London: Gaskell.

Ritchie, J. H., Dick, D. & Lingham, R. (1994) *The Report of the Inquiry into the Care and Treatment of Christopher Clunis.* London: HMSO.

Ritter, S. A. H. (1992) The multi-disciplinary clinical team. In *Textbook of Psychiatric and Mental Health Nursing* (eds J. I. Brooking, S. Ritter & B. L. Thomas), pp. 27–35. Edinburgh: Churchill Livingstone.

Royal College of Psychiatrists (1977) The responsibilities of consultants in psychiatry with the National Health Service. *Bulletin of the Royal College of Psychiatrists,* September, 4–7.

—— (1984) The responsibilities of consultants in psychiatry within the National Health Service. *Psychiatric Bulletin,* **8**, 123–126.

—— (1989*b*) Patient advocacy. Report for Public Policy Committee. *Psychiatric Bulletin,* **13**, 715–716.

—— (1989*c*) Preliminary report on medical audit. *Psychiatric Bulletin,* **13**, 577–580.

—— (1990) *Caring for a Community. I. The Model Mental Health Service.* London: Gaskell.

—— (1992) *The Mental Health of the Nation: the Contribution of Psychiatry.* London: The Royal College of Psychiatrists.

— (1992) *Facilities and Services for Patients who have Chronic Persisting Severe Disabilities Resulting from Mental Illness*. Council Report 19. London: Royal College of Psychiatrists.

Sayce, L., Craig, T. K. J. & Boardman, A. P. (1991) The development of community mental health centres in the UK. *Social Psychiatry and Psychiatric Epidemiology*, **26**, 14–20.

Scott, J. (1993) Homelessness and mental illness. *British Journal of Psychiatry*, **162**, 314–324.

— & Seccombe, P. (1976) Community psychiatry – setting up a service on a shoestring. *Mindout*, **17**, 5–7.

Seager, P. (1992) Identifying unmet needs: the NHS Health Advisory Service. In *Measuring Mental Health Needs* (eds G. Thornicroft, C. R. Brewin & J. Wing), pp. 184–191. London: Gaskell.

Secretaries of State for Health, Wales, Northern Ireland and Scotland (1989a) *Working for Patients*. London: HMSO.

— (1989b) *Community Care in the Next Decade and Beyond*. London: HMSO.

Secretary of State for Health (1992) *The Health of the Nation. A Strategy for Health for England*. London: HMSO.

Shaw, C. D. & Costain, D. W. (1989) Guidelines for medical audit: seven principles. *British Medical Journal*, **299**, 498–499.

Shepherd, G., Murray, A. & Muijen, M. (1994) *Relative Values*. London: Sainsbury Centre for Mental Health.

Simmons, S. & Brooker, C. (1986) *Community Psychiatric Nursing – a Social Perspective*. London: Heinemann.

Sims, A. (1991) Even better services: a psychiatric perspective. *British Medical Journal*, **302**, 1061–1063.

— (1992) Beyond the water towers: current demands upon consultant psychiatrists. *Psychiatric Bulletin*, **16**, 321–324.

—, Heard, D. H., Rowe, Gill, M. M. P., *et al* (1993) "Neurosis" and the personal social environment. The effects of a time-limited course of intensive day care. *British Journal of Psychiatry*, **162**, 369–374.

Sladden, S. (1979) *Psychiatric Nursing in the Community*. Edinburgh: Churchill Livingstone.

Slater, V., Linn, M. W. & Harris, R (1982) A satisfaction with mental health care scale. *Comprehensive Psychiatry*, **23**, 68–74.

Social Services Committee 1984/85 Session, Second Report (1985) *Community Care with Special Reference to Adult Mentally Ill and Mentally Handicapped People*. London: HMSO.

Social Services Inspectorate (1991) *Care Management and Assessment. Managers Guide*. London: HMSO.

Soni, S. D., Steers, L., Warne, T., *et al* (1989) Multidisciplinary teams and line management: practical problems and areas of conflict in clinical psychiatry. *Psychiatric Bulletin*, **13**, 657–661.

Stein, L. I. & Test, M. A. (1980) Alternative to mental hospital treatment. I Conceptual model, treatment program, and clinical evaluation. *Archives of General Psychiatry*, **37**, 392–397.

Strathdee, G. & Thornicroft, G. (1992) Community sectors of needs-led mental health services. In *Measuring Mental Health Needs* (eds G. Thornicroft, C. Brewin & J. Wing), pp. 140–162. London: Gaskell.

—— & —— (1993) The principles of setting up mental health services in the community. In *Principles of Social Psychiatry* (eds J. Leff & D. Bhugra), pp. 473–489. Oxford: Blackwell Scientific.

—— & Williams, P. (1984) A survey of psychiatrists in primary care: the silent growth of a new service. *Journal of the Royal College of General Practitioners*, **34**, 615.

Sutherby, K., Srinath, S. & Strathdee, G. (1992) The domiciliary consultation service: outdated anachronism or essential part of community psychiatric outreach? *Health Trends*, **24**, 103–105.

Szmukler, G. I., Bird, A. & Button, E. J. (1981) Compulsory admission in a London Borough. I. Social and clinical features and a follow-up. *Psychological Medicine*, **11**, 617–636.

Talbott, J. A. & Glick, I. D. (1986) The inpatient care of the chronically mentally ill. *Schizophrenia Bulletin*, **12**, 129–140.

Tantam, D. (1985) Alternatives to psychiatric hospitalisation. *British Journal of Psychiatry*, **146**, 1–4.

Taylor, J. & Taylor, D. (1989) *Mental Health in the 1990s. From Custody to Care?* London: Office of Health Economics.

Thornicroft, G. (1991) Social deprivation and rates of treated mental disorder. *British Journal of Psychiatry*, **158**, 475–484.

—— (1994) The NHS and Community Care Act, 1990. *Psychiatric Bulletin*, **18**, 13–17.

—— & Bebbington, P. (1989) Deinstitutionalisation – from hospital closure to service development. *British Journal of Psychiatry*, **155**, 739–753.

——, Margolius, O. & Jones, D. (1992) The TAPS Project 6: New long-stay psychiatric patients and social deprivation. *British Journal of Psychiatry*, **161**, 621–624.

—— & Strathdee, G. (1994) How many psychiatric beds? *British Medical Journal*, **309**, 970–971.

Tyrer, P. (1984) General practice psychiatric clinics. *British Journal of Psychiatry*, **145**, 15–19.

——, Remington, M. & Alexander, J. (1987) The outcome of neurotic disorders after out-patient and day hospital care. *British Journal of Psychiatry*, **151**, 57–62.

——, Turner, R. & Johnson, A. (1989) Integrated hospital and community psychiatric services and use of inpatient beds. *British Medical Journal*, **299**, 298–300.

United Kingdom Consultative Council for Nursing, Midwifery and Health Visiting (1987) Project 2000. Paper 9. London: UKCC.

Varah, C. (1973) *The Samaritans in the '70s. To Befriend the Suicidal and Despairing*. London: Constable.

Waldron, G. (1983) Crisis intervention – is it effective? *British Journal of Hospital Medicine*, **308**, 367–373.

Warner, R. (1994) *Recovery from Schizophrenia*. London: Routledge.

Watts, F. N. & Bennett, D. H. (eds) (1983) Management of the staff team. In *Theory and Practice of Psychiatric Rehabilitation*. Chichester: Wiley.

White, E. (1990) *The Third Quinquennial National Community Psychiatric Nursing Survey*. Manchester: University of Manchester Department of Nursing.

Williams, R. & Travers, R. (1994) The role of the NHS Health Advisory Service. *Psychiatric Bulletin*, **18**, 721–725.

Wilkinson, G. (1991) The role of primary care physicians in the treatment of patients with long-term mental disorders. *International Review of Psychiatry*, **3**, 35–42.

Wing, J. K. (ed) (1989) *Health Services Planning and Research. Contributions from Psychiatric Case Registers*. London: Gaskell.

—— (1992) *Epidemiologically Based Needs Assessment.* London: Royal College of Psychiatrists.

—— & Brown, G. W. (1970) *Institutionalism and Schizophrenia.* London: Cambridge University Press.

—— & Furlong, R. (1986) A haven for the severely disabled within the context of a comprehensive psychiatric community service. *British Journal of Psychiatry,* **149**, 449–457.

Wykes, T. & Wing, T. (1982) A ward in a house: Accommodation for "new" long-stay patients. *Acta Psychiatrica Scandinavica,* **65**, 315–330.

28 Psychiatry in general practice

Greg Wilkinson

Psychiatric illness in general practice • Pathways to care • Diagnosis and classification by GPs • Treatment of major psychiatric disorders by GPs • Drug prescribing • The interface between general practice and psychiatry

---

We are convinced that for the good of general medicine, this particular study of psychological medicine, dealing as it does with so many complex problems should be merged in the general routine of medical practice. (Andrew Wynter, 1875)

The practice notes of the astrological physician Richard Napier (1559–1637) provide a description of the mental illnesses recognised in an era before psychiatry and general practice (MacDonald, 1989). Of the patients consulting Napier, about 5% of the total suffered from symptoms that he and his contemporaries regarded as signs of a psychiatric disorder. The most common of these were: 'troubled in mind' (33% of consultations), 'melancholy' (20%), 'mopish' (15%) and 'light headed' (15%). 'Mad' and 'lunatic' appeared in 5.5% of consultations and 'distracted' in 5.4%. If 'troubled in mind' can be equated with 'anxiety', 'melancholy' with depression and 'lunatic' with psychoses, the figures show a remarkable similarity to some of the more recent studies which use modern diagnostic methods to estimate the prevalence of these disorders in general practice. For example, Casey *et al* (1984) using ICD–9 criteria reported that 7% of all general practice consultations were 'psychiatric'; the main groups were anxiety 20%, depression 30% and schizophrenia 5%.

Loudon (1983) provides a description of the origins of general practice as a profession in Great Britain. Until 1800 medical care was provided by three groups of doctors: the physicians who were a learned profession trained at the universities and who dealt with internal disorders, the surgeons were craftsmen whose sphere was external disorders requiring surgery or other manual interference and, third, the tradesmen apothecaries whose only legal role was to dispense the physicians' prescriptions. After the Rose Case in 1704 (Clark, 1966) apothecaries won the right to 'practise physic' (to visit, advise and prescribe) but even so they could only charge for the medicine they supplied. There was insufficient work for the surgeons and as there was more work to be found in dispensing, many surgeons became surgeon apothecaries. There was also stiff competition from untrained chemists and midwives, and an additional financial pressure came in 1812 with the imposition of the glass tax to help finance the Napoleonic Wars (medicine was always dispensed in glass containers). To defend their position the apothecaries and the surgeon apothecaries formed a trade association in 1812, *The Association of Apothecaries and Surgeon Apothecaries*, and then pressed for protective legislation. The Apothecaries Acts of 1812 and 1815 stipulated that the apothecaries should have a period of training (an attachment of five years to an established apothecary) and if they passed an examination they were qualified to become a Member of the Royal College of Surgeons and a licencate of the Society of Apothecaries (MRCS–LSA). This licence permitted the apothecaries to practise surgery, midwifery and physic. These early apothecaries were the first general practitioners. The later Medical Act of 1858 led to a unification of all medical education.

General practice flourished during the 19th century mainly as a result of the increasing wealth of the middle classes, and by 1840 GPs comprised over 80% of the medical profession, with one GP per 1000 of the population. Marinker (1988) described the competition between the hospital-based physicians and surgeons and the GPs during the 19th century, which eventually led to the exclusion of the GPs from the hospitals, so a patient could only be admitted to hospital if the GP first referred the patient to a physician or a surgeon. The referral system which originally started as a restrictive trade practice to benefit the physicians and surgeons has survived, being cost effective, and with medical logic has helped in the development of a rational hospital service. The referral system permits the GP to act as a gatekeeper to expensive high technology specialist medical care. The gatekeeper has two functions: to contain the majority of care within general practice, and to select the most appropriate specialist advice.

There are some 30 000 GPs in the UK. Almost all (95%) of the UK population is registered with a GP, and 60–70% of these registered patients consult at least once each year; only about 10% will not consult at all in any three year period. Thus, the GP can be regarded as a personal physician who has access to the medical history and social background of patients. By virtue of the continuity of care GPs provide, not only for the patient but often for the whole family, they are in a unique position to manage psychiatric illness.

Psychiatric illness in general practice

General practitioners are likely to become involved early in the detection and treatment of patients in the acute and chronic phases of mental illnesses, as well as when a relapse occurs; they provide a preventive framework, which recognises the patient in the context of family and community, and continuity of mental health care; and they supply comprehensive general health care to a group of patients who tend to consult more often for physical illness (Wilkinson *et al*, 1988).

The GP plays a major role in mental health care, for the following main reasons (World Health Organization, 1973):

(i) patients with psychosocial problems are high users of medical care and are well known to GPs who may utilise this relationship for psychotherapeutic intervention;

(ii) patients with emotional disorders experience less stigma when treated by a GP than by a psychiatrist;

(iii) physical and psychiatric complaints tend to concur and are often difficult to separate in diagnosis and treatment, which makes the GP, who is well-placed to treat the whole person, the first choice as physician;

(iv) GPs are best placed to provide long-term follow-up and be available for successive episodes of illness.

The scientific study of psychological disorders in general practice starts with the classic study *Psychiatric Illness in General Practice*, which describes a large-scale survey carried out in 12 general practices in Greater London between 1961 and 1962 (Shepherd *et al*, 1966 (2nd edn 1981)). The authors demonstrated for the first time that the vast bulk of psychiatric disorders were identified and treated by GPs and not by mental health specialists. The main conclusions were:

(i) Psychiatric morbidity was one of the more common reasons for consulting a GP. About 14% of the population at risk consulted their family doctor at least once over a 12-month period for a complaint diagnosed as entirely or largely psychiatric.

(ii) Conditions given a psychiatric diagnosis made up about two-thirds of all psychiatric morbidity, and these were mainly neurotic conditions with only 5% suffering from psychoses. Although labelled 'minor' the course was often long lasting and disabling, and medical and social factors were strongly linked with psychiatric illness. Patients suffering from psychiatric disorders exhibited higher rates of general morbidity, consulted their doctors more frequently, and appeared to have more marital problems, spend more time off work, or to present permanent incapacity, when compared with the remainder.

(iii) GP treatment consisted largely of drugs and/or discussion, but almost a third of patients with psychiatric disorders received no treatment.

(iv) GPs dealt with the bulk of identified psychiatric morbidity themselves, referring only 5% to specialist psychiatric services.

This work, based on epidemiological inquiry, and replicated worldwide (National Institute of Mental Health, 1979; Harding *et al*, 1980; Wilkinson, 1985, 1989), was a landmark in the study of mental disorders in the community.

What is general practice psychiatry?

The topic of general practice psychiatry is poorly defined, yet it covers a vast area of medical activity with perhaps more than half a million psychiatric consultations in any one week in the UK. It concerns the common psychiatric disorders in general practice and the way they are diagnosed and treated by the primary care team, and the topic can therefore be viewed from a variety of perspectives. A GP, perhaps writing for his or her fellow GPs might adopt a clinical approach focusing on the individual patient, and the common psychiatric syndromes, as described in the earlier chapters of this book, although in rather less detail. An epidemiological approach is also justified because such large numbers of patients are involved: this would focus more on issues of prevalence, outcome and associated socio-demographic features in order to provide information for funding and administrative bodies as well as finding ways of optimising treatments for the community as a whole. The numerical approach of an epidemiologist contrasts with that of the psychotherapist who would focus exclusively on the nature of the doctor–patient relationship and issues revolving around the transference and counter-transference. The social psychologist would focus even more finely on the minutiae of the consultation itself (see Pendelton & Hasler (1983) for review). This chapter assumes the perspective of a psychiatrist, and how the GP functions as a psychiatrist and so concentrates more on issues such as psychiatric diagnosis in general practice, why psychiatric disorder is sometimes recognised but often remains unrecognised and therefore untreated, and the interface between psychiatry and general practice. The psychiatric disorders themselves and their treatments are not described here, the emphasis being on the way GPs use psychiatric treatments such as psychotropic drugs, or work with the various paramedical professions, and how the primary care team deals with common major psychiatric conditions such as depression, schizophrenia, alcoholism and drug addiction.

Pathways to care

Psychiatric morbidity varies in severity from the extremely ill patients who are in hospital through to people in the community who may experience a few psychiatric symptoms but are not sufficiently distressed to seek help. Goldberg & Huxley (1980) employ the concepts of levels and filters to describe this wide range of severity of disorder and the pathways that patients take to reach specialist care, and this model has been influential in research into general practice psychiatry (Table 28.1). It comprises five levels; to move from one level to the next, it is necessary to pass through one of four filters.

Level 1 refers to psychiatric and emotional disorder in the community as measured by community surveys. Investigations using this approach have shown that the probable prevalence of psychiatric disorder in the community is about 20%, while in samples of general practice attendees, rates of 35–40% are obtained (Goldberg & Williams, 1988). A proportion of people with

Table 28.1 Mental illness in community, general practice and specialist settings: Goldberg & Huxley's (1980) pathway to psychiatric care

		Rate/1000/year
Level 1	Mental illness in the community	260–315
	Filter 1: The decision to consult	
Level 2	Total general practice morbidity	230
	Filter 2: GP recognition	
Level 3	Conspicuous general practice morbidity	101.5
	Filter 3: The decision to refer	
Level 4	All psychiatric patients	23.5
	Filter 4: The decision to admit	
Level 5	Psychiatric in-patients	5.71

such a disorder (but not all) in the community will consult a GP, and they pass through filter 1 to reach level 2. Filter 1 is thus the decision made by the patient to seek help and the act of consulting.

Level 2 comprises the total of all psychiatric morbidity that presents to general practitioners. Goldberg & Huxley (1992) gave an estimate of 236/1000 cases per year in Manchester, while Ormel & Giel (1990) in Holland, using the PSE as a case finding instrument estimated a rate of 224/1000 cases per year. Level 2 morbidity includes all cases in level 3 and above in whom the psychiatric disorder is recognised as well as a large number of cases presenting to the GP in whom the psychological nature of the complaint has not been recognised by the GP. This is referred to as 'hidden psychiatric morbidity' (Goldberg & Blackwell, 1970; Marks *et al*, 1979). This group of patients do not pass through filter 2, and so fail to reach level 3.

Level 3 consists of conspicuous psychiatric morbidity, i.e. morbidity identified and recognised by the GP.

Level 4 consists of all the patients that are referred to psychiatric services (both in-patient and out-patients).

Level 5 refers to those patients who are admitted to hospital, and therefore represent the most severe end of the spectrum.

The prevalence of psychiatric disorders in the community (level 1)

Level 1 refers to psychiatric and emotional disorders as measured in community surveys. Goldberg & Huxley (1992) pooled the results of 11 community surveys and found an overall one month prevalence of 164.0/1000 cases per year. The rates for women were 202.3/1000 and for men

121.4/1000. The Epidemiological Catchment Area (ECA) study in the USA is the largest and most detailed epidemiological study (see also chapter 3 for a description of the methods). The results of its main findings are shown in Table 28.2. The results of a UK based study from the Office of Population Censuses and Surveys (1994) is also shown. The UK study is based on ICD–10 diagnoses whereas the ECA is based on DSM–III which is a rather older system. Although not all the categories are the same in each survey the table shows a broad degree of agreement on prevalence for many different psychiatric disorders. A variety of factors described below may affect the overall rates of psychiatric disorders in the community.

Sex ratio

Most, but not all, studies show higher rates for women than for men. The ECA study (Regier *et al*, 1988) showed an almost equal sex ratio because it

Table 28.2 Prevalence rates of psychiatric disorders per 100 persons in the community in the USA and UK

	USA (ECA study)[1]			UK (OPCS, 1994)[2]		
	Male	Female	All	Male	Female	All
Any DIS disorder	14.0	16.6	15.4	–	–	–
Any neurotic disorder	–	–	–	12.3	19.5	16.0
Anxiety disorders	4.7	9.7	7.3	–	–	–
Mixed anxiety & depression	–	–	–	5.4	9.9	7.7
G.A.D.	–	–	–	2.8	3.4	3.1
Phobias	3.8	8.4	6.2	0.7	1.4	1.1
Obsessive–compulsive disorder	1.1	1.5	1.3	0.9	1.5	1.2
Panic	0.3	0.7	0.5	0.8	1.1	0.8
Major depression	1.6	2.9	2.2	1.7	2.5	2.1
Dysthymia	2.2	4.2	3.3	–	–	–
Somatisation	0.0	0.2	0.1	–	–	–
Functional psychoses	0.6	0.6	0.6	0.4	0.4	0.4
Manic episode	0.3	0.4	0.3	–	–	–
Substance use disorder	6.3	1.6	3.8	10.4	3.6	6.9
Alcohol abuse dependency	5.0	0.9	2.8	7.5	2.1	4.7
Drug abuse	1.8	0.7	1.3	2.9	1.5	2.2
Antisocial personality disorder	0.8	0.2	0.5	–	–	–
Severe cognitive impairment	1.3	1.4	1.3	–	–	–

1. Rates are as diagnosed by the Diagnostic Interview Schedule (Robins *et al*, 1981), applying DSM–III (1980) criteria. Date from five sites combined, *n* = 18 571 (Regier *et al*, 1988).
2. Rates are one week prevalence rates for anxiety , affective and neurotic disorders, but 12 month prevalence rates for drug and alcohol abuse, psychoses and cognitive impairment. Diagnosis based on the Composite International Diagnostic Interview applying ICD–10, n=10 108.

included alcoholism, drug dependency and antisocial personality disorder which are all disorders with a male predominance. If these disorders are excluded, then the sex ratio for the ECA study rises to around 2 : 1 which is similar to other studies. Anxiety, and affective disorders, are more common in women and surveys which concentrate on the measurement of these disorders tend to show a female excess. It is possible also that some men with anxiety and affective disorders resort to alcohol and drugs to self-medicate themselves and this may account for some of the differences. The presence of co-morbid physical disease may increase the rate of psychiatric disorder particularly in women. When physical disorder is excluded, Vazquez-Barquero *et al* (1987) found the sex ratio was equal.

Age

Age plays an important role in the prevalence of most mental disorders. Major illnesses such as the functional disorders, personality disorders and substance misuse are more common in those under 45. Affective disorders are common and peak in middle age, while cognitive impairment is most frequent in old age.

Social factors

Some but not all studies show that lower social class is associated with increased rates of psychiatric disorder. Brown & Harris (1978) found that lower social class was associated with 'caseness' while Bebbington *et al* (1981) found only a weak and non-significant relationship between lower social class and 'caseness' in the community. Most studies have shown that unemployment has an adverse effect on mental health, increasing the rates for depression. Surtees *et al* (1983) in their survey of women in Edinburgh found that social class, unemployment, and being separated or divorced, all made an independent contribution to 'caseness'. However, once the adverse financial impact of unemployment is controlled for, unemployed people are no more psychologically distressed than those in work (Kessler *et al*, 1987). For women with children the effects of unemployment are complex; for some the additional strain of caring for children on top of a job increases the burden, but most studies show that employment protects against depression.

The complex interaction between psychiatric disorder, marital status, employment, and gender was studied by Bebbington *et al* (1981). The lowest rates for psychiatric disorder were for employed married men (4.4%), whereas unmarried, non-employed men had much higher rates (36%). For women, rates were lowest for those who were employed and unmarried (11%) and were highest for those who were not employed and married (41%). Further analysis of the latter group showed that most of the women in this group had children and therefore did not work. The higher morbidity in this group was mainly accounted for by the higher rate of non-employment, the effect of children being mediated more through not being employed, and the factor of having children itself did not increase psychiatric morbidity.

Race

The data concerning race from the various epidemiological surveys are complex and difficult to interpret, but there is evidence from the American studies that once social class and other indices of social deprivation are controlled for, the differences between the rates of depression in black and white people disappear (Hirschfeld & Cross, 1982). This does not appear to be the case for the prevalence of psychosis among people of Afro-Caribbean origin in the UK where the increase appears to be real (see page 325). Among those of Asian origin in the UK, there appears to be a significant trend for patients with minor psychiatric morbidity (a high GHQ score) to present more commonly with somatic symptoms than Caucasian patients. Overall morbidity does not differ, although GPs are more likely to recognise psychiatric morbidity in Caucasian rather than Asian patients (Wilson & Macarthy, 1994).

Urban and rural differences

Urban/rural differences have been found in many studies, with anxiety being more prevalent in rural areas and schizophrenia and depression in urban areas (Prudo *et al*, 1984; Vazquez-Barquero *et al*, 1987). Sociodemographic correlates for individual psychiatric disorders are discussed in previous chapters in this book.

Natural history of psychiatric disorders in the community

Tennant *et al* (1981) followed up the cases ascertained in the Camberwell survey and found that one month after the initial diagnosis around half the cases had resolved, and where the disorder had been triggered by a recent threatening life event 80% had resolved. Remission was unrelated to medical factors such as consultation or taking a psychotropic drug, or the severity of the disorder. Neutralising or fresh start events that appeared to give new hope were associated with remission, and the presence of adequate support and the absence of physical disorder appeared to hasten recovery.

Psychiatric morbidity in general practice (level 2)

This consists of all the psychiatric morbidity that presents to the GP. It comprises two groups – those who are recognised and are said to have 'conspicuous' psychiatric morbidity and are on level 3 or above, and those whose morbidity is not recognised by the GP and are said to have 'hidden' psychiatric morbidity.

Hidden psychiatric morbidity (level 2)

Goldberg & Blackwell (1970) used the General Health Questionnaire to screen for 'probable caseness' in a sample of patients attending a GP. Conspicuous psychiatric morbidity as assessed by the GP was calculated to be 20%, while 31% of the patients were found to be 'cases' by the psychiatrist, suggesting that around one-third of the cases who present to the GP and are therefore in level 2 remain unrecognised and fall into the category of hidden psychiatric morbidity.

Recognition of psychological disorder is strongly associated with management and outcome. Ormel & Giel (1990) examined a stratified sample of 296 patients twice using the Present State Examination and the Groningen Social Disability Schedule . GPs missed half of the 'cases' and typically assigned non-specific diagnoses to recognised 'cases'. Depressions were more readily recognised than anxiety disorders and the detection rates for severe disorders were higher than those for less severe disorders. Recognised, as compared with non-recognised, 'cases' were more likely to receive mental health interventions from their GP, and had better outcomes in terms of both psychopathology and social functioning. Better recognition and outcome were related to both initial severity, psychological reasons for encounter, recency of onset, diagnostic category, and psychiatric comorbidity.

In Sweden, Borquist *et al* (1993) administered the Hopkins Symptom Checklist and the Present State Examination to identify cases presenting to the GP and compared the morbidity of the recognised to the unrecognised cases. Of 84 consecutive patients, 25 were identified as having a psychiatric disorder with the PSE but only 10 were recognised by the GP as being a case, and 15 (60%) were hidden cases. In this study those with hidden psychiatric morbidity had more sick leave than those whose disorder was recognised (60 days versus 27 days) although the overall cost for the hidden cases was about the same as those with a recognised disorder because the diagnosed cases were referred to local day hospitals and other treatment facilities. Patients with hidden psychiatric morbidity are also more likely initially to complain of physical symptoms, and have an increased rate of psychotropic drugs prescribed implying at least a tacit recognition of some psychological disorder (Irwin & Cupples, 1986).

The problem of hidden psychiatric morbidity in general practice has been cause for concern because it indicates a large amount of unrecognised and therefore unmet need, although the size of the problem varies widely from one practice to another. A few studies have examined the effect of giving GPs feedback about the psychiatric status of patients in their practice, but as the GPs tended not to act on this information the psychiatric morbidity of the patients was unaltered. Goldberg & Huxley (1992) concluded that this was probably a pointless exercise and suggested that a better option was to provide more and better training for GPs to help sharpen their skills in the detection of the common mental disorders.

Conspicuous psychiatric morbidity (level 3)

This refers to cases of psychiatric morbidity that are recognised by the GP. Psychiatric illness defined by modern research criteria occurs in a quarter to a third of all new episodes of illness seen in general practice. Depression, with or without anxiety, and associated problems comprise the bulk of this morbidity. In addition to these common disorders, the GP is confronted by a wide range of psychological and psychiatric disorders such as the addictions, sleep disorders, psychosexual problems, psychiatric problems in children and so forth. This diverse range of disorders is illustrated in Table 28.3, derived from data based on all consultations at the general practice unit at the Aldermoor Health Centre in Southampton, where 19 766 encounters (9.4% of the total), were recorded for psychiatric, emotional, personality and social problems from 1975 to 1980 (Metcalfe & Edwards, 1981). Although depression and anxiety have the highest overall rates of occurrence in general practice, psychoses and personality disorders also make an impact because these disabilities are more severe, and may make a greater demand on the GP's time.

Studies by psychiatrists using more rigorous methodology and research criteria confirm this picture. Casey *et al* (1984) applied the PSE and CATEGO program to make ICD–9 diagnoses on all the patients that the GP thought had a psychiatric disorder during a one year period. A total of 7% of patients at risk were recognised by the GP as having a psychiatric diagnosis. The frequency of the different diagnostic subgroups among those with 'recognised psychiatric disorder' was neurotic depression 30%, depressive psychosis or retarded depression 11.7%, anxiety and phobias 21.6%, schizophrenia 5%, manic depression 2.3%. Only 14% of those considered by the GP to be cases were not found to be cases by the research psychiatrist. Additional screening instruments detected the presence of alcoholism (11%), and personality disorder (33%) although the GPs had not diagnosed these conditions. A dimensional way of describing the phenomenology of minor psychiatric morbidity in general practice has been described by Goldberg *et al* (1987) who found two highly correlated dimensions of anxiety and depression. The biological symptoms of depression were found in the same dimension as the psychological symptoms but appeared to represent a more severe manifestation of the depression.

How chronic are the neurotic disorders of general practice?

Most illnesses in general practice are probably transient with a natural tendency to remit but a proportion of these cases may become chronic and

Table 28.3 Psychiatric encounters in a general practice (*n* = 19 766; 9.4% of all consultations; Metcalfe & Edwards, 1981)

	Men %	Women %	Total %
Depression	16.3	22.9	20.5
Anxiety	16.0	22.5	20.2
Social problems	12.4	17.1	15.3
Sleep problems	9.4	6.8	7.7
Smoking	17.5	2.0	7.6
Emotional problems	3.0	4.4	3.9
Bereavement	1.7	5.0	3.8
Marital problems	2.3	4.3	3.6
Enuresis	4.1	1.6	2.5
Schizophrenia	3.5	1.9	2.5
Behaviour problems	1.8	2.4	2.2
Personality problems	1.7	2.2	2.0
Other psychiatric disorders	1.3	1.7	1.6
Alcoholism	3.2	0.2	1.3
Overanxious parent	2.1	0.9	1.3
Psychosis, unspecified	1.1	1.1	1.1
Psychosexual problem	0.7	1.1	0.9
Acute paranoia	0.6	0.8	0.8
Manic depressive psychosis	0.2	0.9	0.7
Drug dependence	1.1	0.4	0.6

these patients impose a heavy workload on the GP. Thus Brodaty (1983) found that of those who had a positive GHQ at consultation, only half were still positive four months later and by six months this proportion had fallen to 40%. Mann *et al* (1981) identified 100 cases with conspicuous morbidity as defined by a high GHQ score and reinterviewed them one year later. He found that 52% were no longer cases, a further 23% were improved but 25% showed a more chronic course. Early improvement was associated with a 'good family life' while a more chronic outcome was associated with a more severe initial illness, being older, physically ill, and receiving a prescription for a psychotropic drug. In a similar study, Wright (1990) administered the GHQ to a cohort of GP attenders and repeated the same exercise one year later. Around 65% of the sample had low scores both at the beginning and at the end of the study and were therefore non cases, 19% changed from high to low score, and 8% changed from low to high score; these patients probably had transient disorders. However, for 9% of the subjects high scores were recorded on both occasions indicating a more chronic psychiatric disorder.

These chronic cases have increased rates of comorbid chronic physical illness, and in about half, the psychiatric disorder was unrecognised by the

GP. Even five years prior to the study these patients had higher consultation rates. The combination of an increase in consultation frequency and chronicity extending back over several years may make a considerable demand on a GP's time and emotional resources. Over a three year period patients with personality disorders were found to have a greater morbidity, took more psychotropic drugs particularly benzodiazepines, and had more contacts at all levels of the psychiatric service (Sieverwright *et al*, 1991).

The contrast between general practice (level 3) and hospital-based disorders (levels 4 and 5) is the high frequency of depression, adjustment disorders, and anxiety and somatisation in general practice (Table 28.4). Psychiatric disorder on levels 4 and 5 is described in previous chapters in this book, and in the section below the first three filters in Goldberg & Huxley's (1980) model are described.

Filter 1 – the decision to consult

> The essential unit of medical practice is a consultation and all else in
> the practice of medicine derives from it (Sir James Spence, 1960).

The recognition of any medical disorder hinges critically on two decisions. The first is made by the patient that there is sufficient "discomfort" to consult a doctor and the second is by the doctor that "something is wrong" and in so doing initiates the diagnostic process. Eisenberg (1986) points out that patients are driven to consult a doctor more because of ill defined states of dysphoria and social dysfunction in daily living rather than specific symptoms or any pathology which may underly this. Intra-psychic distress must reach a certain critical level which varies widely between people before help is sought. Although physical illness and illness severity are the main determinants of consultation, sociodemographic and personality factors may also increase the likelihood of consultation.

In order to know precisely which sociodemographic and psychiatric factors underly treatment-seeking behaviour the psychiatric status of a large community sample first needs to be ascertained. This is then compared with general practice consultations made at the same time. During the 1970s, in response to public pressure the government funded a large scale survey in west London to see if the noise from Heathrow airport had any deleterious effect on mental health. Taking advantage of the large database of GHQ scores ($n = 3314$) from this survey, Williams *et al* (1986) also obtained GP case records to see how many subjects had consulted their GP in the two weeks prior to the survey. They found that 14.3% of the men and 17% of the women had consulted the GP, that probable minor psychiatric morbidity (a high GHQ score) doubled the likelihood of consulting (26% for men and 33% for women) and that about one-fifth of all consultations could be attributed to it. Female sex, lower social class and minor psychiatric morbidity all showed a complex interaction increasing the probability of GP consultation.

Although women were found to consult more often than men this could not be explained by illness behaviour because once consultations on behalf of someone else (usually children) were excluded the female excess in consulting behaviour could be wholly accounted for by a female excess in probable minor psychiatric morbidity. Unemployment makes consultation more likely, particularly for men (Williams *et al*, 1986).

In a similar study, Vazquez-Barquero *et al* (1992) ascertained the GHQ status of a stratified sample of 1223 people in the province of Cantabria in Northern Spain. Consultation with a doctor (in any medical setting) was also assessed within the two weeks prior to the survey and as might be expected physical illness was the main determinant of consultation and this was strongly associated with minor psychiatric morbidity. The combination of physical and psychiatric disorder led to very high rates of consultation, 89% for men and 97% for women. In men there was also an interaction with lower educational level, and the combination of physical illness, minor psychiatric morbidity and lower educational level made consultation seven times more likely than for those without these factors. As in the west London study, minor psychiatric morbidity itself appeared to double the likelihood of consultation (54% of those with compared with 23% of those without), and around one-fifth of all female and one-sixth of all male consultations were due to minor psychiatric morbidity. The clinical profile of cases found in community surveys is similar to that found in general practice with the possible exception that somatisation and neurasthenic presentations are more common in the surgery than in the community (Goldberg & Huxley, 1992).

Filter 2 – GP recognition of psychiatric disorders

GPs vary widely in their ability to recognise psychiatric disorder (Whitehouse, 1987). In a large survey of five urban health districts psychosocial disorders were recorded in 8% of consultations, but more significantly the range for individual GPs recording a psychosocial diagnosis was from 1.1% to 24%, with 20% of doctors recording less than 5.1% cases and 20% of the doctors more than 10.4%. Doctors who recorded a higher proportion of psychological diagnoses also appeared to have a longer than average consultation time.

The most important factor associated with GPs, ability to detect psychiatric illness is the ability of the general practitioner to conduct a simple mental state examination in an empathic manner (Marks *et al*, 1979).

More recent studies (Millar & Goldberg, 1992) have shown that GPs skilled in the detection of psychiatric problems elicit more cues from their emotionally distressed patients than those who are poor in recognition. Doctors with fewer skills tend to prevent their patients from giving them verbal and non-verbal cues by conducting a more hurried theory-led interview, while a patient-led interview which clarifies the patient's problem and facilitates discussion is used more often by skilled doctors. Little is known about why some doctors are more skilled than others, but in the study of

Marks *et al* (1979) personality factors appeared to be important; 'Conservatism' and 'interest and concern' accounted for much of the variation. The recognition of psychiatric disorder by the GP, or the operation of filter 2, is of great importance because it is only once their condition is recognised that patients can benefit from the full range of other available medical and social interventions.

Filter 3 – referral to specialist psychiatric service

Kessel (1963) asked the question, who ought to receive psychiatric care in Britain? He restricted his theme to referral between GPs and psychiatrists, arguing that psychiatrists should welcome increasing public demand for their services, and that GPs should be encouraged to refer patients freely to psychiatrists "when they want advice".

However, if GPs were to freely refer any patient who wanted a psychiatric opinion the psychiatric services would soon be overwhelmed. GPs screen out the milder cases of anxiety or depression and only patients with the more severe disorders are referred on to psychiatric services, and clinical severity is therefore the main determinant of permeability through the third filter. Table 28.4 compares morbidity in general practice with that on a psychiatric case register. It demonstrates the extent and relative impact of the neuroses and adjustment disorders which are screened out by the GPs so that these disorders make only a small impression in the hospital-based figures.

A change in the sex ratio between levels 3 and 4 also occurs. The National Morbidity Study showed a sex ratio in general practice (level 3) of 2.38 : 1 whereas in level 4 this was reduced to 1.37 : 1 indicating a relatively greater permeability for men to pass through filter 3 and for men to be referred to psychiatric clinics (Goldberg & Huxley, 1992).

Determinants of psychiatric referral by GPs are shown in Box 28.1. There are wide variations in the referral rates of individual GPs. The reasons for these are not clear (Kessel, 1963; Wilkinson, 1985).

Reasons given by GPs for referring patients to psychiatrists are shown in Box 28.2. Characteristics of GPs, patients and psychiatric services interact in an intricate and enigmatic way. Stigma still remains the most common reason for GPs not referring patients.

The pathways of referral in other countries

The GP screening mechanism probably operates in different ways in different countries. In Holland, Veerhak (1993) described a similar pattern to the UK, and using a large database of doctor–patient contacts found that only 6% of patients presenting with a psychosocial problem during surgery hours were referred to specialist care. An increased probability of being referred was associated with being younger, male, and having a more severe

Table 28.4 Annual rates per thousand of psychiatric disorder from general practice[1] and hospital-based statistics[2]

	General practice	Serious mental illness
Other neuroses[3]	35	2.46
Depression	28	5.35
Adjustment disorders	26	1.74
Affective psychosis	3	1.47
Alcohol, drugs	2.7	1.37
Organic, dementia	2.2	2.75
Schizophrenia	2	4.08
Personality disorder	1.1	1.62

1. Annual rates per 1000 population at risk in primary care. Data from Morbidity Statistics in General Practice 1981–82 (HMSO, 1986).
2. Data from Salford Case Register (Goldberg *et al*, 1982).
3. Mainly somatic presentation of affective illness and anxiety disorders.

psychiatric diagnosis. Urban referral rates were also increased partly because psychiatric morbidity is higher in cities, but also because transport is easier. Doctors with a "limited task perception", with regard to psychiatric treatment also tended to refer more often. Although diagnosis was associated with the facilities to which patients were referred (psychotic conditions to psychiatric services and social problems to social workers), the most prevalent diagnoses, that is neurotic conditions and relationship problems, were more or less randomly distributed over the various services and agencies. Referral preferences appeared to be related to regular contact between GPs and specialists and a positive regard by GPs for the resources concerned.

In a community based service in South Verona, Italy, the referral rate was much higher and 22% of patients identified with conspicuous psychiatric morbidity by GPs were referred to a specialist (Tansella & Williams, 1989). A previous psychiatric history, a psychological presenting complaint, social problems and the GP's psychiatric diagnosis exert positive effects on referral while organic illness had a negative effect. In the presence of a psychological complaint, a psychiatric diagnosis had no influence on the probability of referral but in the absence of a psychological complaint (a more endogenous picture) a GP's diagnosis of depression increased the probability of referral (Arreghini *et al*, 1991). A more recent study of the same service in Italy showed that the pattern was now changing and an increasing number of patients were presenting directly to the community-based service. Of those reaching the service, only 43% presented initially to the GP, 36% presented directly to the service, 11% went through the hospital doctor and a small number of patients reached the service through a variety of other agencies (CPNs, social workers, courts, etc.) indicating that many patients are now bypassing 'filter 3' or GP referral (Balestrieri *et al*, 1994).

Box 28.1 Determinants of referral to the psychiatrist

Characteristics of GP
  High rate of identification of psychiatric disorder
  Older age
  Single-handed practice
Characteristics of patient
  Male sex
  Younger age (between 25 and 45)
  Psychotic disorder
  Chronic disorder (over one year's duration)
The psychiatric service
  Community-oriented services (for patients with psychotic
    disorders)
  Urban and accessible services

After Shepherd *et al* (1966)

Pathways of referral from primary care to specialist services vary widely in different countries. The topic was studied by the World Health Organization and is reviewed by Gater *et al* (1991). Direct referrals from the community to psychiatric services without involving the GP are relatively common in America. This may be a feature of any insurance-based service in which the patients can select their own doctor. A similar pattern was present in Spain, Portugal, Mexico, Pakistan and India.

Diagnosis and classification by GPs

Psychiatric diagnosis in the surgery is a markedly different process and has a different purpose when compared to making a diagnosis in the psychiatric clinic. Sharp & King (1989) highlight some of the differences: "Psychiatric disorder, like most illness, behaves as a continuously distributed variable and a valid question from the general practitioner might therefore be 'how much of it is present?' In psychiatry there is an even more fundamental question – deciding what 'it', the disorder, actually is. The general practice setting further compounds the problem of psychiatric case definition – there is a high incidence of transient morbidity and the illness is often seen in its very early stages, before the full clinical picture has developed. For these reasons in particular the classifications of psychiatric disorder in current use are quite inappropriate for primary care..." (Sharp & King, 1989).

There are three main official classification systems that GPs can use for patients with mental disorders: ICD–10 or DSM–IV, which are both designed primarily for use by psychiatrists; and the International Classification for Primary Care (ICPC). This was derived from earlier versions of the ICD and

---

Box 28.2 Reasons given by GPs for referring patients to a psychiatrist

Common
    Patient failed to respond to GP treatment
    Diagnostic opinion or investigations required
    Patient, relative, hospital doctor or social worker requested
        specialist referral
    Specialist to share or take over management of the patient
Less common
    Need for a specialist form of treatment
    Behavioural disturbance or serious social difficulties
    Risk of suicide
    A member of the patient's family is already being treated by
        a psychiatrist, and it is considered beneficial that the
        patient should also attend
    The GP wishes to recruit the psychiatrist's support in helping
        a patient with legal problems or in negotiating with local
        authority services

After Shepherd *et al* (1966)

DSM systems and was specially designed for use in general practice by the World Organisation of National Colleges, Academics, and Academic Associations (WONCA) of general practitioners; there are tri- or multiaxial classifications, with separate assessments of physical and mental health, social problems, personality and level of stress.

In practice, GPs use a variety of different methods of classification (Sharp & King, 1989). Most GPs proceed directly from symptoms to treatment and may have problem-orientated approaches which are idiosyncratic; official systems of classification as described above are seldom used compared with the use of loose aggregates of symptoms combined with the GP's knowledge of the patient's personality and family circumstances. Although this may be unreliable, traditional diagnosis is inadequate for the majority of complex disorders found in general practice.

General practitioners are less pre-occupied than psychiatrists by questions of phenomenology and psychiatric classification, but tend to be more concerned with the distinction between psychiatric disorder and physical disorder, and psychiatric disorder that merits intervention versus that best left alone.

Jenkins *et al* (1988) conducted an illuminating investigation to test how far official systems in the ICD and the General Practice International Classification of Health Problems in Primary Care (ICHPPC–2) could be applied consistently by GPs to mental disorders presenting in primary care; they found that neither system could be. The overall diagnostic concordance between participants using ICD and ICHPPC was disappointingly low (indicating low inter-rater reliability for these schemes), but there was moderately good agreement on individual observations relating to psychological, physical, personality and social features.

In the absence of useful schemes GPs tend to avoid making a diagnosis and are more likely to resort to symptomatic treatment. GPs usually adopt a pragmatic problem-solving approach based on probabilities, linked to notions of risk as well as assessing the usefulness or otherwise of intervention, and make the management decisions first and a diagnosis afterwards to justify their decisions (Howie, 1972).

Treatment of major psychiatric disorders by GPs

Although GPs treat more 'minor psychiatric disorder' than major illness, they still play an important role in the management of the more serious psychiatric conditions. The sections below cover some of the more recent studies on the ways GPs deal with the major psychiatric disorders. The emphasis is on the frequency and nature of the GP contact and the use of psychiatric treatments in primary care.

Depression

Watts, an early pioneer in the study of depression in general practice, wrote:

> In six years of practice before the War, I diagnosed only one case of endogenous depression and that after the patient had committed suicide. After psychiatric experience in the army I have found the condition comparatively common in general practice. In six months, no fewer than 20 cases came under my care pointing to the prevalence of the complaint (Watts, 1947).

Depression is the most common psychiatric condition treated by the GP. Because patients with psychotic depression, other comorbid disorders such as personality disorder, drug and alcohol abuse, or those with severe suicidal intent, are referred to the specialist services, most studies have found that depression in general practice is less severe.

Recognition and non-recognition of depression

With the advent of effective medical and psychological treatments for depression there is an added impetus to recognise and treat depression in general practice, because the vast majority of episodes occur in the community. However, there is evidence that depression often remains unrecognised in a proportion of these subjects. Certain factors in the patient's presentation, the interview with the doctor, and the doctor's style may make an independent contribution to the failure to recognise depression. In the study of Freeling *et al* (1985) 'unrecognised depressions' were more likely to have lasted for more than one year, patients were less likely to admit to the symptom of depression, were less obviously depressed, and were more likely to show greater reactivity of mood to external events. These patients also had higher scores on an item called 'distinct quality of mood' which refers to the degree to which the patient regarded his subjective mood state as different from the normal experience of depression and sadness (Freeling *et al*, 1985). Patients with unrecognised major depression more often have physical illness and those with serious physical disease are five times more likely not to have their depression recognised compared with those without any physical disease. This may be because physical symptoms lead to a suspicion of organic disorder which results in the GP being preoccupied with physical illness and organic pathology, while in other cases the problem may be one of 'somatisation' (Freeling, 1993).

Videotapes of interviews with patients whose depression was recognised show that early on in the interview, cue words such as 'depressed', 'can't cope', 'nervous breakdown', 'poor sleep' occurred in more than two-thirds of the cases of recognised depression but these cue words only occurred in one-third of those whose depression went unrecognised. GPs were more likely to make the diagnosis of depression if patients stated that they were depressed, reported one other depressive symptom, and the doctor had a 'feeling' that they were depressed which presumably developed in response to non-verbal cues. Only 13% of diagnosed depressed patients gave only one cue. Unrecognised depressions tend to become recognised with the passage of time. By six months 20% were recognised, a further 20% had remitted but 20% will still remain unrecognised (Freeling, 1993).

Does recognising depression in general practice matter and are patients with unrecognised depression worse off than those who receive a diagnosis? Sireling *et al* (1985) found that 12 weeks after consultation patients with unrecognised depression had significantly higher scores on depressed mood, loss of energy, and irritability compared with those with recognised depression. However, Dowrick & Buchan (1995) found that recognition made little difference to outcome when all cases of depression (including both new and chronic cases) were considered. These authors screened consecutive attenders in a Liverpool general practice with the Beck Depression Inventory, and identified 179 cases of depression of which 116 (59%) were not known to the GP. Cases of unrecognised depression were then randomly allocated into two equal groups: in one group the GP was informed about the patient's depressed status, but for the second group the GP was not informed. Disclosure had no effect on outcome 6 and 12 months later, possibly because the GPs tended not to act on the information and the Beck depression scores for the group as a whole fell only slightly over 12 months. Possible reasons for the discrepancy between these two studies is that in the earlier study of Freeling *et al* (1985) GPs were invited to refer only new cases of depression to the study, while in the Liverpool study all cases of depression in the practice (new and chronic) were included. Dowrick & Buchan (1995) concluded that a GP diagnosis of depression was only a marker of severity and that most of the depression in the community was beyond the reach of medical intervention, and mainly due to other intractable medical and social problems.

Management of depression in general practice

Wright (1994) suggests that the key to treating depression in general practice consists of a series of weekly yet brief (10–15 minutes) interviews which can be decreased in frequency as the patient gets better. Support and reassurance as well as antidepressants are essential (see also chapters 4 and 6). A more formal trial for cognitive psychotherapy comparing four treatment groups in general practice was conducted by Scott & Freeman (1992). They compared cognitive–behavioural therapy by a clinical psychologist, case work by a social worker, amitriptyline prescribed by a psychiatrist, and routine treatment by the GP. By 16 weeks all treatment groups had improved and the advantage of specialist treatment over routine GP care was small. Psychological treatment, especially social work was most positively evaluated by patients but as the overall cost of specialised care was double that of routine GP care and involved four times as much therapist time, specialised care of this type is probably not justified.

Around half of the subjects who commit suicide will have consulted their GP in the previous eight weeks, most will have received a diagnosis of depression and a third will have been prescribed an antidepressant. However, as Diekstra & Egmord (1989) point out the event is very rare in general practice. A GP with an average list of 2000 can expect only one suicide every three years, so it is unlikely that a GP would be able to pick up or spot potential cases.

Antidepressant drug trials are usually hospital-based and so the applicability of their findings to general practice is uncertain. Hollyman *et al* (1988) conducted a six week placebo-controlled trial of amitriptyline in general practice and confirmed its effectiveness among a group of mild to moderate depressed patients in general practice. Drug/placebo differences emerged after only two weeks (in studies of psychiatric out-patients this period is usually 3–6 weeks) and drug placebo differences were present in all except the most mildly ill subjects. Drug effects related only to the initial severity of depression and it is of interest that neither endogenous symptomatology nor precipitating stress had any influence on drug effect.

In this trial the compliance rate was high at 80%, but in routine practice the rate is probably far lower. For example, Johnston (1981) found that after one week 16% of depressed patients had stopped their antidepressants, and this figure reached 68% by four weeks. Yet 57% of patients who defaulted from treatment were still seriously depressed at six weeks, with side-effects being the main reason for non-compliance. A recent study of prescriptions for antidepressants in general practice showed that the older tricyclics (amitriptyline, clomipramine and dothiepin) were still the most frequently prescribed drugs (61%) but therapeutic levels were only reached in 13.4% of the prescriptions. Lofepramine was given in 8.5% of the patients but a higher proportion of patients received therapeutic doses (61%) and the SSRIs comprised 16% of all the prescriptions but were prescribed in full therapeutic doses in 98% of the cases (Donoghue & Tylee, 1996).

GP attitudes to depression

The treatment of depression in general practice will in part be dependent on the GP's knowledge and attitude to depression. Botega *et al* (1992) found that GPs clustered into three roughly equal groups with regard to their attitude to depression: those who have a sympathetic and supportive approach to the patient and who are less likely to prescribe antidepressants; those who accept the organic determinants of depression and the advantages of medication over psychotherapy; and those who view the treatment of depression as unrewarding and feel uncomfortable dealing with depressed patients.

To investigate whether an educational programme on depression could influence attitudes and the ability to treat depressive disorders, Rutz *et al* (1989) instituted an educational programme on depression for all the GPs on the island of Gotland. This particular island was selected because it lies in the middle of the Baltic Sea and is quite isolated with a 'natural' catchment area of 56 000 and 18 GPs. The programme consisted of a series of lectures on suicide, depressive illness, old age, psychotherapy and antidepressants. To ensure the GPs had grasped everything the course was repeated twice. Eighteen months later there had been a substantial decrease in the proportion of new cases of depression referred to the clinic (from 25% to 5% of all new patient referrals), admissions for depression to hospital (1138 hospital admission days to 338), number of patients on sick leave for depression (44 to 29), and an increase in the amount of lithium prescribed. In the year following the education programme the number of suicides showed a statistically significant fall from 11 to four but in subsequent years the rate soon reverted to the original rate for Gotland (Rutz *et al*, 1992). Although the teaching programme was gratefully accepted by the GPs and produced useful results in the short term, there is a moderate turnover of GPs on Gotland, and some questions remain as to how long improvements might last. Rutz *et al* (1992) recommend that such programmes need to be repeated every two to three years if their effectiveness is to be maintained. A similar research educational programme in Gotland on sexual and relationship problems had led to a marked reduction in the number of induced abortions but a few years later the rate had returned to the normal overall rate for Sweden (Nilsson, 1981).

Somatisation

Many patients in general practice satisfy research criteria for psychiatric illness but are classified as having physical illnesses by their doctor. These patients are said to be somatising their psychological problems. These patients describe symptoms of psychiatric illness, yet their psychological distress is overlooked by their doctor. The more severe somatisation disorders seen by psychiatrists are described in Chapter 16.

Bridges & Goldberg (1985) produced a four point operational definition of somatisation illnesses in general practice in which a psychiatric disorder is present:

(i)   the patient is seeking help for somatic symptoms
(ii) the patient attributes these symptoms to some physical disorder
(iii) a specific mental disorder defined by standardised diagnostic criteria is present
(iv) the somatic symptoms are not due to physical disease, but can be thought of as part of the mental disorder.

In most somatisation cases found in general practice the underlying psychiatric condition is usually depression or an anxiety state (Goldberg & Huxley, 1992). However, in a somatic presentation the patient is seeking help only for their somatic symptoms which form a part of their mental disorder; the patients do not consider that they have any mental disorder.

Table 28.5 shows that as a type of presentation for psychiatric disorder, somatisation is very frequent. Purely psychological presentations of psychiatric disorder are relatively uncommon and in general practice comprise only 5% of the cases in contrast to the psychiatric out-patient clinic where psychological presentations are more frequent (Bridges & Goldberg, 1985).

Comparisons of those presenting with purely mental symptoms – 'psychologisers' – with 'somatisers' show that the latter are less depressed, have fewer and less severe psychological symptoms, lower levels of social dissatisfaction, and less social stress and dependency on relatives, but were more likely to have received medical in-patient care as an adult as well as being more likely to have an unsympathetic attitude towards mental illness. Somatisers and psychologisers do not differ in sociodemographic and intellectual characteristics or in their attitudes towards the role of the family doctor (Wright, 1990; Bridges *et al*, 1991).

Patients who satisfy research criteria for psychiatric disorder (a high GHQ score, or fulfil diagnostic criteria in a research interview) but the GP classified as having an entirely physical illness form a more disturbing group. Balint (1957) described how patients in this group might be passed from one organic specialist to another without psychological factors even being considered in what he called "a collusion of anonymity". Goldberg & Huxley (1992) also describe how the GP will manage such patients by ordering physical investigations and then prescribe a symptomatic physical remedy.

The doctor colludes with the patient's denial of psychological disorder and both patient and doctor are usually satisfied with encounters of this type and "it ill behoves an outsider to declare that anything is wrong".

Schizophrenia and long-term mental disorder

There are a multitude of organisations concerned with the mentally ill, including statutory bodies and charitable and voluntary groups. Many different professional groups as well as untrained carers are involved in the care of these patients. How well are they working together? Could their efforts be better synchronised so that duplication is avoided and optimum use is made of their resources? The inadequacy of present arrangements is in no doubt and better systems are needed to be developed in order to reduce the unacceptable number who are 'falling through the net' (Horder, 1991).

As the old asylums are disappearing the majority of patients, even those at the more severe end of the spectrum, are now living in the community. A recent survey into the degree of contact GPs had with patients with chronic mental illness in the South West Thames region found that most GPs thought they had around 10 patients with schizophrenia on their list. Practices with higher numbers of patients with schizophrenia were more likely to be in Greater London, were located within three miles of a mental hospital, and had a psychiatrist visiting the practice (Kendrick *et al*, 1991).

Patients with schizophrenia are in frequent contact with their GPs, and are more likely to see their general practitioner than the psychiatrist. Melzer *et al* (1991) found that at one year following discharge 57% had been in recent contact with their GP, 52% had visited an out-patient clinic but only 20% had seen the CPN. Patients with schizophrenia consult their GPs at

Table 28.5 Relationship of mental disorder to reason for consultation in 590 new onsets of illness in primary care in Manchester (from Goldberg, 1994)

	All patients ($n = 590$)	Psychiatric cases only ($n = 195$)
Not mentally ill	67%	N/A
Physical illness with secondary mental disorder	1%	3.2%
Unrelated physical and mental disorder	8%	24.0%
Somatisation	20%	57.0%
Entirely mentally ill	5%	15.0%

around the same rate as other patients with chronic physical disorders and usually present with a physical complaint (Nazareth *et al*, 1993).

Many patients regard the doctor who prescribes their medication to them as the most important member of the treatment team. In this context, Boddington (1992) reported that 45 of a sample of 47 (94%) patients with schizophrenia in an inner city practice received a prescription from their GP. Contact with the practice was frequent and over a two year period there was an average of 43 entries per patient suggesting an entry for each patient every 17 days, mostly for a drug-related intervention such as a depot injection. Liaison with the local psychiatrist in the form of letters was evident in 28 (60%) of the cases but "liaison with other involved parties was haphazard and rare, furnishing little evidence of the teamwork favoured in the literature" (Boddington, 1992). Both Parkes *et al* (1962), and more recently Kendrick *et al* (1991) reported that contact with GPs usually occurred during a crisis, was most intense initially, and it was the GP's task to alert other members of the team. The GP will also often become involved when the Mental Health Act is applied.

Treatment may be started, stopped or changed by the patient, GP or psychiatrist without one party letting the other parties know, and problems in communication frequently arise in the post discharge period. The responsibilities of the different professionals are often ill defined and this kind of confusion has led to the use of shared care cards in antenatal care and for people with diabetes mellitus. Essex *et al* (1990) tried to develop such cards for use in patients with long-term mental illness but found that although the patients liked the system and cooperated well, the professionals hardly used the cards at all.

The general practice team is being increasingly involved in maintenance treatment, particularly in rural areas where there may be difficulties in travelling frequently to hospital. In other cases patients prefer to receive their depot injection from the practice nurse as this is less stigmatising than returning to hospital. Some GPs have also assumed the role of the visiting doctor to the many new hostels springing up in the community which, in effect, are the transposed wards of the old asylums. The carers of patients with schizophrenia are usually the parents and they need support over the long term, and GPs are well placed to fulfil this role. Distressed relatives will usually first turn to the GP when the patient is non-compliant or experiencing other difficulties or requiring readmission.

A preliminary impression of how GPs view the new community psychiatric service came from the Worcester Development Project (Bennett, 1989). Of those who remembered the previous hospital based service most thought that the new services with their emphasis on community care were an improvement and criticisms revolved around difficulties in obtaining emergency admissions as well as the slowness of the social service department in responding to requests for help. A study of the new services in Harlow found that only 32% of the GPs felt satisfied with the new service, 61% of

GPs were dissatisfied and 6% had feelings neither way (Stansfield, 1991). The recent stabbing of a London GP by a patient released by a tribunal and other violent incidents (*Daily Telegraph*, December 14, 1995) may also have led to some loss of confidence in community care at least in the London area. In the future GPs will be expected to play a key role in the coordination of community services but in the Worcester study the majority of the GPs had neither any particular interest nor training in psychiatry and this raises questions about how they may be helped to fulfil such a role.

Alcohol problems

A curious paradox exists concerning alcohol and the medical profession. On the one hand, there is an insistence on the medical concept of alcoholism and the necessity to treat alcoholism as a disease like any other, while on the other hand GPs seem reluctant to diagnose, treat or refer people with problems related to alcohol. Based on national data, Wilson (1980) estimated that in the average general practice list of 2000 there would be 55 (2.75%) people with heavy drinking which had resulted in some harm, and a further 200 (10%) moderate drinkers who are at some risk of harm. The morbidity of heavy drinkers remains high and they consult their GPs twice as often as other patients. Alcoholism contributes to as many as 40 000 deaths per year (smoking contributes to 100 000, cervical cancer 2000) and there are substantial social costs in terms of family disruption, while lost production is estimated to cost £2 billion a year (Wallace & Jarman, 1994).

A survey into the amount of drinking among patients on the lists of two GP practices in a north London housing estate revealed that 11% of the men were heavy drinkers (more than 42 units per week) and 5% of the women drank more than 21 units per week. Primary care has long been recognised as a major setting for the identification of alcohol problems because of its accessibility, avoidance of stigma and because of the diverse presentations of alcohol problems (medical, legal, social, psychiatric). In this section we are only concerned with how GPs diagnose and view patients with drinking problems. The topic of alcoholism and drug addiction is comprehensively covered in *Seminars in Alcohol and Drug Misuse* (Chick & Cantwell, 1994); the neuropsychiatric aspects are described on page 1104 in this volume.

Recognised and unrecognised drinking in general practice

As with minor psychiatric morbidity, much of the moderate and heavy drinking in the community often goes unrecognised by the GP for many years. Wilkins (1974), a GP in a Manchester group practice, in his book *The Hidden Alcoholic in General Practice* described an elegant study he undertook to estimate how many drinkers went unrecognised in general practice. He devised a questionnaire, "The Spare Time Activity Questionnaire", which included questions on eating, smoking, leisure activities and the amount of alcohol consumed. During the course of the year he administered the questionnaire to 544 subjects who had at least one risk factor for an alcohol problem and identified 87 subjects as heavy drinkers, of whom only 11 (7.9%) were known to the practice as 'alcoholics'.

In a similar study in Australia, Reid *et al* (1986) investigated the accuracy with which GPs identified patients with heavy drinking. Patients were interviewed with regard to their drinking habits in the waiting room and then saw their GP who was subsequently asked to indicate the patient's level of alcohol intake. GPs successfully identified only 28% of the high risk drinkers and 45% of those classified as moderate to heavy drinkers.

There are many reasons why GPs fail to recognise people with drinking problems and sometimes have a negative attitude to them, but the phenomenon is of considerable importance because without GP recognition there can be no intervention either through a medical service or some other agency and the morbidity and mortality of alcohol problems are very high. Thom & Tellez (1986) used a series of in depth interviews with 33 GPs and the following themes emerged.

Difficulties in defining the condition

Many GPs expressed difficulty in making the diagnosis because it was impossible to draw the line between social drinking and the quantity of drinking that constituted a medical problem. One GP commented "Who should make the diagnosis? Is it a problem to me or a problem to them, or is it a certain quantity of drink or is it that they cannot stop?" Most GPs took the view that until the patient showed evidence of drink-related harm, alcohol consumption was not a medical matter. This view, which was widespread, mitigates against the Department of Health's preventative approach which seeks to reduce alcohol intake during the pre-symptomatic phase.

A worthwhile diagnosis?

Over half the GPs interviewed thought that their chances of helping their patients were 'poor' or 'very slim' and none could think of a patient who had changed drinking habits as a result of their intervention in the last year. The pattern of recurrent relapses and readmission and the skid-row picture of the more severe cases also coloured GP attitudes. Others commented that when success did come it usually was as a result of the intervention of some other agency, such as Alcoholics Anonymous, and lay beyond the control of the GP. In contrast to the non-recognition of minor psychiatric morbidity such as anxiety and depression by GPs, the non-recognition of drinking problems appears to be a much more active process, or as one GP in the study put it, "one of the things I do not do, is ask too many questions because I do not want to uncover a whole lot of things I cannot deal with. If it were obvious how I could deal with it effectively then I might go looking for a few patients".

Difficulties in confronting the patient

GPs in middle class practices, in which the stigma against alcoholism is high, reported that even informing the patient about a diagnosis of alcoholism was "a delicate affair" and this applied particularly to women. An opposite problem was encountered by a GP working in a docklands practice where drinking 8 pints a day was the norm and the GP found that his comment that drinking so much might be harmful was generally met with derision. Confronting patients often led to antagonism which impaired the doctor–patient relationship with subsequent reluctance to consult over other problems. Blood tests or referrals were sometimes used as a stratagem to jolt the patients into recognising the seriousness of the problem but only a few GPs felt sufficiently courageous to confront their patients directly.

Attempts at treatment

Some GPs expressed negative views of their own failed attempts at treatment while others expressed negative attitudes about the hospital service. Policies which insist on the patient being sober before treatment could start seemed paradoxical while waiting lists also seemed inappropriate for patients whose motivation was transient at best. Advertising and government health programmes failed to emphasise the harmful effects of alcohol enough and many GPs contrasted this with the more helpful government sponsored advertising programme which had been successfully used to combat smoking. Anderson (1985) estimated the frequency of such negative attitudes among GPs in Oxford, and found that only 40% of the GPs felt motivated to work with drinkers and less than a third were satisfied with the way they did so. Although more than half the GPs thought they had a legitimate role in working with alcoholics, only a few doctors (9%) reported any satisfaction from working with patients with drinking problems.

Screening

Alcohol is a great mimic and a common cause for medical and psychiatric presentations to the GP or for hospital admission. Drinking problems should always be suspected in any person presenting frequently at the surgery with a wide variety of medical disorders, and in almost any psychiatric disorder, particularly anxiety and depression, and marital difficulties (or the partner may present), road traffic accidents, and for those in at-risk occupations, such as publicans, seamen, journalists, etc. Screening questionnaires such as the CAGE (Mayfield *et al*, 1974) and MAST (Pokorny *et al*, 1972) and AUDIT (World Health Organization, 1989) have proved useful tools in epidemiological research but have not become established in routine clinical work. Blood tests especially gamma glutamyl transferase and mean corpuscular volume (MCV) are the most commonly used tests if the GP has a suspicion of a drinking problem.

Intervention in general practice

Recently the concept of a rigid categorisation between those who drink as 'alcoholics' and those who drink in a more sociable and controlled fashion as 'social drinkers' and 'non-drinkers' has been questioned and the notion of a continuum of drinking behaviours is thought more probable. At the one end are the heavy drinkers, who if they request treatment are usually referred to the specialist services. In the middle of the range of drinkers are a large number of people who drink moderately; Vaillant (1983) has shown that up to a third of people in this group will treat themselves without any external help and stop drinking, particularly if there is an associated medical problem which deteriorates rapidly with further drinking.

There has been some interest in seeing whether intervention during the pre-symptomatic phase in the form of simple advice from the GP on the harmful effects of alcohol can have any impact on moderate drinking behaviour. A review of six studies which compared the effects of advice versus no advice to moderate drinkers found a favourable effect in three studies but there was no difference in the other three (Wallace & Jarman, 1994). In the Scottish DRAMS study (Drinking Reasonably And Moderately Sensibly) GPs offered advice and gave patients a self-help book entitled *So You Want to Cut Down Your Own Drinking* (Heather *et al*, 1987). There was no difference in the amount of drinking between patients receiving advice and the booklets compared with those who only had routine GP treatment. A study in Oxford found that a ten minute talk by the GP giving advice to the patient led to significant reduction in drinking behaviours six months later in men but not in women, while Anderson & Scott (1992) found that five sessions of advice had more impact than one. The Department of Health is trying to encourage GPs to take a greater interest in alcohol problems and GPs who run specialised alcohol clinics may receive an extra payment. However Anderson (1993) comments that the assumptions made by Department of Health planners in the 1980s that GPs would willingly participate in preventative medicine and that their patients would heed their advice might be questioned.

Drug misuse

Opiate abuse is a problematic area of clinical practice, both for GPs and general psychiatrists, particularly in districts which lack a designated drug abuse service. A survey into opiate abuse in general practice found that during a four week period, one in five GPs had been consulted by an opiate misuser, and in one-third of these cases the patient was not known to the GP, and this suggested an estimate of 30–44 000 new cases of opiate misuse presenting each year in general practice (Glanz & Taylor, 1986). A new case of opiate addiction may also have a high degree of associated medical morbidity such as HIV (Table 28.6) or violence and make considerably more demands on the GP's time and resources than most other categories of psychiatric disorder. In the study of Glanz & Taylor (1986), 66% of the subjects claimed they were seeking help concerning withdrawal and rehabilitation, only 23% wanted a prescription and 20% wanted other types of help. A study of intravenous drug misusers in Scotland found that 60% were also HIV positive (McKeganny & Boddy, 1988).

In this study the GPs thought that 58% of the subjects were primarily using the consultation to obtain drugs even though this usually masqueraded as a request for help. This degree of manipulation and lying by addicts was often distressing and many GPs found this aspect difficult to deal with. There was also a consensus that working with alcoholics was easier than working with drug addicts. McKeganny & Boddy (1988) suggest that difficulties arise in treating addicts in general practice because of the gross distortion of the traditional doctor–patient relationship. In the classical doctor–patient relationship there is a shared assumption that decisions concerning the management of the illness are made by the doctor, that the patient considers the illness to be an undesirable state and that the patient should cooperate with those whose concern is to help them get better. Most consultations with opiate users in general practice do not even remotely fit this description. Drug misusers are entitled to the full range of primary health care and voluntary sector services, and families and friends are equally important secondary sufferers who also need help.

Working with children

Work with children has been estimated to occupy about a third of a doctor's time. Ninety per cent of pre-school children, and 64% of 5–14-year-olds will consult their GP at least once a year (Court Report, 1976). Between 2–5% of children attend their GP with a primary psychological problem such as anxiety, conduct problems, hyperactivity or other psychiatric disorders. Psychosocial factors may also contribute to a substantial additional number of consultations particularly among those with psychosomatic disorders. Giel *et al* (1981) in a study in four European countries found mental disorders were present in 20% of the children presenting to their GPs, while Bailey *et al* (1978) in the UK estimated that 22% of those presenting with mainly physical complaints also had some 'psychological deviance'.

As in adults the vast majority of episodes of ill health in children do not lead to consultation. A variety of social factors mainly relating to the parents may increase the likelihood of consultation with the GP corresponding to 'Filter 1' in Goldberg & Huxley's (1980) model. Consultation is strongly associated with childhood psychiatric disorder, family stress, psychosocial disadvantage, coming from a broken home, parental marital disharmony and maternal mental health problems. Other factors that increase the likelihood of consultation include the paramenstrual period (Tuch, 1975) and a perception that their child has an increased vulnerability or is especially fragile, for example, if there were severe neonatal complications. Garralda (1995) remarks how it is striking that mothers from deprived and disturbed backgrounds experience greatest upset in regard to their children to the relative neglect of other social difficulties such as their marital problems or financial impoverishment. Their failure to control their behaviourally disturbed child is the issue of paramount importance which gives maximal subjective distress and leads to the initial contact with the medical and social services.

Like adults, the somatisation of distress is also common in children and primary psychological presentations are infrequent (3.5%). More classical psychosomatic disorders (insomnia, headache, abdominal pain or other abdominal symptoms) account for 8–10% of the consultations of children attending primary care in a US study (Goldberg *et al*, 1984). In cases of

Table 28.6 Problems associated with drug misuse reported by general practitioners (% of drug misuse cases)

Medical	
Opiate dependence	35
Poor health	32
Hepatitis	30
Infections related to injection	20
Pain/self-medication	15
Dependence on other drugs than opiates	10
Deliberate self-harm	6
Trauma	2
Drug use in pregnancy	1
Not specific	20
Legal	
Theft/deception	15
Offences under Misuse of Drugs Act	8
Prostitution/soliciting	7
Prison during study year	4
Assault	1
Not specified	21
Social	
Relationship difficulties	60
Financial problems	15
Spouse or social group using drugs	15
Work problems	13
Behavioural problems	10
Accommodation problems	8
Children in care	2
School problems	2
User in care	1
Not specified	4

frequent minor illness presenting to the GP, children often miss much school, and this may conceal an undiagnosed school refusal problem. As many as a quarter of the child attenders at a general practice may be regarded as having psychosomatic problems. Psychosomatic presentations to the GP may also be more common at times of psychosocial transition, for boys this may be at the start of school, possibly reflecting the stress of learning, and for girls during early adolescence, as puberty is often a time of major change (Schor, 1986). It should be noted, however, that most children who present with psychosomatic symptoms even if they have some mood changes and relationship difficulties do not fulfil criteria for psychiatric disorder.

Adolescence may also be a time of emotional turmoil and is also commonly associated with psychiatric disorder, but the pattern of disorders in adolescence shows a greater resemblance to adult disorder. Thirty-eight per cent of adolescents who received a psychiatric diagnosis from their GP during adolescence, also received a psychiatric diagnosis as a young adult. Most commonly this was depression but often there were comorbid anxiety states or phobias (Smeeton *et al*, 1992). Eating disorders commonly present initially to the GP and are not always diagnosed.

Referral to the child psychiatrist (Filter 2)

Around one in ten children with psychiatric disorders are referred to child psychiatric clinics. Referrals are associated with high levels of disturbance, and in boys, an excess of antisocial behaviour. Referral to the child psychiatrist is more likely if overt psychological symptoms are displayed in the surgery (Goldberg *et al*, 1984). There is often a background of multiple psychosocial difficulties such as unemployment, marital and mental health problems resulting in family stress. Children with learning difficulties have high rates of psychiatric disorder and the GP is often involved in the long term care of these children. A small number of children are referred who do not have any psychiatric disorder but their referral results from normal exuberant over-activity and rebelliousness occurring in a family context of housing problems, emotional and financial circumstances with which their parents feel unable to cope (Garralda, 1995).

Treatment of children in general practice

The GP will be the main therapist for most of the children who consult with an emotional difficulty whether this has a psychological or somatic presentation. Bailey *et al* (1978) found the most common intervention was simple ventilation of the problem by the mother but around a quarter of the mothers were also offered psychotherapy (a treatment loosely defined in this study as if some change was intended). A surprisingly high number of the children (46%) were prescribed medication, mainly hypnotics for sleep disorders and antidepressants for enuresis, both of which may be better managed behaviourally. Widespread prescribing of stimulant drugs occurs in the USA but not in the UK.

The teaching of child psychiatry during the medical student stage is often rudimentary, and happens at a time when students may be more orientated to biological disorders and may be less receptive to learning about disorders with a large psychosocial component, so further training is required once doctors are in practice. Garralda (1995) makes specific recommendations on the skills GPs should acquire to deal with the mental health of children in primary care. These include:

(i)   an awareness of the importance of psychosocial factors
(ii) skills in interviewing children with, and without their parents
(iii) advice on simple behavioural techniques for treating minor behavioural probelms such as tantrums, oppositional behaviour, bed wetting, and sleep problems
(iv) counselling skills, for example with school and academic worries or family concerns
(v)   the treatment of maternal depression
(vi) knowledge of family dynamics and an ability to spot over concern and over protection
(vii) skills to determine when referral to a child psychiatrist is indicated.

Drug prescribing

The introduction of benzodiazepines in the 1960s which were considerably less toxic than their predecessors the barbiturates led to a steady increase in psychotropic drug prescribing. Parish (1971) reported that 8% of men and 17% of women were being prescribed a psychotropic drug during the course of one year. Trethowan (1975) in his paper *Pills for Personal Problems* raised the alarm of "the relentless march of the psychotropic drug juggernaut". Figures at that time based on general practice data in the UK gave one year prevalences of 9–15% of patients taking psychotropic drugs, while community-based studies in the USA reported higher rates in the 20–40% range (see Williams, 1979 for review). Three groups of psychotropic drugs are commonly used although there is some variation between studies, one finding that of those prescribed psychotropic drugs, 45% were taking hypnotics, 30% minor tranquillisers and 14% antidepressants (Irwin & Cupples, 1986). Female sex emerges as a risk factor; possibly this is due to the higher rates of minor psychiatric morbidity in women, while men have a greater tendency to self-medicate with alcohol and drugs of misuse, rather than seek treatment from their GP.

Increasing age also appears to be associated with higher rates of prescribing in most studies. Thus in a recent Finnish study only 10% of younger patients (18–34 years) compared with 50% of those in the oldest age group (75–89 years) received a drug. Being widowed, unemployed, retired, or living alone were also associated with higher rates of psychotropic drug prescribing. Lower rates of drug prescription were associated with being unmarried, employed and being in social class 1–3 (Joukamaa *et al*, 1995).

Psychotropic drug prescribing and psychiatric diagnoses

The match between having a psychiatric diagnosis and taking a psychotropic drug is often poor. In the west London study, Murray *et al* (1981) ascertained cases with probable minor psychiatric morbidity (a high GHQ score) and correlated this with GP prescriptions for psychotropic drugs. Women with a high GHQ score were 2.7 times more likely to receive a prescription than GHQ negative cases, and for men this ratio was 3.4.

Irwing & Cupples (1986) using a rather more global diagnosis of psychosocial disorder found a ratio of 1.7 : 1 in favour of a psychiatric diagnosis versus no diagnosis being associated with a prescription for a psychotropic drug. Thus around two-thirds of those with a diagnosis were prescribed medication. Compared with the remaining patients with a psychosocial problem, those who received a drug were more likely to be older, to have no children in the household, to have a past history of physical illness, but were less likely to have an acute physical problem or to have a social factor contributing to their psychiatric disorder.

In this study sedative and antidepressant drugs were prescribed with a similar frequency for all age groups although more patients in the over-45 age group were taking psychotropic drugs and 75% of hypnotic drugs were prescribed for the elderly. Neither sex distribution nor social class had any influence on drug prescribing and more significantly the involvement of a social worker, psychologist or psychiatrist was not associated with any reduction in psychotropic drug prescribing.

Psychotropic drug prescribing and physical illness

A strong association with chronic physical disease and psychotropic drug use has been found repeatedly. Williams (1978) suggests several possible mechanisms: rates of psychiatric disorder are probably higher among those with physical disease; in many cases even if the distress is insufficient to fulfil criteria for a psychiatric disorder the GP may still prescribe psychotropic drugs to relieve symptomatic distress; some psychotropic drugs may have effects which are useful in physical disease, for example, diazepam is a muscle relaxant and is widely used in rheumatic conditions, similarly tricyclics have analgesic effects and are sometimes used in cases of chronic pain; many patients with a primary psychiatric disorder may present somatically and in these cases psychotropic drugs may relieve the underlying psychiatric condition even if this is not formally recognised. More recently Irwin & Cupples (1986) have confirmed this association but shown that it only applies to patients with chronic physical disorders and not to those with acute physical conditions where the rate for psychotropic drug prescribing is lower than the average prescribing rate. Possibly in the face of the psychological distress due to a known physical illness of short duration the GP feels better able to resist the pressure to prescribe psychotropic medication because an end is in sight, whereas in cases of chronic physical illness the need to relieve the psychological suffering and 'do something' is ever present.

Duration of psychotropic drug prescribing

Most psychotropic prescribing is short-term. Parish (1971) found that 50% of patients took their drugs for less than one month, 15% for a year and only 5% for more than five years. Williams (1983) also found a similar pattern and showed that longer term drug usage was associated with a social problem, a history of previous psychotropic drug use, and longer previous duration of treatment, but there was considerable variation between doctors. Antidepressants were also more likely to be taken for a longer period than tranquillisers (Williams, 1983).

Repeat prescriptions

A situation of greater concern are those patients who take psychotropic medication for poorly defined reasons often over many years, a group first highlighted by Balint (1957) who suggested that this represented a doctor–patient relationship based on anonymity. In this way the doctor is able to create a distance between himself and some of the more difficult patients by allowing them to collect prescriptions without being seen (Melville, 1980). Such anonymity can act against the patients' best interests; Varnam (1981) found that when drugs were issued as repeat prescriptions and the patients were not being seen, the mean duration of drug use was 4.3 years, but if repeat prescriptions were issued and the patient was seen, the mean duration of prescribing was shortened to 2.7 years.

'Low' and 'high' GP prescribers

Global results can conceal individual differences between GPs which may be wide. The effect of this on patient care is uncertain. Fleming & Cross (1984) found that when GPs were classified in five categories by volume of issuing (low to high), there was a twofold difference between the low and high categories in the prescribing of new psychotropic drug prescriptions; a fourfold difference for continuing prescriptions; and a tenfold difference for repeat prescriptions (51% of all prescriptions were issued as repeats). Higher prescribers issued prescriptions more frequently for patients of all ages, especially the elderly and their prescriptions were more likely to be associated with polypharmacy. Prescribing rates did not vary with GP workload. The authors commented that if the average list size was reduced GPs might find more time for psychiatric counselling but it remained questionable whether this would influence a GP's prescribing habits. In the absence of prescribing guidelines it is uncertain whether the high prescribers are inadvertently giving their patients too many drugs and perhaps increasing the risks for toxicity or the low prescribers are depriving some of their patients of potentially useful treatments.The reasons that lie behind these wide differences in prescribing rates are obscure.

Benzodiazepines

Benzodiazepine prescribing peaked at 18 million prescriptions in the late 1970s. This was followed by a gradual decline to 9 million prescriptions in 1988, accompanied by a move away from new prescriptions towards an increase in repeat prescriptions. Benzodiazepines are prescribed most commonly in general practice for anxiety and insomnia but they are also prescribed for physical illnesses affecting almost every system. The continuing large-scale prescribing of benzodiazepines in general practice is disappointing, given their well-publicised association with dependency and misuse, and especially because simple measures such as an appropriate letter from the GP or a small self-help group in the practice may reduce the prescribing rate (Cormack *et al*, 1989) (see also page 608).

Interface between general practice and psychiatry

GPs' use of psychiatric out-patient clinics

Up to a half of GPs use psychiatric out-patient clinics as a primary source of advice, without first treating or investigating patients, and psychiatrists at out-patients tend to regard themselves as largely responsible for the total care of patients rather than as consultants. Scrutiny of the specialist care provided in out-patient clinics suggests that fewer than half the patients attending need to remain under the direct supervision of consultants, and even fewer require special facilities or treatments available only at hospital sites (Johnson, 1973).

At the out-patient clinic there is a high degree of uniformity in the diagnostic categories recorded, treatments prescribed and disposal arrangements. Kaeser & Cooper (1971) found that the most usual management decision at initial specialist consultation was to continue out-patient treatment, the intended disposal for three-quarters of patients attending. Subsequently, however, some two-thirds of out-patients were seen on fewer than four occasions; this rapid decline in attendance appeared to be due equally to high rates of discharge and to lapse from care. After three months, under a half of patients referred were still attending out-patient clinics, a quarter were receiving psychiatric treatment from their GP, and around a quarter were not receiving any treatment, and those who decided to stop treatment tended to make relatively poor progress. The place of the out-patient clinic in psychiatric services is also discussed on page 1283.

GPs' and psychiatrists' working arrangements in the general practice setting

Much discussion has centred on the possibility of a new type of relationship between GPs (and primary care teams) and psychiatrists (and mental health team members), in which psychiatrists, instead of remaining in hospital, attach themselves to primary care settings in order to develop closer, more effective working relationships (Horder, 1988).

Almost 20% of consultant psychiatrists in England and Wales (or their junior staff) spend some time, usually a morning or afternoon a week, in a general practice setting (Strathdee & Williams, 1984). Regional influences are important with the preponderance of attachments in rural areas (Pullen & Yellowlees, 1988). Three working patterns are apparent.

Shifted out-patient clinic

A shifted out-patient clinic is favoured by the majority of psychiatrists because the format is similar to that used in hospital practice. Four out of five psychiatrists apportion half of their time to seeing one or two new patients and the rest to seeing follow-up patients.

Tyrer (1984) described a service in which patients were seen at five psychiatric clinics in general practice serving an urban population in Nottingham of 78 200. Patients preferred seeing the psychiatrist in a general practice setting because of better access particularly for older people and those with physical illness, and 20% of the patients reported that they would not have attended a hospital clinic, mainly because of the associated stigma. In comparison with a conventional hospital-based service this particular community general practice service involved greater use of the day hospital, more extensive multi-disciplinary care and more involvement with long-term mentally ill patients (Ferguson *et al*, 1992).

Team-work

Liaison-attachment team working is typical of more longstanding attachments, in which psychiatrists have instituted working links and training with other professionals such as social workers, psychologists and community psychiatric nurses.

Consultation

This involves only the assessment of patients, usually in collaboration with the GP, with the treatment being administered by the GP. Creed & Marks

(1989) describe a scheme with the psychiatrist spending a session a week in general practice. The liaison attachment was found to be cost-effective as more patients benefited from the psychiatrist's advice than if the psychiatrist had treated the cases directly, and the diagnostic skills of the GPs and their trainees were enhanced. For psychotherapists this involves giving discussion seminars and focusing on the GP–patient relationship.

A minority of GPs have a regular link of this kind, but many would welcome such arrangements: the type of link most commonly desired by GPs being one in which the GP shares actively in the assessment and treatment of the patient (Brown & Tower, 1990). Stansfield (1991) found that only half the GPs in Harlow wanted the psychiatrist to see their patients in the practice.

Communication between GPs and psychiatrists

Good communication is essential for the practice of good medicine and the communication between GPs and psychiatrists depends almost exclusively on the quality of the letters they write to each other. How useful are these letters, and what items of information should they include? Williams & Wallace (1974) in their survey asked a group of GPs and psychiatrists in Cardiff to rank 12 items in order of relevance for inclusion in a GP referral to a psychiatrist and for the psychiatrist's response to the GP. The five most relevant items of information for each type of letter are shown in Box 28.3 as well as the frequency with which these items were present (Pullen & Yellowlees, 1985). GPs were more likely to include key items and provide a more comprehensive social history in letters that were addressed to a named consultant rather than a letter directed "Dear Doctor".

A patient's social history is generally held to be of importance to understanding a psychiatric case. Adolf Myers' biopsychosocial formulation of psychiatric disorder has been highly influential in the training of psychiatrists and the writing of psychiatric summaries and these often include detailed social histories. However in the Cardiff survey described above GPs rated this item tenth out of 12 items, and psychiatrists rated it 11th out of 12 items (Williams & Wallace, 1974).

In contrast to the lowish relevance of the social history, GPs appear to want more in the way of explanation, for example, Williams & Wallace (1974) found that 79% wanted more explanation of the psychopathology and Margo (1982) found that 70% of GPs wanted more education in terms of differential diagnosis and the rationale of the drug prescribing. Orrel *et al* (1983) rated the "perceived usefulness" of the letters and found this correlated with information concerning the differential diagnosis, prognosis and details of follow up.

Psychiatric summaries used in the case notes are often quite lengthy documents. Craddock & Craddock (1989) found that GPs preferred to have a letter of around one A4 page while psychiatrists preferred to have a 2½ page summary which used the 11 headings recommended by the Institute of Psychiatry. These studies suggest that GPs do not wish to read a lengthy reiteration of a patient's social history, with which they are probably familiar, but are interested in the psychiatrist's diagnosis, suggested management and the recommended drug prescription, and also want to receive some explanation of their patient's disorder.

Notes fit for patients to read

The Access to Heath Records Act 1990 came into force in 1991 and has given patients the right to see any information held in the medical case record. The only exception is for third party information or if the clinician believes that the information may cause serious mental or physical harm to the patient or someone else. Patients must apply to the hospital management for this right. There is therefore an onus on both the GP and psychiatrist to ensure that their letters are well written, jargon is kept to a minimum and potentially offensive remarks are avoided. A diagnosis of personality disorder is often perceived as derogative and therefore comments about a patient's personality and personality traits which may be relevant to the diagnosis must be made with care. A study has shown that the patients who were most upset when they read their own notes were more often younger, male and had a diagnosis of psychosis or personality disorder (Bernadt *et al*, 1991).

Referrals to other personnel in general practice

As psychiatric services move into the community there has been an increasing trend for paramedical workers, such as CPNs, social workers, psychologists and counsellors to be attached to general practices. This trend started in the mid 1970s and is well documented in one inner London practice (Jarman, 1992) which shows an increasing number of internal referrals to practice-based paramedical staff with a corresponding decrease in the number of referrals to the psychiatric out-patient department. Prior to 1970 almost all consultant psychiatrists and paramedical staff were hospital-based and it has been the recently accelerating trend of placing psychiatric paramedical staff in general practice that has been an essential element in the development of community care.

A study of five group general practices in Manchester (Whitehouse, 1987), found that when all patients with a psychosocial diagnosis were considered, 5% were referred to a consultant, 0.6% to social services, 0.5% to the nursing services (mainly CPNs). However in one of the districts of this study, where the GPs could refer directly to the CPN service without having to make an initial referral to the local psychiatric services there were three times as many referrals to the CPNs (1.3% of the total versus 0.4% in the other districts) and with the increasing number of CPN attachments to general practice this is likely to increase further.

> **Box 28.3 Key items required in letters from GPs and
> psychiatrists**
>
> Items required by psychiatrists (*n*=120) in referral letters (%)
> Medication   62
> Family history   37
> Main symptom/problem   100
> Reason for referral   88
> Psychiatric history   72
> Items required by GPs (*n* = 120) in letters from psychiatrists (%)
> Diagnosis   88
> Treatment   92
> Follow up   95
> Prognosis   23
> Concise explanation   60
>
> After Pullen & Yellowlees (1985)

Kendrick *et al* (1991) have reported on the numbers of the various different paramedical professionals attached to GPs in the South West Thames region in 1991 (Table 28.7). There is considerable regional variation, and as the position is changing rapidly and there is a greater emphasis on primary care the figures now may be higher than the 1991 data. Most of those referred to paramedical professionals usually have a variety of neurotic, personality and relationship, sexual and other non-psychiatric disorders while patients suffering from psychoses continue to be referred to the psychiatrist. In spite of the increased investment in primary care the impact of this type of intervention on the total psychosocial morbidity is probably not large. Whitehouse (1987) reported that out of 3405 consultations for anxiety, minor psychogenic and other neuroses, marital and social problems there were only 93 (2.8%) referrals to counsellors, social workers, clinical psychologists and CPNs. For those with a primary diagnosis of anxiety (*n* = 1729), 75% received a prescription, and 2% were referred to another agency or paramedical therapist. Even for the 306 subjects given a diagnosis of marital or social problems only 25 (8%) were referred to another agency while 40% were given a prescription.

Community psychiatric nurses (CPNs)

The remarkable growth of the CPN service is described on page 1291. Although the initial role of CPNs was to support people with severe mental illness in the community, in an increasing number of districts the CPNs receive referrals directly from the GP. Data from the Salford case register show that CPNs are increasingly treating general practice patients (those with minor psychiatric morbidity) rather than patients with more serious psychiatric disorders and are not reducing the demands on traditional psychiatric services (Wooff *et al*, 1988). The present position of the CPN service is controversial; both GPs and psychiatrists want to work closely with them, each competing for precious CPN time, each with their distinctive diagnostic group of patients; whether they will do more general practice psychiatry or more psychiatry in general practice remains to be seen.

Counsellors

Counselling is the newest of the caring professions and is growing at an explosive rate. In 1980 there were only 1000 counsellors registered with the British Association of Counsellors but by 1993 this figure had risen to 13 000 (British Association of Counselling, 1994). Most are employed in non-medical settings, for example, in the universities where around 6% of all students per year attend a counsellor (Stein, 1995). Commissioning authorities in the NHS are increasingly favouring the employment of counsellors on a sessional basis in general practice because their use may be more cost effective than the use of other NHS paramedical professionals or the psychiatric services.

Counselling is developing its own theoretical framework and three broad schools are recognised: the psychodynamic, the humanistic (based on Rogerian methods), and the cognitive–behavioural. In recent years the Egan model has proved influential as a theoretical basis for counselling. It consists of three stages, with obvious parallels with brief psychotherapy (Egan, 1986):

  (i)   Stage 1 – problem exploration and clarification. The counsellor helps clients explore their problems. This stage requires giving attention, active listening skills, interviewing with a degree of empathy, the use of paraphrasing and summarising, reflecting feelings, non-critical acceptance and helping the client to be specific.
 (ii)   Stage 2 – clients are helped to see themselves and their situation in new perspectives, develop new understanding to find solutions and set realistic goals.
(iii)   Stage 3, action and resolution. Here clients are encouraged to consider ways in which they are going to act and to examine the costs and consequences of any action they are going to take.

Most counsellors are usually drawn from other caring professions, such as teaching or nursing; they complete a one or two year university course which will include some supervised counselling, and are then able to register with the British Association of Counsellors.

Sheldon (1994) uses the term medical counselling to refer to the specialist nurses attached to hospital clinics who provide advice and counselling for patients with illnesses such as diabetes, cancer, colostomies. The CPN has an analogous role in relation to people with psychiatric illness, and they are gradually becoming the psychiatric advisors to the GP and other practice staff.

Many general practices now employ counsellors, funded in part by purchasing and commissioning agencies, but the impact of counselling as a distinctive professional activity in general practice is controversial (Anderson & Hasler, 1979; Mugatroyd, 1983). Martin & Mitchell (1983) described the outcome of including a counsellor within the professional staff of a practice of 11 000 patients. The counsellor worked for five hours a week and during a 12 month period counselled 89 patients in 197 sessions. The problems dealt with most frequently were anxiety, depression, stress, bereavement, marital troubles, sexual problems and abortion. In response to a follow-up survey 93% of the patients said they found the service 'useful' or 'very useful' and 88% thought the doctor was right to suggest that they saw the counsellor. The work appeared to be focused and time limited as most of those referred for counselling had acute or transitory disorders with the average number of sessions being 2.3 per patient, and there was no evidence that patients were being drawn into long-term psychotherapeutic relationships.

General practitioners do informal counselling much of the time, particularly over relationship problems and adjustment to illness. At the same time, GPs need to be prescriptive and to give information and advice with authority, and treat the more serious medical conditions that their patients may have. As a result of this many patients see their GP as a 'parent' figure rather than as an equal, or have memories of the GP giving them injections as a child which may have caused pain, or intervening during some serious medical crises for themselves or members of their family. Accepting the doctor in the counselling role may then be difficult for both parties. General practitioners do not, in general, have sufficient time to undertake lengthy counselling sessions as they have more pressing demands on their time, and so patients in a crisis will often miss out unless there is a designated counsellor.

GPs and counsellors need to collaborate closely, particularly if more serious cases of psychiatric disorders are not to be missed (Sheldon, 1994). The effectiveness of counselling has still to be demonstrated. The most detailed evaluation of mental health counselling in general practice is the Leverhulme Counselling Project (Ashurst & Ward, 1983), which examined a random sample of patients presenting to their GPs with minor neurotic disorder. There was no difference at one year between counselled patients and those who only saw the GP, although it should be noted that most patients with transitory disorders tend to improve regardless of any intervention, and it has always been extremely difficult to 'prove' that any form of psychotherapy is effective.

Social workers

The role of the social worker in the psychiatric services is described on page 1293. Today, there are very few psychiatric social work attachments in general practice, but an earlier study by Corney (1984) is of interest because it demonstrates a sound methodology for evaluating the effectiveness of paramedical personnel in general practice.

Seven doctors from one practice were invited to refer all female patients aged between 18–45 years who had either acute or acute on chronic depression, to an experienced psychiatric social worker. Before seeing the social worker the patients were assessed by a psychiatrist using the Standardised Psychiatric Interview (Goldberg, 1970) and received a social maladjustment interview which covered the domains of current physical health of the family, housing, occupation, financial, social and leisure activities and relationships with spouses and children. The social workers in the study were given a copy of the social assessment and told to proceed with whatever intervention they thought appropriate. Patients were divided into subgroups according to whether the patient had (i) acute or acute on chronic depression, (ii) was cohabiting or not, (iii) aged 18–29 or 30–45. Within each sub-group patients were randomly allocated to an experimental group who were seen by the social worker and a control group who had routine GP treatment. At six months there were no overall differences in psychiatric morbidity or social dysfunction between the two groups. However one subgroup, women with acute on chronic depression and marital problems, appeared to benefit from social work intervention. Forty per cent of all the subjects also received some practical help and among these patients the combination of practical help and counselling was superior to counselling alone. Two-thirds of the patients thought the social worker had been helpful in alleviating their depression. The implication of this work is that a policy of referring every client with a psychiatric disorder to a paramedical person is probably an inefficient use of resources but selective referral which optimises the skills of particular therapists may be a more cost-effective strategy.

Clinical psychologists

The profession is small in the UK with only 1500 practitioners (see page 1288) and it is unlikely, therefore, to have any major impact on morbidity through direct attachment to GPs. However, GPs are high users of district clinical psychology services and in most districts refer directly to the psychologist without referring to the psychiatric services. Milne & Souter (1988) described the service provided by a psychologist attached to a general practice and examined 30 consecutive GP referrals over a one year period. Most of the patients had longstanding psychological difficulties, rather than transient situational reactions and they seemed to be appropriate. The main diagnostic groups were anxiety states, phobias, depression, obsessive–compulsive disorder and sexual dysfunction. At referral only 25% had 'probable minor psychiatric morbidity' as measured by a high GHQ score, and by the end of the study this figure had fallen to 9%. Therapeutic interventions were mainly behavioural, including exposure *in vivo*, relaxation therapy, and cognitive restructuring. Patients received 6–18 sessions and 74% were thought to have had a satisfactory outcome.

A quite different type of attachment is described by Deys *et al* (1989) in which a psychologist from the Tavistock Clinic with a psychodynamic orientation acted either as a consultant to the GP or conducted joint interviews together with the GP. Family trees or genograms were used extensively and these revealed high rates of unresolved grief as well as frequent earlier histories of abuse in many patients. Patients with somatic presentations appeared to respond well to this approach and began to talk at length about their family problems with the psychologist.

Several studies (Ashurst, 1982) have examined whether the rate of psychotropic drug prescribing fell during a period of consultation with clinical psychologists or counsellores and some have found a short-term effect. However Earll & Kincey (1982) found that seven months after the intervention of a psychologist had ceased the number of prescriptions for psychotropic drugs was similar to that prior to the psychologist's intervention.

Two controlled studies give favourable results for the use of cognitive therapy in the treatment of depressive disorders in general practice (Blackburn *et al*, 1981) but two studies of anxiety management produced discrepant findings (Kiely & McPherson, 1986; Trepka *et al*, 1986).

Other paramedical staff

Practice nurses are a valuable and often under-utilised resource as they have been an important part of the primary care team for a long time. Their training is usually in general nursing and they are, therefore, in a good position to administer physical treatments such as depot injections and in many practices they are gradually taking over this role from the CPNs. Wilkinson *et al* (1993) described how a suitably trained practice nurse is able to assist the supervision of antidepressant medication in general practice although this should always be done in close collaboration with the GP. Most practices have a health visitor attached, and as health visitors must visit every woman who has recently given birth they are well placed to detect cases of postnatal depression. Holden *et al* (1990) demonstrated that health visitors could be taught how to use the Edinburgh Postnatal Depression Scale (Cox *et al*, 1987) which aids in the detection of postnatal depression and so reduces the total morbidity due to postnatal depression. District nurses are in a similar position with regard to the detection of depression in the elderly, and this often responds well to treatment. A specialist behavioural nurse can treat phobias and obsessive–compulsive disorder in the primary care situation as patients preferred being treated in this setting (Marks, 1985). Brook & Temperley (1976) have also demonstrated the value of a psychoanalyst offering a consultative service in general practice. While all these studies are of interest, only the CPNs are sufficiently numerous to make any impact on a national scale. There are too few social workers, clinical psychologists, psychotherapists or nurse therapists to make anything more than a token contribution in a few practices (Table 28.7).

How effective are paramedical attachments in general practice?

General practitioners and their patients have welcomed the attachment of other staff to general practice but measuring how effective they are is a more complex matter. Three areas require evaluation:

(i)   is psychological distress decreased among the patients?
(ii) is the demand on the traditional psychiatric service decreased to a sufficient extent to justify the transfer of resources?
(iii) is the work load and stress on GPs lowered?

Balestrieri *et al* (1988) conducted a meta-analysis of 11 controlled studies in the UK which compared specialist mental health treatment to routine GP treatment in a general practice setting: they estimated that specialist help was 10% more effective than routine treatment by a GP, which was a small enough margin to raise questions of the cost–benefit ratio.

Can the additional psychiatric input in general practice decrease admission to hospital? Williams & Balestrieri (1989) examined hospital admission statistics over an 18-year period and found a steeper fall in non-psychotic admissions in those parts of the country where psychiatry was well established in general practice although admissions were gradually decreasing throughout the country during this period. Tyrer (1984) reported a 20% reduction in admissions for a service if psychiatric clinics were held in general practice. However, both these studies were conducted at a time when the majority of the admissions were for non-psychotic disorders and there were many more hospital beds than today. A more recent study by Jackson *et al* (1993) of a psychiatric team operating closely with GPs found no reduction in admissions but rather an increase in referrals to the local psychiatric day hospital. Lawrence *et al* (1990) in the conclusion to their study on the Worcester project remarked "there is a bedrock of psychiatric illness which will always need in-patient care however comprehensive the community resources".

Stansfield (1991) reporting from a district where half of the GPs had attached CPNs found that all the remaining GPs in the district wanted this type of attachment and they all also wanted direct access to the CPN service without having to initially refer to the local psychiatric service. This suggests some degree of satisfaction with the new services, and that GPs value the contribution of the CPNs.

Stress among GPs

General practice is thought to be a stressful occupation. Around 60% of the referrals to the National Counselling Service for Sick Doctors are for GPs, and 50% of these referrals concern alcoholism and 25% depressive illness. Doctors, as a group, are known to have higher rates of alcohol dependence. Murray (1976) found that the rate for first admissions among doctors was 2.7 times more than among comparable controls of the same social class.

Table 28.7 Psychiatric personnel visiting 369 general practices in the South West Thames region (Kendrick *et al*, 1991)

Community psychiatric nurse	218 (59% of practices)
Consultant psychiatrist	138 (37% of practices)
Social worker	103 (26% of practices)
Clinical psychologist	69 (19% of practices)

The standardised mortality ratio (SMR) of illnesses known to be linked to stress is raised for doctors as a group (the SMR for suicide is 335; for cirrhosis 311; and for accidental poisoning 818; HMSO, 1986). The mortality for myocardial infarction among GPs is twice as high as in other members of the profession of comparable age (Morris *et al*, 1952). The psychiatric health of GPs was investigated by Cooper *et al* (1989) who used the Middlesex Hospital Questionnaire in a survey of a large cohort of GPs. They found that male GPs had raised levels of anxiety but women GPs were less depressed and less anxious than normal population controls. With regard to health behaviours, doctors seem to be able to take their own advice on smoking as only 1.6% of GPs smoked more than 20 cigarettes a day, but have not been able to heed their own counsel on drinking: 5.4% of GPs drank 3–6 pints daily (or alcohol equivalent) which was similar to the rate for heavy drinking among patients who were on a GP list in the same survey (Anderson, 1985).

Several studies have tried to pinpoint the main sources of anxiety and stress among GPs. Most studies concur that neither the practice of medicine nor work with patients were the major stressors but that certain associated factors were stressful. These were interruptions, involvement with the administrative workload, the work–home interface and routine medical work (Makin *et al*, 1988). Although the type of work encountered in general practice may not be the major stressor, the quantity of work or workload may be. Porter *et al* (1985) undertook a detailed study of 18 GPs and found that 83% of the allocated work time was spent in direct patient care. This comprised 28 hours per week in direct patient contact of which 16 hours were in surgeries, 11 hours on visits, and one hour in specialised clinics. Two hours were spent in practice meetings and a further two and a half hours in other non-practice medical activity. The average consultation rate based on 66 surgeries was 7.0 patients per hour (range 3.8–11.5) and the average time for each was 7.2 minutes (range 3.7–12.5). A six point scale measuring 'subjective pressure' (1 = idle/bored, 6 = frenetic activity) was found to correlate with a faster consultation rate (8 or more patients per hour) and measures of stress, while 'low pressure scores' were associated with slower consultation rates (5.9/hour).

In a detailed hourly analysis of the mood of 44 GPs, Rankin *et al* (1987) found the uncertain nature of the work was the main cause of dissatisfaction.

Thus factors of 'hassle' and 'lack of time' accounted for 54% of the reasons given for a drop in mood, as opposed to worries concerning the patients' health and response to treatment which accounted for only 7% of lowering of mood. Improvement in mood was largely explained by domestic happiness (34%) while pleasure over improvement in patients' health only accounted for 6%. Sutherland & Cooper (1992) measured work satisfaction in 1987 and 1990 using the same scale, the Warr, Cook and Wall job satisfaction scale (Warr *et al*, 1979) on both occasions, and observed a significant decrease in work satisfaction which they attributed to the new general practice contract.

In the study of Makin *et al* (1988) job satisfaction among most GPs was generally high and was strongly associated with a feeling of being able to choose their method of working, choose the amount of responsibility they had, and the amount of variety in their daily work. These items correspond to Karasek's (1979) concept of "job decision latitude" where a subjective feeling of latitude is correlated with job satisfaction. Extrinsic factors, such as hours of work or rates of pay, did not appear to correlate with ratings of job satisfaction. Rankin *et al* (1987) tried to assess which types of clinical work were the most satisfying by asking GPs to rate 14 clinical tasks. The most satisfying intervention was treating a patient with acute asthma, and the second diagnosing a child with acute appendicitis. The third item which gave most satisfaction was having morning coffee with a partner. The two least popular activities were both psychiatric, talking to the wife of an alcoholic, and admitting a patient with schizophrenia under a section.

In spite of the high prevalence of psychiatric problems in the surgery, they do not appear to be a major cause of stress among GPs. Makin *et al* (1988) found that only two out of 31 items which contributed to GP stress (fear of assault during a night visit, and dealing with difficult patients) had any possible psychiatric bearing. None of the other 29 items were related to mental disorder, nor do other studies on GP stress suggest that working with psychiatric patients is a major stress, although occasional patients are undoubtedly difficult to manage. Rankin *et al* (1987) concluded that much of the day to day stress in general practice was associated with time pressure and voluntarily taking on an excessive workload, and with better time management at least some of this might be corrected.

The physical and mental health of older GPs was studied by Allibone *et al* (1981) who found a high incidence of self-treatment, delay in seeking medical care and inadequate follow-up of chronic disorders. In this study, GPs often expressed the view that consulting another GP, who may be a partner or a friend, might be seen as a sign of weakness especially when the problem was emotional or psychological in origin. Richards (1987) found 33% of 500 GPs reported personal distress and anxiety about making personal disclosures concerning their own emotional difficulties. There is also often the worry that the consultation could result in loss of their own professional credibility or even their livelihood (Chambers, 1989).

General practitioner training

> They (general practitioners) are faced with undifferentiated illness and discover that unlike in the psychiatric out-patient department the patient does not necessarily present with emotional distress if he/she has a psychiatric problem. They are understandably more concerned about how to help the patient in the limited time available to them (Gask, 1994).

Psychological understanding – the work of Michael Balint

Almost the most critical step in psychiatric treatment is the initial recognition of the presence of a psychiatric disorder. This will depend crucially on the GP's ability to respond to emotional cues and to psychological distress. The first serious attempt to increase the degree of psychological mindedness among GPs was made by Michael Balint, a Hungarian psychoanalyst who emigrated to England before the Second World War. His seminal book *A Doctor, his Patient and the Illness* (Balint, 1957) had a profound effect on general practice and even some 30 years later remains controversial. Balint ran weekly seminars for GPs at the Tavistock Clinic, where the possible underlying psychopathology and management strategies of patients that the GPs presented to the group were discussed as well as focusing on the doctors' own feelings about their patients. He believed that the GPs themselves were the most important therapeutic agents and used the metaphor of a drug to convey this notion to a medical audience:

> By far the most frequently used drug in general practice is the doctor himself. No guidance is contained in any textbook as to the dosage in which the drug doctor should prescribe themselves in what form, how frequently and what is the curative and what the maintenance dose should be, and so on (Balint, 1957).

The 'drug doctor' could have both positive and negative effects but above all the doctor had a very powerful influence on the patient and he referred to this as the doctor's "apostolic function", by which he meant "the urge to prove to the patient, to the whole world, above all to himself that he is good, kind, knowledgeable and helpful". Pietroni (1986) in a reassessment of Balint noted that the apostolic function was described in the 1950s when doctors adopted a more authoritarian position and frequently gave their patients direct advice on personal matters in a manner which would be unthinkable today.

Balint also tried to convey some important general psychotherapeutic principles in his groups, such as the importance of listening rather than simply asking questions, the use of empathy, and the significance of transference and the counter-transference. He believed that a limited, though definite, change in the doctors' personality was needed to acquire any degree of psychological mindedness. Possibly as a consequence of this unpalatable requirement many of the earlier Balint groups had drop-out rates in the order of 60% although later this fell to 25–30%. Through the medium of these groups he also tried to examine the psychopathology which underlay a variety of presentations in general practice, such as multiple somatic complaints, repeat prescribing, night calls and children who consulted with excessive frequency.

The extensive use of psychoanalytic theory in a general practice setting was criticised by Sowerby (1977) while Zigmond (1978) felt that focusing on psychodynamic factors led to a distorted emphasis on psychological curiosity rather than care, and wrote that "to Balint means to compulsively offer interpretations to patients who have not asked for them". There has generally been some reaction to the overuse of psychoanalytic concepts in general practice psychiatry.

Current training methods

More recent developments in psychiatric training for GPs have been summarised by Gask (1994). The Medical Act (1983) stipulated that doctors entering general practice must complete a three year training course, of which two years must be spent in hospital posts and one year working with a recognised general practitioner trainer. The Act does not specify any further what the hospital training should consist of, but it has led to more GP trainees taking a hospital post in psychiatry. Continuous experience with clinical responsibility for a wide variety of cases for a six month period is likely to create a rather deeper and more long lasting impression than any series of lectures and seminars can. Two independent studies suggests that around 20% of all GPs have worked in a psychiatric department (Kendrick *et al*, 1991; Stansfield, 1991) but as this figure includes GPs entering general practice prior to the 1983 Medical Act, the proportion may be even higher. However, as noted previously the spectrum of cases dealt with on an in-patient psychiatric unit is very different from that found in general practice.

Gask (1994) has outlined the syllabus and teaching methods used in one vocational training scheme in the northwest of England. The topics covered should bear some resemblance to the profile of disorders seen in general practice with relatively less emphasis on the more severe functional psychosis but more on minor psychiatric morbidity. The most relevant topics are shown in Box 28.4.

Marks *et al* (1979) have described a way of measuring a GP's ability to recognise psychiatric disorder. Patients are asked to complete the 60-item GHQ and are then interviewed by the GP who completes a six point rating scale which measures the severity of any psychiatric disorder present. The correlation between the patient's GHQ score and the doctor's ratings are then used to compute an "identification index" for each doctor, which gives an estimate of his or her ability to recognise psychiatric disorder. Goldberg *et al* (1980) have shown that if GPs who are poor at identifying psychiatric disorder are then given short training courses (no more than four individual sessions) their ability to recognise psychiatric disorder can be greatly improved. This type of training has also been shown to be helpful for training medical students (Gask *et al*, 1988). Self-report questionnaires have also been used to help improve the recognition of psychiatric illness by GPs but the results are conflicting (Wright & Perini, 1987). Training in the more practical aspects of the recognition of psychiatric disorder requires more active participation and the use of videos. Teaching from videos is an art in itself (Lesser, 1985).

Counselling and psychotherapy are also essential skills for good general practice psychiatry but acquiring these skills is a much more protracted affair. Gask (1994) points out that counselling cannot be taught in a few sessions and to suggest otherwise might be harmful to both patients and doctors leading some over-enthusiastic or inexperienced doctors into deep emotional waters. It also undervalues the skill of the professional therapist (Gask, 1994).

Training for established GPs

Only a third of GPs have any interest in psychiatry with roughly equal numbers among both older and younger GPs (Bennett, 1989). Most postgraduate training today is through local postgraduate centres which receive funding to support an education programme for GPs. Only a limited amount of this funding is available for psychiatry. This generally takes the form of a guest expert lecture, but the effectiveness of this type of teaching is uncertain. The only other regular and consistent input that most GPs receive is from pharmaceutical representatives. Their information is biased, most obviously towards any particular company's product but there is also a more subtle bias towards the biological model of psychiatry which may not be the most appropriate model for the psychiatric and emotional disorders commonly found in general practice. Practitioners with a particular interest may obtain training in a variety of different settings, such as Balint groups, of which there are about 20 in the UK, in formal psychotherapy training, family therapy and other specialised treatments but the proportion of GPs who seek this additional training is small.

Conclusion

As the old asylums close and there is increased emphasis on community care, general practice psychiatry is likely to become an increasingly important area of medical activity. This means that strengthening the GP's role remains as pertinent today as it was 30 years ago when Shepherd *et al* (1966), following their major study into general practice, concluded that "the cardinal requirement for the mental health service in this country is not a large expansion of the number of psychiatrists and psychiatric agencies, but rather strengthening the role of the family doctor in his therapeutic role".

Over the last 30 years two strategies have evolved to help accomplish this. First, there have been attempts to increase the skill of the established GP in diagnosing and treating psychological disorder, as described above. However, even the most well educated and enthusiastic GP is unlikely to invest much additional time and energy into treating psychiatric disorder unless more resources are provided. In this respect the decision by the Department of Health to place psychiatric paramedical personnel, such as CPNs, counsellors, and psychologists, in the primary care setting is to be welcomed and there are many patients now receiving treatment from paramedical psychiatric professionals who would not have been treated a generation ago.

The case for more intensive investigation has been established in this major but poorly developed field of enquiry (Shepherd, 1982; Cooper & Eastwood, 1992). A range of studies are required to clarify the cost-effective contributions that may be made by mental health specialists, non-medical health professionals, and voluntary and private agencies in the management of mental disorders in general practice (Wilkinson & Wright, 1994).

References

Allibone, A., Oakes, D. & Shannon, H.S. (1981) The health and health care of doctors. *Journal of the Royal College of General Practitioners*, **31**, 728–734.

Anderson, A. & Hasler, J. C. (1979) Counselling in general practice. Journal of the *Royal College of General Practitioners*, **29**, 352–356.

Box 28.4 Psychiatric topics for a GP vocational training scheme (after Gask, 1994)

Anxiety and depression
Somatisation
Dealing with a new episode of psychotic illness
Chronic psychotic illness; the role of the GP
Common psychiatric disorders in childhood
Problems related to pregnancy and childbirth
Confused elderly patients
Alcohol problems
Drug problems
Sexual and marital problems
Dealing with suicidal behaviour
In addition, certain topics which are important for general
    medical practice, such as bereavement counselling and how
    to break bad news

Anderson, P. (1985) Managing alcohol problems in general practice. *British Medical Journal*, **290**, 1873–1875.

—— (1993) The interaction between research and policy – alcohol and general practice. *Addiction*, **Suppl. 88**, 1215–1275.

—— & Scott, E. (1992) The effect of general practitioners' advice to heavy drinking men. *British Journal of Addiction*, **87**, 891–900.

Arreghini, F., Agostini, C. & Wilkinson, G. (1991) General practitioner referral to specialist psychiatric services. A comparison of practices in North and South Verona. *Psychological Medicine*, **21**, 485–494.

Ashurst, P. (1982) Counselling in general practice. In *Psychiatry in General Practice* (eds A. W. Clare & M. Lader), pp. 77–89. London: Academic Press.

—— & Ward, D. F. (1983) *An Evaluation of Counselling in General Practice*. Final report of the Leverhulme Counselling Project. Unpublished report available from the Mental Health Foundation, London.

Bailey, V., Graham, P. & Boniface, D. (1978) How much child psychiatry does a general practitioner do? *Journal of the Royal College of General Practitioners*, **28**, 621–626.

Balestrieri, M., Williams, P. & Wilkinson, G. (1988) Specialist mental health treatment in general practice: a meta-analysis. *Psychological Medicine*, **18**, 711–718.

——, Bon, M. G., Rodriguez-Sa Criston, A. & Tansella, M. (1994) Pathways to psychiatric care in South Verona in Italy. *Psychological Medicine*, **24**, 641–649.

Balint, M. (1957) *The Doctor, His Patient and the Illness*. London: Pitman.

Bebbington, P., Hurry, J., Tennant, *et al* (1981) Epidemiology of mental disorders in Camberwell. *Psychological Medicine*, **11**, 561–569.

Bennett, C. (1989) The Worcester Development Project. General practitioner satisfaction with a new community service. *Journal of the Royal College of General Practitioners*, **39**, 106–109.

Bernadt, M., Gunning, L. & Quenstedt, M (1991) Patients' access to their own psychiatric records. *British Medical Journal*, **303**, 967.

Blackburn, I., Bishop, S., Glen, I. M., *et al* (1981) The efficacy of cognitive therapy in depression: a treatment trial using cognitive therapy and pharmacotherapy, each alone and in combination. *British Journal of Psychiatry*, **139**, 181–189.

Boddington, J. (1992) Role of general practitioners in the care of long-term mentally ill patients. *British Journal of Psychiatry*, **160**, 568–569.

Borquist, L., Hansorson, L., Nethlblad, G., *et al* (1993) Perceived health and high consumers of care: a study of mental health problems in a Swedish primary health care district. *Psychological Medicine*, **25**, 763–770.

Botega, N., Mann, A. & Wilkinson, G. (1992) General practitioners and depression – first use of the Depression Attitude Questionnaire. *International Journal of Methods in Psychiatric Research*, **2**, 169–180.

Bridges, K. & Goldberg, D. (1985) Somatic presentations of DSM–III psychiatric disorders in primary care. *Journal of Psychosomatic Research*, **29**, 563–569.

——, ——, Evans, B., *et al* (1991) Determinants of somatisation in primary care. *Psychological Medicine*, **21**, 473–483.

British Association of Counselling (1994) *Annual Report of the British Association of Counselling*.

Brodaty, H. (1983) Brief Psychotherapy in General Practice: A controlled prospective intervention study. Unpublished MD thesis. University of New South Wales, Australia.

Brook, A. & Temperley, J. (1976) Contribution of psychotherapists to general practice. *Journal of the Royal College of General Practitioners*, **26**, 86–94.

Brown, L. M. & Tower, J. E. C. (1990) Psychiatrists in primary care: would general practitioners welcome them? *British Journal of General Practice*, **40**, 369–371.

Brown, G. W. & Harris, T. (1978) *Social Origins of Depression: a Study of Psychiatric Disorder in Women*. London: Tavistock.

Casey, P. R., Dillon, S. & Tyrer, P. J. (1984) The diagnostic status of patients with conspicuous psychiatric morbidity in primary care. *Psychological Medicine*, **14**, 673–581.

Chambers, R. M. (1989) The health of general practitioners: a cause for concern. Editorial. *Journal of the Royal College of General Practitioners*, **39**, 179–181.

Chick, J. & Cantwell, R. (eds) (1994) *Seminars in Alcohol and Drug Misuse*. London: Gaskell.

Clark, G. (1966) *A History of the Royal College of Physicians*. Vol. 2, 476–479. Oxford: Oxford University Press.

Cooper, B. & Eastwood, R. (1992) Primary Care and Psychiatric Epidemiology. London: Tavistock/Routledge.

Cooper, C. L., Rout, U. & Faragher, B. (1989) Mental health, job satisfaction and job stress among general practitioners. *British Medical Journal*, **298**, 366–370.

Cormack, M. A., Owens, R. G. & Dewey, M. E. (1989) The effect of minimal intervention by general practitioners on long term benzodiazepine use. *Journal of the Royal College of General Practitioners*, **39**, 408–411.

Corney, R. (1984) The effectiveness of attached social workers in the management of depressed female patients in general practice. *Psychological Medicine Monograph Supplements*, **6**.

Court Report (1976) *Fit for the Future*. London: HMSO.

Cox, J. L., Holden, J. M. & Sagovsky, R. (1987) Detection of postnatal depression. Development of the 10-item Edinburgh Postnatal Depression Scale. *British Journal of Psychiatry*, **150**, 782–786.

Craddock, N. & Craddock, B. (1989) Psychiatric discharge summaries: differing requirements of psychiatrists and GPs. *British Medical Journal*, **299**, 1382.

Creed, F. & Marks, B. (1989) Liaison psychiatry in general practice: a comparison of the liaison-attachment scheme and the shifted outpatient clinic models. *Journal of the Royal College of General Practitioners*, **39**, 514–517.

Daily Telegraph (1995) Doctor stabbed by released mental patient. December 14th.

Deys, C., Dowling, E. & Golding, V. (1989) Clinical psychology: a consultation approach in general practice. *Journal of the Royal College of General Practitioners*, **39**, 342–344.

Diekstra, R. F. W. & Egmord, M. V. (1989) Suicide and attempted suicide in general practice, 1979–1986. *Acta Psychiatrica Scandinavica*, **79**, 268–275.

Donoghue, J. M. & Tylee, A. (1996) The treatment of depression: prescribing patterns of antidepressants in primary care in the UK. *British Journal of Psychiatry*, **168**, 164–168.

Dowrick, C. & Buchan, I. (1995) Twelve month outcome of depression in general practice: does detection or disclosure make any difference. *British Medical Journal*, **311**, 1274–1276.

Earll, L. & Kincey, J. (1982) Clinical psychology in general practice: a controlled trial evaluation. *Journal of the Royal College of General Practitioners*, **32**, 32–37.

Egan, G. (1986) *The Skilled Helper* (3rd edn). Pacific Grove, C.A.: Brooks/Cole.

Eisenberg, L. (1986) Mindlessness and brainlessness in psychiatry. *British Journal of Psychiatry*, **148**, 497–508.

Essex, B., Doig, R. & Renshaw, J. (1990) Pilot study of records of shared care for people with mental illnesses. *British Medical Journal*, **300**, 1442–1446.

Ferguson, B., Cooper, S., Brothwell, J., *et al* (1992). The clinical evaluation of a new community psychiatric service based on general practice psychiatric clinics. *British Journal of Psychiatry*, **160**, 493–497.

Fleming, D. M. & Cross, K. W. (1984) Psychotropic drug prescribing. *Journal of the Royal College of General Practitioners*, **34**, 216–220.

Freeling, P. (1993) Diagnosis and treatment of depression in general practice. *British Journal of Psychiatry*, **163** (suppl. 20), 14–19.

——, Rao, B. M., Paykel, E. S., *et al* (1985) Unrecognised depression in general practice. *British Medical Journal*, **290**, 1880–1883.

Garralda, M. E. (1995) Primary care psychiatry. In *Child and Adolescent Psychiatry. Modern Approaches* (3rd edn) (eds M. Rutter, E. Taylor & L. Hersov), pp.1055–1069. Oxford: Blackwell Scientific.

Gask, L. (1994) Training for general practitioners in psychiatry. In *Psychiatry and General Practice Today* (eds I. Pullen, G. Wilkinson, W. Wright, *et al*), pp. 337–359. London: Royal College of Psychiatrists and Royal College of General Practitioners.

——, Goldberg, D., Lesser, A., *et al* (1988) Improving the psychiatric skills of the general practice trainee: an evaluation of a group training course. *Medical Education*, **22**, 132–138.

Gater, R., de Almeida e Sousa, R., Caraveo, J., *et al* (1991) The pathways to psychiatric care: a cross-cultural study. *Psychological Medicine*, **21**, 761–774.

Giel, R., de Arango, M. V., Climent, C. E., *et al* (1981) Detection of childhood mental disorders in primary health care: results of observations in 4 developing countries. *Paediatrics*, **68**, 677–683.

Glanz, A. & Taylor, C. (1986) Findings of a natural survey of the role of general practitioners in the treatment of opiate misuse: extent of the contact with opiate misusers. *British Medical Journal*, **293**, 427–430.

Goldberg, D. (1994) Epidemiology of mental disorder in general practice. In *Psychiatry and General Practice Today* (eds I. Pullen, G. Wilkinson, A. Wright, *et al*), pp. 36–44. London: Gaskell.

—— & Blackwell, B. (1970) Psychiatric illness in general practice. A detailed study using a new method of case identification. *British Medical Journal*, **ii**, 439–443.

——, Cooper, B., Eastwood, M. R., *et al* (1970) A standardised interview useful for use in community surveys. *British Journal of Preventative Social Medicine*, **24**, 18–20.

—— & Huxley, P. (1980) *Mental Illness in the Community. The Pathway to Psychiatric Care*. London: Tavistock.

——, Steele, J. J., Smith, C., *et al* (1980) Training family doctors to recognise psychiatric illness with increased accuracy. *Lancet*, **ii**, 521–523.

——, Bridges, K., Duncan Jones, P., *et al* (1987) Dimensions of neurosis seen in primary care settings. *Psychological Medicine*, **17**, 461–470.

—— & Williams, P. (1988) *A User's Guide to the General Health Questionnaire*. Oxford: Nfer–Nelson.

—— & Huxley, P. (1992) *Common Mental Disorders – A Biosocial Model*. London: Routledge.

——, Roghmann, K. J., McInerny, T. K., *et al* (1984) Mental health problems among children seen in pediatric practice prevalence and management. *Pediatrics*, **73**, 278–292.

Harding, T., De Arango, M., Baltazar, J., *et al* (1980) Mental disorders in primary care: a study of their frequency in four developing countries. *Psychological Medicine*, **10**, 231–242.

Heather, N., Campion, P. D., Neville, R. G., *et al* (1987) Evaluation of a controlled drinking minimal intervention for problem drinkers in general practice (the DRAMS scheme). *Journal of the Royal College of General Practitioners*, **37**, 358–363.

Her Majesty's Stationery Office (1986) *Morbidity Statistics from General Practice*. London: HMSO.

Hirschfeld, R. & Cross, C. (1982) Epidemiology of affective disorders. Psychosocial risk factors. *Archives of General Psychiatry*, **35**, 46–50.

Holden, J. M., Sagovsky, R. & Cox, J. L. (1989) Counselling in a general practice setting, controlled study of health visitor intervention in treament of postnatal depression. *British Medical Journal*, **298**, 223–226.

Hollyman, J., Freeling, P., Paykel, E., *et al* (1988) Double-blind placebo controlled trial of amitriptyline among depressed patients in general practice. *Journal of the Royal College of General Practitioners*, **38**, 393–397.

Horder, J. (1988) Working with general practitioners. *British Journal of Psychiatry*, **153**, 513–521.

—— (1991) Care for patients discharged from psychiatric hospitals (Editorial). *British Journal of General Practice*, **41**, 399–400.

Howie, J. G. R. (1972) Diagnoses - The Achilles heel? *Journal of the Royal College of General Practitioners*, **22**, 310–315.

——, Porter, A. M. D., Heaney, D. J., *et al* (1991) Long to short consultation ratio: a proxy measure of quality of care for general practice. *British Journal of General Practice*, **41**, 48–54.

Irwin, W. G. & Cupples, M. E. (1986) A survey of psychotropic drug prescribing. *Journal of the Royal College of General Practitioners*, **36**, 366–368.

Jackson, G., Gater, R., Goldberg, D., *et al* (1993) A new community health team based on primary care. A description of the service and its effect on service use in the first year. *British Journal of Psychiatry*, **162**, 375–384.

Jarman, B. (1992) Psychiatric illness and services in a UK health centre. In *Primary Health Care and Psychiatric Epidemiology* (eds Brian Cooper & Robin Eastwood), pp. 99–108. London: Tavistock/Routledge.

Jenkins, R., Smeeton, N. & Shepherd, M. (1988) Classification of mental disorder in primary care. *Psychological Medicine Monograph Supplements*, **12**.

Johnson, D. A. (1973) An analysis of outpatient services. *British Journal of Psychiatry*, **153**, 513–521.

Johnston, D. A. W. (1981) Depression: treatment compliance in general practice. *Acta Psychiatrica Scandinavica*, **63** (suppl.), 447–453.

Johnstone, A. & Goldberg, D. (1976) Psychiatric screening in general practice. *Lancet*, **i**, 605–608.

Joukamaa, M., Sohlman, B. & Lehtinen, V. (1995) The prescription of psychotropic drugs in primary health care. *Acta Psychiatrica Scandinavica*, **92**, 359–364.

Kaeser, A. C. & Cooper, B. (1971) The psychiatric patient, the general practitioner and the outpatient clinic. An operational study and a review. *Psychological Medicine*, **1**, 312–325.

1388   *Wilkinson*

Karasek, R. A. (1979) Job demands, job decision latitude and mental strain: Implications for job redesign. *Administrative Science Quarterly*, **24**, 285–308.

Kendrick, T., Sibbald, B., Burns, T., *et al* (1991) Role of general practitioners in care of long-term mentally ill patients. *British Medical Journal*, **302**, 508–510.

Kessel, W. I. N. (1963) Who ought to see a psychiatrist. *Lancet*, *i*, 1092–1095.

Kessler, R., House, J. & Turner, J. (1987) Unemployment and health in a community sample. *Journal of Family Practice*, **16**, 319–324.

Kiely, B. G. & McPherson, I. G. (1986) Stress and self help in primary care: a controlled trial evaluation. *Journal of the Royal College of General Practitioners*, **36**, 307–309.

Lawrence, R. E., Copas, J. B. & Cooper, P. W. (1990) Community care: does it reduce the need for psychiatric beds. A comparison of two different styles of service in three different hospitals. *British Journal of Psychiatry*, **159**, 334–340.

Lesser, A. (1985) Problem-based interviewing in general practice. *Medical Education*, **19**, 200–204.

Loudon, I. S. L. (1983) James McKenzie lecture. The origin of the general practitioner. *Journal of the Royal College of General Practitioners*, **33**, 13–18.

McKeganny, N. P. & Boddy, F. A. (1988) General practitioners and opiate-abusing patients. *Journal of the Royal College of General Practitioners*, **38**, 73–75.

Macdonald, M. (1989) Psychiatric disorders in early modern England. In *The Scope of Epidemiological Psychiatry* (eds. P. Williams, G. Wilkinson & K. Rawnsley), pp. 145–147. London: Routledge.

Makin, P. J., Rout, U. & Cooper, C. L. (1988) Job satisfaction and occupational stress among general practitioners – a pilot study. *Journal of the Royal College of General Practitioners*, **38**, 303–306.

Mann, A., Jenkins, R. & Belsey, E. (1981) The 12-month outcome of patients with neurotic illness in general practice. *Psychological Medicine*, **11**, 535–550.

Margo, J. L. (1982) Letters from psychiatrists to general practitioners. *Bulletin of the Royal College of Psychiatrists*, **6**, 139–141.

Marinker, M. (1988) The referral system. *Journal of the Royal College of General Practitioners*, **38**, 487–491.

Marks, I. (1985) Controlled trial of psychiatric nurse therapists in primary care. *British Medical Journal*, **290**, 1181–1183.

Marks, J., Goldberg, D. & Hillier, V. (1979) Determinants of the ability of general practitioners to detect psychiatric illness. *Psychological Medicine*, **9**, 337–353.

Martin, E. & Mitchell, H. (1983) A counsellor in general practice in a one year survey. *Journal of the Royal College of General Practitioners*, **33**, 366–367.

Mayfield, D., McCleod, G. & Hall, P. (1974) The CAGE questionnaire. Validation of a new alcohol screening instrument. *American Journal of Psychiatry*, **131**, 1121–1123.

Melzer, D., Hale, A. S., Malik, S. J., *et al* (1991) Community care for patients with schizophrenia one year after hospital discharge. *British Medical Journal*, **303**, 1023–1026.

Melville, A. (1980) Reducing whose anxiety? A study of the relationship between repeat prescribing of minor tranquillisers and doctors' attitudes. In *Prescribing Practice and Drug Usage* (ed. E. Mapes). London: Croom Helm.

Metcalfe, C. & Edwards, G. (1981) Psychiatry and primary care. In *Psychiatry in General Practice* (ed. Guy Edwards), pp. 1–12. Southampton: University of Southampton.

Millar, T. & Goldberg, D. P. (1991) Link between the ability to detect and manage emotional disorders: a study of general practitioner trainees. *British Journal of General Practice*, **41**, 357–359.

Milne, D. & Souter, K. (1988) A re-evaluation of the clinical psychologist in general practice. *Journal of the Royal College of General Practitioners*, **38**, 457–460.

Morris, J. N., Heady, J. A. & Barley, R. G. (1952) Coronary heart disease in medical practitioners. *British Medical Journal*, *ii*, 503–520.

Murgatroyd, S. (1983) Counselling and the doctor (Editorial). *Journal of the Royal College of General Practitioners*, **33**, 323–325.

Murray, J., Dunn, G., Williams, P., *et al* (1981) Factors influencing the consumption of psychotropic drugs. *Psychological Medicine*, **11**, 551–560.

Murray, R. M. (1976) Alcoholism amongst male doctors in Scotland. *Lancet*, *ii*, 729–733.

National Institute of Mental Health (1979) *Mental Disorder and Primary Care: An Analytical Review of the Literature* (authors J. Hawkins & J. S. Oktay). Series D. No 5 DHEW, Pub. no. ADM 78–661. Washington, DC: National Academy of Sciences.

Nazareth, I., King, M., Haines, A., *et al* (1993) Care of schizophrenia in general practice. *British Medical Journal*, **307**, 910–911.

Nilsson, A. (1981) Alt arbeta med sex-och samlevnad. En handbok: abortforebygyande upplysning. Stockholm Liber Forlag.

Office of Population Censuses and Surveys (1982) *Morbidity Statistics from General Practice. Second National Study 1970–71*. London: HMSO.

Ormel, J. & Giel, R. (1990) Medical effects of non-recognition of affective disorders in primary care. In *Psychological Disorders in General Medical Settings* (eds N. Sartorius, D. Goldberg, G. de Girolamo, *et al*). Bern: Huber, Hogrefe.

Parish, P. A. (1971) The prescribing of psychotropic drugs in general practice. *Journal of the Royal College of General Practitioners*, **21** (Suppl. 4), 1–77.

Parkes, C. M., Brown, G. W. & Monck, E. M. (1962) The general practitioner and the schizophrenic patient. *British Medical Journal*, **1**, 972–976.

Pendleton, D. & Hasler, J. (1983) *Doctor–Patient Communication*. London: Academic Press.

Pietroni, P. C. (1986) Would Balint have joined the British Holistic Medical Association? *Journal of the Royal College of General Practitioners*, **36**, 171–173.

Pokorny, A. D., Miller, B. A. & Kaplan, H. B. (1972) The brief MAST: a shortened version of the Michigan Alcohol Screening Test. *American Journal of Psychiatry*, **129**, 342–344.

Porter, A. M. D., Howie, J. G. R. & Levinson, A. (1985) Measurement of stress as it affects the work of the general practitioner. *Family Practice*, **2**, 136–146.

Prudo, R., Harris, T. & Brown, G. W. (1984) Psychiatric disorders in a rural and in an urban population: 3. Social integration and the morphology of affective disorder. *Psychological Medicine*, **14**, 327–364.

Pullen, I. & Yellowlees, A. (1985) Is communication improving between general practitioners and psychiatrists. *British Medical Journal*, **290**, 31–33.

— & — (1988) Scottish psychiatrists in primary health care settings: a silent majority. *British Journal of Psychiatry*, **153**, 663–666.

Rankin, H. J., Serieys, N. M. & Elliott-Binns, C. P. (1987) Determinants of mood in general practice. *British Medical Journal*, **294**, 618–620.

Regier, D., Boyd, J., Burke, J., *et al* (1988) One-month prevalence of mental disorders in the United States. *Archives of General Psychiatry*, **45**, 977–985.

Register General (1978) *Decennial Supplement for England and Wales*. London: HMSO.

Reid, H. L. A., Webb, G. R., Hennrikus, D., *et al* (1986) Detection of patients with high alcohol intake by general practitioners. *British Medical Journal*, **295**, 735–737.

Richards, C. (1987) A survey of ten health care needs of doctors. MSc. Dissertation. Exeter: Exeter University.

Rutz, W., Walinder, J., Eberhard, G., *et al* (1989) An educational programme on depressive disorders for general practitioners. *Acta Psychiatrica Scandinavica*, **79**, 19–26.

——, Knorring, V. L., Walinder, J., et al (1992) Long term effects of an educational programme for general practitioners given by the Swedish Committee for the Prevention and Treatment of Depression. *Acta Psychiatrica Scandinavica*, **85**, 83–88.

Schor, E. L. (1986) Use of health care services by children and diagnoses received during presumably stressful life transitions. *Pediatrics*, **77**, 834–841.

Scott, A. I. & Freeman, C. (1992) Edinburgh primary care depression study: treatment outcome, patient satisfaction and cost after 16 weeks. *British Medical Journal*, **304**, 883–887.

Sharp, D. J. & King, M. B. (1989) Classification of psychosocial disturbance in general practice. *Journal of the Royal College of General Practitioners*, **39**, 356–358.

Sheldon, M. (1994) Counselling and psychotherapy. In *Psychiatry and General Practice Today* (eds I. Pullen, G. Wilkinson, A. Wright, *et al*), pp. 280–293. London: Royal College of Psychiatrists and Royal College of General Practitioners.

Shepherd, M. (1982) Psychiatric research and primary care in Britain – past, present and future. *Psychological Medicine*, **12**, 493–499.

——, Cooper, A. B., Brown, A. C., *et al* (1966) *Psychiatric Illness in General Practice*. Oxford: Oxford University Press.

Sieverwright, H., Tyrer, P., Casey, P., *et al* (1991) A three year follow up of psychiatric morbidity in urban and rural primary care. *Psychological Medicine*, **21**, 495–504.

Sireling, L. I., Paykel, E. S., Freeling, P., *et al* (1985) Depression in general practice: case thresholds and diagnoses. *British Journal of Psychiatry*, **147**, 113–119.

Smeeton, N., Wilkinson, G., Stense, D., *et al* (1992) A longitudinal study of general practice consultations for psychiatric disorder in adolescence. *Psychological Medicine*, **22**, 709–715.

Sowerby, P. (1977) The doctor, his patient and the illness: a reappraisal. *Journal of the Royal College of General Practitioners*, **27**, 583–589.

Spence, J. (1960) The need for understanding of individuals as part of the training and function of doctors and nurses. In *The Purpose and Practice of Medicine*. Oxford: Oxford University Press.

Stansfield, S. (1991) Attitudes to developments in community psychiatry among general practitioners. *Psychiatric Bulletin*, **15**, 542–543.

Stein, S. (1995) Student Counselling Services. Annual Report, University of Greenwich.

Strathdee, G. & Williams, P. (1984) A survey of psychiatrists in primary care: the silent growth of a new service. *Journal of the Royal College of General Practitioners*, **34**, 615–618.

Surtees, P. G., Dean, E., Ingham, J. G., *et al* (1983) Psychiatric disorders in women from an Edinburgh community association with demographic factors. *British Journal of Psychiatry*, **142**, 238–246.

Sutherland, V. J. & Cooper, C. L. (1992) Job stress, satisfaction and mental health among general practitioners before and after the introduction of the new contract. *British Medical Journal*, **304**, 545–547.

Tansella, M. & Williams, P. (1989) The spectrum of psychiatric morbidity in a defined geographical area. *Psychological Medicine*, **19**, 765–770.

Tennant, C., Bebbington, P. & Hurry, J. (1981) The short term outcome of neurotic disorders in the community. The relation of remission to clinical factors and to neutralising events. *British Journal of Psychiatry*, **139**, 213–220.

Thom, B. & Tellez, C. (1986) A difficult business detecting and managing alcohol problems in general practice. *British Journal of Addiction*, **81**, 405–418.

Trepka, C., Laing, I. & Smith, S. (1986) Group treatment of general practice anxiety problems. *Journal of the Royal College of General Practitioners*, **35**, 86–88.

Trethowan, W. H. (1975) Pills for personal problems. *British Medical Journal*, **3**, 749–751.

Tuch, R. H. (1975) The relationship between a mother's menstrual status and her response to illness in her child. *Psychosomatic Medicine*, **37**, 388–394.

Tyrer, P. (1984) Psychiatric clinics in general practice: an extension of community care. *British Journal of Psychiatry*, **145**, 9–14.

—— (1986) What is the role of the psychiatrist in primary care? *Journal of the Royal College of General Practitioners*, **36**, 373–375.

Vaillant, G. E. (1983) *The Natural History of Alcoholism*. Cambridge, Mass: Harvard University Press.

Varnam, M. (1981) Psychotropic prescribing. What am I doing? *Journal of the Royal College of General Practitioners*, **31**, 480–483.

Vazquez-Barquero, J. L., Diez-Manrique, J. F., Saite, L., *et al* (1992). Why people with probable minor psychiatric morbidity consult a doctor. *Psychological Medicine*, **22**, 495–502.

Veerhak, P. (1993) Analysis of referrals of mental health problems by general practitioners. *British Journal of General Practice*, **43**, 203–208.

Wallace, P. & Jarman, B. (1994) Alcohol: strengthening the primary care response. *British Medical Bulletin*, **50**, 211–220.

Warr, P., Cook, J. & Wall, T. (1979) Scales for the measurement of some work attitudes and aspects of psychological well being. *Journal of Occupational Psychology*, **52**, 129–148.

Watts, C. A. H. (1947) Endogenous depression in general practice. *British Medical Journal*, **1**, 11–14.

Whitehouse, C. R. (1987) A survey of the management of psychosocial illness in general practice in Manchester. *Journal of the Royal College of General Practitioners*, **37**, 112–115.

Wilkins, R. H. (1974) *The Hidden Alcoholic in General Practice*. London: Elek Science.

Wilkinson, G. (1985) Mental health practices in primary care settings: An annotated bibliography 1977–1985. London: Tavistock.

—— (1989) Referrals from general practitioners to psychiatrists and paramedical mental health professionals. *British Journal of Psychiatry*, **154**, 72–76.

——, Smeeton, N., Skuse, D., et al (1988) Consultation for physical illnesses by patients diagnosed and treated for psychiatric disorders by a general practitioner: 20 year follow up study. *British Medical Journal*, **297**, 776–778.

——, Allen, P., Marshall, E., *et al* (1993) The role of the practice nurse in the management of depression in general practice: treatment adherence to antidepressant medication. *Psychological Medicine*, **23**, 229–237.

—— & Wright, A. (1994) Research potential in general practice. In *Psychiatry in General Practice Today* (eds I. Pullen, G. Wilkinson & A. F. Wright), pp. 360–370. Royal College of Psychiatrists and Royal College of General Practitioners.

Williams, P. (1978) Physical ill health and psychotropic drug prescription. A review. *Psychological Medicine*, **8**, 683–693.

—— (1979) The extent of psychotropic drug prescribing. In *Psychosocial Disorders in General Practice* (eds P. Williams & A. Clare), pp. 151–160. London: Academic Press.

—— (1983) Factors influencing the duration of treatment with psychotropic drugs in general practice: a survival analysis approach. *Psychological Medicine*, **13**, 623–633.

—— & Wallace, B. B. (1974) General practitioners and psychiatrists – do they communicate? *British Medical Journal*, *i*, 505–507.

—— & Balestrieri, M. (1989) Psychiatric clinics in general practice; do they reduce admissions?, *British Journal of Psychiatry*, **154**, 67–71.

——, Tarnopolsky, A., Hand, D., *et al* (1986) Minor psychiatric morbidity and general practice consultations: the West London Survey. *Psychological Medicine Monograph Supplements*, **9**.

Wilson, M. & Macarthy, B. (1994) GP consultation as a factor in the lower rate of mental health service use by Asians. *Psychological Medicine*, **24**, 113–119.

Wilson, P. (1980) *Drinking in England and Wales*. London: HMSO.

WONCA (World Organisation of National Colleges, Academies and Academic Associations of General Practice) (1979) ICHPPC–2 (International Classification of Health Problems in Primary Care – 2nd edn). Oxford: Oxford University Press.

Wooff, K., Goldberg, D. & Fryers, T. (1988) The practice of community psychiatric nursing and mental health social work in Salford: some implications for community care. *British Journal of Psychiatry*, **153**, 30–37.

World Health Organization (1973) *Psychiatry and Primary Medical Care*. Copenhagen: WHO Regional Office for Europe.

World Health Organization (1989) The Alcohol Use Disorders Identification Test. AUDIT. Geneva: WHO.

Wright, A. F. (1990) A study of the presentation of somatic symptoms in general practice by patients with psychiatric disturbance. *British Journal of General Practice*, **40**, 459–463.

—— (1994) Depression. In *Psychiatry and General Practice Today* (eds I. Pullen, G. Wilkinson, A. F. Wright, *et al*), pp. 93–110. London: Royal College of Psychiatrists and Royal College of General Practitioners.

—— & Perini, A. F. (1987) Hidden psychiatric illness: use of the General Health Questionnaire in general practice. *Journal of the Royal College of General Practitioners*, **37**, 164–167.

Wynter, A. (1875) The role of the general practitioner. In *The Borderlands of Insanity*. London: Robert Hardwicke.

Zigmond, D. (1978) When Balinting is mind rape. *Update*, **16**, 1123–1126.

Index

Compiled by Nina Boyd